IAPSM's Textbook on
National Health Programs and Policies of India in a Nutshell

Disclaimer

The information presented in this medical book titled *IAPSM's Textbook on National Health Programs and Policies of India in a Nutshell* has been compiled by all authors and is intended for general educational purposes only. The authors have made reasonable efforts to ensure that the information included in this book is accurate, up to date, and reflective of the current understanding of national health programs and policies of India. While every effort has been made to ensure the accuracy and reliability of the content, the authors and publishers cannot be held responsible for any errors, omissions, or outcomes arising from the use of this information. However, it is important to note that medical knowledge is constantly evolving, and best practices may change over time. Readers are strongly encouraged to consult current guidelines, peer-reviewed research, and professional healthcare providers for specific medical advice or treatment plans. Individuals should always exercise caution and discretion when implementing any medical advice or recommendations found within this book. This book is designed to provide guidance for medical students and healthcare professionals on the national health programs and policies of India.

The editor-in-chief, editors, contributors, and publishers of this book have exerted reasonable efforts to ensure that the information provided is accurate and reliable. However, they disclaim any legal responsibility for any errors or omissions that may be present, as this book is a compilation of notes and personal content from various authors, derived from scientific facts and research. In the event that the content shows similarity with someone's personal content, it should be regarded as a coincidental similarity of thoughts. The flowcharts in the book are a creative reflection of the experiences of the aforementioned representatives with the assistance of artists and designers. By reading and utilizing the information in this book, readers acknowledge and accept the terms of this disclaimer and release the authors and publishers from any claims or liabilities, known or unknown, arising from the use of the information contained herein.

IAPSM's Textbook on National Health Programs and Policies of India in a Nutshell

For Medical Undergraduates, Postgraduates, Public Health Experts & Nursing Community

Editor-in-Chief

Purushottam Giri
MBBS MD (PSM) MIPHA FIAPSM CCEBDM (Diabetes)
Professor and Head
Department of Community Medicine
Indian Institute of Medical Science and Research (IIMSR) Medical College
Badnapur, Jalna, Maharashtra, India

Editors

Parul Sharma
MBBS MD (Community Medicine) PGDHM
ACME Fellow ACMDC
Professor and Head
Department of Community Medicine
GMERS Medical College, Patan, Gujarat, India

Shaili Vyas
MBBS MD (Community Medicine) PGDHM
Professor
Department of Community Medicine
Himalayan Institute of Medical Sciences (HIMS)
Dehradun, Uttarakhand, India

Forewords

Sanjay Zodpey
Suneela Garg
AM Kadri

Annarao Kulkarni
Ashok Bhardwaj

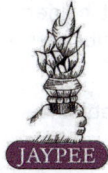

JAYPEE BROTHERS MEDICAL PUBLISHERS
The Health Sciences Publisher
New Delhi | London

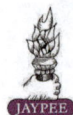

Jaypee Brothers Medical Publishers (P) Ltd

Headquarters
Jaypee Brothers Medical Publishers (P) Ltd
EMCA House, 23/23-B
Ansari Road, Daryaganj
New Delhi 110 002, India
Landline: +91-11-23272143, +91-11-23272703
+91-11-23282021, +91-11-23245672
Email: jaypee@jaypeebrothers.com

Corporate Office
Jaypee Brothers Medical Publishers (P) Ltd
4838/24, Ansari Road, Daryaganj
New Delhi 110 002, India
Phone: +91-11-43574357
Fax: +91-11-43574314
Email: jaypee@jaypeebrothers.com

Overseas Office
J.P. Medical Ltd
83 Victoria Street, London
SW1H 0HW (UK)
Phone: +44 20 3170 8910
Fax: +44 (0)20 3008 6180
Email: info@jpmedpub.com

Website: www.jaypeebrothers.com
Website: www.jaypeedigital.com

© 2025, Jaypee Brothers Medical Publishers

The views and opinions expressed in this book are solely those of the original contributor(s)/author(s) and do not necessarily represent those of editor(s) and publisher of the book.

All rights reserved. No part of this publication may be reproduced, stored or transmitted in any form or by any means, electronic, mechanical, photocopying, recording or otherwise, without the prior permission in writing of the publishers.

All brand names and product names used in this book are trade names, service marks, trademarks or registered trademarks of their respective owners. The publisher is not associated with any product or vendor mentioned in this book.

Medical knowledge and practice change constantly. This book is designed to provide accurate, authoritative information about the subject matter in question. However, readers are advised to check the most current information available on procedures included and check information from the manufacturer of each product to be administered, to verify the recommended dose, formula, method and duration of administration, adverse effects and contraindications. It is the responsibility of the practitioner to take all appropriate safety precautions. Neither the publisher nor the author(s)/editor(s) assume any liability for any injury and/ or damage to persons or property arising from or related to use of material in this book.

This book is sold on the understanding that the publisher is not engaged in providing professional medical services. If such advice or services are required, the services of a competent medical professional should be sought.

Every effort has been made where necessary to contact holders of copyright to obtain permission to reproduce copyright material. If any have been inadvertently overlooked, the publisher will be pleased to make the necessary arrangements at the first opportunity.

Inquiries for bulk sales may be solicited at: jaypee@jaypeebrothers.com

IAPSM's Textbook on National Health Programs and Policies of India in a Nutshell

First Edition: **2025**

ISBN: 978-93-6616-763-3

Printed at: Samrat Offset Pvt. Ltd.

Dedicated to

All past Presidents and past Secretary Generals who nurtured IAPSM to reach this level

Contributors

AK Srivastava
Himalayan Institute of Medical Sciences
Swami Rama Himalayan University (SRHU)
Dehradun, Uttarakhand, India

Abhay Srivastava
Himalayan Institute of Medical Sciences
Swami Rama Himalayan University (SRHU)
Dehradun, Uttarakhand, India

Abhishek Gope
Noida International Institute of Medical Sciences
Greater Noida, Uttar Pradesh, India

Abhishek Raut
Mahatma Gandhi Institute of Medical Sciences
Wardha, Maharashtra, India

Ajeet Singh Bhadoria
All India Institute of Medical Sciences
Rishikesh, Uttarakhand, India

Akash Krishali
Himalayan Institute of Medical Sciences
Swami Rama Himalayan University (SRHU)
Dehradun, Uttarakhand, India

Akhil Dhanesh Goel
All India Institute of Medical Sciences
Jodhpur, Rajasthan, India

Amit Sachdeva
Indira Gandhi Medical College
Shimla, Himachal Pradesh, India

Amrita Srivastava
GSVM Medical College
Kanpur, Uttar Pradesh, India

Anamika Tomar
RUHS College of Medical Sciences
Jaipur, Rajasthan, India

Ankit Yadav
Teerthankar Mahaveer Medical College and Research Centre
Moradabad, Uttar Pradesh, India

Ashish Pundhir
All India Institute of Medical Sciences
Kalyani, West Bengal, India

Bhautik Modi
All India Institute of Medical Sciences
Rajkot, Gujarat, India

Bhavna Jain
SMMH Medical College
Saharanpur, Uttar Pradesh, India

Chaitali Borgaonkar
Dr DY Patil Medical College, Hospital and Research Centre
Pune, Maharashtra, India

Chhaya Mittal
SMMH Medical College
Saharanpur, Uttar Pradesh, India

Deepak Upadhyay
Rohilkhand Medical College and Hospital
Bareilly, Uttar Pradesh, India

Ghanshyam Ahir
Government Medical College
Bhavnagar, Gujarat, India

Girish Jeer
All India Institute of Medical Sciences
New Delhi, India

Hariom Kumar Solanki
Maulana Azad Medical College
New Delhi, India

Harshal Ramesh Salve
All India Institute of Medical Sciences
New Delhi, India

Huma Khan
Shri Ram Murti Smarak Institute of Medical Sciences
Bareilly, Uttar Pradesh, India

Immanuel Joshua E
Postgraduate Institute of Medical Education and Research (PGIMER)
Chandigarh, India

Janki Bartwal
Veer Chandra Singh Garhwali Government Institute of Medical Science and Research, Srinagar Garhwal, Uttarakhand, India

Jyotsana
Post Graduate Institute of Medical Sciences
Rohtak, Haryana, India

Kajal Srivastava
Dr DY Patil Medical College, Hospital, and Research Centre
Dr DY Patil Vidyapeeth
Pune, Maharashtra, India

Kartik Prajapati
Bhagyoday Medical College
Kadi, Gujarat, India

Kartikey Yadav
Hamdard Institute of Medical Sciences and Research
New Delhi, India

Kavita Vishwakarma
Dr DY Patil Medical College, Hospital and Research Centre
Pune, Maharashtra, India

Krishna M Jasani
All India Institute of Medical Sciences (AIIMS)
Rajkot, Gujarat, India

Krupal J Joshi
All India Institute of Medical Sciences (AIIMS)
Rajkot, Gujarat, India

Lakshay Beri
MM Institute of Medical Sciences and Research
Ambala, Haryana, India

M Swathi Shenoy
Public Health Foundation of India
Gurugram, Haryana, India

Mahendra Singh
All India Institute of Medical Sciences
Rishikesh, Uttarakhand, India

Malatesh Undi
Karawar Institute of Medical Sciences
Karawar, Karnataka, India

Manish Kumar Singh
Dr Ram Manohar Lohia Institute of Medical Sciences
Lucknow, Uttar Pradesh, India

Manoj Kumar Gupta
All India Institute of Medical Sciences
Jodhpur, Rajasthan, India

Mansi Kala
Himalayan Institute of Medical Sciences
Swami Rama Himalayan University (SRHU)
Dehradun, Uttarakhand, India

Medhavi
Autonomous State Medical College
Shahjahanpur, Uttar Pradesh, India

Mital Rathod
Pandit Deendayal Upadhyay Government Medical College
Rajkot, Gujarat, India

Mohammad Waseem Faraz Ansari
ESIC Medical College and Hospital
Chennai, Tamil Nadu, India

Neha Gawarle
Dr DY Patil Medical College, Hospital and Research Centre
Pune, Maharashtra, India

Niharika Verma
Himalayan Institute of Medical Sciences
Swami Rama Himalayan University (SRHU)
Dehradun, Uttarakhand, India

Nitesh Kumar
All India Institute of Medical Sciences
Vijaypur, Jammu (J&K), India

Nitin Kumar Joshi
All India Institute of Medical Sciences
Jodhpur, Rajasthan, India

Pallavi Singh
MM Institute of Medical Sciences and Research
Mullana, Ambala, Haryana, India

Pankaj Bhardwaj
All India Institute of Medical Sciences
Jodhpur, Rajasthan, India

Parth Takkar
GMERS Medical College and Hospital
Patan, Gujarat, India

Parul Sharma
GMERS Medical College and Hospital
Patan, Gujarat, India

Pradeep Aggarwal
All India Institute of Medical Sciences
Rishikesh, Uttarakhand, India

Pragya Tripathi
Himalayan Institute of Medical Sciences
Swami Rama Himalayan University (SRHU)
Dehradun, Uttarakhand, India

Prerna Verma
Dr DY Patil Medical College, Hospital and Research Centre
Pune, Maharashtra, India

Priya Ranjan Avinash
Himalayan Institute of Medical Sciences
Swami Rama Himalayan University (SRHU)
Dehradun, Uttarakhand, India

Puneet Ohri
Shri Guru Ram Rai School of Management and Commerce Studies
Dehradun, Uttarakhand, India

Purushottam Giri
IIMSR Medical College
Badnapur, Jalna, Maharashtra, India

Rajendra Singh
Himalayan Institute of Medical Sciences
Swami Rama Himalayan University (SRHU)
Dehradun, Uttarakhand, India

Rakhee Khanduri
Himalayan Institute of Medical Sciences
Swami Rama Himalayan University (SRHU)
Dehradun, Uttarakhand, India

Ranjana Singh
Noida International Institute of Medical Sciences
Greater Noida, Uttar Pradesh, India

Ranjitha R
All India Institute of Medical Sciences
Jodhpur, Rajasthan, India

Ritesh Singh
All India Institute of Medical Sciences
Kalyani, West Bengal, India

Rohit Katre
MM Institute of Medical Sciences and Research
Mullana, Ambala, Haryana, India

Rudresh Negi
Government Medical College
Haldwani, Nainital, Uttarakhand, India

Sadhna Singh
Teerthanker Mahaveer Dental College and Research Centre
Moradabad, Uttar Pradesh, India

Sanjeet Panesar
Atal Bihari Vajpayee Institute of Medical Sciences and Dr RML Hospital
New Delhi, India

Sanjeev Pandey
Himalayan Institute of Medical Sciences
Swami Rama Himalayan University (SRHU)
Dehradun, Uttarakhand, India

Satabdi Mitra
KPC Medical College and Hospital
Kolkata, West Bengal, India

Shaili Vyas
Himalayan Institute of Medical Sciences
Swami Rama Himalayan University (SRHU)
Dehradun, Uttarakhand, India

Shalki Mattas
Shri Guru Ram Rai School of Management and Commerce Studies
Dehradun, Uttarakhand, India

Sharon Baisil
MOSC Medical College
Kolenchery, Kerala, India

Shweta Gangurde (Chauhan)
Dr DY Patil Medical College, Hospital and Research Centre
Pune, Maharashtra, India

Shyambhavee
Hamdard Institute of Medical Sciences and Research
New Delhi, India

Soumya Swaroop Sahoo
All India Institute of Medical Sciences
Bathinda, Punjab, India

Surabhi Mishra
Himalayan Institute of Medical Sciences
Swami Rama Himalayan University (SRHU)
Dehradun, Uttarakhand, India

Suraj Kapoor
Armed Forces Medical Services
Pune, Maharashtra, India

Surendra Singh Negi
Veer Chandra Singh Garhwali Government Institute of Medical Science and Research
Srinagar, Garhwal, Uttarakhand, India

Suseendar Shanmugasundaram
All India Institute of Medical Sciences
Jodhpur, Rajasthan, India

Sushant Khanduri
Himalayan Institute of Medical Sciences
Swami Rama Himalayan University (SRHU)
Dehradun, Uttarakhand, India

Swati Ghonge
DY Patil Medical College
Pune, Maharashtra, India

Thamizhanban A
All India Institute of Medical Sciences
Jodhpur, Rajasthan, India

Thej Kiran Reddy
State Health System Resource Centre
Gandhinagar, Gujarat, India

Varsha Chaudhary
Subharti Medical College
Swami Vivekanand Subharti University
Meerut, Uttar Pradesh, India

Varun Vijay Gaiki
Regional Office for Health and Family Welfare
Government of India
Hyderabad, Telangana, India

Vikram Kumar Gupta
Dayanand Medical College and Hospital
Ludhiana, Punjab, India

Vineet Kumar Pathak
Institute of Medical Sciences
Banaras Hindu University
Varanasi, Uttar Pradesh, India

Vinod Chayal
Pandit Bhagwat Dayal Sharma University of Health Sciences
Rohtak, Haryana, India

Vinothini J
All India Institute of Medical Sciences (HMR)
Bibinagar, Telangana, India

Vipul Nautiyal
Himalayan Institute of Medical Sciences
Swami Rama Himalayan University (SRHU)
Dehradun, Uttarakhand, India

Reviewers

- Akhil Dhanesh Goel
- Anjali Modi
- Ashwin Ramana
- Bharti Koria
- Bhautik Modi
- Bhavesh Kanabar
- Deepika Aggarwal
- Ganesh Lokhande
- Ghanshyam Ahir
- Gneya Bhatt
- Harsha Solanki
- Hathila
- Hetal Rathod
- Hinal Baria
- Jagruti Prajapati
- Jaydeep Ghevaria
- Kajal Srivastava
- Kalpita Shringarpure
- Kapil Gandha
- Kavita
- Kinnari Gupta
- Krupal J Joshi
- Mallika Vasantbhai Chavada
- Margi Sheth
- Nilesh Fichdiya
- Nilesh Thakor
- Padmaja Kanchi
- Pallavi Singh
- Parul Katara
- Parul Sharma
- Praveena P
- Pritesh Patel
- Priti Solanki
- Rashmi Bhujade
- Rivu Basu
- Rudresh Negi
- Rupesh Kumar
- Sadhana Singh
- Santosh Kumar
- Shaili Vyas
- Sudeep Bhavsar
- Surendra Singh
- Veidehi
- Venu Shah
- Yash Shah

Foreword

I am happy to write foreword for the book titled *IAPSM's Textbook on National Health Programs and Policies of India in a Nutshell* under the leadership of Professor (Dr) Purushottam Giri, Secretary General of IAPSM. Having spent four decades in public health service, I have witnessed first-hand the evolution of India's healthcare landscape. This textbook comes at a crucial time when our nation is undergoing significant transformation in healthcare, steadily progressing toward Universal Health Coverage while simultaneously facing unprecedented challenges in public health delivery.

The IAPSM's initiative to create this concise yet comprehensive compilation highlights the urgent need for healthcare professionals to access accurate and up-to-date information about our national health programs. As we move through the postpandemic era, understanding and effectively implementing these programs is more important than ever. This textbook serves as an invaluable resource for undergraduate and postgraduate medical students, practicing physicians, and healthcare administrators alike.

This publication is notable for its practical approach to complex policy frameworks and program guidelines. The authors effectively balance academic rigor with practical utility, making it a vital resource for learning and reference. The inclusion of recent policy changes, particularly those influenced by the COVID-19 pandemic, adds to its relevance. As we pursue goals like the Ayushman Bharat Digital Mission and enhance our primary healthcare infrastructure, this textbook will be an essential guide for future public health professionals, reflecting our commitment to improving India's healthcare system and outcomes.

I praise the editorial team for their thorough efforts in assembling this extensive resource. I hope this textbook motivates and directs our healthcare professionals in their honorable mission of addressing the health requirements of the nation.

Sanjay Zodpey
President, Public Health Foundation of India (PHFI), New Delhi
National President (2020–21), Indian Association of Preventive and Social Medicine (IAPSM)

Foreword

It is a matter of great privilege for me to write foreword for the book titled *IAPSM's Textbook on National Health Programs and Policies of India in a Nutshell* by Professor (Dr) Purushottam Giri. The IAPSM's initiative to create this concise yet comprehensive compilation highlights the urgent need for healthcare professionals to access accurate and up-to-date information about our national health programs. Public health is a vital pillar of national development, influencing the quality of life, economic productivity, and overall well-being of a population. India, with its vast and diverse demographic landscape, has implemented numerous National Health Programs and Policies to tackle critical health challenges, including maternal and child health, infectious and noncommunicable diseases, nutrition, mental health, environmental health, and emerging public health threats. These programs are aligned with global health objectives, including the Sustainable Development Goals (SDGs), and are guided by key national institutions, such as NITI Aayog, ensuring a structured and evidence-based approach to public health governance. However, despite their significance, navigating through these policies, strategies, and their real-world implications can be daunting for students, healthcare professionals, and policymakers. This textbook is designed to provide a comprehensive yet concise understanding of these programs, presenting them in an organized, student-friendly manner that is both academically relevant and practically useful.

This book stands out for its clear and structured presentation, making complex policies easier to grasp. Each chapter provides a succinct explanation of national programs, breaking down their objectives, implementation strategies, target populations, and expected outcomes. To further aid students and professionals preparing for exams, each chapter includes a detailed question bank with MCQs and short-answer and long-answer questions, reinforcing key concepts and enhancing retention. Designed to bridge the gap between policy and practice, this book serves as a ready reference for medical undergraduates, postgraduates, public health experts, and aspirants preparing for competitive exams.

I trust that this book will serve as an invaluable resource, enabling readers to gain an in-depth and practical understanding of India's national health programs and their crucial role in shaping the healthcare system.

Suneela Garg
National President (2021–22), Indian Association of Preventive and Social Medicine (IAPSM)
Chair Programme Advisory Committee, National Institute of Health and Family Welfare (NIHFW), New Delhi

Foreword

It is a great privilege for me to write the foreword for the book titled *IAPSM's Textbook on National Health Programs and Policies of India in a Nutshell* by Professor (Dr) Purushottam Giri. Public health has always been a cornerstone of national development, and India's commitment to improving healthcare is reflected in its numerous National Health Programs and Policies. These initiatives play a crucial role in disease prevention, health promotion, and healthcare accessibility across the country. However, understanding these programs in a structured and comprehensive manner can often be challenging for students and professionals alike. This *IAPSM's Textbook on National Health Programs and Policies of India in a Nutshell* aims to bridge that gap by providing a well-organized, concise, and exam-oriented approach to these essential programs. It serves as a one-stop reference guide, making complex policies and strategies easy to comprehend and apply.

What makes this book unique is its systematic and student-friendly approach. Each program is explained in a nutshell, ensuring a quick and clear grasp of key concepts. Additionally, a well-structured question bank, including MCQs, short questions, and long questions, is provided at the end of each chapter, making it highly beneficial for students and professionals preparing for exams. The book ensures comprehensive coverage of all national programs and policies, leaving no essential initiative overlooked.

With chapters covering the history and evolution of health programs, RMNCAH+N initiatives, disease-specific programs, nutrition, digital health, and emerging public health concerns, this book serves as a ready reference for medical undergraduates, postgraduates, public health experts, nursing community and aspirants preparing for various competitive exams. The content is designed to provide clarity, relevance, and easy access to information, making it a valuable tool for both academic learning and practical application in healthcare.

I am confident that this book will serve as a comprehensive and indispensable resource for all those seeking to understand and implement health programs effectively.

AM Kadri
National President (2023–24), Indian Association of Preventive and Social Medicine (IAPSM)
Executive Director, State Health System Resource Centre (SHSRC), Gujarat

Foreword

Health programs and policies are the backbone of a nation's well-being, shaping the quality of life for its people and driving socioeconomic progress. India, with its vast population and diverse healthcare challenges, has witnessed the evolution of numerous national health programs aimed at addressing critical public health issues. National Health Programs and Policies in India is a valuable contribution to the understanding of these initiatives, offering a detailed analysis of their development, implementation, and impact.

From the early efforts to combat communicable diseases to the more recent push for universal healthcare under Ayushman Bharat, India's health policies have continuously evolved to meet emerging challenges. Programs targeting maternal and child health, immunization, tuberculosis control, and noncommunicable diseases have played a transformative role in improving health indicators across the country. However, despite commendable progress, significant gaps remain in accessibility, affordability, and quality of healthcare services.

This *IAPSM's Textbook on National Health Programs and Policies of India in a Nutshell* meticulously examines the successes and shortcomings of India's health policies, providing readers with a comprehensive understanding of their scope and effectiveness. By offering insights into policy frameworks, implementation strategies, and real-world outcomes, it serves as an essential resource for policymakers, public health professionals, researchers, and students.

As India strives toward achieving Sustainable Development Goals (SDGs) and strengthening its healthcare infrastructure, informed discussions on national health programs become crucial. I believe this textbook will inspire meaningful dialogue and contribute to the ongoing efforts to create a more equitable and efficient healthcare system for all.

I commend the authors for their thorough research and insightful analysis and hope this work will serve as a guiding light for future health policy improvements in India.

Annarao Kulkarni
National President (2024–25), Indian Association of Preventive and Social Medicine (IAPSM)

Foreword

It gives me immense pleasure to write foreword for the book titled *IAPSM's Textbook on National Health Programs and Policies of India in a Nutshell* by Professor (Dr) Purushottam Giri. This textbook serves as an invaluable resource for students, researchers, and healthcare professionals seeking a concise yet thorough understanding of India's diverse and intricate healthcare landscape.

The book expertly distills the complex web of national health programs and policies into a readily accessible format, making it an ideal resource for those seeking a quick yet informative overview. It covers a wide spectrum of topics, from primary healthcare initiatives to specialized interventions, providing a holistic perspective on the evolution and current state of India's healthcare system. Working on different domains of learning, this book is of interest to MBBS undergraduate students, public health postgraduates, nursing postgraduates, and community wellness experts.

The "nutshell" approach adopted by the authors is particularly commendable. It allows readers to grasp key concepts and information efficiently, making it an ideal resource for busy professionals and students. Furthermore, the book serves as an excellent foundation for those who wish to delve deeper into specific areas of public health policy and program implementation.

I am confident that this textbook will serve as a valuable tool for students, teachers, researchers, and policymakers alike. It will not only enhance their knowledge of India's health programs and policies but also foster critical thinking and informed discussions on improving the nation's healthcare system.

Ashok Bhardwaj
National President (2025–26), Indian Association of Preventive and Social Medicine (IAPSM)

Preface

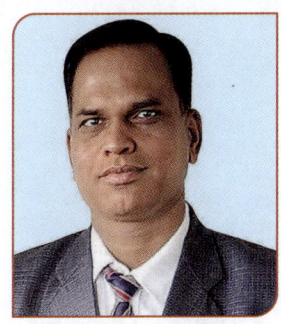

Public health is the backbone of national development, and India's health programs are instrumental in disease prevention, health promotion, and ensuring equitable healthcare access. However, navigating these initiatives in a structured and comprehensive manner can be challenging.

This *IAPSM's Textbook on National Health Programs and Policies of India in a Nutshell* is designed to simplify complex policies and health programs through a well-organized, concise, and exam-oriented approach. Covering fundamental health programs, policies, and emerging public health challenges, it bridges the gap between theoretical knowledge and practical implementation. For this, community medicine physicians from all over the country were approached and a team of enthusiast physicians came forward to put their individual effort toward this book in a very short period of time.

What makes this book unique is its concise and methodical presentation, ensuring that national programs are easy to comprehend. Each chapter systematically outlines key concepts, program objectives, implementation strategies, and expected health outcomes, making learning more effective. To facilitate academic preparation, by presenting key concepts clearly and systematically, the book includes a comprehensive question bank at the end of each chapter, featuring MCQs and short-answer and long-answer questions, aiding both exam readiness and deeper understanding. With a structured and well-organized format, this book serves as an essential reference for medical students, postgraduates, public health professionals, and nursing community and aspirants preparing for competitive exams.

I extend my sincere gratitude to the Indian Association of Preventive and Social Medicine (IAPSM) for its unwavering support in strengthening public health education. This book is the result of collective efforts of many experts in the field of community medicine from all over the country. I deeply appreciate the contributions of all the authors and reviewers who have played a crucial role in shaping this book into a comprehensive and practical reference for understanding national health programs and policies of India. Definitely, there is a scope of improvement. So, we all are eager to have your valuable feedback and suggestions for improving this textbook in subsequent editions.

Purushottam Giri

Acknowledgments

The creation of this book *IAPSM's Textbook on National Health Programs and Policies of India in a Nutshell* has been a collaborative and rewarding journey, and I am deeply grateful to all the individuals who have contributed to this project. Without their support, guidance, and expertise, this book would not have been possible.

First and foremost, I would like to express my heartfelt thanks to my colleagues and mentors in the field of community medicine. Their invaluable insights, dedication to public health, and encouragement have significantly shaped the content and direction of this book. Their commitment to advancing the discipline of community medicine has been a constant source of inspiration.

Having an idea and turning it into a book has not been an easy task. This simply could not have been possible without the great helping hands around me. While I was committed as Secretary General of the National Indian Association of Preventive and Social Medicine (IAPSM) and President of IAPSM Maharashtra Chapter, I had been procrastinating the completion of this book. I would first of all like to thank the induction battery of this project, Professor Dr Parul Sharma who made sure to continuously supervise the progression and completion of all chapters on time. I will not forget to thank enough Professor Dr Shaili Vyas, who with her utmost dedication gave most of her time and skills to finely do this book-writing project and complete it before deadline. She has always strived to grow and help others grow too.

Being the Secretary General of National IAPSM, I would like to thank all the Presidents with whom I have closely worked, namely Dr Suneela Garg (2021–22), Dr Harivansh Chopra (2022–23), and Dr AM Kadri (2023–24), for their constant guidance and unwavering support. I would also like to show my gratitude toward the current President Dr Annarao Kulkarni (2024–25) and President Elect Dr Ashok Bhardwaj (2025–26), for their immense support.

I deeply appreciate the contributions of all the authors, editors, and reviewers who have played a crucial role in shaping this book into a comprehensive and practical reference for understanding national health programs and policies of India.

My sincere appreciation goes to the entire team of M/s Jaypee Brothers Medical Publishers (P) Ltd, New Delhi, for their tremendous effort and unwavering support, Shri Jitendar P Vij (Group Chairman), Mr Ankit Vij (Managing Director), Mr MS Mani (Group President), Dr Madhu Choudhary (Director-Educational Publishing), Ms Pooja Bhandari [Director-Production (Books and Journals)], Mr Ajay Kumar Sharma [Deputy General Manager (Books and Journals)], Ms Sunita Katla (Executive Assistant to Group Chairman and Publishing Manager), Ms Samina Khan (Executive Assistant to Director-Educational Publishing), Dr Upma Tomar (Senior Development Editor), Mr Vijay Kumar Bhatia (Manager–Production), Ms Seema Dogra (Cover Visualizer), Ms Neha Verma (Graphic Designer–Cover), Mr Vakil Khan (Proofreader), Mr Mahesh Chand Joshi (Typesetter), Mr Ratan Lal (Graphic Designer). Without their cooperation, I could not have completed this project. We also extend our special thanks to Dr Akhil Goel, Additional Professor, Community Medicine from AIIMS, Jodhpur, Rajasthan, India, for final shaping of the book.

At last, my sincere thanks go to the Almighty God for providing me with a blessed team who contributed their best in turning this dream into reality.

Contents

Section I: Understanding National Health Program Framework

Chapter 1:	Evolution of Health Programs in India	3
Chapter 2:	Logos of All National Health Programs	5
Chapter 3:	Planning a National Health Program	13
Chapter 4:	Evaluating National Health Programs: A Crucial Endeavor	17
Chapter 5:	Mastering India's Healthcare Delivery System for Effective Program Implementation	24
Chapter 6:	Health Committees in India	35
Chapter 7:	National Institution for Transforming India Aayog	38
Chapter 8:	Sustainable Development Goals	43

Section II: Health Policies

Chapter 9:	National Health Policy	51
Chapter 10:	National Nutrition Policy	60
Chapter 11:	National Population Policy	64
Chapter 12:	National Policy for Rare Diseases	67
Chapter 13:	National Policy for Older Persons	73

Section III: National Health Mission

Part A: RMNCAH+N (Reproductive Maternal Newborn Child Adolescent Health Plus Nutrition)

Chapter 14:	National Health Mission—NRHM and NUHM	83

i. R: Reproductive Health

Chapter 15:	Mission Parivar Vikas National Family Planning Indemnity Scheme	89

ii. M: Maternal Health

Chapter 16:	LaQshya—Labor Room Quality Improvement Initiative	93
Chapter 17:	Janani Suraksha Yojana	98
Chapter 18:	Janani Shishu Suraksha Karyakram	101
Chapter 19:	Pradhan Mantri Surakshit Matritva Abhiyan	103
Chapter 20:	Pradhan Mantri Matru Vandana Yojana	106
Chapter 21:	Surakshit Matritva Aashwasan	109
Chapter 16:	Dakshata	114
Chapter 23:	Maternal and Child Death Surveillance and Response	117

iii. M: Maternal Health

Chapter 24:	Facility-based Newborn Care	123
Chapter 25:	Navjaat Shishu Suraksha Karyakram	129
Chapter 26:	Home-based Newborn Care	134
Chapter 27:	Home-based Care for Young Child	138
Chapter 28:	Rashtriya Bal Swasthya Karyakram	146
Chapter 29:	Universal Immunization Programme and Mission Indradhanush	151
Chapter 30:	Integrated Management of Neonatal and Childhood Illnesses	156
Chapter 31:	Social Awareness and Action to Neutralize Pneumonia Successfully	170
Chapter 32:	MusQan: Ensuring Child-friendly Services in Government Health Facilities	174

iv. A: Adolescent Health

Chapter 33:	Rashtriya Kishor Swasthya Karyakram	179
Chapter 34:	School Health Program and Menstrual Hygiene Scheme	186
Chapter 35:	Adolescent-friendly Health Clinics	191
Chapter 36:	Peer Education Program	196
Chapter 37:	Scheme for Adolescent Girls	199
Chapter 38:	Weekly Iron Folic Acid Supplementation Program and National Deworming Day	201

v. N: Nutrition

Chapter 39:	Anemia Mukt Bharat	206
Chapter 40:	National Nutrition Mission: POSHAN 2.0	213
Chapter 41:	Mothers' Absolute Affection	219
Chapter 42:	Infant and Young Child Feeding	223

Part B: Communicable Diseases

Chapter 43: National Vector Borne Disease Control Programme — 229
Chapter 44: National Tuberculosis Elimination Programme — 236
Chapter 45: National AIDS Control Programme — 241
Chapter 46: National Leprosy Eradication Programme — 246
Chapter 47: National Viral Hepatitis Control Programme — 253
Chapter 48: National Rabies Control Programme — 260
Chapter 49: Endgame Strategy for Poliomyelitis — 264
Chapter 50: Integrated Disease Surveillance Programme and Integrated Health Information Platform — 269

Part C: Noncommunicable Diseases

Chapter 51: National Programme for Prevention and Control of Noncommunicable Diseases — 275
Chapter 52: Integration of NAFLD into NP-NCD — 279
Chapter 53: National Programme for Healthcare of the Elderly — 283
Chapter 54: National Programme for Control of Blindness and Visual Impairment — 289
Chapter 55: National Programme for Prevention and Control of Deafness — 293
Chapter 56: National Mental Health Programme — 301
Chapter 57: National Tobacco Control Programme — 310
Chapter 58: National Oral Health Programme — 318
Chapter 59: National Sickle Cell Anemia Elimination Programme — 321
Chapter 60: National Programme for Prevention and Management of Trauma and Burn Injuries — 324
Chapter 61: Pradhan Mantri National Dialysis Programme — 328
Chapter 62: National Programme for Palliative Care — 332

Part D: Nutrition

Chapter 63: Integrated Child Development Services Scheme — 339
Chapter 64: PM—Poshan Scheme/Mid-Day Meal—Pradhan Mantri Poshan Shakti Nirman — 347
Chapter 65: National Iodine Deficiency Disorders Control Programme — 350
Chapter 66: National Programme for Prevention and Control of Fluorosis — 353
Chapter 67: Antyodaya Anna Yojana — 357

Part E: Digital Health Initiatives

Chapter 68: National Digital Health Mission/Ayushman Bharat Digital Mission — 363
Chapter 69: eSanjeevani—National Telemedicine Service — 372
Chapter 70: e-Health Initiatives in India — 378

Part F: Miscellaneous

Chapter 71: Ayushman Bharat Programme — 385
Chapter 72: Pradhan Mantri Bhartiya Janaushadhi Pariyojana — 391
Chapter 73: Beti Bachao Beti Padhao — 396
Chapter 74: Kayakalp — 399
Chapter 75: National Jal Jeevan Mission — 404
Chapter 76: Swachh Swasth Sarvatra Initiative — 408
Chapter 77: Pradhan Mantri Ujjwala Yojana — 412
Chapter 78: Ujjawala Scheme for Prevention of Trafficking and Rescue, Rehabilitation and Reintegration of Victims of Trafficking — 415
Chapter 79: National Programme on Climate Change and Human Health — 418
Chapter 80: Voluntary Blood Donation Programme — 425
Chapter 81: National Organ Transplant Programme — 430
Chapter 82: National Programme for Control and Treatment of Occupational Diseases — 434
Chapter 83: National Programme on Containment of Anti-Microbial Resistance — 439
Chapter 84: Social Security Schemes for Unorganized and Organized Sectors — 446
Chapter 85: Schemes for Intellectual Disability — 455
Chapter 86: Pradhan Mantri Swasthya Suraksha Yojana — 460
Chapter 87: Affordable Medicines and Reliable Implants for Treatment — 463
Chapter 88: National Action Plan for Prevention and Control of Snakebite Envenoming — 465

Index — 471

SECTION I: Understanding National Health Program Framework

Section Outline

Chapter 1: Evolution of Health Programs in India
Chapter 2: Logos of All National Health Programs
Chapter 3: Planning a National Health Program
Chapter 4: Evaluating National Health Programs: A Crucial Endeavor
Chapter 5: Mastering India's Healthcare Delivery System for Effective Program Implementation
Chapter 6: Health Committees in India
Chapter 7: National Institution for Transforming India Aayog
Chapter 8: Sustainable Development Goals

CHAPTER 1

Evolution of Health Programs in India

Pallavi Singh, Rohit Katre, Bharti Koria

Program	Timeline
NITI Aayog	1st January 2015
National Health Mission	12th April 2005
RMNCHA+N	February 2013
LaQshya	14th April 2016
Janani Suraksha Yojana	12th April 2005
JSSK	1st June 2011
PMSMA	31st July 2016
Surakshit Matritva Aashwasan	10th October 2019
HBNC	2011
HBYC	2018
IMNCI	2003
SAANS	November 2019
MAA	8th August 2016
IYCF	2004
RBSK	February 2013
RKSK	7th January 2014
Dakshta Training	30th April 2015
Menstrual Hygiene Scheme	2011
UIP/Mission Indradhanush	1985/December 2014
NVBDCP	2003–4
NTEP	1962
NACP	1992
NLEP	1983
IDSP	November 2004
IHIP	26th November 2018
National Viral Hepatitis Control Program	28th July 2018
National Programme for Prevention and Control of Deafness	2006–2007
National Mental Health Programme	August 1982
National Oral Health Programme	2014–2015
National Sickle Cell Anemia Elimination programme	1st July 2023

Section I: Understanding National Health Program Framework

Program	Timeline
POSHAN	8th March 2018
ICDS	2nd October 1975
National Iodine Deficiency Disorder Control Programme	December 1989
PM- POSHAN/Mid-day Meal Scheme	15th August 1995
National Programme for Prevention and Control of Fluorosis	2008–2009
Antyodaya Anna Yojana	25th December 2000
Ayushman Bharat	23rd September 2018
Swach Bharat Mission	2nd October 2014
Kayakalp	15th May 2015
Pradhan Mantri Ujjwala Yojana	1st May 2016
Ujjwala Scheme	2007
Pradhan Mantri Jan Aushadhi Yojana	November 2008
National Programme on Climate Change and Human Health	2019
National Rabies Control Programme	2013
National Organ Transplant Programme	2019
National Programme for Palliative Care	2012
Pradhan Mantri National Dialysis Programme	7th April 2016
NPPMBI	6th February 2014
National Programme on Containment of Antimicrobial resistance	2012
National Jal Jeevan Mission	August 2019
National Tobacco Control Program	2007–08
NP-NCD	2010–11
National Programme for Control of Blindness and Visual Impairment	1976

CHAPTER 2

Logos of All National Health Programs

Pallavi Singh, Rohit Katre, Bharti Koria

Program	Logo
NITI Aayog	
National Health Mission	
LaQshya	
Janani Suraksha Yojana	
JSSK	

Section I: Understanding National Health Program Framework

Program	Logo
PMSMA	Pradhan Mantri Surakshit Matritva Abhiyaan – 9th of Every Month
Surakshit Matritva Aashwasan	SUMAN
MDSR	Maternal Death Surveillance and Response (MDSR)
HBNC HBYC	Home Based Care of New Born and Young Child – HBNC & HBYC
IMNCI	IMNCI – Integrated Management of Neonatal and Childhood Illness
SAANS	SAANS – निमोनिया नहीं, तो बचपन सही

Chapter 2: Logos of All National Health Programs

Program	Logo
MAA	
RBSK	
RKSK	
Dakshta Training	
UIP/Mission Indradhanush	
NVBDCP	

Section I: Understanding National Health Program Framework

Program	Logo
NTEP	
NACO	
NLEP	
IDSP	
Pradhan Mantri Digital Saksharta Abhiyan	
National Viral Hepatitis Control Programme	

Chapter 2: Logos of All National Health Programs

Program	Logo
National Programme for Prevention and Control of Deafness	
National Mental Health Programme	
National Oral Health Programme	
National Sickle Cell Anemia Elimination Programme	
POSHAN	
ICDS	

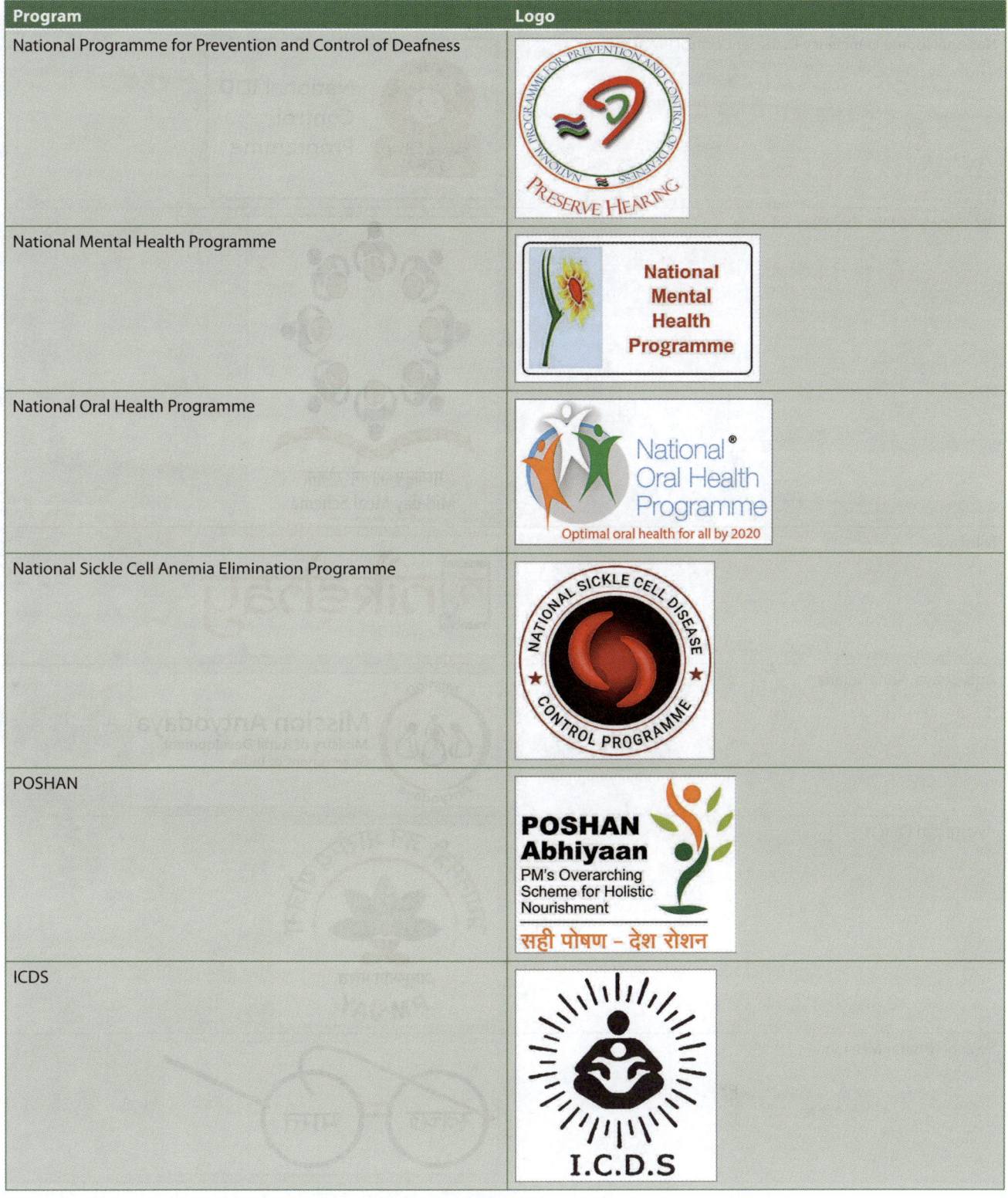

Section I: Understanding National Health Program Framework

Program	Logo
National Iodine Deficiency Disorder Control Programme	National IDD Control Programme
PM-POSHAN/Mid-day Meal Scheme	मध्याह्न भोजन योजना Mid-day Meal Scheme
Nikshyay	nikshay
Antyodaya Anna Yojana	Mission Antyodaya, Ministry of Rural Development, Government of India
Ayushman Bharat	प्रधानमंत्री जन आरोग्य योजना आयुष्मान भारत PM-JAY
Swachh Bharat Mission	स्वच्छ भारत

Chapter 2: Logos of All National Health Programs | 11

Program	Logo
Kayakalp	
Pradhan Mantri Ujjwala Yojana	
Pradhan Mantri Jan Aushadhi Yojana	
National Program on Climate Change and Human Health	
National Rabies Control Programme	

Section I: Understanding National Health Program Framework

Program	Logo
National Organ Transplant Programme	
National Programme for Palliative Care	
National Jal Jeevan Mission	
National Tobacco Control Program	
NP-NCD	
National Programme for Control of Blindness and Visual Impairment	

CHAPTER 3
Planning a National Health Program

Shyambhavee, Kartikey Yadav, Rudresh Negi

Background	Health program is a totality of *"an organized structure designed for provision of a fairly discrete health-focused intervention, where that intervention is designed for a specific target audience".*[1] Health programs are one of the pillars of the public health system in India. These are the key to disease prevention and control and addressing health disparities. They are prime in achieving better health outcomes, promoting health equity in providing health for all. Development of a health program is a process of continuous organized motivated efforts towards optimal utilization of available resources in achieving the desired health related goal, with selection of the best available alternative. Before understanding the development and evolution of a health program, making an informed decision regarding selection of disease of public health concern, to be considered for inclusion as a national health program, is of major concern, given the limitation of resources. Numerous factors are involved while deciding the inclusion of a health problem as a disease of public health importance. Following conditions needs to be assessed while deciding the same: • **Burden of the disease:** The magnitude of the disease in terms of mortality and morbidity. Majority of the developing and developed nations are currently undergoing epidemiological transition. This has led to an increase in the burden of non-communicable diseases (NCDs), which has further led to significant morbidity and mortality across the globe. The government of India later developed the National Program for prevention and control of cancer, diabetes, cardiovascular disease and stroke addressing an umbrella of noncommunicable diseases. Apart from noncommunicable diseases, communicable diseases which poses a significant healthcare burden like, tuberculosis, malaria, were considered for inclusion in the healthcare programs. • **Public health impact:** The disease should have a substantial impact on the economic and social status of the community as whole. Diseases like NCDs impose a significant economic burden on the healthcare system as well as is one of the reasons behind catastrophic health expenditure at individual level. Also, diseases like HIV/AIDS and tuberculosis still have a profound social impact apart from economic and health related burden. • **Availability of preventive and curative services:** The disease must have an effective, accessible, acceptable, and affordable prevention and treatment options available. Understanding the disease epidemiology, in order to assess their control and elimination potential is also one of the important considerations. Availability of vaccination and good potential for elimination in terms of the disease transmission rate, agent and host factors were one of the few pillars towards elimination of polio across major geographic areas. • **Concordance with global health priorities:** The health issue should be in concordance with the national health priorities and must address the challenges based on the local country's need, and in alignment with the sustainable development goals. Emphasis has been given to the upcoming burden of NCDs in the national program for prevention and control of NCDs and also to the maternal and child health under the India's National Health Mission. • **Addressing health equity among the vulnerable:** With the disproportionate distribution of diseases among the vulnerable, consideration to be taken while addressing the disparities in healthcare utilization. • **Evidence-based decision making:** Availability of scientific evidence describing the disease burden and its impact using adequate health assessment tools is of importance, while deciding the health priorities.

Planning a health program	Planning a health program in India is a comprehensive and multifaceted process which includes involvement of multiple disciplines. The central government of India lays down the guidelines for all the health programs and the implementation takes place at the state level, with strategies and approaches that are suitable as per the local needs. The development of a national health program also follows the basic principle of planning cycle which includes the following: • Situational analysis • Problem identification and selection of the priorities • Setting goals objectives • Strategy formulation • Identification of resources • Program implementation • Monitoring and evaluation
Steps in planning a national health program	The beginning of a health program usually takes place in the form of a pilot phase. This stage involves program development and need assessment. With the program maturity, it may evolve as a model program. Later the program evaluation helps in assessment of program efficacy and implementation barriers. The planning and evaluation cycle involves four basic stages including, community assessment, planning, implementation, and effect evaluation. 1. **Situational analysis:** This stage involves collection of information regarding the health problem in terms of the associated burden, mortality, distribution, socioeconomic impact in the community, current prevailing prevention and control strategies. The same can be assessed using data from the available scientific reports, research articles, and national or subnational levels surveys. This stage also involves assessment of the target beneficiaries, status of the current health related agencies, already available health infrastructure, etc. 2. **Problem identification and selection of priorities:** Based upon the situational analysis, perceived lacunae between what is there and what further needs to be done, is identified. Identifying the problem and its plausible is the key in setting goals and objectives of the program. The identified problems can be in terms of present disease morbidity and mortality burden, nonavailability of desired data for action, suboptimal functional infrastructure and human resource, poor intersectoral coordination, high out-of-pocket expenditure incurred by the community, etc. Given the resource limitation and an exhaustive list of healthcare problems, prioritizing the needs becomes essential. This can be done with the help of multiple assessment methods including cost-effective analysis, comprehensive assessment of disease morbidity and mortality using disability adjusted life years (DALY), health technology assessment, etc. 3. **Setting goals and objectives:** An overarching open-ended broad vision and goal needs to be made before defining clear objectives for any health program. Goal is the broad statement that is related to the impact that is to be achieved. The aim provides as nonmeasurable direction towards the desired goal. Based on the desired goal, clear objectives are defined which are **S**imple, **M**easurable, **A**ttainable, **R**ealistic, and **T**ime bound (SMART). The objectives are the essential precursor of designing the control strategies. Targets are the desired level of performance for a specific indicator. These are key in defining the performance indicators that enables objective monitoring and evaluation. 4. **Strategy formulation:** It includes detailed descriptive plan of the program process in terms of strategies and detailed intervention plan, in order to achieve the desired goals and objectives. This will include the program timeline in terms of geographical implementation, detailed description of all the intervention, and enumeration of the key stakeholders. 5. **Identification of resources:** Following formulation of the program strategy, resources that are required to implement the formulated strategies needs to be identified. Resources can be in terms of manpower, material, and money. 6. **Program implementation:** Inter-sectoral coordination and commitment of the concerned stakeholders is required for a successful program implementation. Program implementation in India, usually follows a decentralized approach. 7. **Monitoring and evaluation:** A robust monitoring and evaluation system is the final pillar of a functional program. It is vital for tracking the program progress. Key Performance indicators (KPIs) are made in line with the program objectives and strategic plans, to assess the input, process, output and outcome, in a defined objective manner.

Chapter 3: Planning a National Health Program

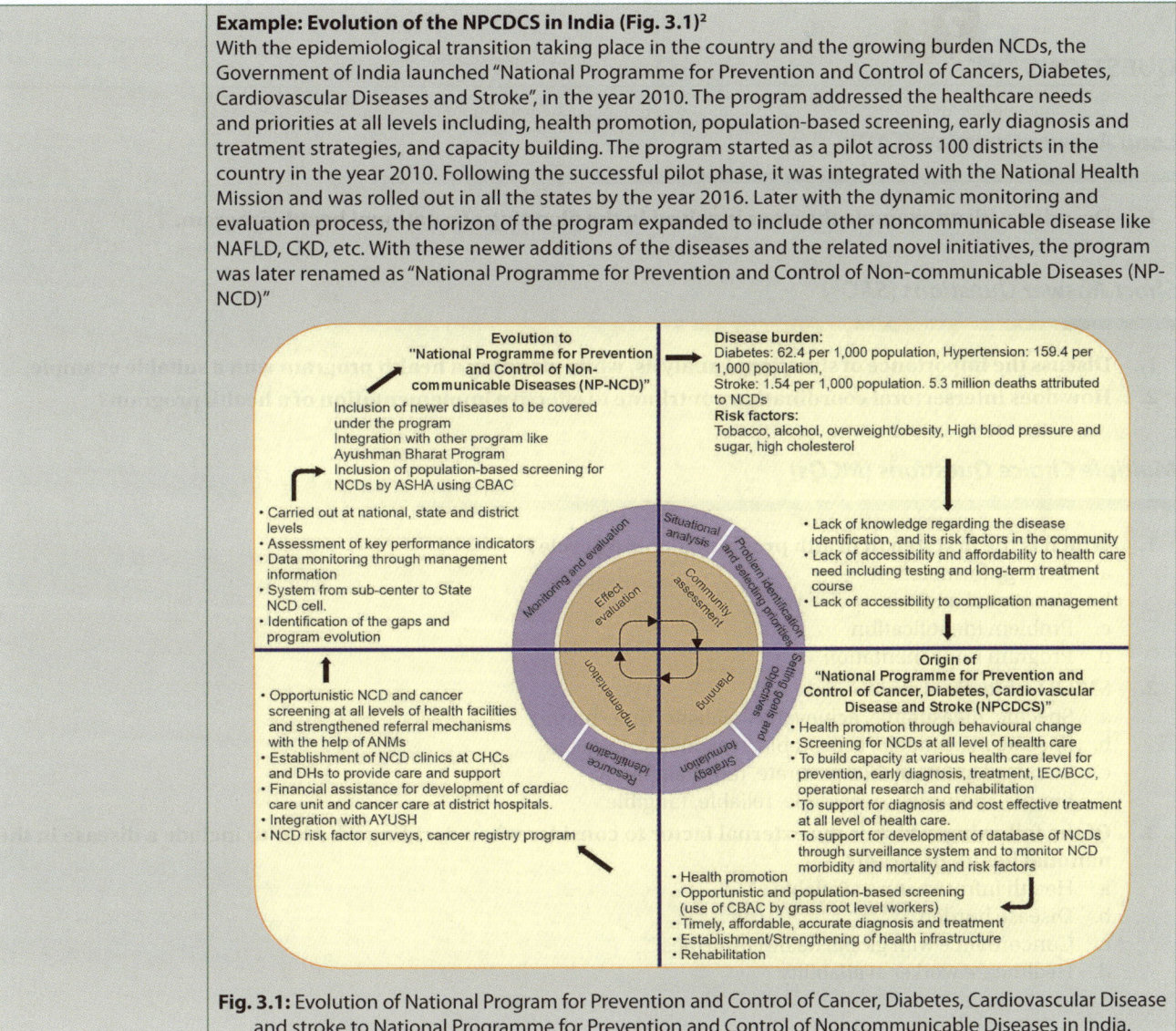

Example: Evolution of the NPCDCS in India (Fig. 3.1)[2]

With the epidemiological transition taking place in the country and the growing burden NCDs, the Government of India launched "National Programme for Prevention and Control of Cancers, Diabetes, Cardiovascular Diseases and Stroke", in the year 2010. The program addressed the healthcare needs and priorities at all levels including, health promotion, population-based screening, early diagnosis and treatment strategies, and capacity building. The program started as a pilot across 100 districts in the country in the year 2010. Following the successful pilot phase, it was integrated with the National Health Mission and was rolled out in all the states by the year 2016. Later with the dynamic monitoring and evaluation process, the horizon of the program expanded to include other noncommunicable disease like NAFLD, CKD, etc. With these newer additions of the diseases and the related novel initiatives, the program was later renamed as "National Programme for Prevention and Control of Non-communicable Diseases (NP-NCD)"

Fig. 3.1: Evolution of National Program for Prevention and Control of Cancer, Diabetes, Cardiovascular Disease and stroke to National Programme for Prevention and Control of Noncommunicable Diseases in India.

References

1. Michele Issel L, Wells R. Health program planning and evaluation: A practical, systematic approach for Community Health. 4th ed. Burlington: Jones & Bartlett; 2018
2. National Programme for prevention and control of cancer, cardiovascular diseases and stroke, Operational guidelines (2013-17) [Internet]. India: Ministry of Health and Family Welfare, Government of India; 2013 [cited 23 July, 2024]. Available from: https://main.mohfw.gov.in/sites/default/files/Operational%20Guidelines%20of%20NPCDCS%20%28Revised%20-%202013-17%29_1.

QUESTIONS

Long Answer Question (LAQ)

1. Describe with an example the steps involved in the planning of a national health program.

Short Answer Questions (SAQs)

1. Discuss the importance of situational analysis, while planning a health program with a suitable example.
2. How does intersectoral coordination contribute to effective implementation of a health program?

Multiple Choice Questions (MCQs)

1. Which is the first step in health program planning cycle?
   a. Strategy formulation
   b. Situational analysis
   c. Problem identification
   d. Program implementation
2. SMART objectives are:
   a. Specific, measurable, achievable, realistic, time-bound
   b. Special, measurable, acceptable, reasonable, targeted
   c. Standard, manageable, accurate, rational, timely
   d. Simple, motivated, accessible, reliable, tangible
3. Of the following, which is the external factor to consider when deciding whether to include a disease in the national health program?
   a. Health infrastructure available
   b. Disease burden
   c. Concordance with global health priorities
   d. Healthcare worker availability

Answers

1. b   2. a   3. c

CHAPTER 4

Evaluating National Health Programs: A Crucial Endeavor

Varun Vijay Gaiki, Thej Kiran Reddy, Rudresh Negi

Background

National health programs play a pivotal role in ensuring citizens' well-being by providing essential healthcare services. These programs aim to provide comprehensive and equitable access to healthcare services for all citizens, regardless of their socioeconomic status. A thorough evaluation of the effectiveness and efficiency of such programs is essential to ensure they are meeting the healthcare needs of the population. This critical appraisal will analyze the key aspects of the national health program, including its objectives, implementation, and outcomes, to identify areas for improvement and inform future policy decisions. Evaluating these programs is essential to gauge their impact and efficiency. Let's delve into the key aspects of program evaluation:

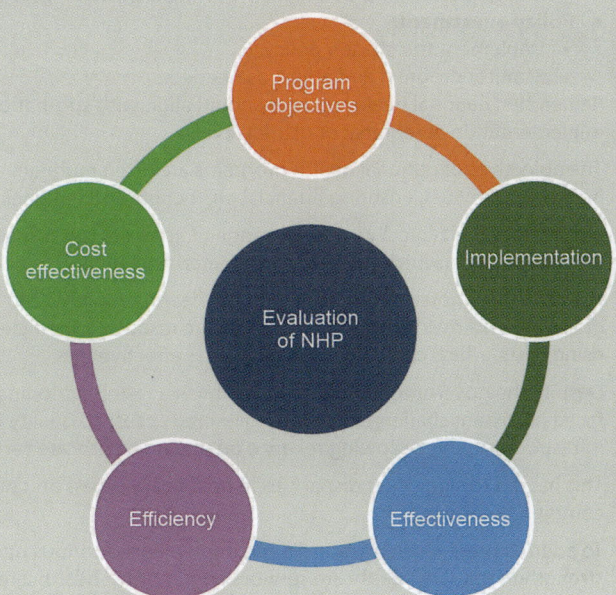

Fig. 4.1: Key aspects of program evaluation.

- **Program objectives:** First, we assess whether the program is achieving its intended goals. Are healthcare services accessible, equitable, and effective? We scrutinize whether the program aligns with its stated objectives.
- **Implementation:** We examine whether the program activities are carried out as originally intended. Is there fidelity to the program design? Are resources effectively utilized?
- **Effectiveness:** The crux of evaluation lies in determining whether the program achieves its desired outcomes. Are health indicators improving? Is disease prevention effective? We measure success against predefined benchmarks.
- **Efficiency:** Efficient use of resources is crucial. We analyze whether the program optimally utilizes budget, staff time, and other resources. Efficiency ensures maximum impact for every resource invested.

	• **Cost-effectiveness:** Beyond efficiency, we assess whether the benefits gained from the program outweigh the costs incurred. Is the value delivered commensurate with the investment? Remember, program evaluation is not an isolated exercise; it occurs within real-world constraints. Practicality, ethics, and accurate findings guide our assessments. By evaluating national health programs rigorously, we pave the way for informed policy decisions and better healthcare outcomes.

Formulation of NHP	To understand how to do program appraisal, we need to focus on steps, on how a program is formulated. Formulating a **National Health Program** involves a systematic process that considers various factors. Let's explore the key steps:[1,2]
	• **Problem identification:**
	  ✦ Define the health issue or problem affecting the population.
	  ✦ Collect relevant data (e.g., frequency, severity, causes).
	  ✦ Identify gaps in information.
	  ✦ Frame the problem for potential policy solutions
	• **Policy analysis:**
	  ✦ Explore different policy options.
	  ✦ Evaluate each option.
	  ✦ Health impact (morbidity, mortality).
	  ✦ Costs (implementation vs benefits).
	  ✦ Feasibility (political and operational factors).
	• **Strategy and policy development:**
	  ✦ Based on analysis, choose the most effective, efficient, and feasible policy.
	  ✦ Develop a comprehensive plan with clear goals, targets, and intersectoral alignment.
	• **Policy enactment:**
	  ✦ Implement the chosen policy.
	  ✦ Monitor progress and adjust as needed.
	Remember, national health policies should align with sub-national operational plans to ensure effective implementation at regional or district levels.
	
	The objectives of national health programs are often multifaceted, ranging from improving access to healthcare services, ensuring financial protection, and enhancing the quality of care.
	
	These programs typically involve a range of activities, such as service delivery, financing, resource generation, and governance, which must be coordinated and aligned to achieve the desired outcomes.
	
	However, the implementation of national health programs can be fraught with challenges, as countries often grapple with a maldistribution of healthcare resources, inefficient medical care delivery systems, and rapidly rising costs, which can hinder the program's effectiveness.
	
	Despite the government's efforts to establish a well-functioning public healthcare system, India has faced persistent challenges, including limited access to quality care in rural areas, a lack of public health infrastructure, and a growing reliance on private healthcare services.
	
	This has led to significant disparities in healthcare access and outcomes, particularly among marginalized communities.
	
	To address these challenges, India has implemented various national health programs, which aims to strengthen primary healthcare services and improve healthcare access in underserved areas.
	
	However, the effectiveness of these programs has been limited by factors such as inadequate funding, weak governance, and the inability to address the underlying social determinants of health.
	
	The critical appraisal of national health programs must also consider the broader social, economic, and political context in which they operate.
	
	Factors such as socioeconomic status, cultural beliefs, and political priorities can all influence the design, implementation, and outcomes of these programs.
	
	For instance, the parallel systems of public and private healthcare in India have created a complex landscape that requires a nuanced approach to policy-making and implementation.
	
	Knowing the steps involved in planning any National Health Program, it now becomes relatively easy to do critical appraisal of an NHP.

Chapter 4: Evaluating National Health Programs: A Crucial Endeavor

We simply need to target each component of the program, with thinking that, is the parameter considered in all its possible aspects or any important dimension if it is missing?

World Health Organization, in its publication, Innov8 approach[7] for reviewing National Health Programs to leave no one behind: technical handbook, mentions of typical eight steps, to evaluate a National Health Program, in order for a program to be all inclusive.

Step 1: Complete the diagnostic checklist;
Step 2: Understand the program theory;
Step 3: Identify who is being left out by the program;
Step 4: Identify the barriers and facilitating factors that subpopulations experience;
Step 5: Identify mechanisms generating health inequities;
Step 6: Consider intersectoral action and social participation as central elements;
Step 7: Produce a redesign proposal to act on the review findings;
Step 8: Strengthen monitoring and evaluation.

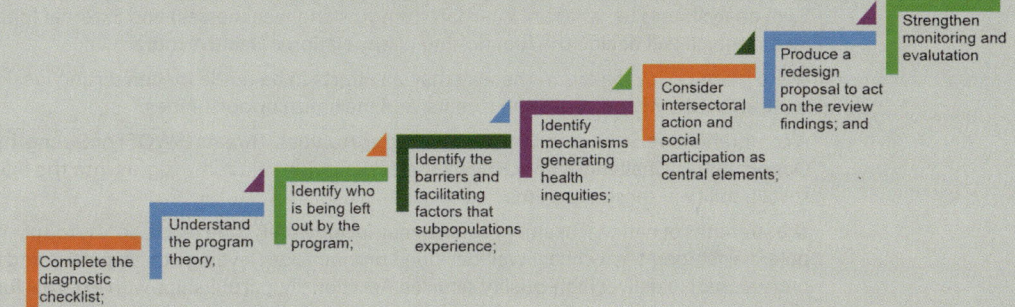

Fig. 4.2: Steps involved in reviewing National Health Program.

Another way routinely used to do situational analysis (situational assessment) is use of SWOT and SWOC analysis. Where, S stands for strengths, W stands for Weaknesses, O for Opportunities T for threats which is sometimes replaced by C in challenges.
(Please note that, there are some minor variations of SWOT, and SWOC being the commonest, others are Strengths-opportunities-aspirations-results and strengths-vulnerabilities-opportunities-risks)
Typical swot analysis is done in a 2 × 2 table as shown in **Figure 4.3**.

Strengths	Weaknesses
Opportunities	**Threats**

Fig. 4.3: Showing typical structure of 2 × 2 table for SWOT analysis.

SWOT analysis	A **SWOT analysis** is a valuable tool for assessing the internal and external factors that can impact a program or organization. Let's break it down:[2,3] <ul><li>**Strengths (internal):**<ul><li>Characteristics of the organization that contribute to success.</li><li>Resources and capabilities that help achieve goals.</li><li>Past successes and positive aspects.</li></ul>Consider how you can leverage these strengths.</li></ul>

- **Weaknesses (internal):**
  - Characteristics that might hinder success.
  - Absence of strengths.
  - Factors contributing to past failures.
  - Areas to improve or avoid.
- **Opportunities (external):**
  - Environmental factors that can positively influence outcomes.
  - Unfulfilled niches or unmet customer needs.
  - Upcoming changes (regulatory, political, social, etc.).
  - How unique strengths can capitalize on opportunities.
- **Threats (external):**
  - Environmental factors that may prevent success.
  - Upcoming changes (regulatory, political, social, etc.).
  - Consider political, economic, sociocultural, and technological factors.

Swot analysis tells us, what are internal (strengths and weaknesses) and External (opportunities and threats) factors which will decide the functioning of any National Health Program.[4]

It also helps policy makers in the way that, all efforts to be made for converting weaknesses into strengths, use these strengths to overcome threats, and maximize opportunities.[5]

A comprehensive Strengths, Weaknesses, Opportunities, Threats (SWOT) or Strengths, Weaknesses, Opportunities, Challenges (SWOC) analysis can provide valuable insights into the effectiveness and sustainability of these programs.[3,5]

The strengths of national health programs may include their wide reach, access to substantial resources, and potential for long-term impact Well-designed programs can leverage the expertise and dedication of healthcare professionals to deliver high-quality services. Additionally, partnerships with external funding institutions can bolster the programmers' financial resources and enable them to tackle complex healthcare challenges.

However, National Health Programs may also face weaknesses, such as poor spatial organization, lack of specifically trained personnel, and inadequate sanitary facilities. Centralization of health services and professionals can hinder the programmers' responsiveness to local needs.[6]

Opportunities for National Health Programs include the potential to expand coverage, improve health information systems, and enhance economic support for healthcare.

Let's have a couple of examples of SWOT analysis of national health programs. Remember these are just for representational purposes and not complete SWOT of any program.

SWOT analysis of NVBDCP:

Strengths	Weaknesses
Integrated approach: NVBDCP cover.' multiple vector-borne diseases (malaria, dengue, etc.) under one umbrella program, allowing shared strategies for vector control and management **Existing infrastructure:** Utilizes existing healthcare infrastructure, including primary health centers (PHCs). Sub-district hospitals (SDKs), and hospitals operating 24 x 7 **ASHA workers:** Over 1.400 accredited social health activists (ASHA) workers contribute to community-level awareness and surveillance.	**Resource constraints:** Limited funding and resources may hinder program implementation. **Fragmentation:** Despite integration, challenges in coordination between different disease-specific components. **Human resource gaps:** Shortage of trained personnel for vector control activities.
Opportunities	*Threats*
Community engagement: Strengthening community participation can enhance vector control efforts. **Research and innovation:** Explore new technologies, insecticides, and surveillance methods.	**Climate change:** Alters vector distribution and disease patterns. **Insecticide resistance:** Growing resistance to insecticides affects control measures. **Urbanization:** Rapid urban growth increases exposure to vectors.
Collaboration: Partner with other health programs and stakeholders for synergies.	

SWOT analysis for NP-NCD

Strengths	Weaknesses
Integrated approach: The NCD program collaborates with existing healthcare services, leveraging infrastructure such as hospitals and clinics. **Health workforce:** Trained healthcare professionals contribute to prevention, early detection, and management of NCDs. **Public awareness:** The program emphasizes health education and awareness campaigns.	**Resource constraints:** Limited binding and staffing may hinder program implementation. **Fragmentation:** Challenges in coordinating efforts across different NCDs (e.g., diabetes, cardiovascular diseases). **Data gaps:** Insufficient data on NCD prevalence and risk factors.
Opportunities	**Threats**
Community engagement: Strengthening community involvement can enhance prevention and control efforts. **Research and innovation:** Explore new technologies. treatments, and preventive strategies. **Policy advocacy:** Advocate for policies that promote healthy lifestyles and NCD prevention.	**Changing demographics:** Aging populations increase NCD burden. **Lifestyle trends:** Unhealthy habits (sedentary lifestyle, poor diet) contribute to NCD risk. **Health inequities:** Address disparities in access to care and resources.

SWOT of RMNCHA+

Strengths	Weaknesses
Integrated approach: RMNCHA- combines services across life stages (reproductive, maternal, newborn, child, and adolescent health), addressing interdependencies. **Health workforce:** Trained professionals contribute to effective service delivery. **Public awareness:** The program emphasizes health education and community engagement.	**Resource constraints:** Limited funding and staffing may hinder program implementation. **Fragmentation:** Challenges in coordinating efforts across different health services. **Data gaps:** Insufficient data on health outcomes and service utilization.
Opportunities	**Challenges**
Community participation: Strengthening community involvement can enhance prevention and control efforts. **Technological advances:** Explore digital health solutions for better service delivery. **Policy advocacy:** Advocate for policies that prioritize RMNCHA+.	**Changing demographics:** Aging populations and population growth impact health needs. **Health inequities:** Address disparities in access to care and resources. **Global health trends:** Consider emerging diseases and health threats.

References

1. Skinner K, Hanning RM, Sutherland C, Edwards-Wheesk R, Tsuji LJS. Using a SWOT Analysis to Inform Healthy Eating and Physical Activity Strategies for a Remote First Nations Community in Canada. Am J Health Promot. 2012;26(6):e159-e70. doi:10.4278/ajhp.061019136
2. Muhammad RP, Meditya W. Business Escalation Strategy Using Time Series Forecasting for Hotel X in Yogyakarta. Int J Curr Sci Res Rev. 2023;6(8):5600-17.
3. Paschalidou A, Tsatiris M, Kitikidou K, Papadopoulou C. Methods (SWOT Analysis). In: Using Energy Crops for Biofuels or Food: The Choice. Green Energy and Technology. Springer: 2018, Cham. https://doi.org/10.1007/978-3-319-63943-7_6
4. Ahsan Siddiqui. SWOT Analysis (or SWOT Matrix) Tool as a Strategic Planning and Management Technique in the Health Care Industry and Its Advantages. Biomed J Sci & Tech Res. 2021; 40(2). BJSTR. MS.ID.006419.
5. Ebrahim EMA, Ghebrehiwot L, Abdalgfar T, Juni MH. Health Care System in Sudan: Review and Analysis of Strength, Weakness, Opportunity, and Threats (SWOT Analysis). Sudan Med J Sci. 2017; 12(3): 133-50. https://doi.org/10.18502/sjms.v12i3.924
6. World Health Organization (WHO) Consultation Document: A Framework for National Health Policies, Strategies and Plans, 2010.
7. Facilitator's manual for the Innov8 approach for reviewing national health programmes to leave no one behind. Working draft 2017: Version for further piloting. World Health Organization 2017.

QUESTIONS

Long Answer Questions (LAQs)

1. Discuss process for deciding priorities in National Health Program. Do swot analysis of National AIDS control Programme.
2. Discuss the significance of conducting a SWOT analysis for a national health program. How can each component of the Strengths, Weaknesses, Opportunities, Threats (SWOT) analysis be utilized to enhance the effectiveness of the program?
3. Analyze how a National Health Program can use its strengths to capitalize on opportunities and overcome threats. Provide examples of specific strategies that could be employed.
4. Examine the potential weaknesses of a national health program and propose strategies for converting these weaknesses into strengths. What role does innovation play in this process?
5. Reflect on the role of opportunities in the expansion and improvement of a national health program. How can a SWOT analysis guide the strategic decision-making process to maximize these opportunities?
6. Evaluate the impact of external threats on the success of a national health program. How can a SWOT analysis help in developing contingency plans to address these threats?

Short Answer Questions (SAQs)

1. What does SWOT stand for in the context of strategic analysis?
2. How can identifying strengths in a national health program benefit its implementation?
3. What is an example of a weakness in a national health program, and how can it affect the program's success?
4. Explain how opportunities in a SWOT analysis can influence the future direction of a national health program.
5. Why is it important to identify threats in a national health program's SWOT analysis?
6. Describe a situation where a national health program's strength can also present a weakness.
7. How can a SWOT analysis assist policymakers in improving a national health program?
8. What role do external factors play in the "Opportunities" and "Threats" components of a SWOT analysis?
9. Give an example of how a national health program can turn a weakness into an opportunity.
10. How can a national health program use its strengths to address identified threats in a SWOT analysis?

Multiple Choice Questions (MCQs)

1. What does the "S" in SWOT analysis stand for?
   a. Strengths
   b. Strategies
   c. Solutions
   d. Successes
2. In the context of a national health program, which of the following is an example of a "Weakness"?
   a. High-quality medical staff
   b. Inadequate funding
   c. Strong government support
   d. Technological advancements
3. What type of factor would the availability of advanced medical technology in a national health program be considered in a SWOT analysis?
   a. Strength
   b. Weakness
   c. Opportunity
   d. Threat

4. Identifying new healthcare delivery models that can be implemented is an example of which component of a SWOT analysis?
   a. Strength
   b. Weakness
   c. Opportunity
   d. Threat
5. Which of the following would be considered a "Threat" in a SWOT analysis of a national health program?
   a. Increasing public awareness of health issues
   b. Rise in chronic diseases
   c. Government policy support
   d. Availability of funds for research
6. In a SWOT analysis, the introduction of a new health technology that could improve patient outcomes falls under which category?
   a. Strength
   b. Weakness
   c. Opportunity
   d. Threat
7. Which of the following is an example of a "Strength" in a national health program's SWOT analysis?
   a. Lack of trained personnel
   b. Strong network of primary health centers
   c. High prevalence of disease
   d. Inconsistent policy enforcement
8. In the context of a national health program, inadequate infrastructure would be categorized under which aspect of SWOT analysis?
   a. Strength
   b. Weakness
   c. Opportunity
   d. Threat
9. The emergence of new health challenges, such as pandemics, would most likely be classified as a:
   a. Strength
   b. Weakness
   c. Opportunity
   d. Threat
10. A SWOT analysis of a national health program reveals strong international collaboration. This would most likely be classified as a:
    a. Strength
    b. Weakness
    c. Opportunity
    d. Threat

Answers

1. a
2. b
3. a
4. c
5. b
6. c
7. b
8. b
9. d
10. a

5 CHAPTER

Mastering India's Healthcare Delivery System for Effective Program Implementation

Thej Kiran Reddy, Varun Vijay Gaiki, Rudresh Negi

Introduction	India's healthcare system is one of the most complex and multifaceted healthcare delivery system in the world. It caters for about 1.41 billion people, which in itself is challenging at the level of program implementation. Clear understanding is necessary for effective implementation of large scale public health programs. This chapter provides an in-depth look at the structure, components, challenges, and opportunities within the Indian healthcare system, offering essential insights for students, program planners and implementers.
Structure	India's healthcare system is a hierarchical model. This is based on the 1946 Bhore committee recommendation to Government of India. The rationale behind this is to give access to primary healthcare to all irrespective of their socioeconomic background. In the federalized system of India, the health is a state subject and the union ministry provides the technical and financial assistance to the state. However some programs are implemented on a national scale by the Union Ministry of health and family welfare (NACP, NTEP, etc.). Public health system in India can be dissected into various sections, for clear understanding, starting from national level to village level. **National level:** The Ministry of Health and Family Welfare (MoHFW) is the apex body responsible for health policy formulation, planning, and funding. MoHFW has two departments, Department of Health and Family welfare and Department of health research (Indian Council of Medical Research). There are several autonomous bodies under MoHFW like JIPMER, AIIMS, FSSAI, etc. Key agencies under MoHFW include the National Health Mission (NHM), which encompasses the DHGS, NHA, National Rural Health Mission (NRHM) and the National Urban Health Mission (NUHM), NHSRC, PM ABHIM.[1] **Directorate General of Health Services (DGHS):** The Directorate General of Health Services (DGHS) is a vital component of India's healthcare system. Let's delve into its role and functions: • *Technical advice*: DGHS provides expert guidance on all matters related to medical and public health. This includes advising on policies, programs, and strategies to improve health outcomes. • *Implementation*: DGHS actively participates in the implementation of various health services across the country. It collaborates with state and district health authorities to ensure effective delivery of healthcare. • *Coordination*: As an attached office of the Department of Health and Family Welfare, DGHS plays a crucial role in coordinating efforts at the national level. It bridges the gap between policy formulation and on-ground execution. • *Subordinate offices*: DGHS has subordinate offices spread throughout India. These offices work closely with local health institutions, monitor programs, and facilitate communication between central and state levels. In short, DGHS serves as a linchpin in India's healthcare machinery, providing technical expertise, facilitating implementation, and ensuring a coordinated approach to health services. • **National Health Authority (NHA):** The National Health Authority (NHA) plays a pivotal role in India's healthcare landscape. Let's explore its functions and the flagship scheme it oversees: ✦ **Ayushman Bharat Pradhan Mantri Jan Arogya Yojana (PM-JAY):** – Launched in September 2018, PM-JAY is the world's largest health assurance scheme. It aims to provide health coverage of ₹5 lakhs per family per year for secondary and tertiary care hospitalization.

        – PM-JAY targets that 40% of population, which is most marginalized and lies in the bottom of Indian population. It covers over 12 crore poor and vulnerable families making approximately 55 crore beneficiaries. Eligibility is determined based on the Census 2011 (SECC 2011) criteria.
        – This scheme replaced the earlier Rashtriya Swasthya Bima Yojana (RSBY) and covers a wide range of medical services.
    + **Health and Wellness Centers (HWCs):**
        – As part of Ayushman Bharat, the government announced the creation of 1,50,000 Health and Wellness Centers by transforming existing sub-centers and primary health centers.
        – These centers deliver Comprehensive Primary Healthcare (CPHC), including maternal and child health services, non-communicable disease management, essential drugs, and diagnostic services.
        – The focus is on health promotion, prevention, and community engagement.
    + **National Digital Health Mission:**
        – NHA is entrusted with designing the strategy and building the technological infrastructure for the **National Digital Health Ecosystem**.
        – This mission aims to create a seamless digital platform for health records, telemedicine, e-pharmacies, and other health services.

    NHA's multifaceted role encompasses health insurance, primary care, and digital health initiatives, all contributing to India's vision of **Universal Health Coverage** and leaving no one behind.

- **National Health Mission (NHM)** is a crucial initiative by the Government of India to address health needs across the country. It encompasses two vital sub-missions:
    1. **National Rural Health Mission (NRHM):**
        – NRHM focuses on providing healthcare services to underserved rural areas.
        – It aims to strengthen health systems, ensuring equitable, affordable, and quality care for all.
        – Key components include Reproductive-Maternal-Neonatal-Child and Adolescent Health (RMNCH+A), communicable and non-communicable disease management, and health system strengthening.
    2. **National Urban Health Mission (NUHM):**
        – NUHM, a newly launched sub-mission, targets urban areas.
        – It aims to enhance healthcare access and quality in cities and towns.
        – NUHM focuses on urban health centers, preventive services, and community engagement.

    Together, NHM strives for universal health coverage, making healthcare accountable and responsive to people's needs.

- **National Health Systems Resource Centre (NHSRC):** The National Health Systems Resource Centre (NHSRC) is a vital institution established in 2007 by the Government of India. As a premier think tank for the Ministry of Health and Family Welfare (MoHFW), its mission is to:
    + Enable technical support and capacity building for strengthening of public health systems.
    + Generate evidence from the field to formulate and evaluate policies and strategies.
    + Focus on decentralization, equity, and quality to align with the goals of the National Health Policy 2017. NHSRC plays a crucial role in improving health outcomes by facilitating governance reform, health system innovations, and information sharing among stakeholders at various levels—national, state, district, and sub-district. Its work areas cover a wide range of topics, including healthcare financing, human resources for health, quality and patient safety, and more. The center's vision is to ensure universal access to equitable, affordable, and quality healthcare that is accountable and responsive to the people of India.[1] If you need further information, you can visit the.

- **Pradhan Mantri Ayushman Bharat Health Infrastructure Mission (PM-ABHIM)**
    For strengthening the Public Health Infrastructure effectively, manage and respond towards any future pandemics and outbreaks, PM-Ayushman Bharat Health Infrastructure Mission (PM-ABHIM) is announced in union budget for 2021-2022. The PM-ABHIM is a centrally sponsored scheme with central sector components, for implementation of the Atmanirbhar Bharat (self-reliant India) package for health sector.
    + **Centrally sponsored components:**
        – Support for 17,788 rural health and wellness centers in 10 high focus states.
        – Establishment of 11,024 urban health and wellness centers across all states.
        – Setting up 3,382 Block public health units in 11 high focus states.

- Support for other states/UTs under XV Finance Commission Health Sector Grants and NHM.
- Integrated public health labs in all districts.
- Critical care hospital blocks in districts with a population of more than 5 lakhs.
  - **Central sector components:**
    - 12 Central Institutions as training and mentoring sites with 150-bedded critical care hospital blocks.
    - Strengthening the National Centre for Disease Control (NCDC) and establishing new regional NCDCs.
    - Expanding the Integrated Health Information Portal to all states/UTs.
    - Operationalizing new public health units at points of entry (airports, seaports, and land crossings).
    - Setting up health emergency operation centers and container-based mobile hospitals.
    - Establishing a national institution for One Health, new National Institutes for Virology, and Bio-Safety Level III laboratories.
- **State level:** In the context of health services management, autonomy plays a crucial role in ensuring effective and responsive healthcare delivery. Based on regional needs, states have complete autonomy in implementing the national policies. States have autonomy in managing health services, including funding, program execution, and human resource management. Health at state level is managed by the state ministry of health and family welfare.

For effective health planning, state health society is formed. At the state level, the mission would function under the overall guidance of the State Health Mission headed by the Chief Minister of the State. The functions under the mission would be carried out through the State Health and Family Welfare Society.[2]

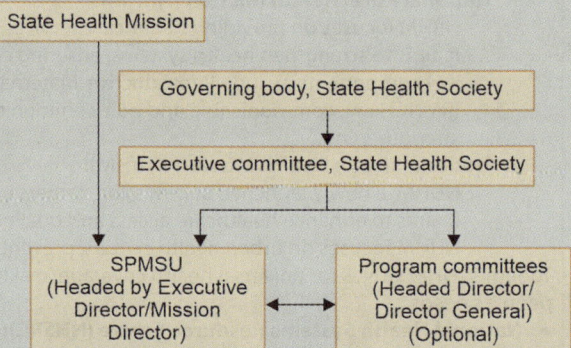

Fig. 5.1: Composition of state health mission.

There are three major divisions under the state health ministry (for the sake of explanation Telangana state is considered here):[3]

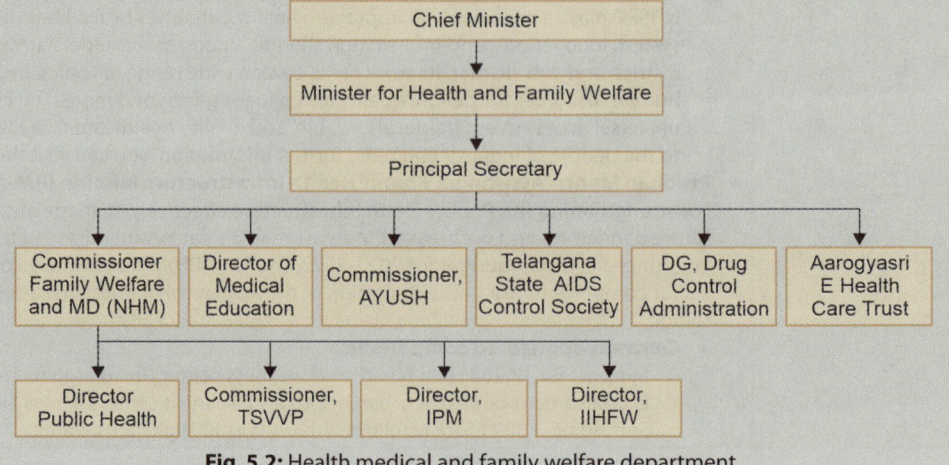

Fig. 5.2: Health medical and family welfare department.

Chapter 5: Mastering India's Healthcare Delivery System for Effective Program Implementation

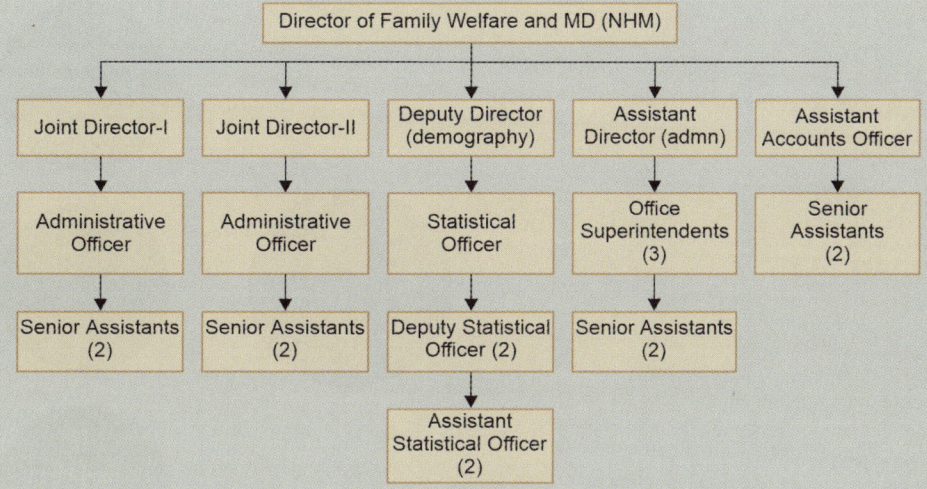

Fig. 5.3: Commissionerate of health and family welfare.

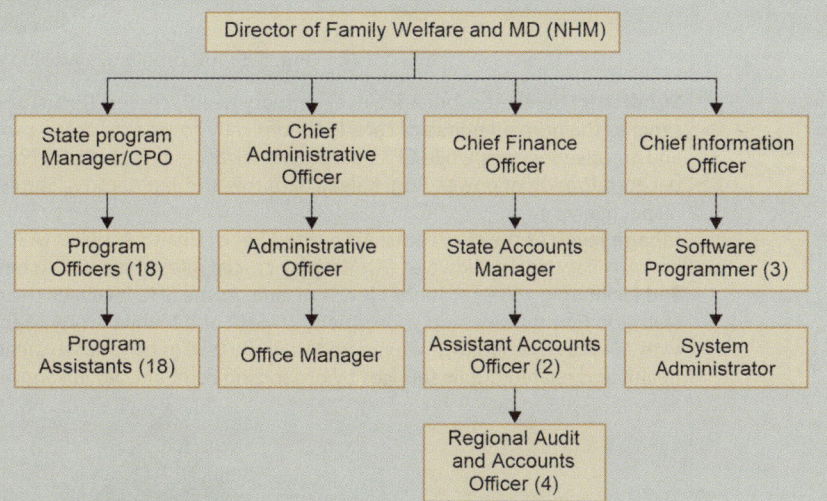

Fig. 5.4: State program management unit (state health mission).

District level:
- At the district level, health system is lead and directed by CMO/DMHO/CDMO/CS. It is the most challenging level in the implementation of the programs. From this level one can notice the change over from policy perspective to people perspective. National health programs are managed and monitored by Nodal officers/Program officers along with district programmatic management unit.[4]
- Similar to the State Health Mission, each district will establish a District Health Mission led by the Chairperson of the Zila Parishad. The District Collector will serve as the Co-Chair, and the Chief Medical Officer will be the Mission Director.
- To support the District Health Mission, each district will form an integrated District Health Society (DHS). This DHS will consolidate all existing societies that function as vertical support structures for various national and state health programs. The DHS will be responsible for planning and managing all health and family welfare programs in the district, covering both rural and urban areas.
- This structure has two significant implications. First, DHS planning must consider both treasury and non-treasury funding sources, even though it may not directly manage all of them. Second, the DHS's geographical jurisdiction will extend beyond the boundaries of the Zila Parishad and Urban Local Bodies (ULBs) within the district.

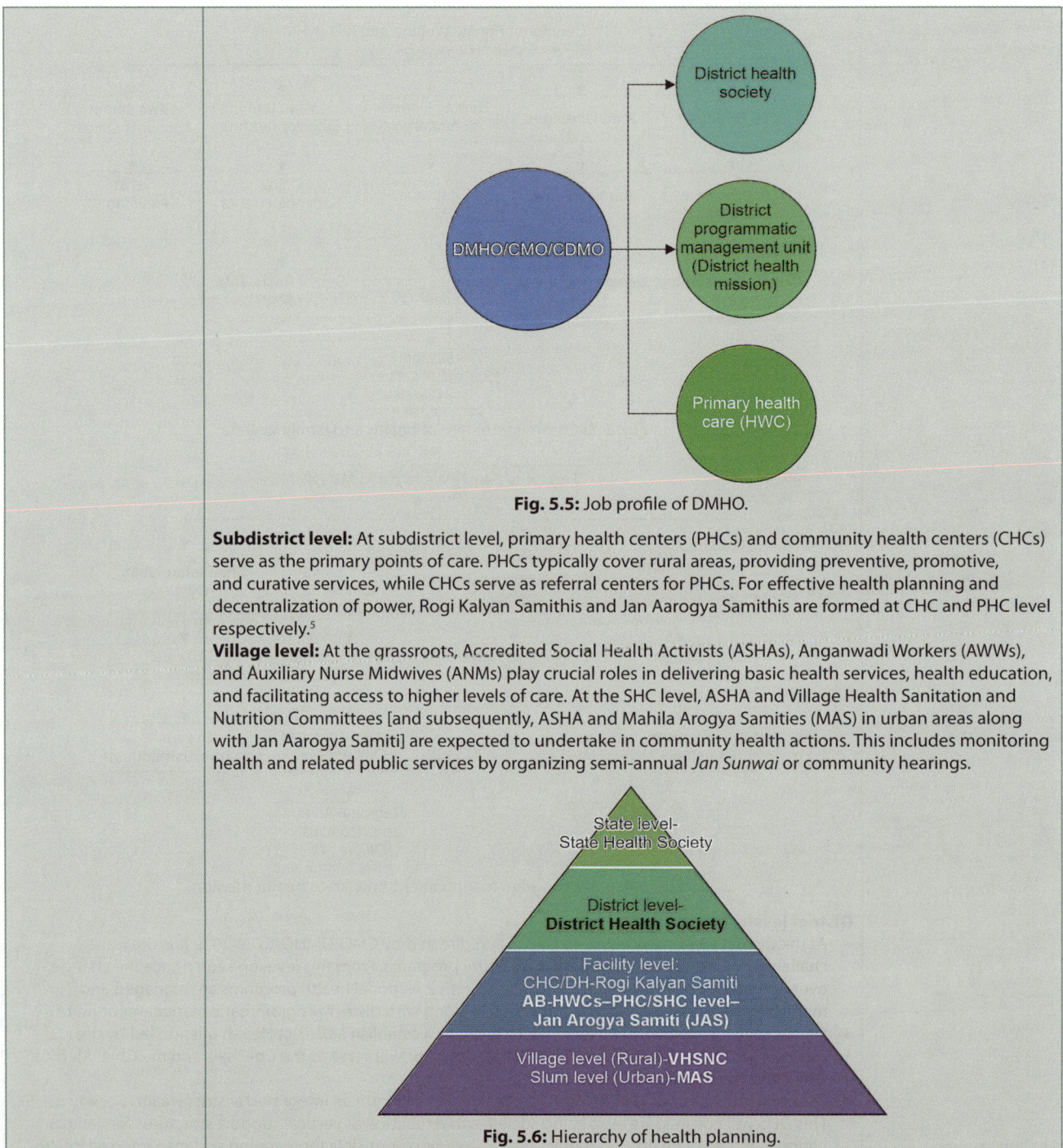

Fig. 5.5: Job profile of DMHO.

Subdistrict level: At subdistrict level, primary health centers (PHCs) and community health centers (CHCs) serve as the primary points of care. PHCs typically cover rural areas, providing preventive, promotive, and curative services, while CHCs serve as referral centers for PHCs. For effective health planning and decentralization of power, Rogi Kalyan Samithis and Jan Aarogya Samithis are formed at CHC and PHC level respectively.[5]

Village level: At the grassroots, Accredited Social Health Activists (ASHAs), Anganwadi Workers (AWWs), and Auxiliary Nurse Midwives (ANMs) play crucial roles in delivering basic health services, health education, and facilitating access to higher levels of care. At the SHC level, ASHA and Village Health Sanitation and Nutrition Committees [and subsequently, ASHA and Mahila Arogya Samities (MAS) in urban areas along with Jan Aarogya Samiti] are expected to undertake in community health actions. This includes monitoring health and related public services by organizing semi-annual *Jan Sunwai* or community hearings.

Fig. 5.6: Hierarchy of health planning.

Goal	The PM-ABHIM aims to strengthen critical healthcare infrastructure across various levels (e.g., villages or blocks) over the next five years, ensuring equitable, accessible, and high-quality healthcare for all

Objectives	• Strengthen public health institutions and deliver comprehensive primary healthcare. • Expand the technology-based surveillance system and develop surveillance laboratories. • Increase research on infectious diseases.

Components of healthcare delivery system in India	India has a three tier system for healthcare delivery. It is divided as primary, secondary and tertiary care services.
	• **Primary**
	  ✦ Primary healthcare forms the foundation of the Indian healthcare delivery system. The primary healthcare approach is grounded in principles of social equity, nationwide coverage, self-reliance, intersectoral coordination, and active community participation in the planning and implementation of health programs to achieve common health goals. The Declaration of Alma-Ata emphasized that primary healthcare is crucial for attaining an acceptable level of health for all by the year 2000. As a signatory to this declaration, the Government of India has committed to providing primary healthcare.
	  ✦ In 2005, the National Rural Health Mission (now the National Health Mission) was launched with the goal of achieving universal access to equitable, affordable, and quality healthcare services that are accountable and responsive to people's needs. This initiative also aimed to foster effective inter-sectoral convergent action to address the broader social determinants of health.
	  ✦ More recently, the Astana Declaration of October 2018 reaffirmed the critical role of primary healthcare globally. The declaration aims to refocus efforts on primary healthcare to ensure that everyone, everywhere, can attain the highest possible standard of health. To meet these national and international commitments, it is essential for public health facilities to deliver quality services.
	  ✦ In order to provide a full range of services, primary healthcare is essential. Health and wellness centers play a significant role in the prevention of many diseases, including both communicable and non-communicable diseases, in addition to providing primary care patients with the fundamental curative services.[6]
	  ✦ Through population enumeration, facility-based and outreach services, frequent home-based and community visits, and improved engagement, they aim to provide a people-centered, holistic, equity-sensitive response to people's health needs. A community-based participatory approach, which ensures preventive and promotive actions, considered as a priority for health, is the primary objective of these centers.
	  ✦ Bringing services closer to the community and closely monitoring them will enhance coverage and help address the marginalization and exclusion of specific population groups.
	The twelve packages envisaged under comprehensive primary healthcare services (CPHC) are:
	  1. Care in Pregnancy and Childbirth
	  2. Neonatal and Infant Healthcare Services
	  3. Childhood and Adolescent Healthcare Services
	  4. Family Planning, Contraceptive Services, and other Reproductive Healthcare Services
	  5. Management of Communicable Diseases: National Health Programs
	  6. General Out-patient Care for Acute Simple Illnesses and Minor Ailments
	  7. Screening, Prevention, Control and Management of Non-communicable Diseases
	  8. Care for Common Ophthalmic and ENT Problems
	  9. Basic Oral Healthcare
	  10. Elderly and Palliative Healthcare Services
	  11. Emergency Medical Services including Burns and Trauma
	  12. Screening and Basic Management of Mental Health Ailments
	Primary Health care is delivered through HWC- primary health centers (1 per 30,000-50,000 population) along with their subsidiary HWC-sub-centers (1 per 5000 population).
	Flow of services at PHC, enquiry-registration-waiting area-doctor's consultation room-injection room/dressing room-laboratory-doctor's consultation room-pharmacy-exit.
	The provision of health services includes, early identification, basic management, counseling, ensuring treatment adherence, follow-up care, ensuring continuity of care by appropriate referrals, optimal home and community follow-up, and disease surveillance.
	• **Secondary care**
	  ✦ Secondary healthcare is delivered through community health centers. They are acting as bridge between primary and tertiary care. Service delivery at secondary level is through Non-FRU-CHC and FRU-CHCs.

- **Non-FRU-CHCs (rural):** Non-FRU-CHCs offer essential services, including preventive, promotive, curative, palliative, and rehabilitative care. Curative services include normal deliveries and the stabilization of common emergencies. These CHCs in rural areas will have 30 essential beds.
- **FRU-CHCs (rural and urban):** In addition to the services provided by Non-FRU-CHCs, FRU-CHCs offer specialized care through specialists such as physicians, surgeons, obstetricians, pediatricians, and anesthesiologists. They are equipped with the necessary infrastructure, including functional operation theaters and blood storage units. Both elective and emergency surgical services of secondary level care are provided, extending beyond obstetric services to include a wide range of surgical interventions.
- **Block public health units (BPHUs):** All CHCs at the block headquarters level, both in rural and urban areas, are to be developed into BPHUs. Every block in the country is envisioned to have a CHC, block PHC, or SDH at the block headquarter (HQ), serving as a referral hub for the SHCs and PHCs within the block. However, the implementation varies across states—in some states, the Block CHC functions merely as another PHC, while in others, it serves as a first referral unit. Currently, the block health facility provides selected clinical services, a limited range of public health functions, and administrative control over the health institutions within the block.
- BPHUs are expected to focus on four functional areas: clinical service delivery, public health functions, a block public health laboratory to support both clinical and public health functions, and a health management information system (HMIS) unit. Clinical and diagnostic services will be delivered according to Indian Public Health Standards (IPHS), with efforts to enhance the quality and timeliness of reporting on service delivery and public health data. BPHUs will also promote decentralized planning and the preparation of block health plans that integrate into district health plans.
- Community health center in rural areas (CHC) is to be established for a population norm of 80,000 (in hilly and tribal areas) and 1,20,000 (in plains) and/or time to care approach. Community health centre in urban areas serve for about 5,00,000 population with a bed capacity of 100. These centers provide 98 services under their purview.

Work flow at a CHC: Enquiry—Registration—Waiting—Nursing Station—Clinic—Dressing room/Injection Room—Diagnostics (lab/imaging)—Drug dispensation—Appraisal by the patient through *Mera Aspataal feedback*—Exit.

- **Tertiary care**
  - Tertiary care is delivered at district hospitals, sub-district hospitals and medical colleges. They are the end point in care at district level.
  - In every district in the country, at least one bed per 1000 population is essential and two beds per 1000 population is desirable. If we consider an example of a district with 10 lakh population, 1000 beds are essential (including all the beds in all facilities from PHC to DH) and 2000 beds are desirable.
  - To achieve the 'Desirable' number of beds, the contribution of the private sector (based on the access to private healthcare in the local area), Railways, Armed Forces, Power Grid, Coal fields, Employees' State Insurance (ESI) and other Public Sector Undertaking (PSU) hospitals may also be considered while continuing to strengthen and increase bed provision at public health facilities.
  - District hospital services are built on three pillars—clinical care, a knowledge hub for capacity development of health human resources, and public health programs to ensure the continuum of care and reduce the disease burden.
  - Clinical care encompasses curative, palliative, and rehabilitative services, along with the implementation of national programs, provision of drugs, diagnostic services, administrative/maintenance services, and other support services. In addition to curative services, district and sub-district hospitals should strongly emphasize health promotion, prevention, palliation, and rehabilitation.
  - District hospitals should strive to become the knowledge hubs of their respective districts by offering a range of services, such as medical courses including the Diplomate of National Board (DNB), nursing schools, ANM training centers, district training centers for various programs, and a resource center equipped with computers, information resources, and telemedicine capabilities. This can be achieved through partnerships with universities.[7]
- **Medical colleges**
  - Major role of medical education is to provide medical education in terms of under graduate education for MBBS, nursing and para-medical students and post-graduate education for MD/MS, nursing, physiotherapists and pharma D students.

	<ul><li>Teaching hospitals often provide specialized care to the local population that may not be available in other hospitals, including advanced surgical procedures, complex diagnostics, and treatment for rare conditions.</li><li>They engage in community outreach programs, including health camps, vaccination drives, and public health awareness campaigns, addressing local health issues and promoting preventive healthcare.</li><li>Medical colleges are hubs for medical research, contributing to advancements in medical knowledge, treatments, and technologies. Research conducted in these institutions helps improve healthcare practices and policies (operational and implementational research).</li></ul><ul><li>**Clinical skills training:**<ul><li>Simulation labs: Use of advanced mannequins and simulation technology to practice procedures and patient interactions in a controlled environment through NELS center.</li><li>Hands-on training in various medical specialties, including internal medicine, surgery, pediatrics, obstetrics and gynecology, and psychiatry.</li><li>Skills training: Regular capacity building of human resource at different levels of healthcare delivery system, through workshops on essential clinical skills like suturing, intravenous access, and cardiopulmonary resuscitation (CPR). Trainings of ASHAs and ANMs on various health conditions are also conducted through medical colleges in the state. Trainings of various program managers and program directors under various NGOs and Mother NGOs also facilitated through medical colleges.</li><li>Medical colleges also do supportive supervision in terms of health system strengthening , this will help improving patient care, enhanced professional competence, better resource utilization and overall community health improvement. They also provide mentorship and guidance to healthcare staff working for primary healthcare.</li><li>Medical colleges often play a vital role during epidemic outbreaks by deploying Rapid Response Teams (RRTs). These teams are composed of healthcare professionals and students trained to provide immediate and effective responses to health emergencies.</li><li>Apart from the three tier public healthcare delivery system, India also has a large scale private healthcare model in place.[8]</li></ul></li></ul>
Role of the private sector in implementing India's National Health Programs	The private sector, which still caters more than 2/3 of population plays a crucial role in India's national health programs, complementing public efforts and addressing critical gaps.<ul><li>**Expertise and infrastructure:**<ul><li>The private sector provides **58% of hospitals** and **81% of doctors** in India, primarily in urban areas.</li><li>Their expertise and infrastructure contribute significantly to healthcare delivery.</li></ul></li><li>**Public-private partnerships (PPPs):**<ul><li>Fight of India against HIV had emphasized need of PPP model and its potential in healthcare, which was restressed by COVID-19 pandemic.</li><li>Collaborations between public and private sectors in diagnostics, technology, and treatment saved lives during the pandemic.</li></ul></li><li>**Affordability and accessibility:**<ul><li>The private sector can help address affordability and accessibility challenges.</li><li>By leveraging their expertise and last-mile infrastructure, they can extend quality healthcare to rural communities.</li></ul></li><li>**Research and innovation:**<ul><li>Private healthcare providers collaborate with international institutions, fostering knowledge exchange and research.</li><li>These partnerships enhance medical practices and benefit the Indian healthcare system.</li></ul></li></ul>Private sector, had played a crucial role in implementation of various national health programs like RMNCH, Universal Immunization Program, National Blindness Control Programs, National Tuberculosis Elimination Program (earlier known as revised National Tuberculosis Control Program), etc. Another important player in delivery of healthcare system in India is the use of involvement of AYUSH. The Ministry of AYUSH regulates the educational standards of the Indian Systems of Medicine and Homoeopathy colleges in the country, as well as in collaboration with Ministry of Health and Family Welfare, takes care of healthcare delivery at grassroot, along with involvement in NHPs. Here's how they contribute to the implementation of national health programs:<ul><li>**National AYUSH Mission (NAM):**<ul><li>The **Ministry of AYUSH** implements NAM, aiming to provide cost-effective AYUSH services.</li></ul></li></ul>

> - **Key objectives include:**
>   - Upgrading AYUSH hospitals and dispensaries.
>   - Co-locating AYUSH facilities at primary health centers (PHCs), community health centers (CHCs), and district hospitals (DHs).
>   - Strengthening AYUSH educational institutions.
>   - Establishing integrated AYUSH hospitals and health and wellness centers.
>   - Empowering self-care through AYUSH principles.
> - **Holistic wellness model:**
>   - AYUSH systems emphasize holistic well-being, combining traditional knowledge with modern practices.
>   - By upgrading existing dispensaries and sub-health centers, AYUSH health and wellness centers offer comprehensive primary healthcare rooted in AYUSH principles.
> - **Local health traditions:**
>   - AYUSH revitalizes local health traditions, bridging gaps in rural healthcare delivery.
>   - These systems, with their low-cost, natural approaches, cater to under-served, remote, and tribal areas.
>
> AYUSH contributes to a **healthy India** by integrating traditional systems, promoting wellness, and ensuring accessible healthcare for all.
>
> In summary, involvement of the private sector, along with involvement of traditional healers from various pathies and their active participation, expertise, collaborative efforts are essential for achieving universal healthcare in India. By working together, we can bridge gaps and improve health outcomes for all.

References

1. Home | Ministry of Health and Family Welfare | GOI . https://main.mohfw.gov.in/.
2. Composition of SHM and SHS https://nhm.gov.in/index1.php?lang=1andlevel=3andsublinkid=1137andlid=143 (accessed July 25, 2024).
3. Organogram of Health, Medical and Family Welfare https://www.telangana.gov.in/departments/health-medical-family-welfare/ (accessed July 25, 2024).
4. Composition of DHS and DHM https://nhm.gov.in/index1.php?lang=1andlevel=3andsublinkid=1136andlid=144 (accessed July 25, 2024).
5. Community ownership of health and wellness centres—Guidelines for Jan Arogya Samiti.
6. Indian Public Health Standards Health And Wellness Centre - Primary Health Centre 2022.
7. Indian Public Health Standards Sub District Hospital And District Hospital 2022..
8. Role of Medical Institutions in RCH Programme - Dr. Pawan Kumar, Additional Commissioner, MoHFW.

QUESTIONS

Long Answer Questions (LAQs)

1. Discuss in detail how healthcare system works at state level.
2. Explain in detail components of healthcare delivery system in India.
3. Critically analyze the strengths and weaknesses of India's three-tier healthcare delivery system. How do these strengths and weaknesses impact the implementation of national health programs?
4. Evaluate the role of the National Health Mission (NHM) in strengthening India's healthcare delivery system. What have been the key achievements and challenges of the NHM in improving health outcomes?
5. Discuss the impact of the Ayushman Bharat Scheme on India's healthcare delivery system. How does this program address the healthcare needs of economically vulnerable populations, and what are the challenges in its implementation?
6. Examine the role of technology in enhancing the efficiency of India's healthcare delivery system. How can digital health initiatives contribute to more effective implementation of health programs?

Chapter 5: Mastering India's Healthcare Delivery System for Effective Program Implementation

7. Analyze the role of public-private partnerships (PPPs) in strengthening India's healthcare delivery system. What are the potential benefits and risks associated with PPPs in the context of implementing national health programs?

Short Answer Questions (SAQs)

1. Write a short note on National Health Authority.
2. Write in detail about components of PM ABHIM.
3. Write a short note on NHSRC.
4. What are the main components of India's three-tier healthcare delivery system?
5. How does the Ayushman Bharat Scheme aim to improve healthcare access in India?
6. What role do Primary Health Centers (PHCs) play in the healthcare delivery system of rural India?
7. Identify a key challenge in implementing healthcare programs in remote areas of India.
8. How do Accredited Social Health Activists (ASHAs) contribute to the effectiveness of healthcare programs in India?

Multiple Choice Questions (MCQs)

1. Which of the following is the primary healthcare delivery model in rural India?
   a. Tertiary care hospitals
   b. Primary health centers
   c. Private clinics
   d. Urban health centers

2. What is the role of Accredited Social Health Activists (ASHAs) in India's healthcare system?
   a. To manage tertiary care hospitals
   b. To provide financial assistance to patients
   c. To act as community health workers at the grassroots level
   d. To regulate private healthcare facilities

3. Which of the following is a key objective of the National Health Mission (NHM) in India?
   a. To promote medical tourism
   b. To improve maternal and child health
   c. To increase privatization of healthcare
   d. To establish more super-specialty hospitals

4. The Ayushman Bharat program aims to provide:
   a. Free primary education to children
   b. Health insurance coverage to economically vulnerable families
   c. Employment opportunities in the healthcare sector
   d. Free electricity to rural households

5. Which of the following is a challenge in implementing effective healthcare programs in India?
   a. High literacy rates across the country
   b. Well-distributed healthcare infrastructure
   c. Limited access to healthcare in remote areas
   d. Excessive government funding

6. What is one of the primary responsibilities of the Directorate General of Health Services (DGHS) in India?
   a. Supervising private hospitals across the country
   b. Conducting medical entrance examinations
   c. Formulating and implementing public health policies
   d. Managing pharmaceutical production in government facilities

7. Which of the following is a key function of the Directorate General of Health Services (DGHS) concerning epidemic control?
   a. Approving new vaccines for market release
   b. Overseeing the national program for epidemic prevention and control
   c. Regulating food and drug safety standards
   d. Conducting medical research on infectious diseases
8. Which of the following is a primary objective of the National Health Mission (NHM)?
   a. To provide universal health insurance coverage
   b. To ensure universal access to equitable, affordable, and quality healthcare services
   c. To promote medical tourism in India
   d. To establish private healthcare facilities in rural areas
9. Which of the following programs is a key component of the National Health Mission aimed at reducing maternal and infant mortality?
   a. Pradhan Mantri Jan Arogya Yojana
   b. Integrated Child Development Services (ICDS)
   c. Janani Suraksha Yojana (JSY)
   d. Mid-Day Meal Scheme
10. The National Health Mission (NHM) includes the National Rural Health Mission (NRHM) and which other mission?
    a. National Urban Health Mission (NUHM)
    b. National Maternal Health Mission (NMHM)
    c. National Child Health Mission (NCHM)
    d. National Nutrition Health Mission (NNHM)

Answers

1. b
2. c
3. b
4. b
5. c
6. c
7. b
8. b
9. c
10. a

CHAPTER 6

Health Committees in India

Parul Sharma, Parth Thakkar

INTRODUCTION

Health committees in India have played a pivotal role in shaping the country's healthcare policies and programs. These committees have laid the foundation for major public health initiatives, policy frameworks, and infrastructural improvements in the healthcare sector.

KEY HEALTH COMMITTEES AND THEIR RECOMMENDATIONS

Committee	Year	Key Recommendations
Bhore committee[1]	1946	• Proposed a three-tier healthcare system (PHCs, Secondary Health Centers, District Hospitals). • Recommended free healthcare services and emphasis on preventive care. • Advocated for a district-based health planning approach. • Suggested increasing health expenditure to improve accessibility.
Mudaliar committee[2]	1962	• Recommended increasing the number of healthcare professionals. • Emphasized strengthening district hospitals. • Suggested reducing the doctor-population ratio to 1:3000. • Proposed improving medical education quality.
Chadha committee[3]	1963	• Suggested utilizing basic health workers for National Malaria Eradication Programme (NMEP). • Emphasized house-to-house surveys for disease control. • Proposed integrating malaria control into general health services. • Recommended improving surveillance and monitoring systems.
Mukherjee committee[4]	1966	• Reviewed the functioning of NMEP. • Recommended integration of malaria control with general healthcare. • Highlighted the need for interdepartmental coordination.
Jungalwalla committee[5]	1967	• Advocated for unification of health services under a single authority. • Suggested integration of health and family planning services. • Recommended decentralized healthcare administration. • Stressed the need for better health infrastructure.
Kartar singh committee[6]	1973	• Recommended training multi-purpose health workers (MPWs). • Suggested linking MPWs with PHCs to improve outreach. • Proposed redefining roles of health supervisors. • Emphasized community participation in health programs.
Shrivastav committee[7]	1975	• Proposed a cadre of community health workers (CHWs). • Suggested task-sharing between doctors and paramedics. • Emphasized primary healthcare strengthening. • Recommended better rural healthcare delivery mechanisms.
Bajaj committee[8]	1986	• Focused on medical education reforms. • Recommended increasing medical colleges. • Emphasized training healthcare professionals for rural services. • Proposed linking health training institutions with service delivery.

Lentin commission[9]	1988	• Investigated medical negligence cases. • Recommended stricter medical regulations. • Suggested improved drug control policies. • Highlighted the need for enhanced hospital accountability.
National commission on macroeconomics and health[10]	2005	• Assessed economic aspects of healthcare. • Suggested increased public health investment. • Proposed financing mechanisms for healthcare expansion. • Emphasized the economic impact of health policies.
High-level expert group on universal health coverage[11]	2011	• Recommended increasing public healthcare spending to 2.5% of GDP. • Suggested strengthening primary healthcare. • Advocated reducing out-of-pocket expenses. • Proposed universal health coverage for all citizens.

Health committees in India have significantly influenced the evolution of the healthcare system. Their recommendations have led to improvements in healthcare infrastructure, workforce development, and service delivery. Continuous evaluation and implementation of these recommendations remain crucial for achieving better health outcomes in the country.

References

1. Bhore J. Report of the Health Survey and Development Committee. Government of India; 1946.
2. Mudaliar A. Health Survey and Planning Committee Report. Government of India; 1962.
3. Chadha VK. National Malaria Eradication Programme Report. Government of India; 1963.
4. Mukherjee Committee. Report. Government of India; 1966.
5. Jungalwalla PN. Report on the Unification of Health Services. Government of India; 1967.
6. Kartar Singh Committee. Report. Government of India; 1973.
7. Shrivastav Committee. Report. Government of India; 1975.
8. Bajaj JS. Report on Medical Education and Manpower Development. Government of India; 1986.
9. Lentin Commission. Report. Government of India; 1988.
10. Ministry of Health and Family Welfare, Government of India. National Commission on Macroeconomics and Health Report. 2005.
11. Planning Commission of India. High-Level Expert Group Report on Universal Health Coverage. 2011.

QUESTIONS

Long Answer Questions (LAQs)

1. Discuss the role of various health committees in shaping India's healthcare system.
2. Explain the recommendations of the Bhore Committee and its impact on public health in india.
3. Compare and contrast the recommendations of the Mudaliar Committee and the Shrivastav Committee.
4. Evaluate the significance of the high-level expert group on universal health coverage in India's health policy.

Short Answer Questions (SAQs)

1. What were the key recommendations of the Chadha Committee?
2. How did the Mukherjee Committee contribute to malaria control policies?
3. Why was the Jungalwalla Committee formed, and what were its major suggestions?
4. What was the focus of the Bajaj Committee in 1986?
5. Explain the significance of the Kartar Singh Committee in improving rural healthcare services.

Chapter 6: Health Committees in India

Multiple Choice Questions (MCQs)

1. The Bhore Committee was established in which year?
   a. 1948
   b. 1946
   c. 1951
   d. 1962
2. The Mudaliar Committee recommended reducing the doctor-population ratio to:
   a. 1:2000
   b. 1:5000
   c. 1:3000
   d. 1:4000
3. Which committee proposed the creation of a cadre of community health workers (CHWs)?
   a. Shrivastav Committee
   b. Chadha Committee
   c. Kartar Singh Committee
   d. Bhore Committee

Answers

1. b
2. c
3. a

CHAPTER 7

National Institution for Transforming India Aayog

Vikram Kumar Gupta, Shaili Vyas, Bhavesh Kanabar

Background/Need of program/ Scheme	NITI stands for "National Institution for Transforming India". In the Sanskrit language, the term "NITI" encompasses concepts such as ethical conduct, proper behavior, and principled guidance. It is the India's premier policy-making institution that is expected to bolster the economic growth of the country. Its objective is to foster a robust governmental framework that contributes to the development of a vibrant and powerful nation. This approach aids India in its journey to become a significant player in the global economic landscape.[1] The establishment of NITI Aayog incorporates two primary components: the "Team India Hub" and the "Knowledge and Innovation Hub." These elements are integral to the organization's structure and purpose. NITI Aayog have replaced the previous 'Planning Commission' having a legacy of 65 years after India attained its Independence since year 1947. For quite some time, the effectiveness and importance of the Planning Commission had been under scrutiny. NITI Aayog appears to be better aligned with and more adaptable to the current economic climate and requirements of the nation. India's diverse landscape is characterized by states at varying stages of economic growth, each with its distinct advantages and challenges. Given this complexity, applying a uniform approach to economic planning is no longer feasible. Such a strategy is ill-equipped to enhance India's competitiveness in the contemporary global marketplace. NITI Aayog is a pivotal organization that is bound to play a vital role in the country's development process. NITI Aayog has identified 117 Aspirational districts for transformation through development of education, health and nutrition, agriculture and water resources, skill development, financial inclusion and basic infrastructure. It could emerge as an agent of change over time and contribute to the government's agenda of improving governance and implementing innovative measures for better delivery of public services. Since its inception, NITI Aayog has established itself as a paragon of effective, open, and responsible governance in India. The organization is characterized by its commitment to innovation and its adherence to exemplary professional standards. As a think tank, it continues to embody the principles of transparency and accountability, setting a benchmark for governance practices across the nation. NITI Aayog's approach to policymaking and implementation reflects a modern, dynamic vision for India's development. By consistently demonstrating high ethical standards and efficient operation, it has reinforced its role as a crucial institution in shaping India's governance landscape.[1]
Implemented since	The NITI Aayog, India's premier policy think tank, came into existence on January 1, 2015. This date marks a significant milestone in the evolution of India's approach to national development planning and policy formulation.
Goal	• As India have entered into Amrit Kaal period in 2022–23, goal is to define national priorities for the next 25 years (Year 2047, 100th years of Independence) and to enhance macroeconomic level growth along with its focus on microeconomic level all inclusive welfare. • Emphasis on 'Bottom–Up' approach to envisage the vision of maximum governance, minimum government, echoing the spirit of 'Cooperative Federalism'. • To be a state-of-the-art resource center with the necessary knowledge and skills that will enable it to act with speed, promote research and innovation, provide strategic policy advice for the government, and deal with contingent issues.[1]

Chapter 7: National Institution for Transforming India Aayog

Targets	The **seven pillars** of effective Governance: 1. **Effective governance** is citizen-centric, fulfilling the aspirations and needs of both society and individuals. 2. It demonstrates **proactivity** by anticipating and swiftly responding to the needs of citizens. 3. Good governance encourages **active participation** and involvement of the citizenry in decision-making processes. 4. It focuses on **empowering** all segments of society, with a special emphasis on enhancing women's capabilities in all aspects of life. 5. **Inclusive governance** ensures that all people are represented and included, regardless of their caste, creed, or gender. 6. It promotes **equality** by providing equal opportunities to all, with a particular focus on youth development. 7. **Transparency** is a key feature, making governmental operations visible and responsive to the public.
Objectives	• Facilitate state involvement in achieving national goals and develop a framework for a 'national agenda'. • Foster cooperative federalism through continuous support initiatives and mechanisms with states. • Develop methodologies for creating credible plans at the village level and progressively aggregating them at higher governmental levels. • Integrate national security concerns into economic policy formulation. • Ensure special focus on societal segments at risk of inadequate benefit from economic progress. • Develop and review long-term policy frameworks, program initiatives, and their effectiveness. • Provide advisory services and promote collaborations among key stakeholders, think tanks, and educational institutions, both nationally and internationally. • Establish a support system for knowledge creation, innovation, and entrepreneurship through a network of experts. • Create a platform for resolving intersectoral and interdepartmental issues to accelerate development agenda implementation. • Maintain a cutting-edge resource center for research on good governance and sustainable development practices, facilitating their dissemination. • Monitor and evaluate program implementation, including resource allocation, to enhance success probability. • Focus on technological advancements and capacity building for effective program execution. • Undertake additional activities necessary for implementing the national development agenda and achieving set objectives.[1]

Organogram	**Chairperson:**
	• The Prime Minister of India
	  Key positions
	  ✦ **Vice-Chairperson**
	    – Appointed by the Prime Minister
	  ✦ **Members**
	    – Full-time and part-time positions
	    – Up to two members from leading universities, research organizations, or innovative institutions (ex-officio)
	    – Part-time members serve on a rotational basis
	  ✦ **Ex officio members**
	    – Up to four members from the Council of Ministers
	    – Nominated by the Prime Minister
	  ✦ **Chief Executive Officer (CEO)**
	    – Appointed by the Prime Minister for a fixed tenure
	    – Holds rank equivalent to Secretary to the Government of India
	  ✦ **Special invitees**
	    – Eminent experts and specialists with relevant domain knowledge
	    – Nominated by the Prime Minister
	Present formation
	• **NITI Aayog Chairman**—Narendra Modi

	• **NITI Aayog Vice-Chairman**—Shri Suman Bery (May 1, 2022 – present) is the current Vice-Chairman of the NITI Aayog. Shri Parameswaran Iyer joined NITI Aayog as Chief Executive Officer on 10th July 2022. D. Arvind Virmani assumed the role of a full-time Member in NITI Aayog on July 16, 2022.
	• **Governing council**
	  ✦ Composition: Chief Ministers of all States and Lieutenant Governors of Union Territories in India
	  ✦ Purpose: Serves as a national platform for collaborative federalism.
	• **Regional councils**
	  ✦ Purpose: Address specific issues and opportunities affecting multiple states
	  ✦ Key features:
	  ✦ Established for a fixed term
	  ✦ Convened by the Prime Minister
	  ✦ Membership includes Chief Ministers of States and Lieutenant Governors of Union Territories
	  ✦ Chaired by the Chairperson of NITI Aayog or their nominated representative
	  ✦ Function: Facilitate regional cooperation and problem-solving.[2]

Beneficiaries	• **Promote cooperative federalism:** Foster collaboration between the central government and states through ongoing, structured support initiatives. • **Strengthen states:** Operate on the principle that robust states contribute to a strong nation. • **Provide policy guidance:** Offer strategic advice on various aspects of governance and development.
Components	NITI Aayog's operations are supported by several specialized verticals. These verticals are crucial for the efficient execution of the organization's diverse responsibilities. They include: • Administration and Support Units • Agriculture and Allied Sectors • Aspirational Districts Program Cell • Communication and Social Media Cell • Data Management and Analysis, and Frontier Technologies • Economics and Finance Cell • Education • Governance and Research • Governing Council Secretariat and Coordination • Industry-I • Industry-II • Infrastructure-connectivity • Infrastructure-energy • Micro, small and medium enterprises • Natural Resources and Environment, and Island Development • Project Appraisal and Management Division • Public–private Partnership • Rural development • Science and technology • Social Justice and Empowerment, and Voluntary Action Cell • Social Sector-I (Skill development, Labor and Employment, and Urban Development) • Social Sector-II (Health and Nutrition, and Women and Child Development) • State Finances and Coordination • Sustainable Development Goals • Water and Land Resources **TWO HUBS OF WORKING**: • **Team India:** It leads to the participation of Indian states with the central government. • **The knowledge and innovation hub:** It builds the institution's think tank capabilities.
Strategies/ Deliverables under the program	• 'One District, One Product Policy': It is a recent agenda of the NITI Aayog Governing Council. It intends to boost exports at the district level. • NITI Aayog to commission a study on the select judgments and verdicts of Supreme Court and National Green Tribunal on the economy of India.

	• National Action Plan for Migrant Workers is underway and for the same NITI Aayog is a responsible authority.
	• The NITI Aayog has drafted a prototype legislation concerning definitive property ownership. This proposed Act is intended for state-level adoption and execution. The primary objectives of this initiative are:
	  ✦ Simplifying farmers' access to financial resources
	  ✦ Decreasing the volume of property-related legal disputes
	  ✦ Enhancing transparency in real estate deals
	  ✦ Streamlining land acquisition processes for infrastructure projects.
	• NITI Aayog proposal to introduce the production-linked incentive (PLI) scheme for more sectors to boost domestic manufacturing. The objective of the PLI scheme is to incentivize investors in this country to put up globally comparable capacity in scale and competitiveness. The Government of India has already introduced the PLI scheme for pharmaceutical, medical devices, mobile phones and electronic manufacturing companies. It is now considering extending the scheme to other sectors as well.

Activities at various level or package of services	NITI Aayog is working on: 1. Fifteen-year vision 2. Seven-year strategy 3. Three-year action agenda
Monitoring and evaluation of program	• The Development Monitoring and Evaluation Office (DMEO), an attached unit of NITI, envisions to institutionalize the application and use of monitoring and evaluation at all levels of government policy and programs and help improve the efficiency, effectiveness, equity, sustainability, and achievement of results. • Evidence based policy making, strengthening data systems and architecture, and strengthening M&E ecosystem are the key pillars of the DMEO. • In addition, NITI Aayog has also developed several indices and dashboards by focusing on effective management and better outcomes backed by data analysis.
Initiatives and Achievements (2022–23 Report):	The agricultural division of the national planning body hosted a country-wide seminar focused on "Agricultural Innovation" on April 25, 2022. This event, held at Vigyan Bhawan in New Delhi, was part of the national independence celebration. The seminar attracted over 1,250 attendees from diverse sectors, including: • Federal ministries • State administration • Commercial enterprises • Farming community • Educational and scientific institutions • Agricultural extension centers • Nongovernmental organizations • Global agencies The event was also broadcast online for remote participation. In a separate initiative, the planning body orchestrated a digital financial technology conference titled 'Fintech Open'. This three-week event ran from February 7 to 28, 2022. The conference served as a platform to unite various stakeholders in the fintech ecosystem, including: • Regulatory bodies • Financial technology experts and enthusiasts • Industry leaders • Emerging businesses • Software developers • The primary aim was to foster collaboration, facilitate knowledge exchange, and promote innovation in the financial technology sector.[1]

References

1. Annual Report 2022-23 NITI Aayog. https://www.niti.gov.in/sites/default/files/2023-02/Annual-Report-2022-2023-English_06022023_compressed.pdf
2. Website NITI Aayog: https://www.niti.gov.in/

QUESTIONS

Long Answer Questions (LAQs)

1. Outline NITI Aayog's organizational structure and its role in promoting cooperative federalism.
2. Discuss five key objectives of NITI Aayog and their alignment with India's development goals.

Short Answer Questions (SAQs)

1. Write a short note on the two primary hubs of NITI Aayog.
2. Briefly describe the leadership structure of NITI Aayog.
3. Explain the concept of 'Amrit Kaal' in the context of NITI Aayog's goals.

Multiple Choice Questions (MCQs)

1. What does NITI stand for in the context of NITI Aayog?
    a. National Institute for Technological Innovation
    b. New India Transformation Initiative
    c. National Institution for Transforming India
    d. National Integration and Territorial Improvement
2. When was NITI Aayog established?
    a. January 1, 2014
    b. January 1, 2015
    c. January 1, 2016
    d. January 1, 2017
3. Which of the following is NOT one of the two primary components of NITI Aayog?
    a. Team India Hub
    b. Knowledge and Innovation Hub
    c. Policy Implementation Hub
    d. Both A and B are primary components

Answers

1. c 2. b 3. c

CHAPTER 8

Sustainable Development Goals

Suraj Kapoor, Shaili Vyas

Need of scheme	The Sustainable Development Goals (SDGs), established by the United Nations in 2015, are essential for addressing the most pressing global challenges and promoting a better, more equitable future. The need for SDGs arises from the complex, interrelated issues the world faces.
Implemented since	The Sustainable Development Goals (SDGs) were officially implemented on January 1, 2016, adopted by all United Nations Member States as part of the 2030 Agenda for Sustainable Development
Goal	The overall goal of the Sustainable Development Goals (SDGs) is to create a blueprint for achieving a better and more sustainable future for all by addressing global challenges such as poverty, inequality, environmental degradation, and ensuring peace and prosperity.
Targets	The Sustainable Development Goals (SDGs) have a total of 169 targets across the 17 goals with salient features as follows:[1] 1. **SDG 1 (no Poverty):** Targets include eradicating extreme poverty reducing the proportion of people living in poverty and ensuring equal access to economic resources and services. 2. **SDG 2 (zero Hunger):** Targets focus on ending hunger and malnutrition, doubling agricultural productivity, ensuring sustainable food production systems, and maintaining the genetic diversity of seeds and plants. 3. **SDG 3 (good health and well-being):** Targets aim to reduce global maternal mortality, end preventable deaths of newborns and children, combat communicable diseases, such as AIDS and malaria, and achieve universal health coverage. 4. **SDG 4 (quality education):** Targets include ensuring all children complete free, equitable, and quality primary and secondary education, promoting lifelong learning, and eliminating gender disparities in education. 5. **SDG 5 (gender equality):** Targets include ending all forms of discrimination and violence against women and girls, ensuring full participation in leadership and decision-making, and achieving universal access to sexual and reproductive health. 6. **SDG 6 (clean water and sanitation):** Targets focus on achieving universal access to safe and affordable drinking water, adequate sanitation, and improving water quality through reducing pollution. 7. **SDG 7 (affordable and clean energy):** Targets aim to ensure universal access to affordable, reliable, and modern energy services, and significantly increase the share of renewable energy in the global energy mix. 8. **SDG 8 (decent work and economic growth):** Targets include promoting sustained economic growth, achieving full and productive employment for all, especially youth and persons with disabilities, and ensuring decent work conditions. 9. **SDG 9 (industry, innovation, and infrastructure):** Targets include developing resilient infrastructure, promoting inclusive industrialization, and enhancing scientific research and technological innovation. 10. **SDG 10 (reduced inequality):** Targets focus on reducing income inequality, promoting social, economic, and political inclusion, and ensuring equal opportunities regardless of age, sex, disability, race, ethnicity, or religion. 11. **SDG 11 (sustainable cities and communities):** Targets aim to ensure access to adequate housing, improve urban planning, reduce the environmental impact of cities, and provide access to safe and sustainable public transportation. 12. **SDG 12 (responsible consumption and production):** Targets include sustainable management of natural resources, halving global food waste, encouraging companies to adopt sustainable practices, and reducing waste generation through recycling and reuse.

	13. **SDG 13 (climate action):** Targets include strengthening resilience to climate-related disasters, integrating climate change measures into national policies, and improving education and awareness on climate change mitigation.
14. **SDG 14 (life below water):** Targets include reducing marine pollution, protecting marine ecosystems, regulating fishing practices to prevent overfishing, and conserving marine and coastal areas.
15. **SDG 15 (life on land):** Targets include protecting terrestrial ecosystems, halting deforestation, combating desertification, conserving biodiversity, and preventing poaching and trafficking of protected species.
16. **SDG 16 (peace, justice, and strong institutions):** Targets include reducing violence, ending abuse and exploitation, promoting the rule of law, reducing corruption, and building effective, accountable institutions at all levels.
17. **SDG 17 (partnerships for the goals):** Targets focus on strengthening global partnerships, mobilizing financial resources, improving access to technology, and promoting fair trade and investment policies.
Objectives	The objective of the Sustainable Development Goals (SDGs) is to establish a global framework for enhancing the quality of life for all individuals, ensuring environmental sustainability, promoting peace, and fostering equitable economic growth.
Figure	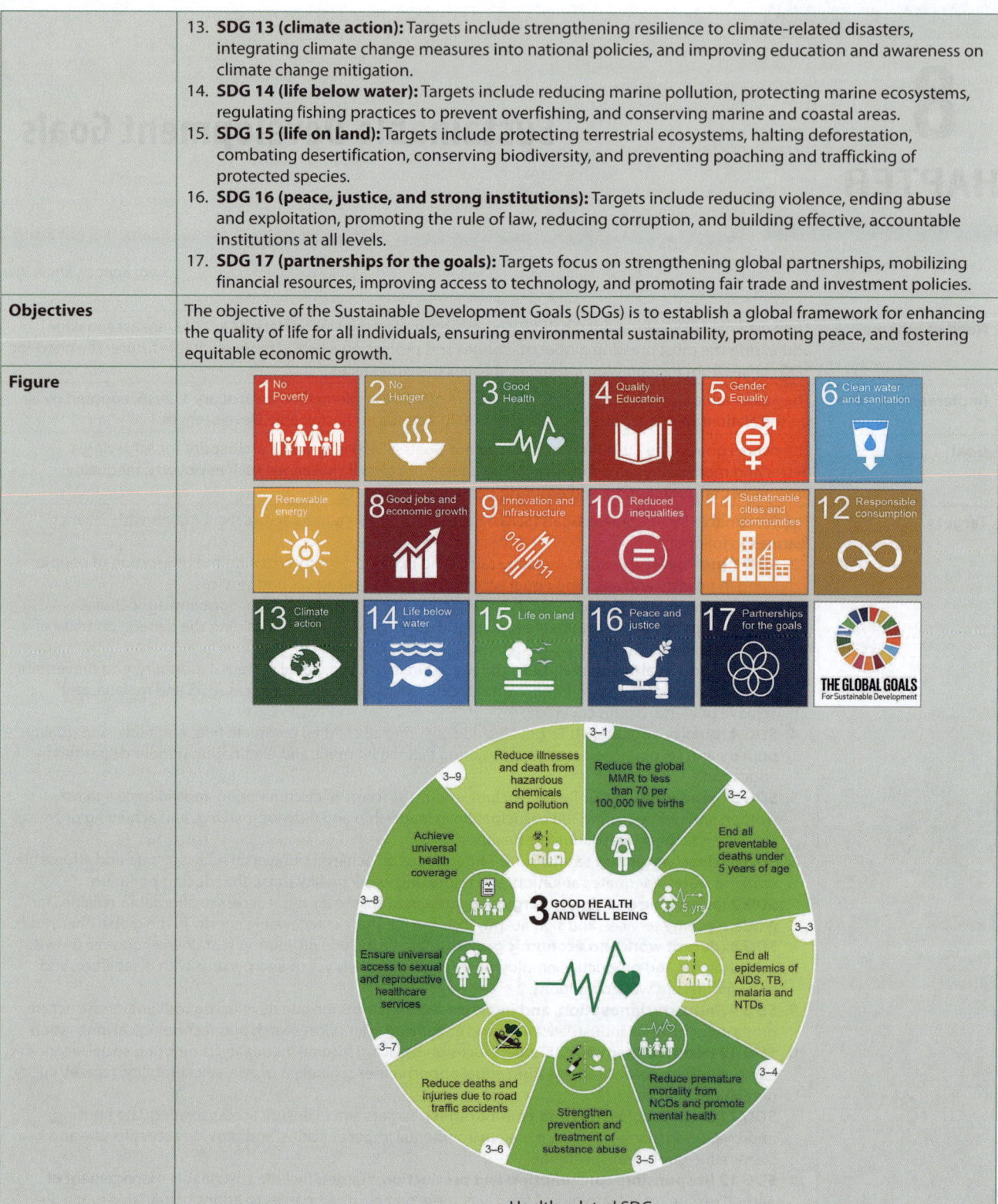 Health-related SDG.

Chapter 8: Sustainable Development Goals   45

Beneficiaries	The SDGs are designed to benefit everyone, with a particular focus on the most vulnerable and marginalized populations.

Components/ Strategies/ Monitoring and evaluation	The Sustainable Development Goals (SDGs) are composed of several key components that work together to provide a comprehensive framework for sustainable development. Here are the main components of the SDGs:[2]
	• **Goals:** Seventeen Global Goals—The SDGs consist of 17 distinct goals that address various aspects of sustainable development, including poverty, inequality, health, education, gender equality, clean water, climate action, and more.
	• **Targets:** 169 Specific Targets—Each SDG is accompanied by specific, measurable targets (169 in total) that define the outcomes to be achieved under each goal. These targets provide a clear focus and guide for countries and stakeholders in their implementation efforts.
	• **Indicators:** 231 Indicators: The targets are monitored through a set of indicators that provide measurable data to track progress. These indicators help assess whether countries are on track to meet their goals and targets.
	• **Themes and areas of focus:** Social, Economic, and Environmental Dimensions: The SDGs encompass three interrelated dimensions of sustainable development:
	  1. **Social:** Goals that focus on ending poverty, improving health, and promoting education and gender equality.
	  2. **Economic:** Goals that promote inclusive economic growth, decent work, and innovation.
	  3. **Environmental:** Goals that aim to protect ecosystems, combat climate change, and ensure sustainable resource use.
	• **Universal and inclusive nature: Global applicability**—The SDGs are applicable to all countries, regardless of their level of development. They aim to address the needs of both developing and developed nations, promoting a global partnership for sustainable development.
	• **Leave no one behind: Equity and inclusivity**—A fundamental principle of the SDGs is the commitment to leaving no one behind. This means addressing inequalities and ensuring that marginalized and vulnerable groups have access to resources, opportunities, and benefits.
	• **Partnerships: Multi-stakeholder collaboration**—Achieving the SDGs requires collaboration among various stakeholders, including governments, civil society, the private sector, and international organizations. Partnerships are essential for mobilizing resources, sharing knowledge, and fostering innovation.
	• **Monitoring and reporting: Accountability mechanisms**—The SDGs include mechanisms for monitoring progress and reporting on achievements. Countries are encouraged to establish national frameworks for data collection, analysis, and reporting, contributing to the global monitoring efforts.
	• **Integration and synergies: Interconnected goals**—The SDGs recognize the interlinkages between different goals and targets. Achieving one goal often supports progress in others, emphasizing the need for integrated approaches to sustainable development.
	• **Implementation strategies: Action plans and policies**—Countries are encouraged to develop national strategies, policies, and action plans that align with the SDGs. This includes setting priorities, allocating resources, and mobilizing support for sustainable development initiatives.

SDG INDIA INDEX

SDG India Index 2023-24 measures and tracks national progress of all States and UTs on 113 indicators aligned to the Ministry of Statistics and Programme Implementation's (MoSPI) National Indicator Framework (NIF). The SDG India Index computes goal-wise scores on the 16 SDGs for each State and UT. Overall State and UT scores or Composite Scores are generated from goal-wise scores to measure the aggregate performance of the sub-national unit based on its performance across the 16 SDGs. These scores range between 0–100, and if a State/UT achieves a score of 100, it signifies it has achieved the targets. The higher the score of a State/UT, the greater the distance covered to the target. The Index represents the articulation of the comprehensive nature of the Global Goals under the 2030 Agenda while being attuned to the national priorities.[1]

Key highlights and results from the fourth edition of the SDG India Index:
- The composite score for India improved from 57 in 2018 to 66 in 2020-21 to further to 71 in 2023–24.
- India has taken significant strides in accelerating progress on the SDGs between the 2020–21 and 2023–24 editions of the Index. Noteworthy advancements have been observed in Goals 1 (No Poverty), 8 (Decent Work and Economic Growth), 13 (Climate Action). These are now in the 'Front Runner' category (a score between 65–99).

- Among these, Goal 13 (Climate Action) has shown the most substantial improvement, with its score increasing from 54 to 67. Goal 1 (No Poverty) follows closely, with its score rising significantly from 60 to 72. The progress underscores the effects of the focused programmatic interventions and schemes of the Union and State Governments in improving the lives of citizens.
- Key interventions facilitating SDG achievements include:
  - Over 4 crore houses under the PM Awas Yojana (PMAY).
  - 11 crore toilets and 2.23 lakh Community Sanitary Complexes in rural areas.
  - 10 crore LPG connections under PM Ujjwala Yojana.
  - Tap water connections in over 14.9 crore households under Jal Jeevan Mission.
  - Over 30 crore beneficiaries under Ayushman Bharat -Pradhan Mantri Jan Arogya Yojana.
  - Coverage of over 80 crore people under the National Food Security Act (NFSA).
  - Access to 150,000 Ayushman Arogya Mandir which offer primary medical care and provide affordable generic medicines.
  - Direct Benefit Transfer (DBT) of ₹ 34 lakh crore made through PM-Jan Dhan accounts.
  - The Skill India Mission has led to over 1.4 crore youth being trained and upskilled and has reskilled 54 lakh youth.
  - PM Mudra Yojana sanctioned 43 crore loans aggregating to ₹ 22.5 lakh crore for entrepreneurial aspirations of the youth besides Funds of Funds.
  - Start Up India and Start Up Guarantee schemes assisting the youth.
  - The Saubhagya scheme for access to electricity.
  - Emphasis on renewable energy resulted in an increase in solar power capacity from 2.82 GW to 73.32 GW in the past decade.
  - Between 2017 and 2023, India has added around 100 GW of installed electric capacity, of which around 80% is attributed to non-fossil fuel-based resource.
  - Improvement in digital infrastructure with reduced internet data costs by 97% which has in turn positively affected and fostered financial inclusion.[2]

References

1. THE 17 GOALS | Sustainable Development (un.org) https://sdgs.un.org/goals#:~:text=At%20its%20heart%20are%20the%2017%20Sustainable%20Development%20Goals%20(SDGs),
2. https://www.undp.org/sustainable-development-goals#:~:text=The%20Sustainable%20Development%20Goals%20(SDGs),%20also%20known%20as%20the%20Global

QUESTIONS

Long Answer Question (LAQ)

1. Describe in detail about Sustainable Development Goals (SDSGs). Describe relevance of SDG in public health.

Short Answer Question (SAQ)

1. Describe in brief health-related SDGs.

Multiple Choice Questions (MCQs)

1. Sustainable climate and city is related to which goal of SDg?
    a. 10
    b. 11
    c. 12
    d. 13
2. Reducing maternal mortality SDG:
    a. 3-1
    b. 3.2
    c. 3.3
    d. 3.4
3. Goals/Targets/Indicators of SDG:
    a. 17/121/ 217
    b. 17/169/231
    c. 19/169/232
    d. 17/176/231

Answers

1. b   **2.** a   **3.** b

SECTION II

Health Policies

Section Outline

- **Chapter 9:** National Health Policy
- **Chapter 10:** National Nutrition Policy
- **Chapter 11:** National Population Policy
- **Chapter 12:** National Policy for Rare Diseases
- **Chapter 13:** National Policy for Older Persons

CHAPTER 9

National Health Policy

Kartik Prajapati, Parul Sharma, Thamizhanban A, Ranjitha R, Bharti Koria

NATIONAL HEALTH POLICY 1983

Need of program/ Scheme	In order to address India's pressing healthcare requirements, the National Health Policy (NHP) of 1983 placed a strong emphasis on attaining universal access, particularly in rural areas that were underserved. With an emphasis on maternity and child health (MCH) and increasing vaccination coverage, the strategy promoted an integrated model that combined preventive, promotive, and curative care. It highlighted safe drinking water, sanitation, and nutrition as essential elements of public health, acknowledging the significance of social determinants of health (Ministry of Health and Family Welfare, 1983).[1] Prioritizing community involvement encouraged local volunteers to support the provision of basic healthcare and promote community ownership of health programs. In order to guarantee safe medical procedures and stop food adulteration, the NHP 1983 also placed a strong emphasis on quality control for medications and food (Govt of India, 1983).[2] It encouraged the integration of traditional and alternative medicine systems into the larger health framework and set up a referral system for expedited access to advanced care. In order to fill the shortage of human resources, it was crucial to train health professionals in preventative and community-oriented treatment (Ministry of Health and Family Welfare, 1983). The ultimate goal of the program was to create a fair and well-coordinated health system that connected primary, secondary, and tertiary care facilities across India. Eventually, new demands and ongoing health issues prompted policy changes with the NHP 2002.
Implemented since	Following parliamentary approval, India began implementing the National Health Policy (NHP) of 1983. Throughout the 1980s and 1990s, it acted as the fundamental framework that directed India's healthcare system, propelling efforts in disease prevention, community health programs, and primary healthcare. Up to the National Health Policy of 2002, which brought changes to address new health issues and improve India's healthcare delivery systems, this policy served as the major national health framework.[1]
Goal	The NHP of 1983 has as its main objective "Health for All by the Year 2000," in accordance with the Alma Ata Declaration. This objective was to guarantee that all residents, especially those living in rural and underserved areas, had access to high-quality healthcare services. Among the main goals were:<ul><li>Building a network of easily accessible primary health clinics (PHCs) to offer necessary medical services is known as "expanding primary healthcare."</li><li>**Promoting public and preventive health:** To lower the burden of disease, prioritize immunization, sanitation, preventive care, and mother and child health.</li><li>**Enhancing community involvement:** Including local volunteers and community people to promote a sense of ownership and enhance health results.</li><li>Combining other medical systems into the healthcare system to offer a holistic approach to treatment is known as "integrating traditional medicine."</li><li>Reducing differences in healthcare access across various demographic groups and geographical areas is one way to improve health equity.</li></ul>The ultimate goal was to improve the health of all citizens through a well-integrated healthcare system that gave priority to preventive, promotional, and curative services.[1,3]
Targets	<ul><li>Reducing infant mortality rate (IMR) to below 60 per 1,000 live births by 2000.</li><li>Lowering maternal mortality rate (MMR) to improve maternal health outcomes, particularly through expanded maternal health services.[4]</li></ul>

	• Controlling communicable diseases such as malaria, tuberculosis, and leprosy by increasing immunization and public health efforts. • Improving nutrition among vulnerable populations, especially children and mothers, to decrease malnutrition rates. • Ensuring safe drinking water and sanitation access to reduce waterborne diseases across all communities. • Expanding immunization coverage to achieve universal immunization for preventable diseases, including measles, polio, and diphtheria. • Strengthening the primary health care Network, aiming to provide health facilities accessible to every rural and urban community. • Increasing life expectancy by reducing preventable mortality rates across all age groups.[1]
Objectives	• **Achieve health for all:** Provide fair access to healthcare in order to achieve "Health for All by the Year 2000". • **Boost primary health care:** Create a thorough network of primary healthcare centers in underprivileged and rural areas. • **Enhance maternal and child health care:** By providing prenatal, postnatal, and vaccination care, we can improve the health of mothers and children. • **Encourage public health and preventative initiatives:** Put an emphasis on health education, nutrition, and sanitation as preventive measures. • **Promote community involvement:** Give local communities a say in the development and execution of health initiatives. • **Integrate different medical systems:** Acknowledge and include alternative and traditional medicine in addition to contemporary procedures. • Establish guidelines for food safety, environmental health, and medication quality to guarantee the quality of healthcare services. • **Develop human resources for health:** Educate and retrain medical staff in community-focused and preventative methods. • **Put in place a productive referral system:** Establish a methodical referral process to gain access to more advanced care. • **Strengthen health infrastructure:** For integrated service delivery, create and maintain a strong health infrastructure.[1]

NATIONAL HEALTH POLICY 2002

Need of program/ Scheme	To address the healthcare issues that have surfaced since the NHP 1983, the NHP 2002 was created. By 2002, India's health profile had changed significantly, necessitating a reassessment of national health goals due to factors like the rise in noncommunicable diseases, demographic trends, and population growth. The following are the main reasons why NHP 2002 had to be implemented: • **Epidemiological transition:** In addition to the ongoing burden of infectious diseases, there was a noticeable increase in noncommunicable diseases (NCDs), such as diabetes, cardiovascular disease, and cancer. The goal of NHP 2002 was to integrate the prevention and management of infectious and noncommunicable diseases into national health policy. • **Inadequate healthcare infrastructure:** Inadequate referral systems and a chronic lack of healthcare facilities, especially in rural and isolated areas, persisted despite efforts made under the NHP 1983. With a focus on rural healthcare and better-trained medical staff, NHP 2002 aimed to enhance service delivery and grow the health infrastructure. • **Need for public health investment:** The private sector provides a significant amount of healthcare services, yet health spending has remained low. This program sought to guarantee fair access to reasonably priced healthcare services and boost public sector investment in health. • **High maternal and child mortality rates:** When compared to worldwide standards, maternal and child health indicators continued to be subpar. To fill these deficiencies, NHP 2002 concentrated on growing maternal and child health services. • **Population growth and health resources:** As the population grew, so did the need for health services, which brought attention to a shortage of resources, especially human resources. Strategies for increasing healthcare training and human resources were part of the NHP 2002. • **Emerging health threats:** The resurgence of tuberculosis and HIV/AIDS are two examples of emergent health threats that have highlighted the need for comprehensive policies that can change to meet evolving health needs.[5]

Chapter 9: National Health Policy

Implemented since	In 2002, the Indian Government formally launched the NHP 2002. The population's evolving healthcare needs and the gaps found since the 1983 policy prompted the introduction of this strategy. A framework for tackling emerging health issues was established by the NHP 2002, with an emphasis on boosting public spending on healthcare, developing infrastructure, and enhancing access to high-quality medical care.[5]
Goal	A number of particular objectives were outlined in the NHP 2002 with the intention of enhancing the health of the Indian populace and establishing an accessible and sustainable healthcare system. The main objectives are listed below with specifics: • Eradicate Polio and Yaws by 2005. • Eliminate Leprosy by 2005. • Eliminate Kala Azar by 2010. • Eliminate Lymphatic Filariasis by 2015. • Achieve zero-level growth of HIV/AIDS by 2007. • Reduce mortality by 50% due to TB, malaria, and other vector and water-borne diseases by 2010. • Reduce the prevalence of blindness to 0.5% by 2010. • Reduce Infant Mortality Rate (IMR) to 30 per 1,000 live births and Maternal Mortality Ratio (MMR) to 100 per lakh live births by 2010. • Increase utilization of public health facilities from <20% to <75% by 2010. • Establish an integrated system of surveillance, National Health Accounts, and Health Statistics by 2005. • Increase government health expenditure as a percentage of GDP from 0.9% to 2.0% by 2010. • Increase the share of central grants to at least 25% of total health spending by 2010. • Increase state sector health spending from 5.5% to 7% of the budget, with a further increase to 8%.[5]
Targets	The 2002 NHP established clear goals to enhance the health and welfare of the Indian populace, emphasizing the development of general health infrastructure as well as illness prevention. Important goals were as follows: • **Lower the maternal mortality ratio (MMR) and infant mortality rate (IMR):** By 2010, emphasis on better maternal and child health services to lower the MMR to less than 100 per 100,000 live births and the IMR to less than 30 per 1,000 live births. • Increasing access to vaccination programs, especially in underprivileged areas, can help achieve universal immunization, which aims to guarantee 100% immunization coverage for diseases that can be prevented by vaccination. • Increase efforts to control major communicable illnesses, such as eradicating lymphatic filariasis, cutting malaria mortality by 50%, and significantly lowering the incidence of leprosy and tuberculosis. • **Enhance sanitation and safe drinking water:** To lower the prevalence of waterborne illnesses, strive for universal access to safe drinking water and sanitary facilities, particularly in underserved and rural areas. • **Increase health expenditure:** In order to lower out-of-pocket costs and improve access to necessary health treatments, public health spending should be increased to at least 2% of GDP. • **Reduce prevalence of blindness:** By increasing access to preventive and curative eye care treatments, especially cataract procedures, the prevalence of blindness can be reduced to 0.5%. • **Encourage population stabilization:** Implement family planning programs, provide access to contraception, and raise awareness in order to work toward a total fertility rate (TFR) of 2.1.[5]
Objectives	• **Universal access to healthcare:** To lessen health inequities, all individuals, particularly those from underprivileged backgrounds, should have fair access to reasonably priced healthcare services. • **Enhancing primary healthcare:** To make sure that basic medical treatments are accessible and available at the local level, the primary healthcare system should be strengthened. • The goal is to lower rates of morbidity and death by implementing efficient disease control strategies, especially for noncommunicable diseases, maternity and child health, and communicable diseases. • **Emphasis on preventive healthcare:** To enhance general public health, promote preventive and promotional health measures, such as nutrition, immunization, sanitation, and health education. • **Improving health infrastructure:** To improve health infrastructure, especially in underserved and rural areas, by building and renovating healthcare institutions at all levels. • The goal of human resource development in the health industry is to train and retain qualified medical personnel in order to address the population's healthcare demands. • **Encourage research and development:** To support health and healthcare delivery research in order to generate innovations and enhance health outcomes. • **Integration of traditional medical systems:** To encourage and incorporate traditional medical systems (AYUSH) into the country's healthcare delivery system in order to provide a comprehensive approach to health.[5]

Section II: Health Policies

Organogram	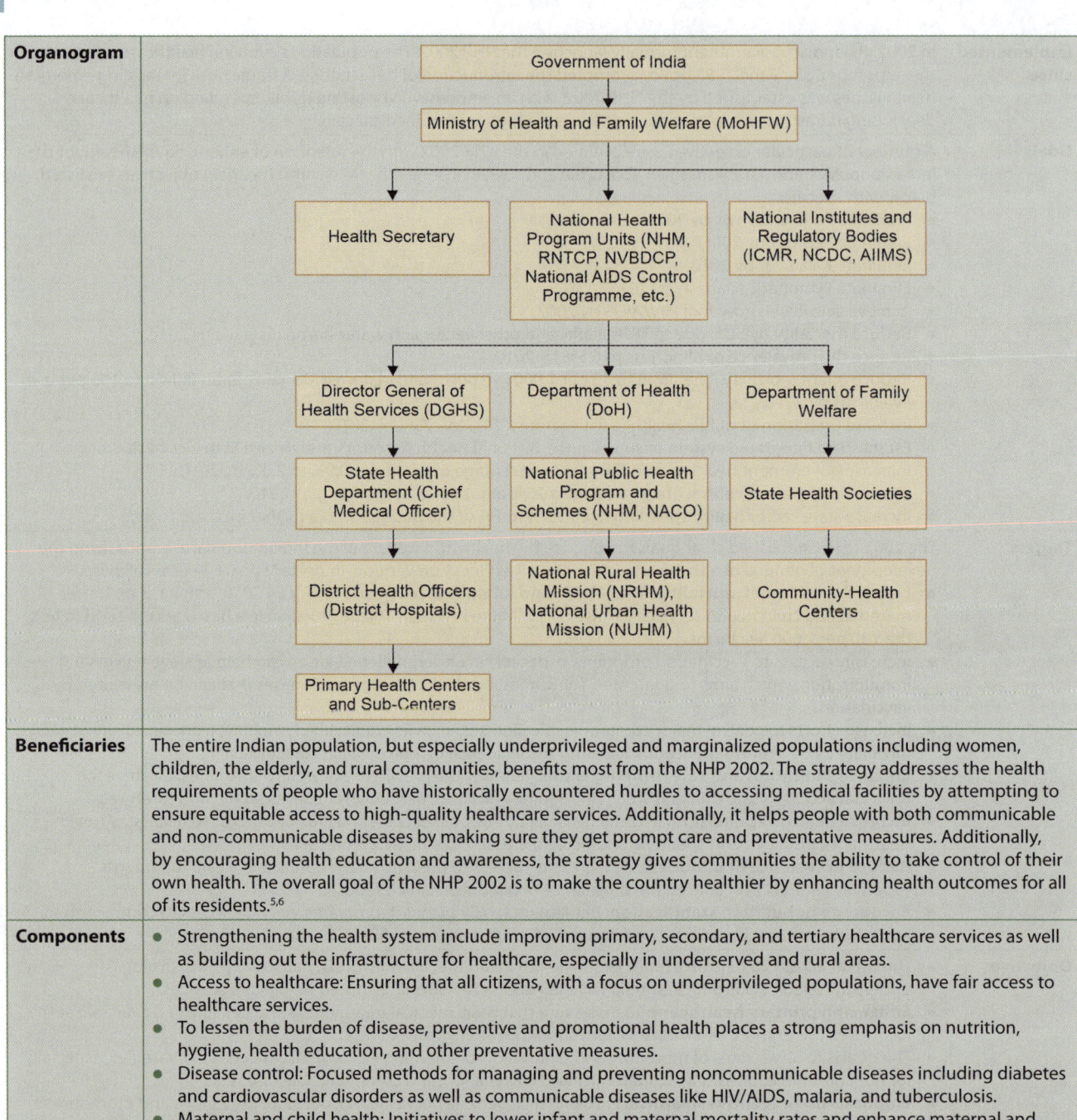
Beneficiaries	The entire Indian population, but especially underprivileged and marginalized populations including women, children, the elderly, and rural communities, benefits most from the NHP 2002. The strategy addresses the health requirements of people who have historically encountered hurdles to accessing medical facilities by attempting to ensure equitable access to high-quality healthcare services. Additionally, it helps people with both communicable and non-communicable diseases by making sure they get prompt care and preventative measures. Additionally, by encouraging health education and awareness, the strategy gives communities the ability to take control of their own health. The overall goal of the NHP 2002 is to make the country healthier by enhancing health outcomes for all of its residents.[5,6]
Components	• Strengthening the health system include improving primary, secondary, and tertiary healthcare services as well as building out the infrastructure for healthcare, especially in underserved and rural areas. • Access to healthcare: Ensuring that all citizens, with a focus on underprivileged populations, have fair access to healthcare services. • To lessen the burden of disease, preventive and promotional health places a strong emphasis on nutrition, hygiene, health education, and other preventative measures. • Disease control: Focused methods for managing and preventing noncommunicable diseases including diabetes and cardiovascular disorders as well as communicable diseases like HIV/AIDS, malaria, and tuberculosis. • Maternal and child health: Initiatives to lower infant and maternal mortality rates and enhance maternal and child health outcomes. • Human resource development is the process of educating and retaining qualified medical personnel to address the population's healthcare needs. • **Integration of traditional medicine:** The advancement and incorporation of traditional medical systems (such as homeopathy, yoga, Unani, siddha, and ayurveda) into the healthcare system. • Public health research: Supporting public health research to enhance healthcare delivery and guide policy decisions. • Community participation is the involvement of nongovernmental organizations (NGOs) and communities in the execution of health programs and initiatives aimed at promoting health.

	• Increasing public health spending to guarantee the sustainability and accessibility of healthcare services is known as health financing.
Strategies/ Deliverables under the program	• **Strengthening primary healthcare:** Focusing on the need to build a robust network of primary healthcare facilities in order to offer the community comprehensive health services. • Promoting an integrated approach to health services that incorporates curative, rehabilitative, preventive, and promotional care is known as "integrated health services." • **Community participation:** To guarantee that services are tailored to local requirements, community involvement in health planning and implementation is encouraged. • **Public-private partnerships:** Promoting cooperation between the public and private sectors to enhance infrastructure and healthcare delivery. • **Capacity building:** Improving healthcare workers' abilities and proficiencies via training and ongoing education initiatives. • **Strengthening disease control programs:** Putting into practice focused disease control programs for non-communicable diseases like diabetes and heart disease as well as communicable diseases like HIV/AIDS, TB, and malaria. • **Maternal and child health initiatives:** Creating and growing initiatives to enhance prenatal and postnatal care as well as maternal and child health. • **Access to vital medicines:** Making sure that healthcare supplies and vital medications are available at all levels of healthcare facilities. • **Health promotion and education:** Organizing health education initiatives to increase public knowledge of health concerns, encourage healthy living, and support preventative care. • **Monitoring and evaluation:** Putting in place strong monitoring and evaluation systems to gauge the success of health initiatives and guide changes to policy.
Activities at various level or package of services	**Primary activities:** Primary activities are emphasized as the foundation of healthcare delivery in the National Health Policy (NHP) 2002. These initiatives center on preventative healthcare, which encompasses health education and awareness campaigns meant to encourage populations to adopt healthy lifestyles. Immunization campaigns are put in place to guard against diseases like polio and measles that can be prevented by vaccination. Initiatives for maternal and child health are equally important, including prenatal and postnatal care to protect mothers' and babies' health. With the help of community health workers like accredited social health activists (ASHAs) and auxiliary nurse midwives (ANMs), who offer direct medical care to the community while guaranteeing accessibility and coverage, PHCs are designed to provide vital health services at the local level. **Secondary activities:** The NHP 2002's secondary activities center on curative care and the treatment of illnesses that call for more specialized care. The purpose of district hospitals and community health centers is to treat common ailments, minor wounds, and standard medical care. In order to guarantee that patients may obtain specialized care when required, these institutions are also made to support a referral system. Additionally, monitoring and managing chronic conditions like diabetes and hypertension, where patients receive the care and rehabilitation services they require, are examples of secondary activities. In order for people to receive prompt treatment and have a seamless transition from primary to more specialized healthcare services, this layer is essential. **Tertiary activities:** Advanced medical care and specialized services are the main emphasis of the tertiary activities included in the NHP 2002. Complex medical conditions that call for specialist intervention, like operations, advanced diagnostics, and critical care, are treated by medical schools and specialty hospitals. Ongoing research and training programs that strive to improve healthcare delivery and create novel therapies support this level of care. Tertiary activities can include developing guidelines and regulations based on research findings, which support future health initiatives and enhance healthcare systems. The NHP 2002 seeks to guarantee comprehensive care for everyone, especially those with severe or complex health issues, by focusing on these advanced services.
Monitoring and evaluation of program	The strategy describes the creation of a methodical framework for monitoring the advancement of health initiatives and programs. This entails putting up specialized health information systems that gather information on important health metrics. • **Frequent data collection:** It is required that health-related data be regularly gathered at all levels (local, state, and federal). This include data on the frequency of diseases, the provision of services, the accessibility of healthcare, and the results of medical procedures. • **Performance indicators:** The policy places a strong emphasis on using particular performance indicators to evaluate how well health services are working. Statistics on maternal and child health, vaccination coverage, illness control rates, and patient satisfaction are a few examples of these indicators.

- **Periodic evaluations:** Planned assessments are carried out to determine the effectiveness of health initiatives and pinpoint areas in need of development. Both midterm and end-of-program evaluations fall under this category.
- **Including stakeholders:** An essential part of the M&E process is including a variety of stakeholders, such as the public, community organizations, healthcare professionals, and government agencies. Their input aids in improving tactics and successfully meeting regional health demands.
- **Policy changes:** In order to effectively address the evolving health landscape and new issues, the policy framework permits changes and reorientations of health programs based on the results of monitoring and evaluation.
- **Building capacity:** It is also stressed to train stakeholders and healthcare professionals in MandE procedures to improve their abilities in data collecting, analysis, and reporting. This guarantees that the data acquired is precise and useful.
- **Research and development:** To find best practices and cutting-edge methods for delivering healthcare, the policy encourages continuous research. This study contributes to evaluation procedures and aids in the expansion of successful programs.[5,6]

NATIONAL HEALTH POLICY 2017

Background/Need of the program	The National Health Policy of India was developed in 2017 with the aim of tackling the mounting burden of infectious and noncommunicable illnesses, the thriving healthcare sector, rising catastrophic costs, poverty, and economic expansion. India's commitment to universal health coverage, as well as the nation's changing demographic patterns and health goals, are reflected in the policy.
Vision	"Attaining the highest possible level of health and well-being for all at all ages" is the National Health Policy of 2017 vision. This vision highlights a preventative and promotive healthcare strategy incorporated into all developmental strategies and is in line with the Sustainable Development Goals (SDGs).
Goals	The set goals of NHP 2017 were, 1. Progressively achieve Universal Health Coverage 2. Reinforcing Trust in the Public Healthcare System 3. Align the growth of the private healthcare sector with public health goals.[7]

Specific objectives of NHP 2017[7]	• **Health status and program impact**
	  ✦ *Life expectancy and healthy life*
	    – By 2025, aim to raise the life expectancy at birth from 67.5 to 70.
	    – By 2022, implement a systematic monitoring system for the disability adjusted life years (DALY) index to assess the impact of diseases and track their trends across main categories.
	    – Achieve a total fertility rate (TFR) of 2.1 at both the national and sub-national levels by the year 2025.
	  ✦ *Mortality by age and/or cause*
	    – Reduce under-five mortality to 23 by 2025 and MMR from current levels to 100 by 2020.
	    – Reduce infant mortality rate to 28 by 2019.
	    – Reduce neo-natal mortality to 16 and still-birth rate to "single digit" by 2025.
	  ✦ *Reduction of disease prevalence/ incidence*
	    – Achieve the global target of 2020, which is also termed as target of 90:90:90, for HIV/AIDS, i.e,. -90% of all people living with HIV know their HIV status, -90% of all people diagnosed with HIV infection receive sustained antiretroviral therapy, and 90% of all people receiving antiretroviral therapy will have viral suppression.
	    – Achieve and maintain the elimination status of Leprosy by 2018, Kala-azar by 2017, and Lymphatic Filariasis in endemic pockets by 2017.
	    – To achieve and maintain a cure rate of >85% in new sputum-positive patients for TB and reduce the incidence of new cases to reach elimination status by 2025.
	    – To reduce the prevalence of blindness to 0.25/1,000 by 2025 and the disease burden by one-third of the current levels.
	    – To reduce premature mortality from cardiovascular diseases, cancer, diabetes, or chronic respiratory diseases by 25% by 2025.

Chapter 9: National Health Policy 57

	• **Health systems performance**
	   ✦ *Coverage of health services*
	      – Increase utilization of public health facilities by 50% from current levels by 2025.
	      – Antenatal care coverage is to be sustained above 90%, and skilled attendance at birth is to be above 90% by 2025.
	      – More than 90% of newborns are fully immunized by one year of age by 2025.
	      – Meet need of family planning above 90% at the national and sub-national level by 2025.
	      – 80% of known hypertensive and diabetic individuals at the household level maintain 'controlled disease status' by 2025.
	   ✦ *Cross sectoral goals related to health*
	      – Relative reduction in prevalence of current tobacco use by 15% by 2020 and 30% by 2025.
	      – Reduction of 40% in prevalence of stunting of under-five children by 2025.
	      – Access to safe water and sanitation to all by 2020 (Swachh Bharat Mission).
	      – Reduction of occupational injury by half from current levels of 334 per lakh agricultural workers by 2020.
	      – National/State level tracking of selected health behavior.
	• **Health systems strengthening**
	   ✦ *Health finance*
	      – Increase health expenditure by Government as a percentage of GDP from the existing 1.15 to 2.5% by 2025.
	      – Increase State sector health spending to >8% of their budget by 2020.
	      – Decrease in the proportion of households facing catastrophic health expenditure from the current levels by 25%, by 2025.
	   ✦ *Health infrastructure and human resource*
	      – Ensure the availability of paramedics and doctors as per Indian Public Health Standard (IPHS) norm in high-priority districts by 2020.
	      – Increase community health volunteers to population ratio as per IPHS norm, in high-priority districts by 2025.
	      – Establish primary and secondary care facilities as per norms in high-priority districts (population and time to reach norms) by 2025.
	   ✦ *Health management information*
	      – Ensure district-level electronic database of information on health system components by 2020.
	      – Strengthen the health surveillance system and establish registries for diseases of public health importance by 2020.
	      – Establish federated integrated health information architecture, Health Information Exchanges, and National Health Information Network by 2025.

Key components	• **Comprehensive primary healthcare:** The importance of strengthening primary healthcare systems and advocates for expanding health and wellness centers (HWCs) to provide comprehensive primary healthcare, including preventive, promotive, curative, and rehabilitative services. These centers aim to offer a wider range of services, including geriatric care, palliative care, and mental health support. • **Health financing:** The policy proposes to increase public health expenditure to 2.5% of GDP by 2025. It emphasizes reducing out-of-pocket expenditures, which are a significant cause of financial distress for many families. The policy also explores innovative financing mechanisms, including taxes on health-detrimental goods and leveraging corporate social responsibility (CSR) funds. • **Access to medicines and technology:** Ensuring the availability and affordability of essential drugs, diagnostics, and vaccines is a critical component of the policy. The policy supports expanding the production capacity of public sector units for essential medicines and encourages the development of domestic manufacturing of medical devices under the "Make in India" initiative. • **Human resources for health:** The policy recognizes the need to address shortages and improve the distribution of health professionals. It advocates for increasing the number of medical and nursing colleges, enhancing the skills of healthcare workers, and implementing measures to attract and retain healthcare professionals in rural and underserved areas. • **Quality of care:** Ensuring quality standards in healthcare facilities is a priority under NHP 2017. The policy calls for developing and enforcing standards and guidelines for healthcare delivery, promoting accreditation of healthcare facilities, and implementing quality assurance mechanisms to enhance patient safety and care quality.[8,9]

Newer strategies	• **Decentralization:** The policy emphasizes decentralizing healthcare governance by empowering states and local bodies to tailor health interventions to local needs. This approach aims to enhance accountability, improve resource allocation, and foster community participation in health planning, ensuring a bottom-up approach. • **Public-private partnership (PPP):** NHP 2017 encourages public-private partnership models to augment health services, particularly in areas with limited public sector capacity. These partnerships are seen as a way to leverage private sector expertise and resources to improve health outcomes. • **Digital health and innovations:** The policy highlights the role of digital health initiatives, including eHealth, telemedicine, and health information systems, in enhancing healthcare delivery. Establishing a National Digital Health Authority aims to promote the use of digital tools to improve healthcare access, quality, and efficiency.[10]
Challenges and critiques	• Low public spending on healthcare, only 1.15% of GDP. • Poorly developed primary healthcare infrastructure. • Nonavailability of skilled human resources and essential infrastructure. • Less fund allocation for building required infrastructure for primary healthcare services. • Weak commitment to regulations, including establishing an independent drug regulator. • Need for regulatory and accreditation agencies for healthcare providers. • Lack of reconciled health data and limited involvement of the private sector. • High out-of-pocket spending and the need for public institutions to offer free essential medicines and diagnostic tests.[11]

References

1. Ministry of Health and Family Welfare, Government of India. National Health Policy 1983. New Delhi: Government of India; 1983.
2. Government of India. National Health Policy 1983 Report. New Delhi: Ministry of Health and Family Welfare; 1983.
3. World Health Organization. Health in India: Monitoring Progress in Health and Development. Geneva: WHO; 1990.
4. Claeson M, Bos ER, Pathmanathan I. Reducing child mortality in India: keeping up the pace. November 1999.
5. Ministry of Health and Family Welfare, Government of India. National Health Policy 2002. New Delhi: Government of India; 2002 [cited 2024 Oct 25]. Available from: https://main.mohfw.gov.in/documents/policy.
6. Government of India. Report on the National Health Policy 2002. New Delhi: Ministry of Health and Family Welfare; 2002.
7. Ministry of Health and Family Welfare, Government of India. National Health Policy – 2017. New Delhi: MoHFW; 2017.
8. Ministry of Health and Family Welfare, Government of India. Situation Analyses: Backdrop to the National Health Policy – 2017 [Internet] [cited 2024 Aug 01]. New Delhi: MoHFW; 2017. Available from: http://www.mohfw.nic.in/showfile.php?lid=4276
9. Planning Commission of India. Twelfth Five Year Plan (2012-2017).
10. Narayana, Muttur Ranganathan. India's Proposed Universal Health Coverage Policy: Evidence for Age Structure Transition Effect and Fiscal Sustainability., Applied Health Economic Policy, dated 19 August 2016.
11. Sundararaman T. National Health Policy 2017: a cautious move. Indian J Med Ethics. 2017;II(2):69-71.

QUESTIONS

Long Answer Questions (LAQs)

1. Explain the main objectives and guiding principles of the National Health Policy (NHP) of 1983, and discuss how these objectives were aimed at addressing the healthcare needs and challenges of India at that time.
2. Discuss the key goals and strategies of the National Health Policy 2002 in India, highlighting how it aimed to improve public health services, reduce regional health disparities, and address emerging health challenges.
3. Discuss the key objectives of the National Health Policy 2017 and analyze how they align with the Sustainable Development Goals (SDGs).
4. Evaluate the strategies proposed by the National Health Policy 2017 to enhance healthcare financing and reduce out-of-pocket expenditures. What are the potential challenges in implementing these strategies, and how can they be overcome to ensure equitable access to healthcare services across different regions in India?

Short Answer Questions (SAQs)

1. What is the primary vision of the National Health Policy 2017 regarding healthcare access and quality?
2. How does the National Health Policy 2017 aim to integrate digital health technologies into India's healthcare system?
3. What was the primary goal of India's National Health Policy introduced in 1983?
4. How did the National Health Policy 2002 address the issue of preventive healthcare?

Multiple Choice Questions (MCQs)

1. National Health Policy 2017 aims to reduce premature mortality from cardiovascular diseases, cancer, diabetes, or chronic respiratory diseases by:
   a. 10%
   b. 25%
   c. 50%
   d. 65%
2. National Health Policy 2017 aims to reduce neo-natal mortality to:
   a. 8
   b. 16
   c. 24
   d. 32
3. National Health Policy 2017 aims to reduce proportion of households facing catastrophic health expenditure from the current levels by:
   a. 75%
   b. 50%
   c. 25%
   d. 0%
4. What was one of the primary objectives of the National Health Policy 2002?
   a. Increase private sector involvement in healthcare
   b. Achieve universal healthcare coverage by 2005
   c. Reduce maternal mortality and child mortality rates significantly
   d. Shift focus from communicable to non-communicable diseases
5. Which of the following did the National Health Policy of 1983 emphasize for improving rural healthcare?
   a. Investment in luxury healthcare facilities
   b. Primary healthcare centers in rural areas
   c. Restricting healthcare to private sectors only
   d. Increasing medical tourism in rural India

Answers

1. b   2. b   3. c   4. c   5. b

CHAPTER 10

National Nutrition Policy

Thamizhanban A, Ranjitha R, Bharti Koria

Background/Need of the program	The National Nutrition Policy (NNP) of 1993 was introduced by the Government of India as a response to the pervasive problem of malnutrition affecting large segments of the population, particularly women and children. The policy's primary objective was to improve the nutritional status of the country's population through a comprehensive set of direct and indirect interventions. The policy was formulated by the Department of Women and Child Development emphasizing the need for a coordinated approach across various sectors such as agriculture, health, and education to address the multifaceted issue of malnutrition.[1]
Situational analysis of nutritional status in 1980s	• **Nutritional intake of calories and protein:** The aggregate consumption of calories at the household level showed consistent upward trend over years. Throughout the years 1957–79, the overall protein consumption in urban areas exceeded the recommended threshold set by the Indian Council of Medical Research (ICMR) for all income groups, with the exception of slum dwellers and rural residents. • **Micronutrient intake:** Throughout the years 1975–79, the overall intake levels of Iron in urban areas exceeded the recommended threshold set by the ICMR for all demographic categories. Nutritional deficits of vitamin A were present in all demographic groups except the high-income groups. • However, despite a decrease in the percentage of the population living below the poverty line since 1960 (from 56.8 to 29.2% in 1987–88), an astonishing 250 million individuals in India are affected by different levels of malnutrition. The remarkable advancements of the Green Revolution in terms of national food security and efficient early warning systems have completely eliminated famines and instances of severe hunger and starvation.
Key features	The NNP 1993 was designed as a multi-sectoral policy with both direct and indirect interventions. Key features of the policy included: • **Direct nutrition interventions:** Expansion of safety nets such as the integrated child development services (ICDS) to cover all vulnerable children aged 0-6 years, fortification of essential foods, and promotion of low-cost nutritious foods. • **Indirect policy instruments:** Addressing food security through increased food production, improving dietary patterns, and providing income transfers to the poor through poverty alleviation programs. • **Community participation:** Emphasizing the role of community involvement in implementing nutrition-related interventions and generating awareness about the policy.

Implementation mechanism	• **Direct intervention—short-term**
	✦ *Nutrition intervention for especially vulnerable groups:*
	  – Expanding the safety net: The nutrition intervention under the ICDS scheme should be expanded to include all vulnerable children aged 0–6 years. The policy should focus on extending the ICDS program to cover all remaining 2,388 blocks, thereby achieving coverage across a total of 5,153 blocks, an increase from the existing 2,765 blocks.
	  – Reducing severe and moderate malnutrition: The approach to growth monitoring, where mothers are passive observers, must be reformed. Mothers should actively participate in managing their children's nutrition at home, with the goal of reducing severe and moderate malnutrition by half.

- Reaching adolescent girls: All adolescent girls from economically disadvantaged families must be included under the ICDS program in all community developmental blocks.
- Ensuring better coverage of expectant women: Supplementary nutrition should be provided starting from the first trimester and continuing for at least the first year after pregnancy, with the objective of reducing the incidence of low birth weight to 10%.

- *Fortification of essential foods:* Essential food items must be fortified with appropriate nutrients, such as iodine and/or iron in salt. Iodized salt should be distributed to all populations in endemic areas to reduce iodine deficiency.
- *Popularization of low-cost nutritious food:* Efforts should be intensified to produce and promote low-cost nutritious foods made from indigenous and locally available raw materials.
- *Control of micronutrient deficiencies amongst vulnerable groups:* Nutritional blindness must be eradicated, and the National Nutritional Anemia Prophylaxis Program should be expanded and strengthened to reduce anemia in pregnant women to 25%.

- **Indirect policy instruments: long-term institutional and structural changes:**
  - *Food security:* To secure food availability, a per capita supply of 215 kg of food grains per person per year must be achieved, necessitating the production of 250 million tonnes of food grains annually.
  - *Improvement of dietary pattern through production and demonstration:* To enhance dietary patterns and nutritional security, efforts should be directed at boosting the production of nutrient-rich foods such as pulses, oilseeds, vegetables, and fruits. Utilizing modern agricultural techniques, improving crop varieties, and reducing food wastage are key. Addressing policy imbalances and aligning food policy with nutritional needs, including appropriate incentives, pricing, and taxation strategies, will ensure that essential foods are both affordable and accessible.
  - *Policies for effecting income transfers:*
    Improving purchasing power: Revise poverty alleviation programs to enhance the purchasing power of the poor. Ensure that nutritional goals are integrated into these programs and that employment generation provides at least 100 days of work for rural landless families and sufficient opportunities for urban slum dwellers.
    Public distribution system: Expand the public distribution system to provide essential food items at reasonable prices, especially for those below the poverty line. Increase the number of fair price shops and strengthen the system during the monsoon months with special rations for vulnerable populations.
    Land reforms: Implement land reform measures, including tenure reforms and ceiling laws, to reduce the vulnerability of both landless and poor landowners.
  - *Health and family welfare:* Enhance health and immunization services under the "Health for All by 2000 AD" initiative, and improve prenatal and postnatal care. Promote education on family planning to manage family size and ensure adequate nutrition.
  - *Basic health and nutrition knowledge:* Promote basic health and nutrition education, especially concerning infant feeding practices, and integrate these concepts into school curricula and nutrition programs.
  - *Prevention of food adulteration:* Strengthen enforcement mechanisms to prevent food adulteration and ensure food safety.
  - *Nutrition surveillance:* Enhance nutrition surveillance through the National Nutrition Monitoring Bureau (NNMB) and National Institute of Nutrition (NIN) to monitor the nutritional status of vulnerable groups and assess the impact of nutrition programs. The NNMB should also serve as an early warning system for initiating prompt action.
  - *Monitoring of nutrition programs:* Continue monitoring nutrition programs like ICDS through the Food and Nutrition Board, now integrated into the Department of Women and Child Development, ensuring effective technical and field-level support.
  - *Research:* Conduct research to identify malnutrition issues and develop high-nutrition food varieties that are affordable for the poor.
  - *Equal remuneration:* Enforce the Equal Remuneration Act to ensure women receive equal wages and expand employment opportunities for women.
  - *Communication:* Utilize mass and group communication strategies to promote nutrition policies and counter social attitudes affecting women's and children's health. Use media effectively to stabilize markets during crises and support nutrition education.

	• *Minimum wage administration:* Ensure effective minimum wage enforcement and timely revisions, with special legislation to support agricultural women laborers, including adequate leave provisions during pregnancy. • *Community participation:* Foster community involvement in nutrition programs through awareness, participation in management, food production, and demand generation for services. • *Education and literacy:* Promote education and literacy, particularly for women, as they are crucial for better nutritional outcomes. • *Improvement of the status of women:* Focus on improving women's economic status through employment and education, as this directly impacts household nutrition and overall health.
Impact	• Since its implementation, the NNP 1993 has contributed to improvements in several nutritional indicators. The prevalence of severe malnutrition among children has decreased, and there has been progress in the fortification of foods to address micronutrient deficiencies. • NNP was pivotal in expansion of ICDS program, which has played a critical role in reducing child malnutrition. • The introduction of fortified foods, such as iodized salt, has significantly reduced the prevalence of iodine deficiency disorders in the country.
Various nutritional programs and Initiative by Government of India after NNP	• Mid-Day Meal Scheme (MDMS) - 1995[2] • Pradhan Mantri Matru Vandana Yojana (PMMVY) - 2017[3] • National Nutrition Mission (Poshan Abhiyaan) - 2018[4] • Anemia Mukt Bharat (AMB) - 2018[5] • Fortification of Food Grains - 2019[6] • Pradhan Mantri Poshan Shakti Nirman (PM POSHAN) - 2021[7]

References

1. National Population Policy 1993. Ministry of Women and Child Development, Government of India.
2. Government of India, Ministry of Education. Mid-Day Meal Scheme. [Online] Available from: https://www.education.gov.in/en/mid-day-meal [Accessed August 11, 2024].
3. Government of India, Ministry of Women and Child Development. Pradhan Mantri Matru Vandana Yojana. [Online] Available from: https://wcd.nic.in/schemes/pradhan-mantri-matru-vandana-yojana [Accessed August 11, 2024].
4. NITI Aayog, Government of India. National Nutrition Mission (Poshan Abhiyaan). [Online] Available from: https://www.niti.gov.in/poshan-abhiyaan [Accessed August 11, 2024].
5. Government of India, Ministry of Health and Family Welfare. Anemia Mukt Bharat. [Online] Available from: https://anemiamuktbharat.info [Accessed August 11, 2024].
6. Food Safety and Standards Authority of India (FSSAI). Fortification of Food. [Online] Available from: https://ffrc.fssai.gov.in/fortified-foods [Accessed August 11, 2024].
7. Government of India, Ministry of Education. Pradhan Mantri Poshan Shakti Nirman (PM POSHAN). [Online] Available from: https://www.education.gov.in/en/pm-poshan [Accessed August 11, 2024].

QUESTIONS

Long Answer Question (LAQ)

1. How has the National Nutrition Mission (Poshan Abhiyaan) enhanced the effectiveness of India's efforts to curb malnutrition, particularly among women and children?

Chapter 10: National Nutrition Policy

Short Answer Questions (SAQs)

1. What are the key strategies implemented under the Mid-Day Meal Scheme that contribute to both educational outcomes and nutritional security for school-going children in India?
2. In what ways have community-based initiatives like "Poshan Vatikas" (Nutrition Gardens) contributed to improving dietary diversity and nutritional status in rural areas?
3. How does the fortification of food grains, such as the introduction of fortified rice in the Public Distribution System (PDS), address micronutrient deficiencies and support the overall goals of the National Nutrition Policy?

Multiple Choice Questions (MCQs)

1. Which of the following is NOT a key feature of the National Nutrition Policy (NNP) 1993?
   a. Direct nutrition interventions
   b. Indirect policy instruments
   c. Community participation
   d. Private sector involvement
2. What was the primary objective of the National Nutrition Policy (NNP) 1993?
   a. To increase food production
   b. To improve the nutritional status of the population
   c. To promote economic development
   d. To reduce infant mortality rates
3. Which of the following is NOT a direct intervention under the NNP 1993?
   a. Fortification of essential foods
   b. Promotion of low-cost nutritious food
   c. Expansion of the Integrated Child Development Services (ICDS) program
   d. Increased agricultural production

Answers

1. d
2. b
3. d

CHAPTER 11

National Population Policy

Thamizhanban A, Ranjitha R, Nilesh Thakor

Background/Need of program/Scheme	The National Population Policy (NPP) 2000 was introduced in the context of India's rapid increase in population, which had reached a staggering 1 billion by May 2000. The need for this policy arose from recognizing that stabilizing the population was crucial for sustainable economic growth, social development, and environmental protection. In 1952, India being the first country in the world to launch a National Program for Family Planning. However, despite these efforts, the population continued to grow at an alarming rate.
Objectives/Goal/Targets[1]	• **Immediate objective:** To address unmet needs for contraception, healthcare infrastructure, and health personnel. It aimed to provide integrated service delivery for basic reproductive and child health care nationwide, thereby reducing fertility rates to replacement levels by 2010. • **Medium-term objective (by 2010):** To achieve a Total Fertility Rate (TFR) of 2.1 by 2010 through vigorous implementation of intersectoral strategies to address the unmet needs in reproductive health, reduce infant and maternal mortality, and promote delayed marriage and childbearing. • **Long-term objective (by 2045):** To stabilize the population by 2045 through continued efforts in reducing fertility rates, improving health outcomes, and enhancing the overall quality of life for the population.
Organogram	The National Plan for Population 2000 (NPP 2000) is to be implemented and managed at panchayat and urban local bodies in coordination with state/union territory administrations. It requires comprehensive and multispectral coordination. The newer structures formed to implement NPP 2000 were[1] • National Commission on Population, • State/UT Commissions on Population, • Coordination Cell in the Planning Commission and • Technology Mission in the Department of Family Welfare. The National Commission will oversee and review policy implementation, while State/UT Commissions will be established to review policy implementation. The Planning Commission will have a Coordination Cell for intersectoral coordination, particularly in states with adverse demographic and human development indicators. The Technology Mission will provide technology support for designing and monitoring reproductive and child health projects and IEC campaigns.
Components	The following were the key components of the NPP 2000 to be achieved in a decade of efforts by the year 2010 • Addressing Reproductive and Child Health Needs • Make school education free and compulsory until age 14. • Reduce school droupout rate to below 20% for both genders. • Achieve universal immunization against all vaccine-preventable diseases. • Promote delayed marriage for girls. • Achieve 100% deliveries conducted by trained persons. • Ensure universal access to fertility and contraception services and contraception services.

	• Achieve 100% registration of births, deaths, marriages, and pregnancy. • Contain the spread of AIDS and promote integration between RTI and STI management. • Prevent and control communicable diseases. • Integrate Indian Systems of Medicine in reproductive and child health services. • Promote small family norm to achieve replacement levels of TFR. • Converge implementation of related social sector programs for family welfare.
Strategies/Deliverables under the program	• **Decentralized planning and implementation:** Significant roles assigned to local self-government institutions such as Panchayats. These institutions were to be strengthened and empowered to plan and implement programs • **Public-Private Partnerships (PPP):** Involvement of the private sector and NGOs in providing reproductive and child health services, for extending the reach of services, improving service delivery, and ensuring the sustainability. • **Community participation:** The policy encouraging active involvement of communities in planning and implementing population stabilization through awareness campaigns, capacity building, and in promoting small family norms and health-seeking behaviors. • **Convergence of services at the village level:** Convergence of health, nutrition, education, and women's empowerment services to create a coordinated and integrated service delivery system. • **Use of Information, Education, and Communication (IEC):** To raise awareness about population stabilization, reproductive health, and the benefits of small family norms. The policy emphasized using mass media, local languages, and culturally relevant messages to reach all population segments.
Small Family Norm under NPP 2000	The following measures were taken in promoting small family norms and family planning literacy among the population • Panchayats and Zila Parishads are to be rewarded for promoting small family norms, reducing infant mortality and birth rates, and promoting literacy. • Balika Samridhi Yojana will continue promoting the survival and care of the girl child, with a cash incentive of ₹ 500 at birth. • The maternity benefit scheme will continue, with a cash incentive of ₹ 500 for mothers having their first child after 19 years of age. • A family welfare-linked health insurance plan should be established, allowing couples below the poverty line to receive health insurance for hospitalization and personal accident insurance. • Rewarding couples who marry after the legal age of marriage, register the marriage, have their first child after the mother reaches 21, accept the small family norm, and adopt a terminal method after the birth of the second child. • Revolving fund set up for income-generating activities by village-level self-help groups. • Opening crèches and child care centers in rural areas and urban slums to promote women's participation in paid employment. • Expanding facilities for safe abortion and making products and services affordable through innovative social marketing schemes. • Providing soft loans to local entrepreneurs and encouraging ambulance services. • Encouraging increased vocational training schemes for girls leading to self-employment. • Strict enforcement of the Child Marriage Restraint Act, 1976 and the Pre-Conception and Techniques Act, 1994.
Challenges and Criticisms of NPP 2000	• Inadequate funding, lack of trained personnel, and resistance to behavioral change hindered implementation in areas with high fertility rates and poor health infrastructure. • High fertility rates in Bihar and Uttar Pradesh required more intensive efforts than states nearing replacement-level fertility. • The promotion of sterilization incentives and enforcement of small family norms raised concerns about reproductive rights and potential coercion. • Policy inadequately addressed issues related to gender and reproductive rights, particularly in patriarchal societies.

Impact and Achievements of NPP 2000[1]	<ul><li>Significant progress towards immediate and medium-term goals, including increased contraception use, maternal and child health improvements, and fertility rate reduction.</li><li>Uneven progress observed across various states.</li><li>Policy contributed to a gradual decline in fertility rates and slowdown in population growth.</li><li>Challenges remained in achieving long-term population stabilization by 2045.</li><li>Key achievements include improvements in maternal and child health, with reductions in infant and maternal mortality rates.</li><li>Success stories include Kerala and Tamil Nadu, which integrated health, education, and welfare services, improving population stabilization and health outcomes.</li></ul>

Reference

1. National Population Policy 2000. Ministry of Health and Family Welfare, Government of India.

QUESTIONS

Long Answer Question (LAQ)

1. How has the age of marriage in India evolved from years 2000 to 2024, and what impact has this shift had on fertility rates and maternal health outcomes?

Short Answer Questions (SAQs)

1. What are India's key challenges in population control in 2024, despite the measures and strategies outlined in the NPP 2000?
2. How effective have public-private partnerships and community participation been in addressing India's unmet needs for reproductive and child health services in the last two decades?
3. In what ways has the demographic context of India in 2024 diverged from the projections made in NPP 2000, and what new strategies are needed to address these demographic changes?

Multiple Choice Questions (MCQs)

1. National population policy emphasize on reducing school dropout rate to less than:
   a. 10%
   b. 20%
   c. 30%
   d. 50%
2. According to NPP 2000, target TFR to be achieved is:
   a. 1.2
   b. 1.5
   c. 2.1
   d. 3.1

Answers

1. b
2. c

CHAPTER 12

National Policy for Rare Diseases

Anamika Tomar, Purushottam Giri, Akhil Dhanesh Goel

Background	The National Policy for Rare Diseases (NPRD) was introduced by the Ministry of Health and Family Welfare on March 30, 2021, to address the challenges faced by patients with rare diseases, which often receive little attention due to their low prevalence and high treatment costs.

Worldwide, rare diseases affect about **3.5% to 5.9%** of the population, translating to around **300 million people** globally.

In contrast, India's prevalence suggests that nearly **5% to 7%** of its population may be affected by rare diseases which accounts for approximately **one-third of global rare disease cases**.

This prevalence is notably high compared to other countries, particularly due to India's large population of over 1.3 billion and its diverse genetic background, which contributes to a higher incidence of genetic disorders and rare diseases.[2,4]

Definition of rare diseases

There is no universal or standard definition of rare disease. A disease that occurs infrequently is generally considered a rare disease, and it has been defined by different countries in terms of prevalence—either in absolute terms or in terms of prevalence per 10,000 population.

A country defines a rare disease most appropriate in the context of its own population, health care system and resources.

As per **World Health Organization (WHO)** defines rare diseases as those affecting 1 or fewer per 1,000 people. The European Union considers diseases affecting no more than 5 in 10,000 people as rare. In the United States, a disease is classified as rare if it affects fewer than 200,000 patients.

Other Country's Criterion of Classifying Rare Diseases **(Table 12.1)**

TABLE 12.1: Definitions of rare disease in different countries.

S. No.	Country	Per 10,000 population
1.	USA	6.4
2.	Europe	5.0
3.	Canada	5.0
4.	Japan	4.0
5.	South Korea	4.0
6.	Australia	1.0
7.	Taiwan	1.0

Source: The IC Verma Sub-Committee Report 'Guidelines for Therapy and Management'.

India is currently facing challenges in defining rare diseases due to a lack of comprehensive epidemiological data, which is essential for establishing prevalence rates similar to those used in other countries.[2]

To address this gap, the Indian Council of Medical Research (ICMR) has initiated a **hospital-based National Registry for Rare Diseases**.

	This registry aims to gather crucial epidemiological data by collaborating with medical centers across the nation that specialize in diagnosing and managing rare diseases. Until sufficient data is collected and a standardized definition based on prevalence is established, the term "rare diseases" will encompass several groups of disorders as categorized by experts based on their clinical experience.[1,2]
	Group Classifications of Rare Diseases
	Group 1: Disorders with one-time curative treatment
	• **Hematopoietic stem cell transplantation (HSCT)** is applicable for:
	  ✦ Lysosomal storage disorders (LSDs) lacking enzyme replacement therapy (ERT), and severe forms of mucopolysaccharidosis (MPS) type I in infants under two years.
	  ✦ Early-stage adrenoleukodystrophy before neurological symptoms manifest.
	• **Immune deficiency disorders** such as severe combined immunodeficiency (SCID), chronic granulomatous disease, and Wiskott-Aldrich syndrome.
	• **Organ transplantation** cases including:
	  ✦ **Liver transplantation** for metabolic liver diseases like tyrosinemia and glycogen storage disorders (GSDs).
	  ✦ **Renal Transplantation** for conditions like Fabry disease and autosomal recessive polycystic kidney disease (ARPKD).
	Group 2: Long-term treatment needs
	• Diseases requiring ongoing treatment with documented benefits and relatively lower costs, necessitating regular monitoring: Conditions managed with special dietary formulas or food for special medical purposes (FSMP), including Phenylketonuria (PKU) and various organic acidemias.
	• Disorders treated with specific therapies such as NTBC for tyrosinemia type 1 and growth hormone therapy for deficiencies.
	Group 3: Definitive treatment available but high cost
	• Conditions with established treatments that present challenges in patient selection and affordability: Disorders like Gaucher Disease, Hurler Syndrome, and Pompe disease where early diagnosis before complications can lead to better outcomes.
	• High-cost treatments with limited long-term follow-up data or small patient cohorts, such as therapies for cystic fibrosis and Duchenne muscular dystrophy.
	The lists of diseases in groups 1, 2, and 3 are not exhaustive and will be periodically reviewed by a technical committee based on the latest scientific evidence.
	
	Currently, 63 rare diseases are included under National Policy for Rare Diseases on recommendation of Central Technical Committee for Rare Diseases (CTCRD).

Objectives[2]	• **Reducing treatment costs:** Aiming to alleviate the financial burden of rare diseases. • **Promoting indigenous research:** Fostering local medicine production and research for effective treatments. • **Enhancing early detection and screening:** Encouraging early diagnosis to improve treatment outcomes. • **Strengthening healthcare infrastructure:** Enhancing tertiary care facilities for better management of rare diseases.

Implementation strategies	Keeping in view lack of availability of epidemiological data on rare diseases, constraints on resources and competing health priorities, the focus of the Government will be on the following:
	• **Categorization of rare diseases:**[1,2]
	  ✦ **Group 1:** Disorders suitable for one-time curative treatment.
	  ✦ **Group 2:** Conditions needing long-term or lifelong treatment, usually at lower costs.
	  ✦ **Group 3:** Diseases with existing treatments but facing high costs or patient selection challenges.
	• **Financial support mechanisms:**[1,2,3]
	  ✦ **Direct financial assistance:** Up to ₹ 20 lakh for group 1 patients and ₹ 50 lakh for others at designated Centers of Excellence (CoE). Since the launch of the policy, a total number of one thousand one hundred and eighteen (1,118) patients have benefited under NPRD.
	  ✦ **Expanded eligibility:** Assistance extends beyond below-poverty-line families to around 40% of the population under the Pradhan Mantri Jan Arogya Yojana.
	  ✦ **Customs duty exemptions:** Waivers on customs duties for drugs imported for personal use.
	  ✦ **Voluntary crowd-funding for treatment:** A digital platform has been established to facilitate crowdfunding for patients with rare diseases. This platform allows individuals and organizations to contribute financially towards treatments, thereby indirectly supporting R&D through increased funding availability

- **Nidan Kendras:**[2] Nidan Kendras have been set up by Department of Biotechnology (DBT) under Unique Methods of Management and treatment of Inherited Disorders (UMMID) project for genetic testing and counseling services. These Nidan Kendras will be performing screening, genetic testing and counseling for rare diseases.
    - Given the limited resources available, universal screening for all rare disorders in every pregnancy and newborn is not practical.
    - The policy suggests a targeted approach where prenatal screening is offered to pregnant women with a confirmed history of a child diagnosed with a rare disease.
    - This would involve tests such as amniocentesis or chorionic villus sampling. This strategy aligns with the goal of reducing the prevalence of rare diseases in the population. If a diagnosis is not made during pregnancy, newborn screening should be conducted, which would include.
        - Testing for small molecule Inborn Errors of Metabolism using liquid chromatography-tandem mass spectrometry (LC-MS/MS).
        - Screening for Severe Combined Immunodeficiency (SCID) through T cell receptor excision circles (TREC).
        - Testing for lysosomal storage disorders (LSDs) using microfluidics or LC-MS/MS
        - Diagnosing other conditions using newer, cost-effective molecular diagnostic technologies.
        - Five Nidan Kendras have been set up for genetic testing and counseling services as given below:
            1. Lady Hardinge Medical College (LHMC), Delhi
            2. Nizam's Institute of Medical Sciences (NIMS), Hyderabad, Telangana
            3. All India Institute of Medical Sciences (AIIMS), Jodhpur, Rajasthan
            4. Army Hospital Research & Referral, Delhi
            5. Nil Ratan Sircar (NRS) Medical College and Hospital, Kolkata, West Bengal
        - Nidan Kendras possessing the facility for treatment may do so under the guidance and supervision of a CoE.
- **Centers of Excellence (CoEs):**[1,2,3] Designated centers aimed at improving infrastructure for diagnosing, preventing, and treating rare diseases, receiving financial support for upgrades and specialized care. Twelve (12) Centers of Excellence (CoEs) have been identified so far, which are premier Government tertiary hospitals with facilities for diagnosis, prevention and treatment of rare diseases.[8]
- **List of Centers of Excellence (CoEs) is at:**
    1. All India Institute of Medical Sciences, New Delhi
    2. Maulana Azad Medical College, New Delhi
    3. Sanjay Gandhi Postgraduate Institute of Medical Sciences, Lucknow
    4. Postgraduate Institute of Medical Education and Research, Chandigarh
    5. Centre for DNA Fingerprinting and Diagnostics with Nizam's Institute of Medical Sciences, Hyderabad
    6. King Edward Medical Hospital, Mumbai
    7. Institute of Postgraduate Medical Education and Research, Kolkata
    8. Center for Human Genetics (CHG) with Indira Gandhi Hospital, Bengaluru
    9. Institute of Child Health and Hospital for Children (ICH and HC), Chennai
    10. All India Institute of Medical Sciences (AIIMS), Jodhpur
    11. Sree Avittom Thirunal Hospital (SAT), Government Medical College, Thiruvananthapuram
    12. All India Institute of Medical Sciences, Bhopal

Patients can approach any CoE across the country as per their convenience.

    The responsibilities and activities of the COE's are followings:
    - Education and Training at all levels
    - Screening—antenatal, neonatal (specified disorders), High risk screening (both antenatal and in newborns and children)
    - Diagnostics—cytogenetic, molecular, metabolic
    - Prevention by prenatal screening and diagnosis
    - Research in the area of low cost diagnostics and therapeutics.
    - Treatment of rare diseases.
- **Promotion of research and development:** Encouraging local research and production of orphan drugs. As envisaged in the policy, the Department of Health Research has established the National Consortium for Research and Development on Therapeutics for Rare Diseases (NCRDTRD) for streamlining the research activities for rare diseases. Additionally, states are urged to establish Departments of Medical Genetics in medical colleges to enhance education and awareness among healthcare professionals.[2,3]

- **National registry:** The Government is establishing a hospital-based National Registry for Rare Diseases under the Indian Council of Medical Research (ICMR) to compile data on various rare diseases. This initiative aims to gather hospital-based information and assess the disease burden over time.
- **Awareness and preventive strategies:** To enhance awareness, the Government plans to educate healthcare personnel and the public about rare diseases. This effort will promote pre-marital genetic counselling, assist in identifying high-risk couples and families, and facilitate early detection and prevention of rare diseases. Standard protocols for screening and diagnosis will be developed to ensure effective management and minimize missed cases.

Moreover, these treatments can be prohibitively expensive and are not universally accessible. Therefore, prevention must be prioritized for all genetic disorders, and this can be approached at multiple levels. The initial step involves building the capacity of healthcare professionals and raising awareness among the general population about the prevalence of these diseases and preventive measures. Frontline workers will be trained for rare disease screening, and informative materials will be developed and distributed throughout the healthcare system to address the lack of awareness.[2]

- **Primary prevention:** The goal of primary prevention is to prevent the occurrence of genetic disorders, particularly avoiding the birth of affected children. Although this strategy may not always be feasible, it offers significant long-term benefits in reducing the incidence and prevalence of rare disorders. Some strategies include:
    - Avoiding pregnancies in older age.
    - Not marrying carriers of rare monogenic disorders.
    - Carrier couples choosing not to reproduce.

While these options may not always be practical, a more achievable approach is secondary prevention. A checklist will be provided to primary healthcare providers in wellness clinics to help identify couples at risk based on family history of genetic disorders.

- **Secondary prevention:** Secondary prevention aims to prevent the birth of affected fetuses through prenatal screening and diagnosis, as well as early detection and medical intervention.
    - *Prenatal screening:* Common methods include biochemical screenings and ultrasounds to detect chromosomal disorders like Down syndrome, along with assessments for structural defects. For rare diseases, the focus is on identifying high-risk mothers based on family history. Targeted screening for specific disorders or carrier testing for monogenic conditions using next-generation sequencing can be offered, although the latter can be costly.
    - *Prenatal diagnosis:* Invasive testing methods, such as chorionic villus sampling and amniocentesis, can diagnose single-gene disorders or chromosomal abnormalities if the disease-causing variants are known. These tests are typically recommended when there is a history of a known disorder in the family. While these procedures are widely available in India and generally safe when performed by experienced specialists, there is a small risk of fetal loss that must be communicated to families. If a fetus is diagnosed with a disorder, couples have the option to terminate the pregnancy, with the legal limit in India set at 24 weeks.
    - *Newborn screening (NBS):* This is a prime example of secondary prevention, as it allows for early screening of newborns for various disorders before symptoms appear, enabling timely treatment to prevent morbidity and mortality. In many developed countries, NBS is conducted for numerous rare but treatable disorders.
    - *Early postnatal diagnosis and treatment:* This includes diagnosing and treating conditions before severe, irreversible complications arise. Increasing awareness and improving access to diagnostics are essential for timely referrals to appropriate facilities for accurate diagnosis and treatment. Genetic testing will be enhanced through the National Genomics Core, supported by the Department of Biotechnology and institutions like IGIB and CCMB.
- **Tertiary prevention:** Tertiary prevention focuses on providing improved care and medical rehabilitation for patients with advanced disease stages. This includes supportive care for individuals with rare disorders, even when specific treatments are unavailable. Such care aims to enhance the quality of life for affected individuals and their families, encompassing developmental assessments, early interventions, physical therapy, rehabilitation, provision of aids, and emotional and psychological support.
    - *Multi-sectoral collaboration:* Emphasizing the need for collaboration among healthcare providers, government agencies, and patient advocacy groups for a coordinated approach. The Departments of Pharmaceuticals and DPIIT will be asked to promote the local development and production of affordable drugs for rare diseases, alongside legal measures to support indigenous manufacturing. Furthermore, the Ministry of Finance will be approached to reduce customs duties on imported medicines related to rare diseases.

Chapter 12: National Policy for Rare Diseases

Main challenges in implementation	Implementing the NPRD faces several significant challenges:[2,3] • **Lack of clear definition and consensus:** Insufficient epidemiological data complicates the classification of rare diseases, making diagnosis and treatment difficult. • **Inadequate financial support:** While financial aid is provided, it may not fully cover the costs of treatment, particularly for long-term care. • **Limited availability of drugs:** A shortage of domestic drug manufacturing leads to high prices for medications, creating access barriers for many patients. • **Insufficient infrastructure and awareness:** Limited infrastructure at the state level and general public and professional ignorance about rare diseases contribute to delays in diagnosis and treatment. • **Coordination among stakeholders:** A multi-stakeholder approach often suffers from a lack of clarity and coordination, resulting in inefficiencies. • **Absence of comprehensive data:** Slow progress on establishing a national registry makes it hard to assess disease prevalence and develop effective strategies. • **Regulatory challenges:** The absence of strong regulatory frameworks raises concerns about the quality and efficacy of drugs for rare diseases.
Conclusion	The National Policy for Rare Diseases 2021 marks a crucial step towards improving the quality of life for individuals affected by rare diseases in India. Successful implementation of this policy will depend on enhanced funding mechanisms, better infrastructure, improved coordination among stakeholders, and increased awareness.

References

1. Initiatives by the Government for treatment of rare diseases - PIB
2. National Policy for Rare Diseases, 2021
3. National Policy for Rare Diseases, 2021: Provisions and Concerns
4. https://www.ispor.org/raredisease-terms-definitions.pdf

QUESTIONS

Long Answer Question (LAQ)

1. What are the key provisions, challenges, and expected outcomes of the National Policy for Rare Diseases 2021, particularly in terms of its categorization of rare diseases, financial support mechanisms for patients, and the establishment of a national registry for rare diseases, and how do these elements aim to improve healthcare access and treatment options for individuals affected by rare diseases in India?

Short Answer Questions (SAQs)

1. What are the three groups of rare diseases categorized under the National Policy for Rare Diseases 2021?
2. How much financial support does the policy provide for patients with disorders amenable to one-time curative treatment?

Multiple Choice Questions (MCQs)

1. What is the maximum financial support provided under the National Policy for Rare Diseases 2021 for patients in Group 1?
   A. ₹ 10 lakh
   b. ₹ 20 lakh
   c. ₹ 30 lakh
   d. ₹ 50 lakh

Section II: Health Policies

2. **Which group under the National Policy for Rare Diseases includes diseases requiring long-term or lifelong treatment?**
   a. Group 1
   b. Group 2
   c. Group 3
   d. None of the above
3. **What is a significant concern regarding patients classified under Group 3 of rare diseases?**
   a. They have immediate access to treatment.
   b. They are not eligible for any funding.
   c. They require sustainable treatment support but lack long-term funding.
   d. They are all children.
4. **What mechanism has been introduced to assist in funding treatment for rare diseases?**
   a. Government loans
   b. Crowdfunding platform
   c. Insurance coverage
   d. International aid
5. **Which organization is responsible for creating a national registry for rare diseases under the policy?**
   a. World Health Organization (WHO)
   b. Indian Council of Medical Research (ICMR)
   c. Ministry of Health and Family Welfare
   d. National Institute of Health

Answers

1. b
2. b
3. c
4. c
5. b

CHAPTER 13

National Policy for Older Persons

Huma Khan, Varsha Chaudhary, Niharika Verma

Need of program/ Scheme	Everyone wants to live longer but nobody wants to grow older. But it is a harsh reality of life that who so ever lives longer has to become older. All over world, the population of older people is increasing because of improved healthcare facilities, awareness and generation of financially better employment for older people. Population of senior citizens is about to reach **193.4 million by 2031** as was projected in the Report of the Technical Group on Population Projections in July 2020. There is a remarkable increase from the 103.8 million elderly as recorded in the **2011 Census**, in which elders contributed to 8.6% of the total population at that time. This demographic shift highlights the urgency of addressing issues related to healthcare, economic security, and social integration for older adults. India's National Policy for Older Persons (NPOP) was first announced by the Government of India in the year 1999. At that time, it was a vital step in accordance of the UN General Assembly Resolution 47/5 to observe 1999 as International Year of Older Persons and aligning with the assurances to older persons as contained in the Constitution of India. All those of 60 years and above are senior citizens. Constitution of India envisages the well-being of senior citizens under Article 41 which stresses upon the principle "the state shall, within the limits of its economic capacity and development, has to make effective provision for securing the right to public assistance in cases of citizens of old age." **World Senior Citizen Day** is celebrated every year on **August 21st** to underline the contributions of senior citizens. It highlights the need to raise awareness about the issues senior citizens face all over the world. The Right to Equality is promised by the Constitution as a basic right. Social security is an important responsibility shared by the Central and State Governments. The latest version of "National Policy for Senior Citizens 2011" is based on several factors including the demographic explosion among the elderly, the changing economic and social environment, the major achievements in medical research, science and technology and high prevalence of destitution among the olders especially in rural poor population. A comparatively higher proportion of elderly women in comparison to men witness loneliness. Most of them are dependent on their sons and daughters. The experience of Social deprivations and exclusion, increasing privatization of healthcare services and changing pattern of morbidity affect the elderly. The **National Action Plan for the Welfare of Senior Citizens (NAPSrC)** is like an umbrella scheme, came into force since 1st April 2020.[1]
Implemented since	1999
Goal	Ensuring to mainstream and ascertain the role of senior citizens especially older women as an invaluable resource for the country, and bring their concerns into the discussion for national development giving priority to enforce mechanisms like employment in income generating activities by governments, civil society and associations with implementation of the Maintenance and Welfare of Parents and Senior Citizens Act, 2007.[2]
Targets	• To ensure income security in old age • To prioritize the healthcare needs of senior citizens • To provide safety and security for elderly • To promote of productive aging
Objectives	The primary objectives of The National Policy for Older Persons are to: • To encourage individuals to make provision for their old age; • To encourage families to take care of their elderly family members; • To enable and support voluntary and nongovernmental organizations to contribute in the care provided by the family.[2]

	• To provide care and protection to the vulnerable elderly people; • To provide adequate healthcare facility to the senior citizens; • To promote research and training specially focusing on geriatric care givers and • organizers of services for the older people; and • To raise awareness regarding elderly persons to help them leading a productive life where the can enjoy freedom of all sorts.
Organogram	The Ministry of Social Justice and Empowerment is the Nodal Ministry for the welfare of senior citizens. The Aging Division in the Social Defense Bureau of the Department of Social Justice and Empowerment for developing and implementing program and policies for the senior citizens in close association with State Governments, Nongovernmental Organizations and Civil Society.[2]
Beneficiaries	• All those of 60 years and above are senior citizens. Young-old: 60–74 years old • Middle-old: 75–84 years old • Oldest-old: 85 years old or older

Components	• **Rashtriya Vayoshri Yojana (RVY):** It is a scheme to give senior citizens assisted living equipment and physical assistance. This is a scheme of central sector which is financed by the "Senior Citizens Welfare Fund (SCWF)" and executed by the "Artificial Limbs Manufacturing Corporation of India (ALIMCO)", which is a public sector enterprise functioning under the Ministry of Social Justice and Empowerment.
	• **Senior Citizens Welfare Fund (SCWF)** was established in 2016. **SCWF** is made up of funds that are made available under the "Central Government Saving Plans" and which remain unclaimed for seven years or more after the account is officially declared inactive by the banks. This fund is used for initiatives that support the welfare of the elderly, such as for their financial stability, to provide healthcare and nutrition, welfare of the older widows, and other initiatives focusing at well-being of elderly.
	• **Atal Pension Yojana (APY):** APY is a Government of India Scheme with the objectives of creating a social security system for all Indians, especially the poor, the under-privileged and the workers in the unorganized sector.
	• **National Council of Senior Citizens (NCSrC):** To reach the goals of the National Policy for Older Persons (NPOP), the Minister for Social Justice and Empowerment led the creation of the National Council for Older Persons (NCOP) in 1999. Its job was to ensure that the policy was followed and to give the Government the recommendations to make and run policies and programs for the elderly. In 2012, the NCOP was reorganized to get more people from all over the country to take part in it , and it was given the name National Council of Senior Citizens (NCSrC).
	The **NCSrC** gives advice to both the Central and State Governments on all matters related to the well-being and enhancement of standard of life senior citizens. It is made up of representation from Central Ministries, Social Welfare Departments, State governments, Senior Citizens' Associations, Pensioners' Associations, Nongovernmental Organizations, and experts from various backgrounds who can suggest for betterment of life of elder people. Each council member serves for three years, and the group meets once a year.
	• **Other schemes from various central ministries for the welfare of senior citizens**
	  ✦ *National programme for healthcare of the elderly (NPHCE):* Launched by The Ministry of Health and Family Welfare (MoHFW) launched during 2010–11 to address the concerns regarding health problems of older people and to make available the dedicated healthcare facilities to older people at different levels of healthcare.
	  ✦ *Pradhan Mantri Jan Arogya Yojana (PM-JAY):* Under the Ayushman Bharat, launched by Ministry of Health and Family Welfare in 2018, it is the largest health assurance scheme in the world which ensures to provide a health cover of ₹ 5 lakhs per family per year for secondary and tertiary care hospitalization across public and private empaneled hospitals in India to poor and vulnerable families. On September 11, 2024 Prime minister of India announced that **all senior citizens aged 70 and above will receive health coverage, regardless of their income.**
	  ✦ *Indira Gandhi National Old Age Pension Scheme (IGNOAPS):* It was first implemented in 2007. This scheme is especially intended for people , who are aged 60 years and above and fall below the line of poverty. Under **IGNOAPS** , the beneficiary is entitled to a monthly pension. **IGNOAPS** being a non-contributing scheme, the beneficiary is not required to contribute any amount in order to get the pension. The sum of pension aged between 60 to 79 years is of ₹ 200 and for people above 80 years, a sum of ₹ 500 is given.

Chapter 13: National Policy for Older Persons

	✦ *The Pradhan Mantri Vaya Vandana Yojana (PMVVY) PMVVY:* A Pension Scheme launched by Government of India (GoI) in May 2017 to provide social security exclusively for the senior citizens aged 60 years and above. Life Insurance Corporation (LIC) of India has the sole privilege to operate the Pradhan Mantri Vaya Vandana Yojana. ✦ *Ministry of Finance:* Provides the various facilities for senior citizens like, a senior citizen is granted a higher exemption limit compared to non-senior citizens. **Very senior citizen (of age above 80 years)** is granted a higher exemption limit compared to others. *Another scheme is of promoting silver economy:* Which provides financial assistance of up to ₹ 1 crore for entrepreneurs to create innovative solutions for elderly care. ✦ *Ministry of Road Transport and Highways:* Provides the facilities of reservation of two people of geriatric age group in front row of the buses of the State Road Transport Undertakings. Some State Governments also provide fare concession to senior citizens in the their respective State Road Transport Undertaking buses. ✦ *Ministry of Railways:* Provides the facilities to senior citizens like fare concession, facility of separate counters on stations for senior citizens to purchase/booking/cancellation of tickets, wheel chairs for use of elderly, Ramps for wheel chairs movement are ensured at the entry to important stations. ✦ *Ministry of Consumer Affairs, Food and Public Distribution:* Provides the many facilities for senior citizens, namely the "Antyodaya Scheme", for the Below Poverty Line (BPL) families which also include older persons are provided food grains at the rate of 35 kg per family per month. The food grains are issued @ ₹ 3/- per kg for rice and ₹ 2/- per kg for wheat. Another scheme is "Annapoorna Scheme" by the States/UT Administration, under "Annapoorna Scheme" 10 kg of food grains per beneficiary per month are provided free of cost to those senior citizens who remain uncovered under the old age pension scheme. ✦ *Maintenance and Welfare of Parents and Senior Citizens Act, 2007:* Promises to ensure for protection of life and property of senior citizens.[1]
Strategies/ Deliverables under the program	The **National Action Plan for the Welfare of Senior Citizens (NAPSrC)** is an umbrella scheme, effective since 1st April 2020. This plan takes care of the top four needs of the senior citizens viz., financial security, food, healthcare and human interaction/life of dignity. It also envisages the aspects of safety/protection and general wellbeing of the elderly.[1]
Activities at various level Or package of services	The **National Action Plan for the Welfare of Senior Citizens (NAPSrC)** has four sub-schemes under it, namely: • **Scheme of Integrated Programme for Senior Citizens (IPSrC):** The scheme helps state and UT governments with up to 100% of the project costs through Registered Societies, Panchayati Raj Institutions (PRIs), local bodies agencies, nongovernmental/voluntary organizations, institutions or organizations set up by the government as autonomous or subordinate bodies, and government-recognized educational institutions, charitable hospitals/nursing homes, and recognized youth organizations like Nehru Yuva Kendra Sangathan, as long as they follow the rules set by this Ministry. The schemes help run and maintain the various projects like: Senior Citizens' Homes for 25 destitute senior citizens to provide food, care and shelter. • Senior citizens' homes for 50 elderly women, including those who are part of the Sansad Adarsh Gram Yojana (SAGY), to give them food, care, and a place to live. • Long-term care homes and homes for seniors with Alzheimer's disease or dementia for at least 20 seniors who have Alzheimer's disease or dementia or are seriously ill and need continuous nursing care and relief care. • Mobile Medicare Units (MMUs) to help older people who live in rural, isolated, or backward places get medical care. • Physiotherapy clinics for seniors for at least fifty seniors every month. • The Ministry funds Regional Resource and Training Centers (RRTCs), which keep an eye on the centers for the elderly and help them provide better services by offering technical support, lobbying, networking, training, and building up staff. • A number of other actions thought to be appropriate to achieve the scheme's goals • **State Action Plan for Senior Citizens (SAPSrC):** The Government of India perceives an important and vital role of all State Governments in implementing the Action Plan for welfare of senior citizens. The State Action Plan comprises a long-term strategy for five years as well as Annual Action Plans. Department of Social Justice and Empowerment releases funds to the states/UTs for formulation and implementation of their State Action Plans. Under the SAPSrC, the states are expected to put in their own funds to augment the resources available for the purpose.

Section II: Health Policies

	• **Convergence with initiatives of other ministries/departments in Government of India in the field of senior citizens welfare (CWMSrC):** In order to help the old, the NAPSrC has suggested that different government departments take certain coordinated actions. Through these projects departments can work together and come up with Annual Action Plans in alignment to the scheme's goals. • **Media, advocacy, capacity building, research and study, pilots and any other project aimed towards the welfare of the senior citizens and falling under the scope and coverage of the NAPSrC through NISD (NISDSrC):** National Institute of Social Defence (NISD), an autonomous body of this Department, is the resource centre on elderly in the country.[1]
Monitoring and evaluation of program	The following ministries and departments are in charge of putting the policy into action: Home Affairs; Health and Family Welfare; Rural Development; Urban Development; Youth Affairs and Sports; Railways; Science and Technology; Statistics and Program Implementation; Labor; Panchayati Raj; and the Departments of Elementary Education and Literacy; Secondary and Higher Education; Road Transport and Highways; Public Enterprises; Revenue; Women and Child Development; Information Technology; and Personnel and Training. Progress made during the year is shown in these Ministries' and Departments' yearly reports.[2] Block development offices are designated as the nodal officers who will help elderly people get their pensions and take care of their paperwork and physical appearance needs. This is especially true for elderly women. In rural or tribal areas, the policy is carried out by the "gram sabha" or the tribal council or the appropriate Panchayat Raj institution. Toll-free number 14567 for the National Helpline for Senior Citizens-Elderline—to listen to what the older people have to say.

References

1. Elderly in India 2021, Government of India, Ministry of statistics and Programme implementation, National Statisticical Office, social statistics division, www.mospi.gov.in
2. National Policy for Senior Citizens, https://socialjustice.gov.in/writereaddata/UploadFile/dnpsc.pdf

QUESTIONS

Long Answer Question (LAQ)

1. Discuss about the social assistance schemes for elderly in India.

Short Answer Questions (SAQs)

1. Rashtriya Vayoshri Yojana.
2. Indira Gandhi National Old Age Pension Scheme (IGNOAPS).
3. Objectives of the National Policy for Older Persons.

Multiple Choice Questions (MCQs)

1. World Senior Citizen Day is celebrated every year on:
   a. 10th October
   b. 14th November
   c. 21st August
   d. 10th December

Chapter 13: National Policy for Older Persons

2. The name for National Health Programme focusing to provide healthcare services to senior citizens is:
   a. National Programme for Healthcare of Elderly People
   b. National Programme for Healthcare of the Elderly
   c. National Programme for Healthcare of Senior Citizens
   d. National Programme for Healthcare of Older People
3. Which of the following is not the target of National Policy for Older Persons?
   a. To ensure income security in old age
   b. To prioritize the healthcare needs of senior citizens
   c. To provide safety and security for elderly
   d. To provide job opportunities for elderly
4. The Nodal Ministry for the welfare of senior citizens is:
   a. The Ministry of Social Justice and Empowerment
   b. Ministry of Defense
   c. Ministry of Finances
   d. Ministry of Health and Family Welfare
5. Beneficiaries for National Policy for older persons are:
   a. Above 75 yeas of age
   b. Above 70 years of age
   c. Above 60 years of age
   d. Above 65 years of age
6. Atal Pension Yojana is social security system for all Indians, especially for:
   a. The poors
   b. The under-privileged workers
   c. The workers in the unorganized sector
   d. None
7. National Programme for Health Care of Elderly was launched during:
   a. 2008–2009
   b. 2010–2011
   c. 2012–2013
   d. 2014–2015
8. National Programme for Healthcare of Elderly was launched by:
   a. Ministry of Health and Family welfare
   b. Ministry of Law and Justice
   c. Ministry of Rural Development
   d. Ministry of Social justice and Empowerment
9. Pradhan Mantri Jan Arogya Yojana was launched in:
   a. 2015
   b. 2016
   c. 2017
   d. 2018
10. Which organization has been given the sole privilege to operate the Pradhan Mantri Vaya Vandana Yojana (PMVVY)?
    a. Life Insurance Corporation (LIC) of India
    b. General Insurance Corporation (GIC) of India
    c. National Insurance Company Ltd
    d. Oriental Insurance Company Ltd

Answers

1. c   2. b   3. d   4. a   5. c
6. d   7. b   8. a   9. d   10. a

SECTION III

National Health Mission—NRHM and NUHM

Section Outline

- **Chapter 14:** National Health Mission—NRHM and NUHM
- **Chapter 15:** Mission Parivar Vikas; National Family Planning Indemnity Scheme (NFPIS)
- **Chapter 16:** LaQshya—Labor Room Quality Improvement Initiative
- **Chapter 17:** Janani Suraksha Yojana
- **Chapter 18:** Janani Shishu Suraksha Karyakram
- **Chapter 19:** Pradhan Mantri Surakshit Matritva Abhiyan
- **Chapter 20:** Pradhan Mantri Matritva Vandana Yojana
- **Chapter 21:** Surakshit Matritva Aashwasan (SUMAN)
- **Chapter 22:** Dakshata
- **Chapter 23:** Maternal and Child Death Surveillance and Response (MDSR)
- **Chapter 24:** Facility-based Newborn Care
- **Chapter 25:** Navjaat Shishu Suraksha Karyakram
- **Chapter 26:** Home-based Newborn Care
- **Chapter 27:** Home-based Care for Young Child
- **Chapter 28:** Rashtriya Bal Swasthya Karyakram
- **Chapter 29:** Universal Immunization Programme and Mission Indradhanush

- **Chapter 30:** Integrated Management of Neonatal and Childhood Illnesses
- **Chapter 31:** Social Awareness and Action to Neutralize Pneumonia Successfully
- **Chapter 32:** MusQan—Ensuring Child-friendly Services in Government Health Facilities
- **Chapter 33:** Rashtriya Kishor Swasthya Karyakram
- **Chapter 34:** School Health Program and Menstrual Hygiene Scheme
- **Chapter 35:** Adolescent Friendly Health Clinics
- **Chapter 36:** Peer Education Program
- **Chapter 37:** Scheme for Adolescent Girls
- **Chapter 38:** Weekly Iron Folic Acid Supplementation Program and National Deworming Day
- **Chapter 39:** Anemia Mukt Bharat
- **Chapter 40:** National Nutrition Mission—Poshan Abhiyaan
- **Chapter 41:** Mothers' Absolute Affection
- **Chapter 42:** Infant and Young Child Feeding Program
- **Chapter 43:** National Vector Borne Disease Control Programme
- **Chapter 44:** National Tuberculosis Elimination Programme
- **Chapter 45:** National AIDS Control Programme
- **Chapter 46:** National Leprosy Eradication Programme
- **Chapter 47:** National Viral hepatitis Control Programme
- **Chapter 48:** National Rabies Control Programme
- **Chapter 49:** Endgame Strategy for Poliomyelitis
- **Chapter 50:** Integrated Disease Surveillance Programme and Integrated Health Information Platform
- **Chapter 51:** National Programme for Prevention and Control of Noncommunicable Diseases
- **Chapter 52:** Integration of NAFLD into NP-NCD
- **Chapter 53:** National Programme for Healthcare of the Elderly
- **Chapter 54:** National Programme for Control of Blindness and Visual Impairment
- **Chapter 55:** National Programme for Prevention and Control of Deafness
- **Chapter 56:** National Mental Health Programme

Chapter 57: National Tobacco Control Programme
Chapter 58: National Oral Health Programme
Chapter 59: National Sickle cell anemia Elimination Programme
Chapter 60: National Programme for Prevention and Management of Trauma and Burn Injuries (NPPMTBI)
Chapter 61: Pradhan Mantri National Dialysis Programme (PMNDP)
Chapter 62: National Programme for Palliative Care
Chapter 63: Integrated Child Development Services Scheme
Chapter 64: PM-POSHAN Scheme/Mid-Day Meal—Pradhan Mantri Poshan Shakti Nirman
Chapter 65: National Iodine Deficiency Disorders Control Programme
Chapter 66: National Programme for Prevention and Control of Fluorosis
Chapter 67: Antyodaya Anna Yojana
Chapter 68: National Digital Health Mission (NDHM)/Ayushman Bharat Digital Mission
Chapter 69: eSanjeevani—National Telemedicine Service
Chapter 70: e-Health Initiatives in India
Chapter 71: Ayushman Bharat Programme
Chapter 72: Pradhan Mantri Bharatiya Janaushadhi Pariyojana
Chapter 73: Beti Bachao Beti Padhao
Chapter 74: Kayakalp
Chapter 75: National Jal Jeevan Mission
Chapter 76: Swachh Swasth Sarvatra (SSS) Initiative
Chapter 77: Pradhan Mantri Ujjwala Yojana
Chapter 78: Ujjawala Scheme for Prevention of Trafficking and Rescue, Rehabilitation and Reintegration of Victims of Trafficking
Chapter 79: National Programme on Climate Change and Human Health
Chapter 80: Voluntary Blood Donation Programme
Chapter 81: National Organ Transplant Program
Chapter 82: National Programme for Control and Treatment of Occupational Diseases

Chapter 83: National Programme on Containment of Anti-Microbial Resistance (AMR)
Chapter 84: Social Security Schemes for Unorganized and Organized Sectors
Chapter 85: Intellectual Disability-related Schemes
Chapter 86: Pradhan Mantri Swasthya Suraksha Yojana (PMSSY)
Chapter 87: Affordable Medicines and Reliable Implants for Treatment
Chapter 88: National Action Plan for Prevention and Control of Snakebite Envenoming

CHAPTER 14

National Health Mission—NRHM and NUHM

Kajal Srivastava, Prerna Verma, Ghanshyam Ahir, Parul Sharma

Background/Need of program/Scheme	National Health Mission (NHM) was started for universal access to equitable, affordable and quality health care services that are accountable and responsive to people's need.
Implemented since	On 12th April 2005, the National Rural Health Mission (NRHM) was launched by the Prime Minister of India to provide accessible, affordable and quality health care to the rural population, especially the vulnerable groups. Launch of National Urban Health Mission (NUHM) as a submission of an overarching NHM on 1st May 2013.
Targets	**Targets under NHM by 2025:** • Reduce maternal mortality rate to 90 from 113 • Reduce infant mortality rate to 23 from 32 • Reduce under five mortality rate to 23 from 36 • Sustain total fertility rate to 2.1 • Reduce prevalence of Leprosy to <1/10000 population and incidence to zero in all districts • Annual Malaria Incidence to be <1/1000 • Prevent and reduce mortality and morbidity from communicable, non-communicable; injuries and emerging diseases • Reduce household out-of-pocket expenditure on total health care expenditure • Ending the tuberculosis epidemic by 2025 from the country
Objectives of the Mission[1]	• Reduction in child and maternal mortality • Universal access to public services for food and nutrition, sanitation and hygiene and universal access to public health care services with emphasis on services addressing women's and children's health and universal immunization. • Prevention and control of communicable and non-communicable diseases, including locally endemic diseases. • Access to integrated comprehensive primary health care. • Population stabilization, gender and demographic balance. • Revitalize local health traditions and mainstream AYUSH. • Promotion of healthy lifestyles.
Organogram[2]	**At national level** • The Mission Steering Group (MSG) has been the highest policy making and steering institution constituted under National Health Mission (NHM) chaired by union health minister as chair and Secretary (Health and Family Welfare) as convener and Additional Secretary and Mission Director (NHM) as co-convener. • MSG provides broad policy direction to the mission and exercises the main program and governance for the health sector and advises the Empowered Programme Committee of the Mission in policies and operation. • **Empowered Programme Committee (EPC):** Executive committee constituted under NHM is chaired by Secretary (Health and Family Welfare) and Additional Secretary and Mission Director (NHM) as convener.

At state level
- At the state level, the State Health Mission, Chief Minister would be Chairperson, Health Minister of State as Co-chairperson and secretary health and family welfare as a Convener
  - Providing health system oversight,
  - Consideration of policy matters related to health sector (including determinants of good health),
  - Review of progress in implementation of NHM; intersectoral coordination,
  - Advocacy measures required to promote NHM visibility
- State health society is headed by Chief Secretary as Chairperson, a Secretary (health and family welfare) as a Vice-Chair and Mission Director (NHM) as convener in governing body and executive committee is chaired by secretary [health and family welfare and Mission Director (NHM)] as convener.
- Approval/endorsement of Annual State Action Plan for the NHM.
  - Consideration of proposals for institutional reforms in the health and family welfare sector.
  - Review of implementation of the Annual Action Plan.
  - Intersectoral coordination
  - Status of follow up action on decisions of the State Health Mission.
  - Co-ordination with NGOs/donors/other agencies/organizations.

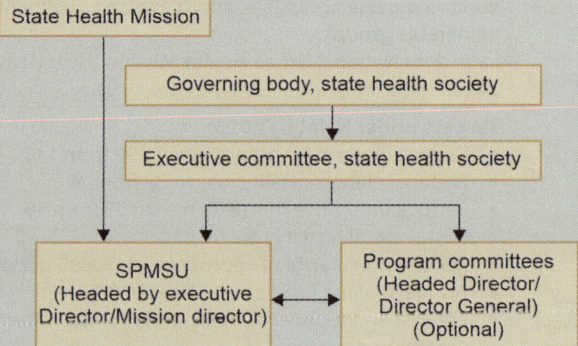

The program committee for health and family welfare sector—state may constitute program committees for the national programs for a more focused planning and review of each activity to be chaired by director and concerned State Program Manager as a member secretary.

At district level
- Every district will have a District Health Mission headed by the Chairperson, Zila Parishad. It will have the District Collector as the Co-Chair and Chief Medical Officer as the Mission Director.
- District health society is headed by District collector as a chair and District CEO as Co-chair and CDMO as Chief Executive Officer in governing body and executive committee is headed by district CEO as chair, CDMO as Co-chair and district RCH Officer/District Program Officer as Convener.

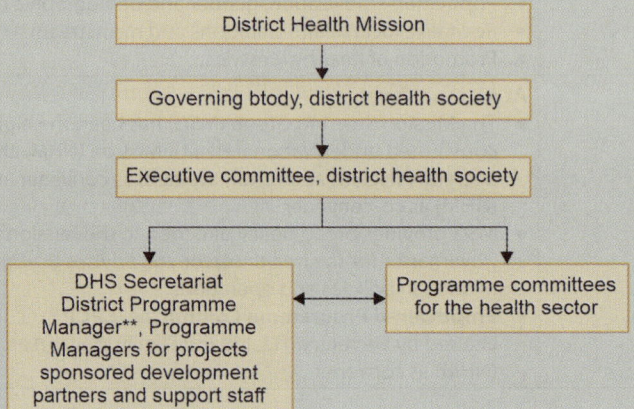

** Key player not only in setting up and operationalizing the DHS secretariat, but also in arranging managerial and supportive assistance to the district health administration, including general management and logistic support.

Beneficiaries	NHM is implemented for universal benefit for entire population, services are offered to everyone visiting the public healthcare facilities with a special focus to vulnerable section of the society.

Components	**National health mission components**
	• **RMNCH+A**
	    ✦ Adolescent Health (RKSK)
	    ✦ Child Health
	    ✦ Maternal Health
	    ✦ Family Planning
	    ✦ Immunization
	    ✦ Aspirational District Program
	• **Health Systems Strengthening (HSS)**
	    ✦ Free Drugs and Diagnostics Service Initiative
	    ✦ ERS/Patient Transport Service
	    ✦ Human Resource
	    ✦ Infrastructure
	    ✦ Mobile Medical Unit (MMUs)
	    ✦ Comprehensive Primary Health Care
	    ✦ Tribal Health
	    ✦ Blood services and blood disorders
	    ✦ District Hospital Strengthening
	    ✦ Other Health Systems Strengthening
	• **Programs/schemes are run by government under National Health Mission:**
	Reproductive, Maternal, Neonatal, Child and Adolescent Health
	    ✦ Janani Shishu Suraksha Karyakaram (JSSK)
	    ✦ Rashtriya Kishor Swasthya Karyakram (RKSK)
	    ✦ Rashtriya Bal Swasthya Karyakram (RBSK)
	    ✦ Universal Immunization Programme
	    ✦ Mission Indradhanush (MI)
	    ✦ Janani Suraksha Yojana (JSY)
	    ✦ Pradhan Mantri Surakshit Matritva Abhiyan (PMSMA)
	    ✦ Navjaat Shishu Suraksha Karyakram (NSSK)
	    ✦ National Programme for Family planning
	    ✦ LaQshya' Programme (Labour Room Quality Improvement Initiative)
	National Nutritional Programmes
	    ✦ National Iodine Deficiency Disorders Control Programme
	    ✦ MAA (Mothers' Absolute Affection) Programme for Infant and Young Child Feeding
	    ✦ National Programme for Prevention and Control of Fluorosis (NPPCF)
	    ✦ National Iron Plus Initiative for Anaemia Control
	Communicable diseases
	    ✦ Integrated Disease Surveillance Programme (IDSP)
	    ✦ National Tuberculosis Control Programme (RNTCP)
	    ✦ National Leprosy Eradication Programme (NLEP)
	    ✦ National Vector Borne Disease Control Programme (NVBDCP)
	    ✦ National AIDS Control Programme (NACP)
	    ✦ Pulse Polio Programme
	    ✦ National Viral Hepatitis Control Program (NVHCP)
	    ✦ National Rabies Control Programme
	    ✦ National Programme on Containment of Anti-Microbial Resistance (AMR)
	Non-communicable diseases
	    ✦ National Tobacco Control Programme (NTCP)
	    ✦ National Programme for Prevention and Control of Cancer, Diabetes, Cardiovascular Diseases and Stroke (NPCDCS)
	    ✦ National Programme for Control Treatment of Occupational Diseases
	    ✦ National Programme for Prevention and Control of Deafness (NPPCD)

Section III: National Health Mission

	+ National Mental Health Programme + National Programme for Control of Blindness and Visual Impairment (NPCBVI) + Pradhan Mantri National Dialysis Programme (PMNDP) + National Programme for Health Care for the Elderly (NPHCE) + National Programme for Prevention and Management of Burn Injuries (NPPMBI) + National Oral Health Programme • **Infrastructure Maintenance** Strengthening of civil works of specialty/GH/DH/CHC's/PHC's/SC's for the transformation to IPHS standards[3]
Monitoring and evaluation of program	Annual Common Review Mission is conducted to Monitor National Health Mission

References

1. [Internet]. [cited 2024 Jun 25]. Available from: https://nhm.gov.in/
2. Union Cabinet informed about progress under National Health Mission (NHM) - 2020-21 [Internet]. [cited 2024 Jul 10]. Available from: https://www.pib.gov.in/PressReleasePage.aspx?PRID=1862938
3. Healthcare Schemes, https://pib.gov.in/pressreleaseshare.aspx?prid=1576128 (accessed July 14, 2024).

QUESTIONS

Long Answer Question (LAQ)

1. Enlist the components of NHM.

Short Answer Questions (SAQs)

1. Who are the target beneficiaries of the National Health Mission (NHM)?
2. What is the primary objective of the Adolescent Health (RKSK) program under NHM?

Multiple Choice Question (MCQ)

1. Which of the following program is not under NHM?
   a. Integrated Disease Surveillance Programme (IDSP)
   b. National Tuberculosis Control Programme (RNTCP)
   c. National Leprosy Eradication Programme (NLEP)
   d. National Programme for Prevention and Management of Trauma and Burn Injuries (NPPMBI)

Answer

1. d

PART A

RMNCAH+N (Reproductive Maternal Newborn Child Adolescent Health Plus Nutrition)

i. **R: Reproductive Health**
  15. Mission Parivar Vikas; National Family Planning Indemnity Scheme (NFPIS)

ii. **M: Maternal Health**
  16. LaQshya—Labor Room Quality Improvement Initiative
  17. Janani Suraksha Yojana
  18. Janani Shishu Suraksha Karyakram
  19. Pradhan Mantri Surakshit Matritva Abhiyan
  20. Pradhan Mantri Matritva Vandana Yojana
  21. Surakshit Matritva Aashwasan (Suman)
  22. Dakshata
  23. Maternal and Child Death Surveillance and Response (MDSR)

iii. **NC: Neonatal and Child Health**
  24. Facility-based Newborn Care
  25. Navjaat Shishu Suraksha Karyakram
  26. Home-based Newborn Care
  27. Home-based Care for Young Child Programme
  28. Rashtriya Bal Swasthya Karyakram
  29. Universal Immunization Programme and Mission Indradhanush
  30. Integrated Management of Neonatal and Childhood Illnesses
  31. Social Awareness and Action to Neutralize Pneumonia Successfully
  32. MusQan—Ensuring Child-friendly Services in Government Health Facilities

iv. **A: Adolescent Health**
  33. Rashtriya Kishor Swasthya Karyakram
  34. School Health including Menstrual Hygiene Scheme
  35. Adolescent Friendly Health Clinics
  36. Peer Education Program
  37. Scheme for Adolescent Girls

38. Weekly Iron Folic Acid Supplementation Program and National Deworming Day
v. **N: Nutrition**
   39. Anemia Mukt Bharat
   40. National Nutrition Mission—POSHAN 2.0
   41. Mothers' Absolute Affection
   42. Infant and Young Child Feeding Program

i. R: Reproductive Health

CHAPTER 15

Mission Parivar Vikas; National Family Planning Indemnity Scheme (NFPIS)

Pallavi Singh, Parul Sharma, Bharti Koria

Background/Need of program

Based on the data from the National Family Health Survey (NFHS) IV, the percentage of individuals with a desire for contraceptives that is not being met is 12.9%. This lack of access to contraceptives is a factor that leads to unwanted pregnancies. Decreasing the Total Fertility Rate (TFR) is crucial since it has a direct correlation with both Maternal Mortality Rate (MMR) and Infant Mortality Rate (IMR). Mission Parivar Vikas (MPV) is an initiative aimed at population control, which aligns with the United Nations' health goals under the Sustainable Development Goals (SDGs). The objective of the Mission Parivar Vikas is to achieve a decrease in TFR by 2025 in areas with high fertility rates, by implementing a range of family planning services and awareness programs. Important methods include enhancing capacity, guaranteeing the availability of essential commodities, and implementing the Reproductive, Maternal, Newborn, Child, and Adolescent Health (RMNCH+A) strategy. SAARTHI, Nayi Pehal, and Saas Bahu Sammelan are initiatives that have the objective of encouraging and advocating for family planning. The implementation has resulted in a decline in the TFR and a rise in the Contraceptive Prevalence Rate. The goal was initiated with the aim of facilitating convenient availability of superior family planning options through dependable services, information, and resources within a rights-based framework.[1]

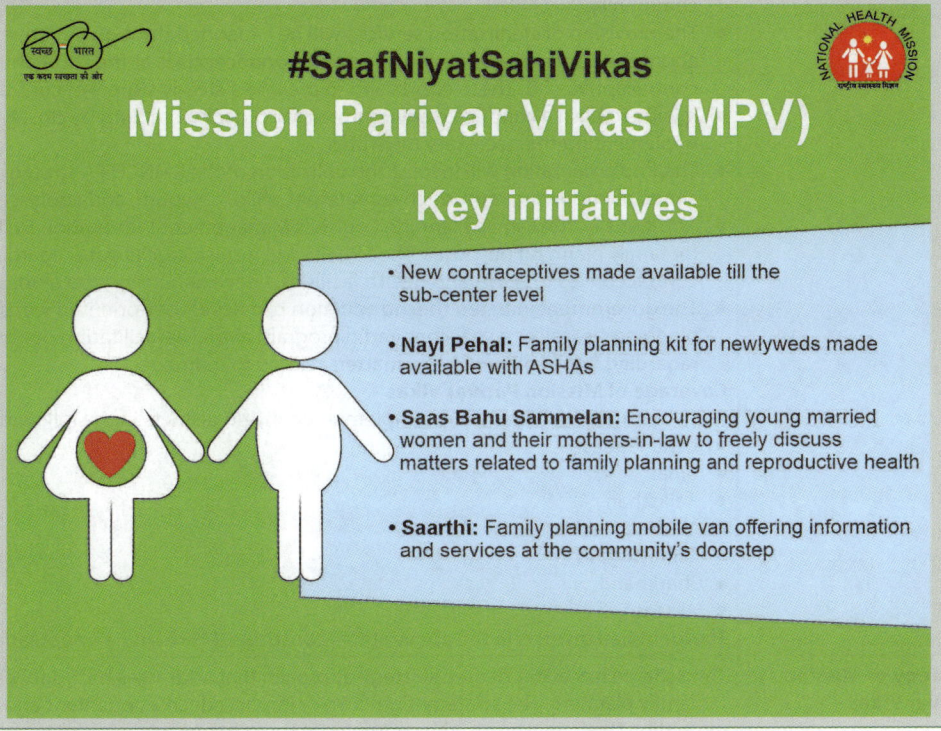

#SaafNiyatSahiVikas
Mission Parivar Vikas (MPV)

Key initiatives

- New contraceptives made available till the sub-center level
- **Nayi Pehal:** Family planning kit for newlyweds made available with ASHAs
- **Saas Bahu Sammelan:** Encouraging young married women and their mothers-in-law to freely discuss matters related to family planning and reproductive health
- **Saarthi:** Family planning mobile van offering information and services at the community's doorstep

Implementation	The government initiated the Mission Parivar Vikas on September 26, 2016, with the aim of significantly enhancing the availability of contraception and family planning services in 146 districts with high fertility rates, specifically those with TFR over three. The 146 districts that have been identified are located in seven high-focus states, namely Assam, Jharkhand, Chhattisgarh, Madhya Pradesh, Rajasthan, Bihar, and Uttar Pradesh.[2]
Objectives	• The objective is to reduce TFR to 2.1 by the year 2025. Our goal is to ensure that individuals have access to credible information, high-quality services, and necessary materials for family planning, all within a framework that respects their rights. • To enhance the availability of contraceptives by providing reliable services through innovative advertising strategies. • To enhance capability, establish a conducive atmosphere with vigilant oversight and execution. • To achieve a population growth rate of 2.1, which is the replacement rate. • To disseminate information regarding the utilization of contraceptives and strategies for family planning. • To alter societal perceptions on the utilization of contraceptive pills, condoms, and other related methods. • The objective is to enhance the quality of life for individuals from economically disadvantaged backgrounds with big families by promoting awareness about the need of not expanding the size of their families. • The objective is to implement injectable contraceptive methods at the sub-center level and enhance sterilization services through the family planning insurance system.
Beneficiaries	• Families with a low income and a large number of family members. • Impoverished and deprived, struggling to support large families. • Individuals belonging to the lower middle-class who exhibit reluctance in utilizing contraceptive devices or oral contraceptives. • Citizens who regard discussing sex as a forbidden or prohibited topic.
Features of Mission Parivar Vikas[1]	• The Parivar Vikas mission is set to introduce a new promotional initiative called 'SAARTHI - Awareness on wheels' to effectively communicate family planning ideas and raise awareness within the community. • The provision of sterilization services will be expanded through initiatives such as raising knowledge about condoms, administering injectable contraceptives at the sub-center level, and distributing contraceptive pills. These efforts aim to provide a steady supply of contraceptives. • It will establish a conducive environment for capacity-building by closely monitoring and implementing the necessary measures. • The implementation will involve the utilization of the RMNCH+A strategy, which is a strategic approach aimed at improving reproductive maternal, child, newborn, and adolescent health. • Additionally, the Family Planning Logistics Management Information System (FPLMIS) will be employed for family planning purposes. The FPLMIS will furnish crucial data regarding the allocation and need for contraceptives to ASHA and health facilities, hence enhancing the management of the supply chain. • The government initiated the introduction of a novel user-oriented website on the topic of family planning, as well as a year-long radio program aimed at facilitating discussions among couples regarding family planning and matters related to marriage. **Coverage of Mission Parivar Vikas** The Mission Parivar Vikas will be implemented in 146 districts in the following states: • Uttar Pradesh • Bihar • Rajasthan • Madhya Pradesh • Chhattisgarh • Jharkhand • Assam The identified districts in the above states constitute 44% of India's population
Strategy of Mission Parivar Vikas	This scheme has a 360-degree strategy approach that addresses the supply and demand side gaps for family planning. The strategy significantly impacts decreasing infant and maternal mortality and morbidity. The following are the strategies of the scheme: • Providing assured services.

Chapter 15: Mission Parivar Vikas; National Family Planning Indemnity Scheme (NFPIS)

	- Maintaining commodity security. - Increasing human resource development/capacity for better service delivery. - Establishing an enabling environment. - Implementing new promotional schemes. **Deliverables** - Introduction of the injectable contraceptive DMPA (Antara) - PPIUCD services should be provided at all distribution sites - Expansion of sterilization services via remuneration programs - Implementation of Condom Dispensers - Social marketing refers to the use of marketing principles and techniques to promote social causes or bring about positive social change. - There are a total of 4 rounds of MPV Campaigns conducted per year in HFD districts, specifically in the months of April, July, October, and January.
Initiatives under Mission Parivar Vikas	**SAARTHI** To increase awareness and disseminate family planning messages throughout this scheme, a completely customized van or bus equipped with interactive communication gadgets, family planning commodities, education, information, and communication materials would be operationalized in the high-fertility districts. **Nayi Pehal** Under this program, newlyweds will receive a family planning kit from Accredited Social Health Activists (ASHA). Condoms, birth control pills, two towels, a mirror, and spouse handkerchiefs are all included in the kit. It comes with a shiny dossier for the wife, a bindi, a nail cutter, and a comb. They will provide family planning knowledge to the recently weds. **Saas Bahu Sammelan** The Saas Bahu Sammelan promotes family planning services by providing an engagement platform for pregnant and new mothers and their mothers-in-law. **Mission Parivar Vikas Implementation** As of 2022, The TFR or the average number of children per woman, reduced from 2.2 to 2.0 between NFHS-5 and NFHS-4. Only five Indian states have TFRs higher than the replacement level of 2.1. India's Contraceptive Prevalence Rate (CPR) has increased significantly from 54% to 67%. **Asha Incentive under MPV**

S. No.	Commodity	Price
1.	Injectable contrecptive MPV (Antara) and non-hormonal weekly centehtoman pill (Chhaya)	₹ 100/dose
2.	MPV campaigns block level activities	₹ 150/ASHA/Round
3.	Nayi Pehal Kit	₹ 100/ASHA/Nayi Pehal Kit
4.	Saas Bahu Sammelan	₹ 100/meeting
5.	Updating of EC Survey before each MPV Campaign	₹ 150/ASHA/quarterly round

References

1. National health Mission
2. https://india.unfpa.org/en/publications/analytical-paper-series-impact-mission-parivar-vikas-programme-evidence-national-family

QUESTIONS

Long Answer Question (LAQ)

1. What is Mission Parivar Vikas and which program is it implemented under? What are the benefits of this mission?

Short Answer Questions (SAQs)

1. Describe various initiatives under Mission Parivar Vikas.
2. What are various strategies and deliverables under MPV?

Multiple Choice Questions (MCQs)

1. Mission Parivar Vikas implemented in .....states.
   a. 5
   b. 6
   c. 7
   d. 8
2. Incentive under Nayi Pahel Kit to ASHA is:
   a. 100
   b. 200
   c. 300
   d. 400
3. Which of the following is *true* about Mission Parivar Vikas?
   a. Launched on World Population Day
   b. A new family planning initiative
   c. Focus on 146 high fertility districts in 7 states with high TFR.
   d. All of these

Answers

1. c
2. a
3. d

ii. M: Maternal Health

Chapter 16: LaQshya—Labor Room Quality Improvement Initiative

Pallavi Singh, Rohit Katre, Nilesh Thakor

Background/ Need of program/ Scheme[1]	• **High maternal mortality on delivery day:** Approximately 46% of maternal deaths occur on the day of delivery, indicating the need for improved care during this critical period. • **Significant newborn deaths and stillbirths:** Over 40% of stillbirths and 40% of newborn deaths also happen on the day of delivery, underscoring the urgent need to enhance delivery and immediate postpartum care. • **Preventable deaths and complications:** Many maternal and newborn deaths are due to preventable complications that arise during labor and immediately after childbirth. Effective interventions can reduce these unnecessary mortalities. • **Gaps in delivery and postpartum care:** There is a need for better quality of care in labor rooms and maternity operating theaters, including timely identification and management of complications, to ensure the safety of both mother and child. • **Need for timely referrals:** Often, complications require referral to higher-level facilities, but delays and lack of coordination can increase the risk of adverse outcomes. A robust referral system is needed to address this. • **Improving patient satisfaction:** Enhancing the quality of care and establishing a reliable two-way follow-up system is essential to increase satisfaction among beneficiaries. • **Ensuring respectful maternity care:** There is a need to ensure that all pregnant women receive dignified, respectful, and compassionate care throughout their childbirth experience in public health facilities. • **Need for trained healthcare providers:** Many healthcare providers require updated skills and training to manage childbirth complications effectively, which is essential to improving overall care quality. • **Lack of standardized procedures:** Standardizing care practices in labor rooms and maternity operation theaters is needed to ensure consistent and high-quality care across all public health facilities. • **Infrastructure and resource gaps:** Many facilities lack adequate infrastructure, essential equipment, and resources. Addressing these gaps is crucial to ensure safe delivery environments.
Implemented since	11th December 2017
Goal[2]	The primary aim of the LaQshya program is to decrease avoidable maternal and newborn deaths, illnesses, and stillbirths that are linked to the care provided during childbirth in the labor room and maternity operation theater. Additionally, the program aims to guarantee the provision of respectful maternity care.
Targets	The LaQshya initiative focuses on improving quality of care in the following healthcare facilities on priority: • **All Government Medical College Hospitals:** Ensuring all government-run medical college hospitals are covered. • **All district hospitals and equivalent health facilities:** Targeting all district-level hospitals and facilities providing similar services. • **Designated First Referral Units (FRUs) and High Case Load Community Health Centers (CHCs)** • **FRUs:** All designated First Referral Units involved in maternal and newborn care. • **High Case Load CHCs:** Community Health Centers with over 100 deliveries per month or 60 deliveries per month in hilly and desert areas.
Objectives	• Decrease maternal and neonatal morbidity and mortality resulting from complications such as retained placenta, preterm birth, hemorrhage, hypertension and eclampsia, obstructed labor, puerperal sepsis, newborn hypoxia, and newborn sepsis, among others. • Enhance the standard of care provided during childbirth and the immediate period following delivery. • The objective is to stabilize any difficulties and ensure that referrals are made promptly, while also establishing an efficient two-way mechanism for follow-up. • Improve the contentment of recipients, ensure a favorable childbirth experience, and deliver Respectful Maternity Care (RMC) to all pregnant women who visit public health institutions.

Organogram	**National Level** • **National Mentoring Group** *Members:* Program Divisions, IEC Division, NHSRC, NIHFW, AIIMS, Medical Colleges, Nursing Colleges, Schools of Public Health, Professional Associations, Hospital Planners, IT Professionals, Development Partners. **Responsibilities:** ✦ Periodic state and health facility visits ✦ Orientation, training, and standardization of skill-based programs ✦ Development of IEC and resource material ✦ Monitoring, evaluation, and recommending corrections ✦ Video-conferencing with QC teams ✦ Review of MDSR/Maternal Near Miss and NMR/Stillbirth review programs **State Level** • **State Mentoring Group:** Chaired by the State Mission Director *Members:* Program Officers, Faculty from AIIMS and other national institutions, Medical Education Department, State Nodal Officers for Quality, IEC, Procurement, Infrastructure, State Level Development Partners, and Eminent Professionals. **Responsibilities:** ✦ Facility visits and on-site support ✦ Training and mentoring of coaching teams ✦ Customization and approval of SOPs and work instructions ✦ Performance monitoring ✦ Mobilization of state-level support and reporting ✦ Identification and promotion of innovations ✦ Conduct MDSR and CDR ✦ Assess and modify referral directories ✦ Track and report indicators **District Level** • **Coaching Team** *Members:* District Family Welfare Officer/RCHO, District/Divisional Quality Consultants, Nursing Instructors/Mentors, Faculty from nearest Medical Colleges, Professional Associations, Development Partners. **Responsibilities:** ✦ Mentor quality circles and support campaigns ✦ Conduct periodic internal reviews and visits ✦ Provide hands-on training on clinical protocols ✦ Monitor availability of diagnostic and blood transfusion services ✦ Conduct OSCE-based staff assessments ✦ Develop referral directories and verify quality indicators ✦ Support National Quality Assurance Standards (NQAS) Certification **Facility Level** • **Quality Circle (Labor Room and OT)** Members: Gynecologist, Pediatrician, Matrons, Nursing Staff, Support Staff, Anesthetists (for OT) **Responsibilities:** ✦ Ensure adherence to protocols and clinical guidelines ✦ Assess labor room and OT using NQAS checklists ✦ Plan and execute rapid improvement cycles ✦ Collate data for monitoring indicators • **Facility Level Quality Team** ✦ Headed by Medical Superintendent or Facility In-charge ✦ Works in coordination with Quality Circles to oversee quality improvement efforts.
Beneficiaries	The beneficiaries of the LaQshya initiative are: • **Pregnant women:** Women delivering in public healthcare facilities, including Medical College Hospitals, District Hospitals, First Referral Units (FRUs), and Community Health Centers (CHCs). • **Newborns:** Infants born in public healthcare institutions who require immediate and high-quality care during and after delivery. • **Healthcare facilities:** Public health institutions that are part of the initiative, including labor rooms and maternity operating theaters, which benefit from improvements in infrastructure, equipment, and quality of care.

Chapter 16: LaQshya—Labor Room Quality Improvement Initiative

	• **Healthcare personnel:** Medical and support staff working in labor rooms and maternity operating theaters, who receive training and resources to enhance their skills and improve patient care.
Components	**Structural Improvement** • **Infrastructure upgradation:** Upgrading labor rooms and maternity operating theaters based on case load and norms. • **Human resource strengthening:** Enhancing staffing levels and upgrading skills through training and capacity building. • **Equipment availability:** Ensuring all necessary, functional, and calibrated equipment is available. • **Supply chain strengthening:** Securing a reliable supply of drugs and consumables for labor rooms and maternity OTs. **Process Improvement** • **Assessment and triage:** Implementing systematic assessment and triage protocols. • **Management of labor and complications:** Improving protocols for labor management, high-risk pregnancies, and third-stage labor. • **Referral and perioperative management:** Strengthening referral systems and perioperative processes for C-sections. • **Newborn care and resuscitation:** Enhancing newborn care, resuscitation, and support services. • **Staff sensitization:** Training staff in respectful maternity care (RMC) and monitoring compliance. **Quality Assurance Interventions** • **Quality circles and rapid improvement cycles:** Establishing teams for problem-solving and conducting targeted campaigns for quality improvement. • **Certification of labor rooms:** Certifying labor rooms based on compliance with established standards. • **Skill assessment and training:** Regular skill assessments (e.g., OSCE) and continuous training using simulations and drills. **Supportive Measures** • **Guidelines and protocols implementation:** Utilizing clinical guidelines, safe birth checklists, and surgical safety checklists. • **Availability of support services:** Ensuring essential services like blood transfusion, diagnostics, water, electricity, and security are always available. • **Use of digital tools:** Implementing digital technology for record-keeping, monitoring, and patient management. • **Feedback and grievance redressal:** Capturing patient feedback through platforms like 'Mera-Aspataal' and addressing concerns promptly. **Monitoring and Evaluation** • **Systematic facility audits:** Conducting regular audits of maternal/neonatal deaths, near misses, and C-sections for continuous learning and improvement. • **Rapid improvement events:** Running focused campaigns in six cycles to enhance specific skills and processes (e.g., electronic partograph use, respectful care, infection prevention).
Strategies/ Deliverables under the program	• The LaQshya initiative aims to enhance the quality of care provided in the labor room and maternity operating theater. • The plan includes a comprehensive approach that involves modernizing infrastructure, assuring the availability of necessary equipment, supplying sufficient Human Resources, enhancing the skills of healthcare personnel, and improving quality processes in the labor room. • Execution of expedited interventions such as NQAS evaluation, training, mentoring, reviews, etc. • Enhancing the capabilities of healthcare professionals through skill-oriented training programs such as Dakshta, and enhancing the quality of processes in the labor room. • As part of the LaQshya program, specialized Obstetric ICUs have been established at Medical College Hospitals and Obstetric HDUs have been set up at District Hospitals to enhance critical care in Obstetrics.
Activities at various level or Package of Services	The Institutional Arrangement of LaQshya initiative spans at the following 4 levels: 1. National level: Under the National Health Mission, the States have been supported in creating institutional framework for the Quality Assurance 2. State Quality Assurance Committee (SQAC), District Quality Assurance Committee (DQAC), and Quality Team at the facility level. The members of the Program Divisions, IEC Division, AIIMS, and Medical Colleges, Nursing Colleges, Schools of Public Health, etc. 3. State level: This includes faculty of AIIMS and other eminent National Institutions and Medical Education Department, State Nodal Officers for Quality

Section III: National Health Mission

	4. District level- Coaching team—an external multidisciplinary team, responsible for mentoring one or more labor rooms, would one or more retired faculty members as a coach for medical college labor rooms and operation theater
Monitoring and Evaluation of program	• New advancements aimed at improving the quality of healthcare services for mothers and newborns. • Enhanced satisfaction of recipients and favorable childbirth experience. • There is a higher need for services from individuals who benefit from public health facilities. • Certification of all health facilities under the LaQshya program. • Persistent endeavors to attain SDG targets and objectives pertaining to maternal and neonatal health. • Sustain and expedite remarkable advancements - eliminate all avoidable maternal, neonatal, and child fatalities.

References

1. LaQshya Guideline-2017. National Health Mission. Ministry of Health and Family Welfare. Available at: https://nhm.gov.in/New_Updates_2018/NHM_Components/RMNCH_MH_Guidelines/LaQshya-Guidelines.pdf
2. LaQshya. National Health System Research Center. Available at: https://qps.nhsrcindia.org/laqshya

QUESTIONS

Long Answer Question (LAQ)

1. Critically analyze LaQshya using SWOT analysis.

Short Answer Questions (SAQs)

1. Describe tools used in LaQshya.
2. Describe the 3 Delay Model with respect to maternal health.

Multiple Choice Questions (MCQs)

1. What is the primary goal of the LaQshya initiative?
   a. To increase the number of C-sections in public hospitals
   b. To decrease avoidable maternal and newborn deaths, illnesses, and stillbirths during childbirth
   c. To promote home births and traditional birthing practices
   d. To provide free contraceptives to all pregnant women
2. What percentage of maternal deaths occur on the day of delivery, as highlighted by the LaQshya initiative?
   a. 20%
   b. 30%
   c. 46%
   d. 60%
3. Which healthcare facilities are prioritized under the LaQshya initiative?
   a. Private hospitals and clinics
   b. All government-run medical college hospitals, district hospitals, designated First Referral Units (FRUs), and high case load Community Health Centers (CHCs)
   c. Only urban hospitals
   d. International healthcare facilities

Chapter 16: LaQshya—Labor Room Quality Improvement Initiative

4. **What is the primary reason for the LaQshya program's emphasis on timely referrals?**
   a. To increase the number of deliveries at private facilities
   b. To ensure complications are managed promptly and effectively, reducing adverse outcomes
   c. To promote hospital revenue
   d. To reduce transportation costs for patients

5. **Which of the following is *not* a component of the LaQshya initiative?**
   a. Infrastructure Upgradation
   b. Human Resource Strengthening
   c. Promotion of Homeopathy for childbirth
   d. Supply Chain Strengthening

6. **Which of the following activities is part of the process improvement under the LaQshya initiative?**
   a. Encouraging natural childbirth at home
   b. Strengthening referral systems and perioperative processes for C-sections
   c. Limiting the use of antibiotics in newborns
   d. Discontinuing the use of electronic records

7. **Which organization is *not* involved in the National Mentoring Group under the LaQshya initiative?**
   a. AIIMS
   b. World Health Organization (WHO)
   c. National Health Systems Resource Centre (NHSRC)
   d. National Institute of Health and Family Welfare (NIHFW)

8. **Which of the following is an objective of the LaQshya program?**
   a. Increase maternal and neonatal morbidity and mortality
   b. Enhance the standard of care provided during childbirth
   c. Promote unassisted childbirth
   d. Disregard feedback from healthcare personnel

9. **Which of the following measures is part of the quality assurance interventions under the LaQshya initiative?**
   a. Disregarding clinical guidelines
   b. Establishing quality circles and rapid improvement cycles
   c. Reducing healthcare personnel training
   c. Eliminating the use of digital tools

10. **Who are the primary beneficiaries of the LaQshya initiative?**
    a. Only newborns
    b. Only healthcare personnel
    c. Pregnant women, newborns, healthcare facilities, and healthcare personnel
    d. Only government officials

Answers

1. b	2. c	3. b	4. b	5. c
6. b	7. b	8. b	9. b	10. c

CHAPTER 17

Janani Suraksha Yojana

Pallavi Singh, Bharti Koria, Yash Shah

Background/Need of program	The Janani Suraksha Yojana is a government-backed program that was introduced in 2005 with the goal of lowering the rates of maternal and newborn death by encouraging hospital deliveries for pregnant women from low-income backgrounds, especially in areas with lower performance levels.
What is Janani Suraksha Yojana (JSY)?[1]	An initiative called the Janani Suraksha Yojana (JSY) was started in 2005 to encourage safe motherhood in India. The objective is to lower the death rates of mothers and babies by promoting the giving of birth in medical facilities among underprivileged women. Prenatal and postpartum care are provided, and pregnant women who fall below the federal poverty threshold can apply for financial help. From 65.5% in 2004–05 to 79.9% in 2015–16, the number of institutional deliveries in India has expanded dramatically due to the JSY.[2]
Vision of the JSY	The vision of the JSY is to provide free, safe, and quality institutional delivery services to all pregnant women in India. The scheme aims to achieve by: • Increasing the number of pregnant women who deliver their babies in health institutions. • Reducing maternal and infant mortality rates. • Improving the quality of maternal and child health services.
Features of Janani Suraksha Yojana	• Healthcare facilities provided by the Janani Suraksha Yojana are accessible across the entire country of India. States are categorized into two groups: Low Performing States (LPSs) and High Performing States (HPSs). This category is based on the rate of institutional delivery. • When implementing the JSY system, the progress of the states in the health sector is considered. The states of Uttar Pradesh, Uttarakhand, Bihar, Jharkhand, Madhya Pradesh, Chhattisgarh, Assam, Rajasthan, Orissa, and Jammu and Kashmir exhibit the lowest levels of performance. States that demonstrate exceptional performance include states other than the ones mentioned. • The Low Performing States category includes Uttar Pradesh, Uttarakhand, Madhya Pradesh, Chhattisgarh, Bihar, Jharkhand, Rajasthan, Odisha, Assam, and Jammu and Kashmir, all of which were previously part of the EAG states. • There are no limitations or constraints in place regarding the age of the mother, the number of children she has, or the specific sort of institution she chooses to give birth in, whether it is a public or permitted private health facility. • The JSY compensation is only available to pregnant women from BPL/SC/ST households in the High Performing States (HPS), when the rates of institutional delivery are sufficient. Furthermore, the initiative provides incentives to Accredited Social Health Activists (ASHAs) based on their success. • The program has established collaborations with private hospitals, nursing homes, and clinics to guarantee the provision of healthcare services to clients, even in areas without the required infrastructure. • About 7% of the money are allocated to the state, while an additional 4% is allocated to the district authorities. There is also a provision to pay administrative expenses. The fund is then utilized to cover the administrative expenses related to the implementation of the Janani Suraksha Yojana. • The program's recipients are required to enroll with the healthcare personnel at the sub-center, Anganwadi, or primary health clinics.
Objectives	The Indian Government has launched the Janani Suraksha Yojana under the National Health Mission with the below-mentioned objectives: • In order to promote the utilization of healthcare facilities for childbirth, especially among economically disadvantaged pregnant mothers, including those belonging to Scheduled Castes, Scheduled Tribes, and Below Poverty Line families.

Chapter 17: Janani Suraksha Yojana

	• The objective of this program is to reduce the number of deaths among mothers and newborns in India by ensuring that affordable and accessible institutional births are accessible to expectant mothers from poor backgrounds.
Eligibility of Janani Suraksha Yojana	Irrespective of the expectant mother's age, the number of previous births, or the health care facility being a government or an accredited private one, the benefits of the JSY scheme are provided.

Eligibility for cash assistance under the JSY scheme	
Category of States	*Eligibility*
Low performing states (LPS)	Pregnant women giving birth in a government health facility, including a subcenter, a primary care clinic, a community health center, a first referral unit, or a common ward of a state or district hospital.
High performing states (HPS)	Expectant mothers belonging to BPL/SC/ST communities who give birth in government health facilities like the SC/PHC/CHC/General wards of district and state hospitals.
Low performing and hHigh performing states	Pregnant women from BPL, SC, or ST communities giving birth in certified private healthcare facilities.

Target Groups of Janani Suraksha Yojana	The JSY is available to all pregnant women in India, irrespective of their income or social status. The scheme is particularly targeted at pregnant women who are 19 years or above from vulnerable groups, such as: • Women from low-income households • Women from rural areas • Women from tribal communities • Women with disabilities
Benefits of Janani Suraksha Yojana	• Pregnant women can avail the benefit of three antenatal visits and institutional delivery under the JSY program. Institutional delivery is connected with the payment of enhanced benefits and cash support. • ASHA-compliant workers also receive incentives. The program trains a number of traditional birth attendants referred to as "Dai." The delivery care systems then incorporate these workers. • Professional help is offered for C-section births. The government provides financial support of up to 1,500 per expectant mother to employ a private expert to execute the cesarean delivery in a healthcare facility in the absence of such government-employed medical professionals. • In accordance with the family welfare scheme, the beneficiary gets compensated if a tubectomy or laparoscopic procedure is suggested. • Every auxiliary nurse, midwife, or any other health worker is given a sum of 5,000 as part of the Janani Suraksha Yojana scheme, subject to a few terms and limitations.[3]
Cash Assistance to ASHA for Institutional Delivery	(see tables below)

Cash assistance provided for rural areas			
	Assistance provided		
State categorization	*Expectant mother*	*ASHA volunteer*	*Total*
High performing states	700	600	1300
Low performing states	1400	600	2000

Cash assistance provided for urban areas			
	Assistance provided		
State categorization	*Expectant mother*	*ASHA volunteer*	*Total*
High performing states	600	400	1000
Low performing states	1000	400	1400

PACS (Panchayats Adhyaksh Sahakari Samiti)	• Providing information about the scheme to pregnant women and their families. • Helping women to register for the scheme. • Assisting women in accessing institutional delivery services. • Monitoring the implementation of the scheme.

References

1. Janani Suraksha Yojana. Available at: https://www.pib.gov.in/PressReleasePage.aspx?PRID=1843841
2. National Health Mission
3. Gupta SK, Pal DK, Tiwari R, Garg R, Shrivastava AK, Sarawagi R, et al. Impact of Janani Suraksha Yojana on institutional delivery rate and maternal morbidity and mortality: an observational study in India. Journal of health, population, and nutrition. 2012;30(4):464.

QUESTIONS

Long Answer Question (LAQ)

1. What is the Janani Suraksha Yojana? What has been its impact? How can its coverage be improved?

Short Answer Questions (SAQs)

1. Describe the monetary benefits provided under JSY.
2. Enlist the beneficiaries of JSY.

Multiple Choice Question (MCQ)

1. **Janani Suraksha Yojana is:**
   a. 100% centrally sponsored scheme
   b. 100% state sponsored scheme
   c. 50% state, 50% central
   d. 70% state, 30% central

Answer

1. a

18 CHAPTER

Janani Shishu Suraksha Karyakram

Pallavi Singh, Rohit Katre, Bharti Koria

Background/Need of program/Scheme	On June 1st, 2011, the Indian government introduced the Janani Shishu Suraksha Karyakaram (JSSK). • Pregnant women who use government health facilities to give birth will benefit from the program. Additionally, it will encourage those who still decide to birth at home to switch to institutional delivery. • The program is now being implemented in all states and UTs. • Exorbitant out-of-pocket costs for medication, user fees, diagnostic testing, food, and C-sections that pregnant women and their families must pay when giving birth in an institution.
Initiative[1]	In order to provide free and cashless services to pregnant women, including normal deliveries and cesarean sections, as well as sick newborns (up to 30 days after birth) in government health institutions in both rural and urban areas, the Ministry of Health and Family Welfare (MoHFW) has launched a major initiative to reach an agreement among all states. The goal of this project is to alleviate the difficulties experienced by expectant mothers and parents of unwell infants, in addition to the substantial out-of-pocket costs associated with delivery and care.
Objective	The JSSK's aim is to remove the need for pregnant women and sick infants receiving treatment at public health institutions to pay out-of-pocket expenses.
Coverage	The JSSK encompasses all government health facilities in both rural and urban areas.
Extension	In 2014, the JSSK was broadened to include all complications during the antenatal and postnatal stages of pregnancy.[2]
Eligibility of pregnant woman	• The applicant must be a pregnant woman. • The applicant must be admitted in a government health facility.
Free entitlements for pregnant women	• Free and cashless delivery • Free C-section • Free drugs and consumables • Free diagnostics • Free diet during stay in the health institutions • Free provision of blood • Exemption from user charges • Free transport from home to health institutions • Free transport between facilities in case of referral • Free drop-back from institutions to home after 48 hours stay
Free entitlements for child	• Free treatment • Free drugs and consumables • Free diagnostics • Free provision of blood • Exemption from user charges • Free transport from home to health institutions • Free transport between facilities in case of referral • Free drop-back from institutions to home
Key features of the scheme	• The program provides free delivery services, including cesarean section, to all pregnant women who deliver in public health institutions. • The benefits include free medications and supplies, free nutrition for up to 3 days after a regular birth and 7 days after a C-section, free diagnostic services, and free blood if needed.

- This project provides free transportation for people from their home to the facility, between different locations if needed, and back home.
- All sick infants receiving care at public health facilities are eligible for the same advantages for up to 30 days after birth.
- The goal of the program is to eliminate the requirement for pregnant women and sick newborns to cover the cost of treatments provided at government healthcare facilities.
- The program is expected to benefit more than 12 million pregnant women who use government health facilities for giving birth.
- Moreover, it will encourage individuals who currently choose homebirths to opt for hospital deliveries instead.
- All the States and union territories have begun implementing the system.

References

1. Janani Suraksha Yojana. Available at: https://www.pib.gov.in/PressReleasePage.aspx?PRID=1843841
2. National Health Mission

QUESTIONS

Long Answer Question (LAQ)

1. Critically analyze the Janani Shishu Suraksha Karyakram.

Short Answer Questions (SAQs)

1. Describe monetary benefits provided under JSSK.
2. Enlist free services under JSSK.

Multiple Choice Questions (MCQs)

1. Consider the following statements regarding Janani Shishu Suraksha Karyakram (JSSK):
   1. The scheme entitles all pregnant women delivering in public health institutions to an absolutely free and no expense delivery except C-section.
   2. Entitlements include free drugs and consumables, etc., for mother as well as sick newborn till 30 days after birth. Which of the above statement(s) is/are correct?
   a. Only 1   b. Only 2
   c. Both   d. None
2. The entitlements consist of complementary medications and consumables, complimentary nutrition for a maximum of .... with a regular birth.
   a. 5   b. 3
   c. 7   d. 21

Answers

1. c   2. b

CHAPTER 19

Pradhan Mantri Surakshit Matritva Abhiyan

Mahendra Singh, Shaili Vyas, Pallavi Singh

Background/ Need of program/ Scheme	India's pursuit of the Sustainable Development Goals (SDGs) and its emphasis on the post 2015 era highlight urgent need to reduce maternal mortality. Each pregnancy is precious, and each expectant mother deserves specialized care. India has made strides in lowering maternal and newborn mortality, yet every year some 44,000 Indian women still pass away from pregnancy-related reasons. It is possible to avert a significant number of these deaths by giving pregnant women excellent care.
Implemented since	The Ministry of Health and Family Welfare (MoHFW), Government of India, started the Pradhan Mantri Surakshit Matritva Abhiyan on June 9, 2016.[1]
Goal/Vision	To enhance the quality and accessibility of Antenatal Care (ANC) including diagnostics and counselling services, as an integral part of the RMNCH+A strategy
Targets	To reach all the pregnant women in 2nd and 3rd trimesters.

Objectives[1]	• Ensure that all the pregnant women in 2nd and 3rd trimesters receive at least one antenatal check up by a physician/specialist.
	• To improve the quality care during antenatal visits, by provision of following services:
	  ✦ To provide all relevant diagnostic services
	  ✦ Screen for applicable clinical conditions
	  ✦ Management of existing clinical conditions appropriately, such as anemia, pregnancy induced hypertension and gestational diabetes
	  ✦ Offer appropriate counselling services and ensure proper documentation of rendered services.
	  ✦ Extend additional service opportunities to pregnant women who have missed antenatal visits.
	• Identifying and line listing of high-risk pregnancies based on existing clinical conditions and obstetric/medical history.
	• Ensure that each pregnant women receives appropriate birth planning and is prepared for potential complications, particularly those identified with risk factors or comorbid conditions.
	• Special emphasis on women with malnutrition by providing adequate, appropriate management and early diagnosis.
	• Special attention to adolescent and early pregnancies as they require additional and specialized care.

Organogram	• Planning for implementation of PMSMA
	  ✦ Planning and execution committees have been established at national, state and district levels.
	  ✦ Facilities/clinics (both public and private sectors) have been identified and mapping was done for implementation of PMSMA
	  ✦ Behavior change communication (BCC) and information, education, communication (IEC) for raising awareness among beneficiaries and service providers must conduct to implement PMSMA.
	  ✦ Logistic requirements are estimated.
	  ✦ Capacity of healthcare providers regarding the service package has been enhanced during PMSMA.
	  ✦ Budget has been allocated.
	• PMSMA has been implemented in public health facilities. On the ninth of every month, OBGY specialists, radiologists, and physicians will deliver a minimum package of antenatal care services to women who are in their second or third trimesters of pregnancy. Private sector doctors will provide support to augment the government sector's efforts. Especially private practitioners/private hospital has been motivated to volunteer for this campaign. State and district authorities will encourage obstetricians/physicians from private sector to provide voluntary services at designated public health facilities. States will take special

	efforts to ensure that enough service providers should be available in the high priority districts. They can also draw on support from donor partners for this activity.
	● Service provider's roles and responsibilities have been defined.
	● Things should be followed at PMSMA site on PMSMA day:
	  ✦ Examination room, waiting area, laboratory area should be properly labelled, etc.
	  ✦ Pregnancy-related eating, drinking water, and restroom arrangements should also be made.
	  ✦ To prevent nosocomial infections, facilities should be kept clean and well-maintained, and infection prevention procedures should be adhered to.
	  ✦ While they wait to visit a doctor, groups of pregnant women can receive counseling on nutrition, rest, and warning signals, breastfeeding, family planning, etc.

Beneficiaries	All pregnant women
Components	● Thorough evaluation of clinical history, physical examination and routine investigations. ● Intervention in the form of prevention, prophylaxis and treatment. ● Promoting health education/counselling and health dissemination.
Strategies/ Deliverables under the program	● Routine antenatal check-up ● Providing relevant diagnostic services ● Identifying and managing high-risk pregnancies ● Counselling on birth preparedness, newborn care, nutrition, postnatal care and family planning
Activities at various level or package of services	● Primary prevention: Screening for gestational diabetes, pregnancy-induced hypertension, anemia, asymptomatic bacteriuria and viral markers (HbsAg, HIV, VDRL). ● Providing iron and folic acid supplementation. Counselling on nutrition and institutional delivery. ● Secondary prevention: Treatment for gestational diabetes and hypertension and anemia. Consultation with specialists like obstetricians and physicians. ● Tertiary prevention: Timely referral services
Monitoring and evaluation of program	● States were required to actively monitor the program rollout for the first six months. State government's assigned one state-level monitor to each district worked with RMNCH+A partners. ● During the initial 3 months, national level monitors were designated to visit districts, ensuring program readiness and effective implementation. ● District monitors will arrive on the 8th day of each month to supervise district preparations, followed by visits to 4-5 PHCs on the 9th day to oversee implementation. ● ASHAs (Accredited Social Health Activists) will maintain beneficiary line list for PMSMA service utilization. ● Services provided during PMSMA should be accurately reported. ● Conduct analysis of services delivered during PMSMA.
Achievement under PMSMA till now	*Component*	**Numbers**
	Volunteer registered	6813
	No. of facilities providing PMSMA services	20,752
	Total Pregnant Women Examined Under PMSMA Scheme	47,346,865
	Top 5 states (In terms of Volunteer Registered till June 2024)	
	1. Maharashtra	1065
	2. Uttar Pradesh	1016
	3. Rajasthan	981
	4. Madhya Pradesh	880
	5. Karnataka	571
	Top 5 states [In terms of no. of pregnant women (in 2nd and 3rd trimesters) received ANC under PMSMA for June 2024]	
	1. Uttar Pradesh	167,769
	2. Bihar	33,304
	3. Andhra Pradesh	27,649
	4. Madhya Pradesh	26,547
	5. West Bengal	21,183

Reference

1. Pradhan Mantri Surakshit Matritva Abhiyan. PMSMA. Mohfw.GOI. https://pmsma.mohfw.gov.in/

QUESTIONS

Long Answer Question (LAQ)

1. Describe goal, objectives, and components of Pradhan Mantri Surakshit Matritva Abhiyan in detail.

Short Answer Question (SAQ)

1. Enlist the key features of Pradhan Mantri Surakshit Matritva Abhiyan (PMSMA).

Multiple Choice Questions (MCQs)

1. Pradhan Mantri Surakshit Matritva Abhiyan (PMSMA) has been launched to improve quality of:
   a. Antenatal care
   b. Postnatal care
   b. Intrapartum care
   c. Newborn care
2. Beneficiaries of Pradhan Mantri Surakshit Matritva Abhiyan (PMSMA) is:
   a. Pregnant women
   c Both
   b. Lactating mother
   d Women of all age group

Answers

1. a   2. a

CHAPTER 20

Pradhan Mantri Matru Vandana Yojana

Shaili Vyas, Pallavi Singh, Parul Sharma, Ganesh Lokhande

Background/ Need of program/ Scheme	Poor nutrition is a widespread issue among Indian women, with one in three being undernourished and one in two suffering from anemia. A malnourished mother is more likely to give birth to a low-birth-weight child. Malnutrition begins in the womb and can cause irreversible changes that last a lifetime. Economic and social pressure often force women to work until the end of their pregnancy to support their families. Despite their physical limitations, many return to work soon after childbirth, which hinders their recovery and makes it difficult for them to breastfeed their newborns for the first six months exclusively.
Implemented since	The Pradhan Mantri Matru Vandana Yojana was implemented nationwide on 01.01.2017. Norms of PMMVY 2.0 under Mission Shakti were implemented from 01.04.2022.
Goal	The goal of the Pradhan Mantri Matru Vandana Yojana (PMMVY) is to improve the health and nutrition of pregnant and lactating women, promote proper rest, encourage institutional deliveries, and support exclusive breastfeeding for the first six months of a child's life by providing partial wage compensation for wage loss during childbirth and childcare. PMMVY seeks to reduce maternal and infant mortality rates and contribute to the well-being of mothers and their newborns.[1]
Targets	The targets of the Pradhan Mantri Matru Vandana Yojana (PMMVY) include: • **Improve maternal health:** Enhance the health and nutrition of pregnant and lactating women by providing financial support during pregnancy and after childbirth. • **Promote institutional deliveries:** Encourage pregnant women to opt for institutional deliveries. • **Support exclusive breastfeeding:** Promote exclusive breastfeeding for the first six months of a child's life by enabling mothers to rest well and care for their newborns. • **Reduce maternal and infant mortality:** Proper care during pregnancy and after delivery, contribute to the reduction of maternal and infant mortality rate. • **Financial assistance for wage loss:** Provide partial wage compensation to pregnant and lactating women during the critical period of pregnancy and early motherhood. • **Promote early registration of pregnancy:** To ensure, that women receive timely antenatal care and health services. • **Enhance nutritional status:** Improve the nutritional status of pregnant and lactating women, reducing the prevalence of malnutrition and anemia among them. • **Raise awareness:** Increase awareness about the importance of nutrition and rest during pregnancy and lactation, and promote healthy practices among women and their families. • **Support first-time mothers:** Focus on providing benefits to first-time mothers, ensuring they receive the necessary financial and healthcare support during their first pregnancy.
Objectives	• Providing partial compensation for the wage loss in terms of monetary incentives so that the mother can take rest well before and after delivery. • The cash incentive provided to the pregnant and lactating mother would lead to improved health-seeking behavior. • To encourage positive girl-child behavior, the initiative offers a financial incentive for the second girl child.
Beneficiaries	The program is available to all pregnant or breastfeeding women, except for those who are full-time employees of the central government, a state government, a public sector undertaking (PSU), or who receive similar benefits under any existing law. PMMVY provides benefits to pregnant and lactating Anganwadi Workers (AWWs), Anganwadi Helpers (AWHs), and Accredited Social Health Activists (ASHAs), provided they meet the scheme's eligibility criteria and conditions.[2]

Chapter 20: Pradhan Mantri Matru Vandana Yojana

	Stillbirth or Miscarriage: In case of abortion/stillbirth, the beneficiary would be treated as a fresh beneficiary in future pregnancy.
Package of services	**Conditionalities and Instalments** • PW&LM will receive a cash benefit of ₹ 5000 in two instalments at the phases listed in the table below:

Instalments	Conditions	Amount
First Instalments	• Women must register for pregnancy and get an antenatal checkup within 6 months of the LMP at the Anganwadi center (AWC) or recognized health facilities identified by the administering state/UT	₹ 3000/-
Second Instalments	• Registration of childbirth • Child has completed first cycle of immunization (14 weeks)	₹ 2000/-

	• The benefit under PMMVY is available to a beneficiary for the first two living children provided the second child is a girl. • If a mother gives birth to more than one baby (twins/triplet/quadruplet) during the second pregnancy and if one or more than one baby is a girl child then the mother is eligible for receiving ₹ 6000. However, registration during pregnancy is mandatory for availing benefits for a second child. This would contribute to improving the Sex Ratio at Birth and to prevent female feticide. • Benefits can be availed based on the Aadhaar Number of the Beneficiary to avoid any duplication or malpractices. • The amount under PMMVY will be transferred directly to the beneficiaries Bank/Post Office account by Direct Benefit Transfer Mode. • Any additional incentives from other schemes, such as the Janani Suraksha Yojana (JSY), will be available. Eligible beneficiaries will also receive prescribed cash incentives for maternity benefits under JSY following institutional births. **Anyone of the following eligibility criteria is required to avail the benefit of PMMVY:[3]** • Women with annual family incomes <₹ 8 Lakh • Women from scheduled castes and tribes • Women with 40% or more disability (Divyang Jan) • Women with BPL ration cards • Ayushman Bharat beneficiaries under PMJAY • Women with E-shram cards. • Kisan Samman Nidhi—women farmer beneficiaries • Female MGNREGA Job Card Holders • Pregnant and lactating AWW/AWH/ASHA • Any other category as may be prescribed by the central government **Newer initiatives** • Self-registration by the citizen through the PMMVY portal and the mobile app has been introduced. • A mobile app has been introduced for Anganwadi workers/ASHA workers as well as for individual beneficiaries.
Monitoring and evaluation of the program	PMMVY is implemented using web-based MIS Software, PMMVY CAS for regular monitoring of the scheme.

References

1. Pradhan Mantri Matru Vandana Yojana (PMMVY). UMANG. Ministry of Electronics and Information Technology. Available at https://web.umang.gov.in/landing/department/pmmvy.html
2. Pradhan Mantri Matru Vandana Yojana (PMMVY). Ministry of Women and Child Development. Available at https://pmmvy.wcd.gov.in
3. https://wcd.nic.in/sites/default/files/FINAL%20PMMVY%20%28FAQ%29%20BOOKELT.pdf

QUESTIONS

Long Answer Question (LAQ)

1. Discuss in detail package of services provided under Pradhan Mantri Matru Vandana Yojana.

Short Answer Questions (SAQs)

1. When was PMMVY launched? Enlist activities under it.
2. Eligibility criteria for PMMVY.

Multiple Choice Questions (MCQs)

1. The Pradhan Mantri Matru Vandana Yojana comes under which Ministry?
    a. Ministry of Home Affairs
    b. Ministry of Women and Child Development
    c. Ministry of Health
    d. None of the above
2. Which one of the following statements is true regarding the Pradhan Mantri Matru Vandana Yojana?
    a. PMMVY provides financial assistance to pregnant women for the first two live births if second baby is girl child.
    b. PMMVY applies only to pregnant women in urban area.
    c. PMMVY provides one time installment of ₹ 6000 to pregnant and lactating mothers if second baby is girl child
    d. PMMVY is solely aims to provide medical treatment during pregnancy
3. Pradhan Mantri Matru Vandana Yojna was launched in year:
    a. 2014
    b. 2015
    c. 2016
    a. 2017
4. In PMMVY when does beneficiary receives first payment (installment) as per guidelines of scheme?
    a. After birth of the child
    b. After completing first checkup of beneficiary
    c. After registration process is complete and first antenatal checkup within 6 months of LMP
    d. After receiving 1st Tetanus Toxoid vaccine
5. Main objective of Pradhan Mantri Matru Vandana Yojana is:
    a. Provides a partial wage compensation to women for wages loss during child birth and child care
    b. Promote health seeking behavior in pregnant women
    c. Improve the nutritional status of pregnant and lactating women
    d. All of the above
6. All of the following are beneficiaries of PMMVY, *except*:
    a. Women with BPL ration card
    b. Women with annual family income <10 lakh
    c. Pregnant and lactating AWW/AWH/ASHA
    d. Women with 40% or more disability

Answers

1. a
2. a
3. d
4. c
5. d
6. b

CHAPTER 21

Surakshit Matritva Aashwasan (Suman)

Shaili Vyas, Pallavi Singh, Sadhna Singh, Parul Sharma

Background/Need of program/Scheme	People who go to public health facilities (PHFs) still have trouble getting all the care they need during pregnancy and childbirth. This is why it's important to come up with a good policy that not only encourages safe birth and respectful maternity care, but also turns rights into a service promise, which is more meaningful for the people who benefit from it. So, GOI decided to write a policy framework to expand maternal health care, including delivery, beyond women's rights to a guaranteed service delivery. This includes more women having access to free, high-quality care services, making sure that women are never turned away from services, and making sure that complications are managed in a way that respects their autonomy, dignity, feelings, choices, and preferences, among other things. All of these can also be used to care for a baby.
Implemented since	The Ministry of Health and Family Welfare started Surakshit Matritva Aashwasan (SUMAN) on October 10, 2019, with the goal of making sure that every woman and newborn gets assured, respectful, high-quality healthcare at no cost, and with no room for denial of services.
Goal	To end all preventable maternal and newborn deaths.[1]
Objectives	<ul><li>To provide high quality medical, surgical and emergency care services in a dignified and respectful manner as per SUMAN service package at no cost to the beneficiaries.</li><li>To leverage institutional and community-based platforms to help create awareness in the community on the entitlements under SUMAN.</li><li>To strengthen Grievance Redressal Mechanism by incorporating client feedback.</li><li>To orient service providers and build their capacity for delivering SUMAN package</li><li>To ensure reporting and review of all maternal and infant deaths.</li></ul>
Organogram	Under RMNCHA+N
Beneficiaries	<ul><li>Women who are pregnant</li><li>All women for six months after giving birth</li><li>Sick babies</li></ul>
Components	**SUMAN initiative**<ul><li>Free care before, during, and after birth</li><li>Free care for babies and young children who are sick</li><li>Secured birth plan for women who are at high risk</li><li>Making sure that high standards are met at all delivery points</li></ul>**Broad pillars of the initiative**<ul><li>**Service guarantee:** JSSK, JSY, PMSMA, LaQshya, MAA, care for sick and small babies, home-based care for mothers and newborn</li><li>**Health system strengthening:** Infrastructure: OT, NBCC, NBSU, SNCU, LDR, Human resources, drugs and diagnostics, referral systems, and establishing centers of excellence.</li><li>**Monitoring and reporting:** Service guarantee charter, grievance resolution (help desk or call center level), Getting feedback from clients.</li><li>**Community awareness:** VHSNC and SHGs are part of SUMAN Volunteer (the best volunteer can be an SUMAN winner).</li></ul>

	• **Incentives and awards:** Honors and awards for Performers
	   ✦ ₹ 1000 will be given to the first person who reports a mother's death.
	   ✦ Identifying and honoring winners
	• **IEC/BCC:** Mega IEC/BCC efforts to support "zero preventable deaths of mothers and babies".
	As part of the SUMAN initiative, all pregnant women and newborns who go to public health centers can get a set of free services. However, because not all facilities can offer all services, each health facility must inform the service guarantee package of their current resources and service availability, along with the steps they are taking to meet all 100% of the expected service standards for their level. There are three types of SUMAN packages: Basic, BemONC, and CemONC. These cover services for both mothers and babies.
	SUMAN service guarantee packages
	1. SUMAN Basic package (HWC-SC/HWC-PHC/PHC/UPHC)
	2. SUMAN BEmONC package (Non-FRU CHC/UCHC/HWC-PHC/other hospitals)
	3. SUMAN CEmONC package (medical college/DH/SDH/CHC-FRU/UCHC)

Activities at various level or package of services[2]	**SUMAN Service Guarantee Packages:** Essential package (to be provided at all level) • Community awareness and participation • Services for family planning, counseling, and pregnancy tests • Clean health centers with water, toilets, and other cleanliness and sanitation measures • Respectful maternity care, such as a birth companion and the freedom to choose how to give birth • Counseling for early initiation of breastfeeding and exclusive breastfeeding. Lactation support at PHF support at community. • Counseling and IEC/BCC for safe motherhood and newborn care • Service delivery by trained personnel (including Midwifery/SBA/NSSK) • Free and zero out of pocket expense services • Conditional cash transfer—JSY PMMVY or any other State scheme. • Safe motherhood booklet, MCP card. **SUMAN Service Guarantee-Basic** *Maternal* • Routine ANC (4+ one PMSMA) • PNC • Finding and treating simple complications • Managing breast problems • Finding, managing, and referring high-risk pregnancies • Skilled Birth Attendants (only in subcenters marked as delivery points) • Pre-referral care for obstetric situations like shock, eclampsia, and pre-eclampsia *Newborn* • Newborn care, including cardiopulmonary resuscitation (NCC) • Birth dose vaccination • Recognizing "at risk" or "sick" newborns and referring them to the hospital immediately • Management of neonatal sepsis • Diarrhea and pneumonia services for babies at the community level *Family Planning* • Providing condoms, over-the counter birth control, and pregnancy test kits • Referring the patients for safe abortions • Offering confidential counselling to patients • Follow-up for any problems that may arise after an abortion and the right referrals **SUMAN Service Guarantee- BEmONC** ALL in basic package + *Maternal* • Vaginal births with assistance • Treatment of minor complications • If necessary, referral after the primary management • Episiotomy and suturing • Keep obstetric emergencies stable and make sure they are sent to CEmONC centers • Postnatal care for mothers that includes a stay of 48 hours

Newborn
- Preterm or PROM antibiotics to prevent babies from getting sepsis
- Non-FRU CHC newborn stabilization units
- Identification and Treatment of LBW Infants >1800 g without any additional complications
- Neonatal phototherapy
- Referral and stabilization of sick and VLBW infants
- Management of a sick neonate at the facility level
- KMC and breastfeeding (expressed)

Family Planning
- Sterilization services (if available)
- PHCs—Comprehensive Abortion Care (CAC) services (including counseling and contraception) for Medical Methods of Abortion (MMA)
- Manual Vacuum Aspiration (MVA) and MMA are available at CHCs under the MTP Act, depending on the availability of trained providers.

SUMAN Service Guarantee-CEmONC

All in BEmONC Package, plus the followings:

Maternal
- Provision of services to prevent the transmission of HIV and syphilis from mother to child, as well as early diagnosis of these infections in infants.
- ART linked to DH.
- Delivery of HIV-positive female patients.
- Signal functions are included in CEmONC services.
- A complete approach to the management of all obstetric emergencies, such as PIH/eclampsia, sepsis, PPH, retained placenta, hypotension, obstructed labor, and severe anemia
- Cesarean section and other surgical operations
- Cross-matching and blood groups done at blood bank or storage center.

Newborn
- SNCU at DH or medical college
- At the SNCU level, the management of LBW neonates
- Managing all ill neonates (excluding those requiring artificial ventilation or extensive surgery)
- Newborn sepsis management
- Sick infant stabilization and level III referral
- Monitor the progress of all infants.

Family Planning
- The MTP Act allows medical and surgical abortions up to 20 weeks.
- Management of incomplete/spontaneous abortions
- Management of any complications that arise following an abortion (subject to the availability of trained providers in the facility)

Grievance Redressal Mechanism
- Under SUMAN, the current 104 GR Mechanism and health helpline will be integrated.
- All 'urgent' issues should be resolved within 24 hours.
- If a facility is unable to resolve a dispute within 7 days, it will be referred to the District/State level.
- Summary of complaints to be brought to the SUMAN committees

Quality Assurance under Suman
- Once SUMAN CEmONC facilities are notified, they must get either full NQAS certification or part NQAS certification from the areas where SUMAN services are being provided.
- SUMAN—compliant HWC—subcenters must meet NQAS minimum criteria.
- All SUMAN—notified facilities should aim for state—level NQAS certification and national—level NQAS certification within six months.

Key Focus Areas for a SUMAN Compliant Facility to Achieve NQAS Certification
- Guaranteed Service Provision in accordance with the scope of service (Basic/BEmONC CEmONC)
- High-Quality care with dignity and respect
- There are no financial barriers to getting services
- Safe, clean, and hygienic facility offering diet options
- The SOP—defined processes are put into practice
- Facility measures, monitors, and uses data for improvement and change sustainability
- A targeted strategy for the enhancement of clinical care processes

	• Referral linkages are clearly defined in both directions • Effective grievance resolution **SUMAN volunteer** Link between the health system and the community to enable the beneficiaries to avail entitlements under various GOI scheme. **Registration and capacity building of volunteers:** STATES/DISTRICT organize half day orientation program for the registered volunteers. Every anganwadi center, sub-centers, HWC and PHC • Conduct a drive to register volunteers • Maintain the village-wise list of volunteers in their area • Display the names of registered volunteers • Share the information with pregnant women and their families • Best performing volunteer can be a SUMAN champion and motivate others.
Monitoring and evaluation of program[2]	SUMAN's National, State, and District Committees are mostly in charge of keeping an eye on and helping to oversee the program. The national and state program divisions must also keep an eye on how the program is being carried out and any problems that come up. They must also help close any gaps in coverage by providing money through their yearly program implementation plans. Under the National Health Mission, different ways of keeping an eye on things have already been set up. These tools should be used to keep an eye on the program, such as: Rogi Kalyan Samiti (RKS) can be very helpful in keeping an eye on how well the health facilities are following the service guarantee charters. These groups can think about and talk about what kind of help the buildings need. Some tools that are already out there are • VHSNC/MAS • Gram/block/Zila Panchayat • Urban local bodies • RKS/DHS/SHS

References

1. SUMAN. Mohfw.GOI. NHP. Available at ttps://suman.mohfw.gov.in
2. Overview of SUMAN initiative. NHSRC. Available on: https://qps.nhsrcindia.org/sites/default/files/2022-01/Overview%20of%20SUMAN.pdf

QUESTIONS

Long Answer Question (LAQ)

1. Given the existing schemes such as JSSK/ PMMVY, justify the rationale behind the need of SUMAN.

Short Answer Questions (SAQs)

1. What is the goal of SUMAN? Ensure the objective to accomplish the goal.
2. Who are SUMAN Champions? What are their roles to accomplish the goal of SUMAN?
3. What are four pillars of SUMAN initiative?
4. Who are the beneficiaries of SUMAN? What are the benefits provided to them?

Chapter 21: Surakshit Matritva Aashwasan (Suman)

Multiple Choice Questions (MCQs)

1. **SUMAN is:**
   a. National Health Program
   b. State Level program
   c. National Scheme/Policy
   d. State Level Scheme/Policy
2. **Component of SUMAN are:**
   a. Free care before delivery and after delivery
   b. Free care for babies and young children
   c. Secured birth plan for women
   d. All of the above
3. **SUMAN is under the:**
   a. MoWCH
   b. MoWCD
   c. MoHFW
   d. ICDS
4. **SUMAN volunteers can be:**
   a. PRI representative
   b. SHG members
   c. School teacher
   d. All of the above

Answers

1. c
2. d
3. c
4. d

CHAPTER 22

Dakshata

Sanjeet Panesar, Shaili Vyas, Pallavi Singh

Background/Need of program/Scheme	Despite efforts by the country to reduce maternal and newborn mortality, the decline observed in Maternal mortality and newborn mortality is lesser than the expected, Hence, to improve the quality of care for maternal and newborn survival at the time of childbirth, Dakshata initiative was launched.
Implemented since	The program was launched on 30th April 2015, by the Government of India as a nation-wide initiative in a phasic manner, to empower the health workforce to impart high quality of care during intra, immediate and postpartum period.[1]
Goal	To improve the quality of maternal and newborn care during the intra- and immediate postpartum period, through providers who are competent and confident.
Targets	The target of Dakshata training is to improve the quality of care for women and newborns during the peripartum period
Objectives	• To strengthen the **competency of providers** of the labor room, including medical officers, staff nurses, and ANMs to perform evidence-based practices as per the established labor room protocols and standards • To implement **enabling strategies to ensure transfer of learning** towards improved adherence to evidence-based clinical practices • To improve the availability of **essential supplies and commodities** in the labor room and the postpartum wards • To improve accountability of service providers through improved **recording, reporting and utilization of data** • **Intermediate term objective:** Implementation of the MNH Tool kit at the delivery points, in a phased manner.[1]
Beneficiaries	Healthcare providers, including medical officers, staff nurses, and ANMs, who work in labor rooms
Components	• Availability of sufficient number of clinically competent health care providers, having an updated knowledge and clinical skills • Availability of essential commodities, supplies and equipment • Strong clinical mentorship and leadership • A comprehensive recording, reporting, analysis and utilization of data to ensure 360 degree accountability of all stakeholders.
Strategies/Deliverables under the program	**Strategies at time of admission** • Use of Safe Childbirth Checklist to improve quality of care • Triaging of the expectant mother based on history, examination and accordingly taking decision for level of care requirement. • Staying prepared for taking Immediate actions to prevent major complications in the mother • Prevention, identification and management of pre-eclampsia and eclampsia among the mothers • Plotting and monitoring the partograph to observe progress of labor • Timely identification and management of prolonged and obstructed labor by standard protocols • Empowerment of birth companions for participation in care of the mother and the baby

	Strategies just before, during and after delivery • Preparing the site for safe delivery • Conducting normal delivery and active management of third stage of labor • Following the principles of essential newborn care (ENBC) • Prevention, identification and management of postpartum hemorrhage (PPH) • Care of mother and newborn, during as well as immediately after birth • Prevention, identification and management of newborn infections • Provision of special and comprehensive care for pre-term and LBW babies **Strategies at the time of discharge** • Preparation for managing postpartum complications in mothers • Providing discharge counselling about danger signs for mother and baby and for the beneficiaries seeking care • Provision of imparting postpartum family planning counseling
Activities at various level or package of services	• Organizing a Sensitization Workshop for district and facility level officials on Dakshata program • Identification and mapping of target facilities simultaneously with assessment of resource availability • Hiring of quality improvement mentor • Rapid assessment of resource availability and practices status • Ensuring availability of essential supplies and other resources • Providing 5 days training of trainers and quality improvement mentor • Preparation of training micro-plan for each facility • Providing 3 days on-site training of labor room staff at district hospital • Post-training follow-up and support to district hospitals • Providing 3 days training of staff from sub-district level facilities at DH • Post-training follow-up and support to SDL facilities by trainers and mentors • Implementation of data recording tools and dashboard indicators
Monitoring and evaluation of program	• **Program management monitoring:** To be done by supervisors, development partners, and other supervisory cadre workers using the GoI's supportive supervision checklist. • **Clinical monitoring by the mentors:** All the trainers and mentors will monitor and report the adherence to quality of care practices at the target institutions apart from providing post-training follow-up and support. • **Dashboard of indicators:** Facilities participating under the program will send monthly reports to districts and districts will send monthly reports to the states for inclusion into the dashboard of indicators.

Reference

1. Dakshata Initiative. Available at: https://nhmmp.gov.in/WebContent/MH/Schemes/Dakshata/Activity%20Report%20Final%20(Sep-15).pdf

QUESTIONS

Long Answer Question (LAQ)

1. Mention the goal and objectives of the Dakshata Initiative. Enumerate and explain the various strategies at various levels in the "Dakshata Initiative".

Short Answer Questions (SAQs)

1. Mention about the monitoring of Dakshata Initiative.
2. Enumerate the various components of Dakshata Initiative and explain in brief the rationale behind these components.

Multiple Choice Questions (MCQs)

1. Among the listed options which is *Not* the beneficiary under the Dakshata Initiative:
   a. Low-risk pregnancies
   b. Mothers before onset of labor
   c. Mothers just before and during childbirth (C-section)
   d. Immediate postpartum (1 hour) mothers and newborn
2. Among the listed options which is/are *Not* correct for monitoring under the Dakshata Initiative (combination answer type):
   a. Program management monitoring shall be done by development partners.
   b. Program management monitoring shall be done by mentors.
   c. Clinical monitoring shall be done by all trainers.
   d. Clinical monitoring shall be done by all beneficiaries.
   Correct answer:
   1. Option a & b only
   2. Option c & d only
   3. Option a & c only
   4. Option b & d only
3. Among the listed options regarding components of Dakshata initiative, which statement is *Not* correct:
   a. Availability of sufficient number of clinically competent health care providers, having an updated knowledge and clinical skills
   b. Availability of essential commodities, supplies and equipment
   c. Strong clinical mentorship and leadership
   d. A comprehensive recording, reporting, analysis and utilization of data to ensure 360 degree accountability of all beneficiaries.

Answers

1. a   2. d   3. d

23 CHAPTER

Maternal and Child Death Surveillance and Response (MDSR)

Medhavi Agarwal, Shaili Vyas, Bharti Koria

Background/Need of program/Scheme	Maternal Death Surveillance and Response (MDSR) is a continuous cycle of identification, notification and review of maternal deaths followed by actions to improve quality of care and prevent future deaths. In the last 7 years, among states regarding the Maternal Death Review process there was varying degree of reporting, review, and action planning and it was found that following gaps were present: • Maternal deaths in India get under reported under the health management information systems.[1] • The institutional mechanisms for reviews have been established, the capacity to undertake quality review at various levels are weak[1] • The translation of key findings into action, in other words the 'mechanism for response' lagged.[1] The guideline also has laid down precise mechanisms for review of deaths of migrant population. Current guidelines have used ICD-10 instead of ICD-9 for classification of maternal deaths.[1] Most importantly, the guidelines reiterate that based on the findings of the maternal death reviews, no disciplinary action is to be initiated against any of the service providers. The key principle to be adopted during the entire process of reviewing is not to blame or find fault with anybody.
Implemented since	Implemented since 2010 and revised in 2017
Objectives	The objectives of the guidelines are: • To strengthen the mechanisms and processes for MDSR • To institute a system of conducting confidential review into maternal deaths
Activities at various level	The first and foremost step of the Maternal Death Review process is preparing a line list of all the maternal deaths in the area following which facility and/or community based maternal death reviews are to undertake. Currently approximately 50% of the estimated maternal deaths across the country are being reported by states/UTs. Improving the surveillance and reporting of maternal deaths is thus critical. State level MDSR Committees must take the following key steps to improve the same: **Monitor whether maternal deaths are being reported:** • By all high delivery facilities (facilities conducting more than 1000 deliveries/year). • Monitor the district-wise number of deaths reported against estimated - identify the number of districts that have zero/poor reporting and focus on improving reporting from these districts. • Analysis of reported maternal death data indicates that approximately 20% of the maternal deaths occur at medical colleges and approximately 15% occur at private hospitals. This would obviously differ across States • Analysis of available data also highlights that approximately 20% of the maternal deaths could happen during transit. States must thus monitor the number of deaths occurring during transit and the mechanism for reporting of deaths occurring during transits (both for private and government vehicles). • Identify areas of high home delivery and monitor whether maternal deaths are being reported from these areas.

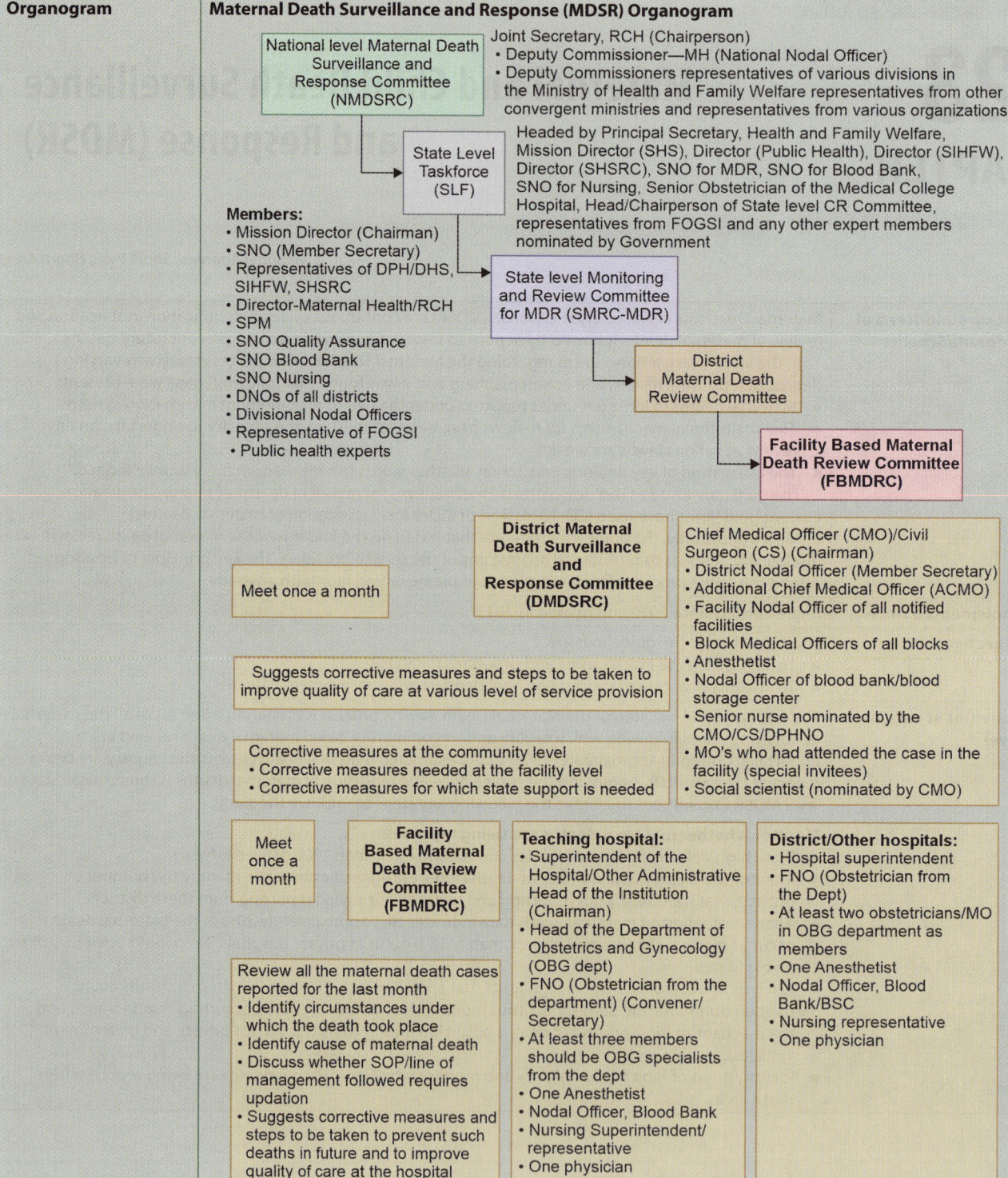

Chapter 23: Maternal and Child Death Surveillance and Response (MDSR)

Community-based MDSR (CBMDSR)	Community Based MDSR is a method of identifying personal, family or community factors that may have contributed to the death by interviewing people such as family members or neighbors who are close to the person and know about the events leading to the death

Steps for Community Based MDSR
A. Notification of maternal death
B. Investigation
C. Data transmission
D. Analysis
E. Review

A. Notification of maternal death

⭐ within 24 hours of death

All deaths of women in the age group of 15 to 49 years irrespective of the cause, i.e. maternal or non-maternal will be notified

⭐ Incentive of ₹ 200

- Primary informant
- Village/coverage area-ASHA
- Urban area-urban ASHA/Link worker

By the primary informant to the ANM and Block Medical Officer/Health Officer-Incharge of a zonal area/equivalent (for urban areas).

- Reporting: ASHA/primary informant will report the death to ANM by filling up the format for all such daths

ANM will counter sign the format before onward submission to BMO office within first week of receiving death information

In-transit death: Deaths occurring during pregnancy or in post-natal period (within 42 days) in ambulance/any recognized patient transport system will be reported by ambulance technician to the DNO

The DNO will further inform the respective BMO for conducting community based investigation. In case the woman has been referred from a facility and dies during transit, facility based review must be conducted at the facility from where the woman was referred as well. In case the woman is a migrant, report will go to respective DNO/SNO

B. Investigation
✦ All the maternal deaths will be investigated using Verbal Autopsy Format within three weeks of reporting maternal death. ASHA or AWW/ANM should ensure the availability of the respondents during the visit of the investigation team and also facilitate the interview process.[2]
✦ *Incentive:* Each member of investigation team is entitled to an incentive of ₹ 150 for conducting the verbal autopsy and a sum of ₹ 200 is available for transport support for the team.
The BMO is overall responsible for the MDSR process at the block. BMO must report all suspected maternal deaths as reported by primary informant to the DNO by telephone within 24 hours of receiving this information (from primary informant) and will provide Supportive Supervision to the investigation team.

	C. Data transmission BMO office will receive notification of death telephonically through primary informant/ASHA/ANM within 24 hours of death of woman aged 15-49 years The primary informant will fill form for each reported death which ANM will verify whether reported death has occurred or not during pregnancy or in postnatal period (within 42 days) and then submit the duly filled form to BMO office within one week of notification of death BMO office will prepare the line list of all women deaths and maternal deaths reported by ANM every month and will send the reported deaths to DNO by the 5th of every month. In case of no death, NIL reporting will be done for the month At DNO office every month all the formats filled for notification, detailed investigation and line listing will be entered in MDSR software, wherever available **D. Analysis** BMO will do the analysis of the data collected and present the findings in the District Level Review being conducted by CMO. BMO will also share the findings in the block level monthly meeting for sensitization of the workers and initiating necessary corrective measures at this level. **E. Review** Review of maternal deaths is the most essential component of this process. Data collected from the community will be reviewed at district level by District MDSR Committee chaired by CMO and then a few selected cases by the District Collector.
Facility Based MDSR (FBMDSR)	**Steps of Facility-based MDSR** **Notification of** All maternal deaths occurring in the hospital, including abortions or within 42 days after termination of pregnancy should be informed immediately by the medical officer who has treated the mother and was on duty at the time of death to the Facility Nodal Officer (FNO) of the institution. The FNO of the hospital should inform the maternal death to the District Nodal Officer (DNO) by telephone within 24 hours of the occurrence of death. **Investigation** Any maternal death which occurred in the hospital should be investigated within 24 hours by the Medical Officer who had treated the mother and was on duty at the time of occurrence of death using the Facility Based Maternal Death Review (FBMDSR) Format. **Data transmission** Office of DNO will receive the notification form (Form 1) from FNO within 24 hours of maternal death. **Analysis** All the deaths reported and investigated will be analyzed every month. The focus of analysis would be to discuss the line of management followed in particular instances.

Chapter 23: Maternal and Child Death Surveillance and Response (MDSR)

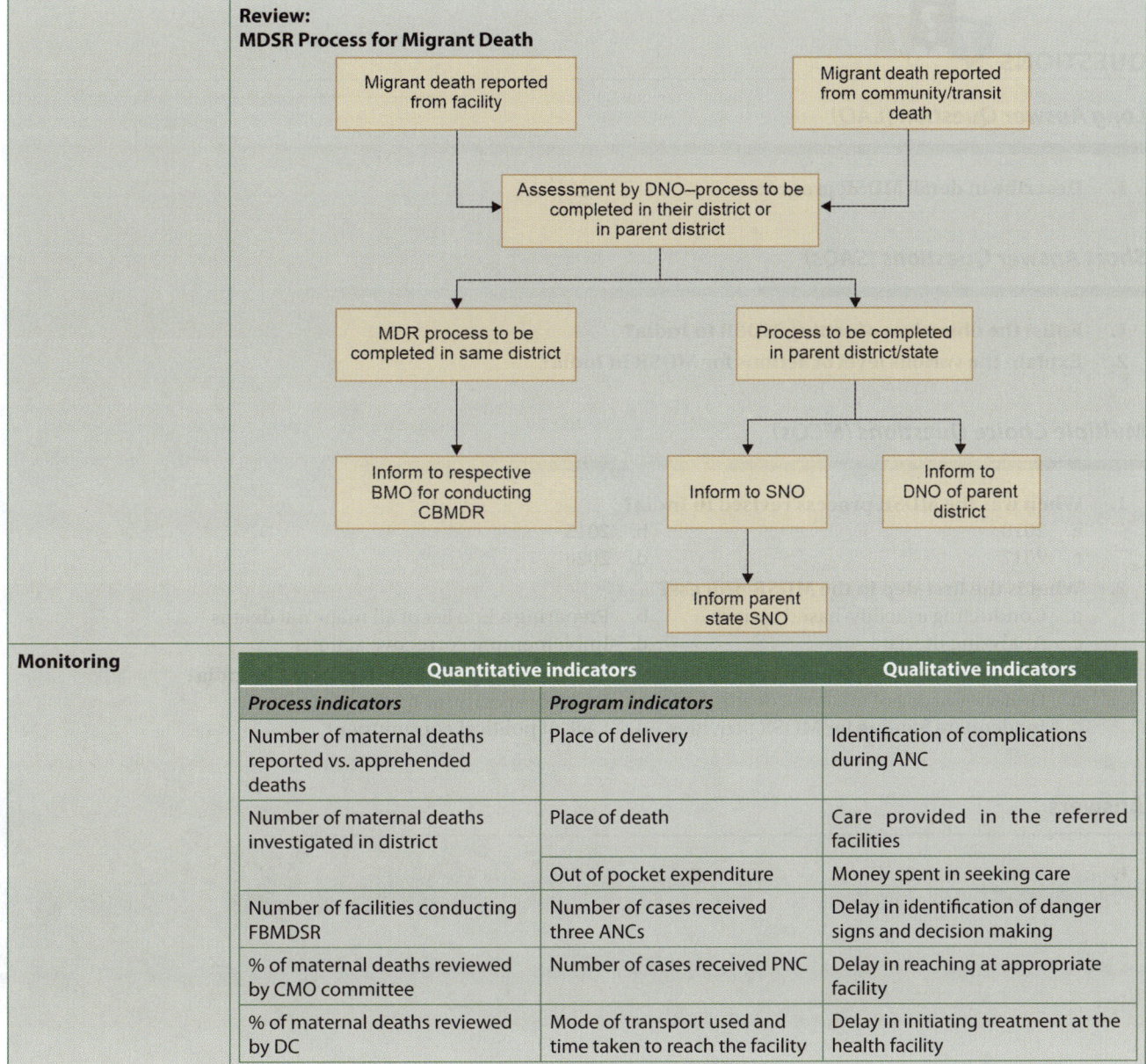

References

1. https://nhm.gov.in/images/pdf/programmes/maternal-health/guidelines/Guideline_for_MDSR.pdf
2. Maternal Death Review Guideline. Available at: http://tripuranrhm.gov.in/Guidlines/MDRGuidelines/MDR_Guidelines_Pg9_36.pdf

QUESTIONS

Long Answer Question (LAQ)

1. Describe in detail MDSR program.

Short Answer Questions (SAQs)

1. Enlist the objectives of setting MDSR in India?
2. Explain the various level of actions for MDSR in India?

Multiple Choice Questions (MCQs)

1. When was the MDSR process revised in India?
   a. 2010
   b. 2015
   c. 2017
   d. 2020
2. What is the first step in the MDSR process?
   a. Conducting a facility-based review
   b. Preparing a line list of all maternal deaths
   c. Analyzing the data
   d. Implementing corrective actions
3. Which of the following is *not* a key challenge in implementing the MDSR process in India?
   a. Underreporting of maternal deaths
   b. Lack of capacity for quality reviews
   c. Inadequate funding for MDSR activities
   d. Lack of political commitment

Answers

1. c
2. b
3. d

iii. NC: Neonatal and Child Health

CHAPTER 24

Facility-based Newborn Care

Ankit Yadav, Shaili Vyas, Priti Solanki

Background/Need of program	As per the Millennium Development Goals (MDGs), the government of India aimed to reduce the infant mortality rate (IMR) and under-five mortality rate (U5MR) to 30 and 38 per 1000 live births respectively.

Indicator	SRS 2004	SRS 2009
Neonatal mortality rate (NMR)	37	34
Infant mortality rate (IMR)	58	50

The data from SRS 2004 and 2009 showed a steady decline in IMR but almost static NMR with a slow decline. NMR contributes to two-thirds of the IMR and almost half of the U5MR, requiring a focus on newborn care to bring down NMR to achieve a significant decline in IMR and U5MR. Major causes of death in the neonatal period are still preventable such as hypothermia, asphyxia, respiratory distress, and infections.

After the introduction of the Janni Suraksha Yojana (JSY) scheme and the Integrated Management of Neonatal and Childhood Illnesses (IMNCI) program, there was increased contact with newborns at the household level along with identification and referral of sick newborns to the health facilities, which highlighted the gap in service delivery to the sick newborns in the existing healthcare system. To fill this gap and accelerate the achievement of desired goals, the government of India implemented this program in 2011 to improve the quality of newborn care services.[1-5]

Goal	To bring down the neonatal mortality rate and improve newborn health status.
Objective	To establish a continuum of newborn care with home-based and facility-based newborn care components, i.e., essential care to the newborn given right from birth till the first 48 hours at the health facility and thereafter home-based care during the first 42 days of life.[1]
Beneficiaries	**Newborns** • Newborn Care Corners (NBCCs) • Special Newborn Care Units (SNCUs) • Newborn Stabilization Units (NBSUs) Essential newborn care to all newborn Care for sick newborns NBCC—Essential newborn care to all newborns SNCUs and NBSUs—Care for sick newborns
Components[1]	**FNBC** → **Newborn care corner (NBCC)** • **Mandatory** for all health centers • Space within the delivery room → **Newborn stabilization unit (NBSU)** • Mandatory for all FRUs/CHCs in **addition to NBCC** • Sick and low birth weight newborns can be given care • Facility within or in close proximity of maternity ward → **Special newborn care unit (SNCU)** • Provide all special care (except assisted ventilation and major surgery) • **Any facility having >3000 deliveries** per year should have SNCU • In vicinity of labor room

Strategies

- **Level of care provided at various facilities**

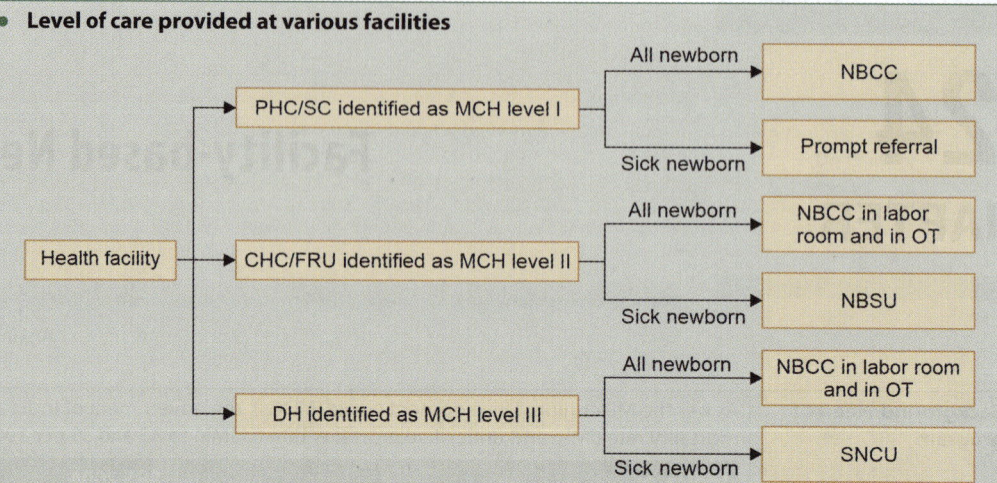

(PHC: primary health center; SC: sub-center, CHC: community health center; FRU: first referral unit; DH: district hospital, OT: operation theater)

- **Human resource for newborn care services**

Component	Required staff/ unit	Training needed
NBCC	1 doctor + 1 staff nurse/ANM (for sub-center)	All should be trained in NSSK
NBSU	1 doctor + 4 staff nurse	All should be trained in F-IMNCI
SNCU	• 3 to 4 trained doctors (proposed to post at least one pediatrician trained in neonatology along with 3-4 trained doctors) - at least 1 trained doctor/pediatrician round-the-clock • 3 staff nurses per shift round-the-clock • Dedicated support staff • Part-time lab technician • Data entry operator	Medical officers and staff nurse' should be trained in FBNC

- **Navjaat Shishu Suraksha Karyakram (NSSK):**
  + Initiated in September 2009 to train all healthcare providers in basic newborn care and resuscitation.
  + 2-day training package for MO, ANMs, and staff nurses
- **Facility-based IMNCI (F-IMNCI)**
  + Due to the non-availability of specialists at most FRUs, F-IMNCI training was designed for MO and staff nurses to improve their skills to provide quality care for normal and sick newborns.
  + This training package is based on the principle of participatory learning approach, using both classroom teaching and hands-on clinical sessions.
  + It is a skill-based training of 11 days, and if medical officers and staff nurses were already trained in IMNCI then a training of 5 days is sufficient.
- **Facility Based Newborn Care (FBNC)**
  + This training package has been developed with the participation of national neonatal experts and facilitated by the National Collaborative Center for Facility Based Newborn Care at Kalawati Saran Children's Hospital under the Ministry of Health and Family Welfare (MoHFW) mandate.
  + This training aims to enhance the psychomotor skills and cognitive knowledge of the medical officers (MO) and staff nurses to provide essential and special newborn care.
  + Duration: 4 days of training, which must be followed by 2 weeks of observership.

- **Empowering frontline health service providers:** The ANMs are now empowered to give a pre-referral dose of antenatal corticosteroid (Injection Dexamethasone) in pregnant women going into preterm labor. The use of antenatal corticosteroids is at all levels of health facilities. ANMs are also trained to administer pre-referral dose of Injection Gentamycin to newborns for sepsis management in young infants (up to 2 months of age).

Package of services at different levels[2,3]

	Newborn care corner (NBCC)	Newborn stabilization unit (NBSU)	Special newborn care unit (SNCU)
Care at birth	• Weighing the newborn • Early initiation of breastfeeding • Provision of warmth • Prevention of infection • Resuscitation	Same as NBCC	Same as NBCC
Care of normal newborn	Breastfeeding/feeding support	Same as NBCC	Same as NBCC
Care of sick newborn	Identification and prompt referral of "at risk" and "sick" newborn	• Management of newborn sepsis • Management of LBW infants ≥1800 grams with no other complications • Stabilization and referral of sick newborns and those with very low birth weight (rooming in) • Phototherapy for newborns with hyperbilirubinemia* • Referral services	• Managing all sick newborns (except those requiring mechanical ventilation and major surgical intervention) • Management of LBW infants <1800 grams • Follow-up of discharged babies and high-risk newborns • Referral services

*Availability of laboratory facilities to estimate bilirubin levels is a prerequisite
Note: Immunization services are provided at all 3 types of facilities

Triage of Sick newborn

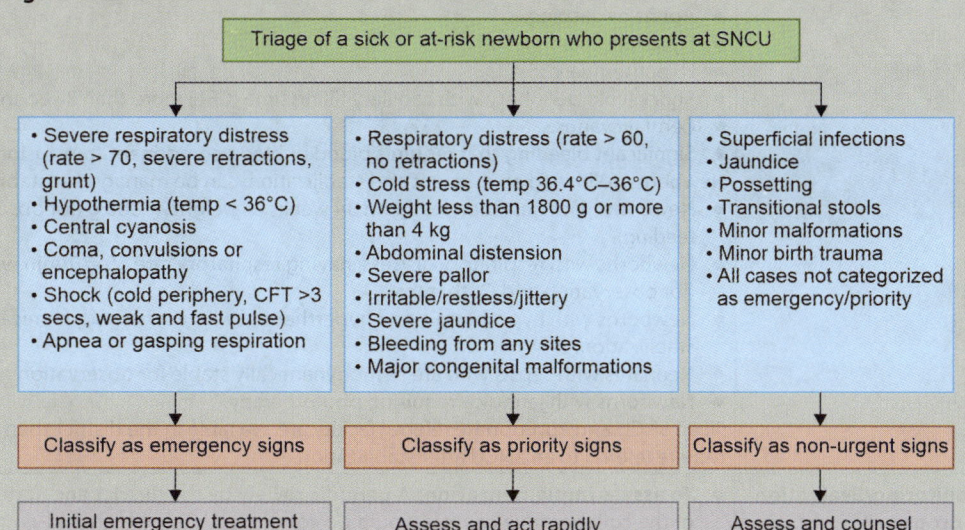

	Criteria for Admission in SNCU *Any newborn with the following criteria should be immediately admitted to the SNCU:* • Diarrhea/dysentery. • Perinatal asphyxia. • Abdominal distension. • Birth weight <1800 g or gestation <34 weeks. • Apnea or gasping. • Bleeding. • Large baby (>4.0 kg). • Refusal to feed. • Severe jaundice (appears <24 hrs/stains palms and soles/lasts >2 weeks). • Respiratory distress (rate >60/min or grunt/retractions). • Hypothermia <35.4°C, or hyperthermia >37.5°C. • Shock (cold periphery with CFT >3 seconds, weak and fast pulse). • Central cyanosis. • Coma, convulsions or encephalopathy. • Major malformations. *Criteria for transfer from SNCU to the Step-Down:* • Newborns admitted for any condition but are now thermodynamically and hemodynamically stable. • Newborn on antibiotics for completion of duration of therapy. • Newborn whose respiratory distress is improving and does not require oxygen supplementation to maintain saturation. • Newborn with jaundice requiring phototherapy but otherwise stable. • Low birth weight newborn (<1800 g), who are otherwise stable (for adequate weight gain). *Criteria for discharge from SNCU:* • Primary illness has resolved. • Newborn is accepting breastfeeds well. • Newborn is able to maintain temperature without radiant warmer. • Newborn is hemodynamically stable (normal CFT, strong peripheral pulse). • Newborn has documented weight gain for 3 consecutive days; and the weight is more than 1.5 kg.
	Criteria for Admission in NBSU Newborn presenting with any of these signs to a facility with NBSU requires admission for initial stabilization and if required, transfer to SNCU: • Respiratory distress (rate >70/min with severe retractions or grunt). • Apnea or gasping. • Hyperthermia >37.5°C • Hypothermia <35.4°C • Shock [cold periphery with capillary filling time (CFT) more than 3 sec and weak and fast pulse]. • Central cyanosis. • Significant bleeding that requires blood or blood component transfusion. Newborns, following assessment and stabilization, can be managed at stabilization unit*: • Newborns with gestation less than 34 weeks or weight <1800 g (for observation and assisted feeding). • Newborns with respiratory distress, having respiratory rate 60–70/min without grunting or retractions (for observation and O_2 therapy). • Newborns with hypothermia and hyperthermia who are hemodynamically stable after initial stabilization. • Neonates with sepsis who are hemodynamically stable for observation and antibiotic therapy. • Newborns with jaundice requiring phototherapy. *If an SNCU and appropriate referral facility are available in the district then other newborns would require referral to an SNCU after stabilization.[2]
Monitoring/Evaluation of program[6,7]	• **To assess implementation:** A periodic review by the district and state officials and the faculty of the collaborative centers would be conducted, after which mid-course corrections can be suggested.

> - **For every SNCU:** A mentoring team will be assigned, which consists of 2 experts from the state, at least for the initial one to two years till the functioning of the units is well established. **This criteria is a must for each SNCU.**
>   - These can be the experts designated by the Indian Academy of Pediatrics (IAP), National Neonatology Forum (NNF), or the Indian Association of Neonatal Nursing (IANN) who will be required to undertake regular monitoring visits and provide mentoring support to the local teams.
>   - Experts should also assist the teams in analyzing the data (case records, death audits, facility assessment, etc.) and accordingly plan and implement steps for improving the quality of service.
>   - Provision for mentoring visits can be built in the PIPs.

References

1. National Health Mission. Facility Based Newborn Care (FBNC) | Ministry of Health and Family Welfare | GOI. Available from: https://nhm.gov.in/index4.php?lang=1&level=0&linkid=484&lid=754
2. National Health Mission. Operational Guide (FBNC). Available from: https://nhm.gov.in/images/pdf/programmes/CH-Programmes/FBNC/Operational-Guide-(FBNC).pdf
3. Child Health Program. Annual report 2013-14. Chapter 5. Ministry of Health and Family Welfare. Available from: https://main.mohfw.gov.in/sites/default/files/Chapter515.pdf
4. Press Information Bureau. Significant decline in child mortality rates in India. Available from: https://pib.gov.in/PressReleasePage.aspx?PRID=1861710
5. Census of India. Sample Registration System Bulletin. Available from: https://censusindia.gov.in/census.website/data/SRSB
6. National Institution for Transforming India (NITI) Aayog. SDA India Index 2023-24. New Delhi: NITI Aayog; 2024. Available from: https://www.niti.gov.in/sites/default/files/2024-07/SDA_INDIA.pdf
7. Park K. Park's Textbook of Preventive and Social Medicine. 27th ed. Jabalpur: Banarsidas Bhanot; 2023.

QUESTIONS

Long Answer Question (LAQ)

1. Discuss the different levels of care provided for newborns under the FNBC program, including the roles of Newborn Care Corners (NBCCs), Newborn Stabilization Units (NBSUs), and Special Newborn Care Units (SNCUs).

Short Answer Questions (SAQs)

1. What are the main causes of neonatal mortality in India as highlighted in the FNBC program?
2. What training are mandatory for doctors under FNBC?

Multiple Choice Questions (MCQs)

1. FBNC Programme was introduced to:
   a. Fill the gap in service provision to sick newborns at health facilities
   b. Establish continuum of care for newborns
   c. Reduce maternal mortality
   d. Only a and b
   e. All of the above

2. **Mandatory component of FBNC for all health centers conducting delivery is:**
   a. Special Newborn Care Unit
   b. Newborn Stabilization Unit
   c. Newborn Care Corner
   d. None of the above
3. **For basic newborn care and resuscitation, the health staff must be trained in:**
   a. Facility based IMNCI
   b. Navjaat Shishu Suraksha Karyakram
   c. Rastriya Bal Swasthya Karyakram
   d. Facility Based Newborn Care
4. **True about Facility-based IMNCI (F-IMNCI) training:**
   a. Post-training observership of 2 weeks is mandatory
   b. In this training, healthcare providers are trained in basic newborn care
   c. If the staff nurse is trained in IMNCI then the duration of F-IMNCI would be 5 days
   d. This training imparts skills for specialized newborn care and clinical management
5. **A newborn baby with a birth weight of 1800 grams and no other complication can be managed at which level of care facility?**
   a. Newborn Stabilization Unit
   b. Primary Health Center
   c. Special Newborn Care Unit
   d. Newborn Care Corner
6. **Tasks of the mentoring team for SNCU include:**
   a. Providing technical support in conducting death audits
   b. Regular monitoring visits and feedback
   c. Guidance in analysis of SNCU data for quality improvement
   d. All of the above

Answers

1. d 2. c 3. b 4. c 5. a
6. d

25 CHAPTER

Navjaat Shishu Suraksha Karyakram

Bhavna Jain, Chhaya Mittal, Akhil Dhanesh Goel

NEED OF THE PROGRAM

- Newborn deaths represent a significant health challenge and contribute substantially to the rates of infant and under-five mortality in low-and middle-income nations, including India.
- In India, over 50% of infant deaths happen within the first month of life, and out of all annual infant deaths, 40% occur during labor or within the first 24 hours following birth. In 2020, India recorded almost one million newborn deaths.
- The National Health Policy (NHP) of India aims to lower neonatal mortality to 16 per 1,000 live births by the year 2025 (Government of India, 2017).
- Sustainable Development Goals (SDGs)—3.2.1 aim to eliminate preventable newborn deaths, with a target for all nations to lower neonatal mortality rates to a maximum of 12 per 1,000 live births by the year 2030 (United Nations, 2018). However, achieving these objectives appears to be challenging.
- Among infants under 29 days old, the leading causes of mortality are prematurity and low birth weight (48%), followed by birth asphyxia and birth trauma (13%), neonatal pneumonia (12%), noncommunicable diseases (7%), and birth defects.
- Having access to trained birth attendants and emergency medical care both during and after delivery can help avert a huge number of these deaths.
- Majority of newborn babies, i.e., 90% make the transition from intrauterine to extrauterine requiring no assistance in breathing while 10% require modest assistance and only 1% require major resuscitation measures.
- To guarantee the best start in life, newborn care and resuscitation are essential first steps in any neonatal program.[1,2]

Implemented Since

Government of India (GoI) launched a program Navjat Shishu Suraksha Karyakram (NSSK) on 15th September 2009 under Ghulam Nabi Azad to address the infant mortality rate (IMR).[3]

Implementing Agency

Ministry of Health and Family Welfare (MoHFW), Government of India.

Goal

To reduce infant/neonatal mortality rates and improve the health outcomes of newborns/infants across the country by improving quality of newborn care.

Targets

To train healthcare providers in essential newborn care and resuscitation measures, ensuring every delivery point has trained personnel capable of providing immediate, quality care to newborns, thereby preventing preventable newborn deaths.

Objectives[4]

- To teach healthcare professionals the fundamentals of newborn care and resuscitation.
- To prevent hypothermia, infection, and asphyxia in newborns.
- To promote early breastfeeding.
- To reduce neonatal mortality.
- To achieve SDGs for child mortality.
- To encourage community involvement and raise knowledge of newborn and infant care through a range of outreach and communication initiatives.

Beneficiaries/Target Group

Newborns and infants, particularly from vulnerable and disadvantaged populations.

About NSSK[3]

NSSK is part of the National Health Mission (NHM) and aims to provide affordable, accesible, high-quality medical services with particular attention to the vulnerable population. With such initiatives NSSK ensures a solid foundation for newborn health and survival, enabling them to thrive and contribute to the nation's future.

Need for NSSK

NSSK acknowledges the:
- High infant mortality rate
- Health disparities
- Vulnerable newborns
- Emphasise need of targeted interventions and equitable distribution of healthcare services
- Strengthen the health care infrastructure

Eligibility Criteria for NSSK

- **Target group:** Newborns and infants, particularly vulnerable ones.
- **Healthcare personnel:** Doctors, nurses, and midwives eligible for NSSK training programs.
- **Geographic coverage:** Underserved areas, including rural and economically disadvantaged regions.
- **Medical needs:** Sick newborns requiring specialized care in SNCUs.

Package of Services[4]

- **Ensuring skilled birth attendance:** Ensures a safe and healthy start for your newborn to ensure that all births are supported by qualified health professionals who can provide adequate care during birth.
- **Enhancing newborn care practices:** Promote essential care practices for newborns immediately after birth, including breastfeeding, thermal care, hygiene practices, and the supply of necessary vaccinations. These practices help protect newborns from infection and improve overall health outcomes.
- **Providing care for sick newborns:** Focus on the creation and strengthening of Sick Newborn Care Units (SNCU) in medical institutions. The SNCU provides specialized medical care for sick newborn patients those with complications or diseases requiring intensive care and treatments.
- **Promoting home-based newborn care:** To highlight the expansion of home-based newborn care services where trained healthcare workers visit newborns and their families at home. This allows newborns to receive essential care, proper monitoring and advice on various aspects of health and well-being.
- **Implementing newborn screening:** To implement newborn screening programmes to identify and address congenital disorders and other health conditions early in a newborn's life.
- **Capacity building and training:** Training medical professionals and frontline workers involved in newborn and infant care (to ensure that they have the skills and knowledge necessary to provide quality care to newborns and infants and can address their medical needs).

How Training is Done

- **Package of training:** According to revised NSSK package training is done for two days which is a clinical update cum skill enhancement training program at selected training sites. (Preferably near SNCU/Newborn Care Unit where the participants can be easily transferred for hands on training).
- **Facilitators:** Trained pediatricians, medical officers and nurse tutors who have undergone master training can conduct this training.
- **Eligibility of participants:** All health personnel working in labor room, involved with care of mother and baby including skilled birth attendants. (mainly doctors, nurses, and ANMs in low-resource areas where immediate medical care for newborns is diificult to provide).
- **Batch size:** Each batch will be of 24–28 participants. Each batch will be divided into four groups having of 6–7 participants in each group. For a batch of 24–28 participants, four facilitators shall be required.
- **Sites of training:** For every district, either district hospital (DH) or high case load subdistrict hospital, community health centers and primary health centers should be the training site.
- **Role of trainers:** The trainers will use interactive training methods to make the training sessions interesting and knowledgeable maintain quality of training also. For competency building trainers will demonstrate skills on anatomic models. Flip charts and four sets of mannequins will be provided to each facilitator for training.
- **Feedback:** Facilitator will give feedback to the participants on their answers, conduct role plays, lead group discussions, organize and supervise skill performing stations.

Types of Skills Imparted in Training[4]

- Training of skilled birth attendant involved in newborn care.
- Preparation of the delivery room following Suman guidelines (Includes favorable ambience, cleanliness, availability of equipment and supplies, readiness at newborn care area and infection prevention practices with biomedical waste management).
- Preparedness of clean and functional equipments before birth.
- Learning infection prevention (Clean birth/safe birth: Water, sanitation and hygiene for maternal and newborn health: WHO "six cleans"—clean hands, clean mother, clean delivery surface, clean cord cut, clean cord tying, clean cord care).
- Learning steps of hand washing (In the following sequence: (1) Palms/fingers/web spaces, (2) Back of hands, (3) Fingers and knuckles, (4) Thumbs, (5) Fingertips, (5) Wrists and forearm up to elbow).
- Following algorithm for neonatal resuscitation
  Key to successful resuscitation:
  - Anticipation preparation
  - Call for help when needed
  - Be able to work quickly in coordination with the helper/team
  - Communicate effectively
  - Be gentle and quick
  - Provide warmth and maintain hygiene
  - Maintain all records
- Actions at the time of birth (Noting time of birth, receiving baby in dry linen, ensuring warmth of baby, ensuring skin to skin contact with mother by placing baby on mother abdomen, turn head to one side and clear all secretions).
- Routine care for babies who cry at birth (Skin to skin care with mother, cover baby and mother together, ensure open airway of mother, clamp and cut cord in 1–3 min, initiate breastfeeding and check color and breathing rate of baby).
- Care of babies who does not cry at birth (Clamp and cut the cord immediately, place the baby under radiant warmer, to open airway position the head so that the neck is slightly extended, suction mouth and nose to clear airway, stimulate baby by rubbing back and reposition by adjusting the neck in the position of slight extension).
- Observational care with mother (Placing baby in prone position between mother breast, covering both mother and baby, initiating breastfeeding, monitoring temperature, colour and heart rate of baby every 15 min in first hour and every 30 min in next one hour).
- Learning to use bag and mask ventilation using room temperature/steps of positive pressure ventilation (Give five ventilatory breaths and look for chest rise still if no chest rise take corrective steps but if adequate chest rise the continue procedure for 30 sec).

❖ Actions if not breathing well even after ventilating for 30 sec Call for help of skilled health personnel for interventions, such as chest compression, intubation and use of medications and continue bag and mask ventilation).
❖ Care after birth (Prevention of hypothermia, prevention of any infection, detection any danger signs, ensuring adequate respiration, ensuring breastfeeding, care of eyes and umbilical cord, administer vitamin K).
❖ Monitoring breathing and temperature in a newborn, continuation of breastfeeding, continuation of kangaroo mother care and immunization
❖ Discharge and follow-up plan (Checklist before discharge: Mother and child free from any illness, baby immunized, breastfeeding started properly, mother explained about MCP card. Child to be followed up for proper growth and development).
❖ Neonatal transport (Babies requiring facility of transport: Those who require PPV for more than 1-minute, sick babies, low birth weight babies <1800 grams and babies requiring orogastric feeds).

References

1. Newborn and child health [Internet]. www.unicef.org. Available from: https://www.unicef.org/india/what-we-do/newborn-and-child-health.
2. Mishra A. What Is The Navjaat Shishu Suraksha Karyakram For Newborns? [Internet]. Jaagruk Bharat (जागरूक भारत). Jaagruk Bharat; 2024 [cited 2025 Feb 12]. Available from: https://www.jaagrukbharat.com/what-is-the-navjaat-shishu-suraksha-karyakram-for-newborns-3411118
3. Darshan Supekar. Goal, Benefits and Need of Navjaat Shishu Suraksha Karyakram(NSSK) [Internet]. Ketto.org. Ketto; 2023. Available from: https://www.ketto.org/blog/navjaat-shishu-suraksha-karyakram-nssk
4. RESUSCITATION AND ESSENTIAL NEWBORN CARE RESOURCE MANUAL NAVJAAT SHISHU SURAKSHA KARYAKRAM 2020 Ministry of Health and Family Welfare [Internet]. Available from: https://nhm.gov.in/images/pdf/programmes/child-health/guidelines/NSSK/NSSK-Resource-Manual.pdf

QUESTIONS

Long Answer Question (LAQ)

1. What is NSSK? Enumerate its objectives and package of services provided by it.

Multiple Choice Questions (MCQs)

1. Which is the program that aimed to train healthcare personnel in basic newborn care and resuscitation?
   a. RBSK
   b. NSSK
   c. IMNCI
   d. HBNC
2. Which of the following is not included in six cleans for safe birth?
   a. Clean hands
   b. Clean mother
   c. Clean doctor
   d. Clean delivery surface
3. Respectful maternity care (as envisaged in Suman guidelines) includes, *all except*:
   a. Privacy, confidentiality
   b. Provision of birth companion
   c. Choice of birthing position
   d. Non cordial congenial

4. All of the following are objectives of NSSK, *except*:
   a. To prevent hypothermia in newborns
   b. To prevent asphyxia in newborns
   c. To promote early breastfeeding
   d. To treat congenital malformations

Answers

1. b   2. c   3. d   4. d

26 CHAPTER

Home-based Newborn Care

Surendra Singh, Shaili Vyas, Nilesh Thakor

Background/Need of program/Scheme	A child is most vulnerable during the neonatal period and mortality during this period accounts for nearly half of all fatalities in children under five. India must therefore prioritize lowering infant and neonatal mortality in children (0–6 years), as these account for 13% of the whole population in India. India has seen a rise in institutional births, but after discharge, infants are still at risk. For mother's who leave hospitals early, home-based infant care is crucial. Home-based infant care is especially important for underprivileged communities or hard to reach areas with few health services. Neonatal death rates have decreased by 4.6 percentage points, according to the NFHS-5 (2019–21). However, there is still a significant urban–rural gap, underscoring the need for high-quality healthcare in underprivileged, disadvantaged, and rural areas.
Implemented since	Home-based Newborn Care (HBNC) as a policy was first mentioned in the XIth plan document (2007–2012). Thereafter, HBNC was approved by Mission Steering Group in June 2011.
Goal	Improve newborn care practices at the community level and for early detection and referral of sick new-born babies.
Objectives	The primary objectives of HBNC are to offer skilled newborn care such that neonatal mortality and morbidity are brought down through: • Ensuring that all newborns receive the necessary care and prevention of complications • Early recognition and tailored care of premature and low birth weight newborn • Prompt diagnosis, appropriate care and referral in case of illness in the newborn • Guidance to new mother and family regarding the adoption of healthy practices in rearing of newborn and build confidence and skill of mother to safeguard both her health and of baby[1]
Beneficiaries	With the exception of Goa and Lakshadweep, HBNC helps mothers and babies. In 2022–2023, ASHAs saw 1.47 crore infants; of those, over 8 lakhs were sent to medical facilities due to illness.
Strategies/ Deliverables under the program[2]	**Newborn care:** ASHAs are required under Home Based Newborn Care to ensure exclusive breastfeeding, prevent hypothermia, and provide home visits for the care of newborns. Along with providing emergency treatment during delivery, they also recognize sepsis symptoms and direct neonates to appropriate facilities. Further visits and weight growth monitoring are required for newborns who are discharged, LBW, or preterm. **Maternal care:** ASHA will provide appropriate prenatal care, assist women in her community who are expecting, identify any issues after giving birth, and offer family planning advice. She will assist with nursing after delivery, provide health promotion techniques, and train mother's of LBW and preterm infants on how to express their breast milk. **Capacity building:** ASHAs undergo four rounds of five-day training, which must be finished in a year, to get training in home-based infant care. Every round is verified after evaluation. In between training sessions, ASHAs get ten to twelve weeks of assistance and mentorship. Checklists for supervisors are employed to guarantee that skills are applied correctly. ASHAs engaged in home-based infant care get mentoring and on-the-job assistance from ASHA facilitators. **Home visit:** The Home-based Newborn Care initiative relies on Accredited Social Health Activists (ASHAs) trained in Modules 6 and 7 to deliver services, with incentives for visiting infants and mothers until 42 days of life. • Six home visits in cases of institutional delivery (days 3, 7, 14, 21, 28 and 42) • Seven home visits whenever there was home delivery (days 1, 3, 7, 14, 21, 28, and 42) • Five visits in the case, woman comes home after a cesarean section after 5–6 days (days 7, 14, 21, 28, 42)

	• For newborn discharged from Special Newborn Care Units (SCNU), the day of discharge is to be taken as day one and ASHAs are required to make the first home visit within 24 hours of discharge (day 1) and complete the remaining home visits as per HBNC schedule till 42 days. However, on completion of specified visits, ASHA will continue to conduct follow up visit once every quarter starting from 3rd month onwards till one year of life, i.e., four home visits at the end of 3rd, 6th, 9th and 12th month with each visit linked with an incentive of ₹ 50 per visit. • In case of LBW or preterm newborn who did not require SNCU admission, ASHAs are required to complete the scheduled HBNC visits, and thereafter she will continue to visit once every quarter starting from 3rd month onwards till one year of life, i.e., four visits and each visit will be incentivized ₹ 50 per visit per quarter. **HBNC kit:** A HBNC kit is provided to ASHA at onset of training so that she can familiarize herself in its use. HBNC kit contains additional contents which facilitate provision of HBNC and include equipment (digital watch, digital thermometer, neonatal weighing scale, sling of the weighing scale, blankets and baby feeding spoon), medications, and consumables. **Health promotion:** ASHA being resident of the same locality, it is expected that she provides to mother one to one inter personal communication and health education to the family and larger community. The aim being adoption of good practices regarding care of the newborn and postpartum mother. **Support to ASHA worker:** ASHA is provided field level support by ASHA facilitator who visits her at least twice a month and facilitates ASHAs in job training, monitoring and support. ANM helps ASHA in developing her technical skills in performance of HBNC and she also reviews the coverage and quality of care provided to newborns by ASHA. Refresher training help in building knowledge and skill retention. MO-PHC supports ASHA in treatment and referral of sick newborns. Regular restocking of the ASHA kit is necessary, and equipment should be inspected and repaired as needed for optimizing work of ASHA. Grievance redressal mechanism helps in prompt redressal and satisfactory outcomes.
Incentives	ASHA will be eligible for the HBNC incentive if they mandatory fill the first examination form and home visit form for each newborn, which are then to be verified by ASHA facilitator/ANM. In addition, the incentive amounts are also subject to fulfilment of the following: • Documentation of newborn's weight in Mother Child Protection (MCP) card • Provides first dose of OPV, BCG and DPT vaccine • Mother and the newborn are cared for and do not suffer any adverse outcome till 42 days of the delivery, and • Registration of birth has been done[2]
Activities at various level or package of services	**Activities at primary/ground level:** The key activities in HBNC performed at primary level include • Throughout the first six weeks of life, an ASHA makes specified home visits to provide care for each newborn. • Provision of health education to the mother and family of every newborn to ensure better health outcomes. • Assessment of every newborn for prematurity and birth weight. • Additional home visits by the ASHA or ANM, with referrals for appropriate care as specified in the guidelines, for preterm and low birth weight babies. • Early detection of the newborn's illness and delivery of suitable at-home treatment or referral in accordance with the standards. • Follow up for sick newborn after they are discharged. • Postpartum care counseling, identifying postpartum problems, and facilitating referrals for the mother. • Counselling and assisting the mother in choosing a suitable family planning strategy. **Actions at district level:** • District Nodal Officer has to be nominated for overall responsibility of HBNC. • Ensure that the support system for ASHA: District community mobilizer, block community mobilizer and facilitators are in place. • Widely publicize free entitlements in public domain. • Establish a grievance redressal mechanism to make sure that the commitments are fulfilled. • Enable and monitor the quality of ASHA training in Modules 6 and 7. • Check the medicine and consumable inventories frequently to make sure that they are available in the ASHA kit.

	• Review referral linkages and their utilization by beneficiaries. • Give block MOs and facility in-charges the necessary funding/authority to use funds for the aforementioned operations, especially in emergency situations or stock outs. • Monitor and report on approved formats on a regular basis at a predetermined intervals. • Review the implementation status at meetings with the block MOs/MOs. **Actions at state level:** • State Nodal Officer has to be nominated for overall responsibility of HBNC. • Establishment of a state-level resource center/centers to offer district and block levels training support in order to guarantee ASHA and facilitators receive quality training. • Assure that ASHA completes her training in Modules 6 and 7 within a year and receives her certification to offer HBNC. • Ensure that the ASHA has the supervision and support systems necessary to carry out HBNC, with at least two monthly on-site mentoring visits from supervisor/facilitator. • Establish a grievance redressal mechanism for ensuring that the commitments are fulfilled. • Ensure that medications and consumables for the ASHA kit and in the public health facilities are regularly purchased and made available. • Establish district wise assured referral linkages. • Provide necessary funding and administrative support for implementation of above activities. • Empower the district and facility in-charges with the financial authority to carry out the aforementioned tasks. • Monitor and report on approved formats on a regular basis at a predetermined intervals. • Review the implementation status of HBNC at district CMO meetings and in quarterly review meetings with district community mobilizers and district nodal officers.
Monitoring and evaluation of program	The progress of implementation of the HBNC program is being monitored at the central level by the Ministry of Health and Family Welfare (MoHFW), Government of India on a quarterly basis. For monitoring purposes states are expected to provide to MoHFW, details of information on following: • The status of ASHA training • Equipment related to HBNC • Particulars of the HBNC visits done and referrals made by ASHAs • Total expenditure on HBNC by the state **Steps of monitoring:** • Every time an ASHA visits a home with a newborn, they are required to fill out the home visit form. The purpose of these home visitation forms is to evaluate the quantity and quality of her visits. • During the monthly meeting with the ASHAs, the ASHA facilitator/ANM confirms and signs the house visit forms completed by ASHA. • The ASHA facilitator/ANM then provides and turns in a signed token/slip to the PHC personnel based on the ASHAs' performance. • Subsequently, during the VHND/village visit, the ANM takes a note of how well each ASHA performed in terms of home visits for newborns, in her subcenter region. • The PHC personnel will pay ASHAs after receiving approval from the MO-PHC, who will monitor the implementation during meetings. • The district nodal officer is responsible for overseeing and monitoring the program's execution at the district level. At the district-level CMO meeting, the CMOs additionally are to assess the progress in HBNC. • The State nodal officer in turn monitors program's efficacy and execution at state level. At the state-level CMOs meeting, the State Mission Director reviews the program's progress. • The Child Health Division of the MoHFW, Government of India, will provide direction and support to the National Health System Resource Center, which is the nodal center **to oversee the program at the national level.**

References

1. World Health Organization (WHO). Newborn mortality [Online]. WHO; 2024 [Accessed 2024 Jul 17]. Available from: https://www.who.int/news-room/fact-sheets/detail/newborn-mortality
2. Ministry of Health and Family Welfare, Government of India. HOME BASED NEWBORN CARE. Operational Guidelines (Revised 2014). New Delhi; 2014 Mar, p. 40.

QUESTIONS

Long Answer Question (LAQ)

1. Describe in detail HBNC program with specific mention of the strategies under the program.

Short Answer Questions (SAQs)

1. Explain the role of ASHA in Home-based Newborn Care.
2. What are the activities performed under HBNC at the district level?

Multiple Choice Questions (MCQs)

1. In case of home deliveries, how many visits are done by ASHA under HBNC?
    a. Five
    b. Six
    c. Seven
    d. Eight
2. Apart from home visits, incentives for ASHAs in HBNC are also based on following, *except*:
    a. Mother and the newborn are cared for and do not suffer any adverse outcome till 42 days of the delivery
    b. Documentation of newborn's weight in Mother Child Protection (MCP) card
    c. Provides last dose of OPV, MR and JE vaccine
    d. Registration of birth has been done

Answers

1. c
2. c

27 CHAPTER

Home-based Care for Young Child

Surendra Singh, Shaili Vyas, Nilesh Thakor

Background/ Need of program/Scheme	**Priority of child health:** • Ensuring the health of children is a top priority for every nation. • Children are particularly vulnerable to diseases, especially when healthcare services are inadequate. **Impact of undernutrition:** • Undernutrition is responsible for about 35% of child deaths. • It affects children's cognitive and physical development and increases the risk of infections. **Inadequate feeding practices:** Poor practices in Infant and Young Child Feeding (IYCF) are a major cause of undernutrition. • Key components of IYCF, such as exclusive breastfeeding for the first 6 months and age-appropriate complementary feeding, need to be reinforced in the community. • Incorrect timing and quality of complementary feeding can lead to inadequate diets, causing growth faltering. **Existing gaps in newborn care:** • The Home-based Newborn Care (HBNC) program launched in 2011, provides care for newborns up to 42 days after birth. • After this period, health workers mainly interact with children only during immunization or if the child is ill. • There is a gap in routine care between the end of HBNC and the beginning of regular Immunization visits. **Purpose of the HBYC program:** • **Bridge the gap**: HBYC aims to fill this gap by ensuring continuous care for children from 3 months to 15 months of age. • **Promote nutrition and growth:** Focuses on promoting exclusive breastfeeding, timely complementary feeding, and regular growth monitoring to detect and address nutritional deficiencies early. • **Manage childhood illnesses**: Helps in the early identification and management of illnesses, with timely referrals for serious cases. • **Support early childhood development:** Provides counseling and support to parents for creating a healthy and stimulating environment for young children. • By providing counseling and support, ASHAs also empower mothers and caregivers to create stimulating environments for their children. Under the program ASHAs counsel mothers on EBF, age appropriate complementary feeding, other aspects of nutrition, immunization, family planning practices, WASH, etc.
Implemented since	**Phased rollout of the program:** • The HBYC program began its rollout in a phased manner during the financial year 2018-19. • First Phase (2018-19): Implemented in all the identified Aspirational Districts across India. **Expansion of the program:** 2022-23: The HBYC program was expanded and approved for 690 districts across all states and Union Territories (UTs), including all Aspirational Districts, except for Goa. **Reach and impact:** In the year 2022-23, over 2.5 crore home visits were conducted by ASHAs to young children aged 3 months to 15 months.
Goal	**Promoting Good Child Nutrition** **Breastfeeding practices:** • Initiate breastfeeding within an hour of delivery. • Ensure exclusive breastfeeding for the first 6 months of life. **Complementary feeding:** • Begin appropriate and sufficient complementary feeding after 6 months while continuing breastfeeding.

	Ensuring age-appropriate immunization: Ensure that all children receive vaccines according to the national immunization schedule, protecting them against preventable diseases. **Ensuring optimal early childhood development (ECD):** Support activities and interventions that promote physical, cognitive, and social-emotional development during early childhood. **Promoting appropriate health-seeking behavior:** Encourage caregivers to seek timely and appropriate medical care to reduce child morbidity and mortality.

Objectives	• **Reduce child mortality and morbidity:** Decrease the rates of child deaths and illnesses by ensuring timely identification, referral, and management of common childhood illnesses during home visits.
	• **Improve nutrition status, growth, and early childhood development:**
	    ✦ Enhance the nutritional status, growth, and overall development of young children through regular, structured, and focused home visits by ASHAs.
	    ✦ Provide counseling on appropriate infant and young child feeding (IYCF) practices, immunization, hygiene, and other key health behaviors.[1]

Organogram	**National level**
	• **Ministry of Health and Family Welfare (MoHFW):**
	    ✦ Secretary
	    ✦ Joint Secretary (RCH)
	    ✦ Deputy Commissioner (Child Health)
	    ✦ National Health Mission (NHM) Director
	• **Ministry of Women and Child Development (MWCD):**
	    ✦ Secretary
	    ✦ Joint Secretary (Anganwadi Services)
	    ✦ Director (Anganwadi Services)
	State level
	• **State Health Department:**
	    ✦ State Health Secretary
	    ✦ State Mission Director (NHM)
	    ✦ State Program Officer (RCH)
	• **State Women and Child Development Department:**
	    ✦ State Commissioner (WCD)
	    ✦ State Mission Director (POSHAN Abhiyaan)
	District level
	• **District Health Department:**
	    ✦ District Health Officer (DHO)
	    ✦ District Program Officer (RCH)
	    ✦ Block Medical Officers (BMOs)
	• **District Women and Child Development Department:**
	    ✦ District Child Development Officer (DCDO)
	    ✦ Child Development Project Officers (CDPOs)
	Community level
	• **Anganwadi Centers (AWCs):**
	    ✦ Anganwadi workers (AWWs)
	    ✦ Anganwadi helpers
	• **Primary Health Centers (PHCs):**
	    ✦ Auxiliary nurse midwives (ANMs)
	    ✦ Accredited social health activists (ASHAs)

Beneficiaries[1]	• **Young children (3–15 months):** The primary beneficiaries are children aged between 3 to 15 months. These children receive five structured home visits by ASHAs to monitor growth, development, nutrition, and overall health. • **Mothers and caregivers:** Mothers and caregivers benefit from the program through counseling and support provided by ASHAs. This includes education on exclusive breastfeeding, complementary feeding, early childhood development, management of common illnesses, and referrals for complications. • **Families of young children:** Families gain awareness and skills to promote better child health and nutrition practices at home, contributing to reduced child morbidity and mortality.

Components[1]	The HBYC program is designed to address gaps in care between the end of Home-based Newborn Care (HBNC) and the regular immunization schedule by ensuring continuous monitoring and support for young children (3 to 15 months). The key components of the HBYC program are: **Home visits by ASHAs and AWWs:** ● *ASHAs (Accredited social health activists):* Responsible for conducting five additional home visits to young children at 3, 6, 9, 12, and 15 months, providing health education and promotion activities. ● This includes exclusive breastfeeding, age-appropriate complementary feeding, immunization checks, growth monitoring, and managing common childhood illnesses. ● *Anganwadi workers (AWWs):* Work in conjunction with ASHAs to provide support during home visits, conduct monthly weighing of infants, and offer supplementary nutrition to underweight children. They also provide counseling on nutrition, health, and hygiene practices. **Growth monitoring and promotion:** Regular weighing and growth chart plotting for children to identify any growth faltering or underweight issues. ASHAs and AWWs will take appropriate actions, such as counseling mothers on exclusive breastfeeding, complementary feeding, and addressing malnutrition. **Nutritional interventions:** ● Promotion of appropriate Infant and Young Child Feeding (IYCF) practices, including exclusive breastfeeding for the first six months, timely introduction of complementary feeding, and ensuring a balanced diet for children. ● Counseling mothers on nutritional needs, distribution of Iron Folic Acid (IFA) supplements, ORS (Oral Rehydration Solution), and Zinc for children as necessary. **Immunization and health check-ups:** ● Ensure age-appropriate immunization for children up to 15 months. ● Identification and management of common childhood illnesses, such as diarrhea and pneumonia, with timely referrals for severe cases. ● Support for Early Childhood Development (ECD) ● Counseling mothers and caregivers on age-appropriate play, communication, and cognitive stimulation to promote optimal early childhood development. ● Focus on creating a stimulating home environment for physical and cognitive growth. **Promotion of wash (water, sanitation, and hygiene)**: Encourage proper handwashing practices, safe drinking water, and improved sanitation to prevent infections and improve child health outcomes. **Capacity building of frontline workers:** ● Additional training sessions for ASHAs, AWWs, and ANMs to reinforce existing skills and provide new skills for HBYC-specific duties. ● Regular refresher training and joint training sessions for better role clarification and synergy in actions. **Supportive supervision and monitoring:** Supervisory support provided by the Anganwadi Services Supervisors and ASHA Facilitators through routine visits and on-the-job mentoring. Regular monitoring and review meetings at the PHC level, using checklists and supervisory tools, to ensure the quality of care provided to young children. **Incentive mechanisms:** ASHAs receive a financial incentive of ₹ 250 for completing the five additional home visits per young child according to the specified schedule, contingent on validated immunization and growth records. **Data collection and program monitoring:** ● Utilization of HBYC cards to document home visits, health checks, and interventions provided by ASHAs. ● Monthly compilation and data entry by Block Data Entry Operators and aggregation at the district, state, and national levels to monitor program progress and assess key indicators.
Strategies/ Deliverables under the program	**Home-based care:** ● Under HBYC, ASHAs will undertake additional five home visits in children, starting from 3rd month with support from Anganwadi workers. ● From 2–3 months onward ASHAs will provide quarterly home visits (3rd, 6th, 9th, 12th and 15th months). ● During the home visits, ASHAs will offer health education and promote health promotion activities including exclusive and continued breastfeeding, adequate complementary feeding, age-appropriate immunization and early childhood development. ● The quarterly home visits schedule for low birth weight babies, SNCU and NRC discharged children will now be synchronized with the new HBYC schedule.

	Capacity building: • ASHAs have already been trained in Modules 6 and 7 during their training for HBNC. The skills developed during these trainings and during the provision of HBNC will help ASHA in HBYC as well. • Additionally, in order to reinforce existing skills and impart new ones, extra training session of 3 days with sufficient hands on experience is envisaged. • Periodic refresher trainings are to be conducted which will help in retention of knowledge and skills. • Furthermore, a collaborative training program involving ASHAs, ANMs, and AWWs will be implemented to enhance role clarification and to foster synergy in action. • The training package's contents shall include new skills needed to complete HBYC-specified duties including encouraging ECD, IFA supplementation and reinforcing ORS use, supplemental feeding, and hand washing, among others. • To improve their supervisory abilities, a two-day combined training program with ASHA, AWW will also be attended by the Anganwadi Services Supervisor and the ASHA Facilitator. **Incentive:** • Financial incentive to ASHA in the form of ₹ 250 for completion of 5 additional home visits for each young child as per the specified schedule. • The payment will be released after validating that age appropriate vaccination is completed and recorded along with the weight in MCP card. • The ANM/ASHA Facilitator will verify at least 10% of the home visits by reviewing the necessary documentation. • Additionally, in accordance with guidelines from MoHFW, ASHAs will also receive their designated portion of the team-based reward under domain of child health and nutrition. **Supportive supervision:** • The supportive supervision to both ASHA and AWW shall be provided by respective supervisors from Anganwadi Services and NHM. • The supervisors are required to carry out routine visit to ASHAs under them and during these visits they should review and provide 'on the job' mentoring support using supervisory checklists. • Every supervisor needs to make sure that every ASHA and AWW in their care receives at least one visit per quarter. This implies that six to seven employees will receive visits on average each month. • During monthly review meetings, planning for joint supportive supervision should also be done in order to create a schedule of villages that each supervisor will visit. • At least 10% of the infants in her subcenter area should receive joint home visits from ANM and ASHAs. • ANM should check the HBYC forms that ASHAs have completed, as well as guide and assist the ASHAs in doing their responsibilities effectively. • ANM should use the Village Health and Nutrition Day platform to assess the coverage and quality of care given to young children by ASHAs. • The Medical Officer should oversee the activities of ANM, and district level evaluation should take place for same. • Monthly review sessions are to be held at PHC level for solving problems and creating referral linkages. • A functioning Village Health, Sanitation and Nutrition Committee (VHSNC) or Women's Health Committee is required to support the ASHA at the village level.
Activities at various level or package of services	• HBYC aims to reduce the burden of child mortality and morbidity in India through specified, focused and effective home visits by ASHAs. • HBYC also tries to fill the gaps in continuum of care, in children post 42 days; since unavailability of quality care to a child till 2 years of age has ramifications on his future life. • HBYC envisages this by additional yet mandatory home visits by ASHAs wherein activities related to interventions delivered in four key domains namely nutrition, health, child development and WASH (water, sanitation and hygiene) is being promoted. These interventions are evidence based and objective. • The services under HBYC are provided by ASHA with the help from AWW. Both of them will visit young children (3 months-15 months) in their locality and provide for the following services:

Home visits	Asha	AWW
At 3rd month	• Support for exclusive breastfeeding • Counsel on hand washing practices • Appropriate play and communication • Check immunization status • Check weight recording in MCP card; identify growth faltering	• Monthly weighing of infants • Recording of weight and plotting of growth chart • Detect underweight children and take further action • Counsel mother for exclusive breastfeeding
At 6th, 9th, 12th and 15th months	• All above activities PLUS • Counsel on initiation of complementary feeding and continued breastfeeding • Provision of age appropriate and adequate complementary nutrition • Encourage age appropriate play and communication • Ensure complete immunization • Prophylactic IFA and ORS distribution • Counseling • Depot holder for ORS and Zinc	• 'Take Home Ration' and nutrition specific counselling to mothers • Monthly recording of weight and provision of supplementary food from AWC • Counseling regarding Complementary feeding • Recording on growth chart; monitoring for underweight children and their management • Measure and record length/height • Advice for deworming in children above 1 year

- At the central level, HBYC is a joint program of MoHFW and MWCD, with technical guidance for the program being provided by NHSRC, which is responsible for developing and dissemination of the HBYC guidelines, training packages, job aids and communication materials. NHSRC is also responsible for capacity building of ASHAs, while budgetary allocation is also disbursed at central level, after receiving PIP from states.
- At the level of District and states, activities/services have been defined so as to bring a clarity in the roles and responsibilities of providers, and to provide uniform, integrated and quality care to the beneficiaries. A summary of activities to be done at state and district level in HBYC program is discussed in the following table:

Activities	State level	District level
Developing joint action plan	• Joint planning by NHM and Anganwadi services regarding schedule of key activities, role clarity of front line workers, joint training plan, and availability of commodities • Orientation of key stakeholders • Printing of training packages, job aides, formats, checklists and reporting formats	Joint planning by district level NHM and Anganwadi services + Orientation of key stakeholders + Joint training and community mobilization plan for the district
Capacity building	• Ensure the preparedness of ASHA resource center to provide support for district and block level trainings of front line workers and supervisors • Advance planning by state team to support the district resource centers for conducting training; ongoing monitoring for quality of training	• District Resource Centre to gear up for training and HBYC related activities • Develop training microplan and accordingly review its own the preparedness for conducting quality trainings • Refresher trainings/reorientation for workers in each quarter
Commodities	• Projection of annual requirement for commodities, budgeting and approvals	• Timely procurement of commodities to avoid stockouts
Funds	• Timely approvals and allocation of funds to districts; ensure smooth fund flow to districts	• Timely payment of incentives
Monitoring/ Supervision	• Regular monitoring of services delivered and children covered during specified period in each district • Share reports at specified periodicity with national counterparts • Review meets to evaluate progress and make mid-course improvements	• Regularly monitor HBYC activities; analyze data; and review at monthly meetings • Develop joint supportive supervision plan • Share data at specified periodicity with state cell/teams

Monitoring and evaluation of program	**Monthly monitoring at the central level:** • The progress of the HBYC program will be monitored by the central authorities on a monthly basis. • States must provide details on the number of training sessions and home visits conducted under the program. • This information will enable child-wise tracking of home visits, which will be integrated with the Reproductive and Child Health (RCH) portal of the Government of India. **Data collection and entry:** • Monitoring starts with ASHA filling out the HBYC card for each child during home visits. • HBYC cards are collected, collated, and compiled into registers by ASHA supervisors/facilitators during their monthly review meetings. • Data from the HBYC cards is entered into a web-based tracking system that links with the RCH portal to ensure accurate monitoring and verification of incentive payments to ASHAs. **Manual data collection approach:** • Until the web-based system is fully operational, manual data collection will be conducted by ASHAs and compiled by their supervisors. • The Block Data Entry Operator will compile data from each ASHA supervisor into an Excel sheet monthly. • The district will compile these Excel sheets for each block, and data will be further compiled at state and national levels. • Regular data analysis will help identify areas needing improvement based on key indicators. **Outcome evaluation:** • The evaluation of the program's outcomes will utilize child health and nutrition indicators, which are part of the Ministry of Health and Family Welfare (MoHFW) team-based incentive program for frontline staff. • The performance of frontline workers, including ASHAs, will be evaluated using the team-based incentive system. **Integration with other evaluation methods:** • HBYC evaluation will be combined with existing evaluation methods such as National Family Health Surveys (NFHS) and National Health Surveys. • Additional need-based evaluations will be conducted in specific geographic areas, like aspirational districts, to provide targeted guidance and strengthen the initiative.

Reference

1. Ministry of Health and Family Welfare and Ministry of Women and Child Development, Government of India. Home Based Care for Young Child (HBYC). Strengthening of Health and Nutrition through Home Visits. Operational Guidelines. New Delhi; 2018 Apr; p. 60.

QUESTIONS

Long Answer Question (LAQ)

1. What is the need for the HBYC Program? Explain in detail the goals, strategies and monitoring mechanisms under the program.

Short Answer Questions (SAQs)

1. Enlist the salient features of HBYC program.
2. What is the need for home-based care in HBYC and how it is related to infant and young child feeding practices?

Section III: National Health Mission

Multiple Choice Questions (MCQs)

1. **What is the primary aim of the HBYC program?**
   a. To provide financial assistance to families
   b. To bridge the gap in care for children between 3 to 15 months
   c. To provide free education to children
   d. To support adult health care services

2. **Which program provides care for newborns up to 42 days after birth before the HBYC program takes over?**
   a. Integrated Child Development Services (ICDS)
   b. Home-based Newborn Care (HBNC)
   c. National Health Mission (NHM)
   d. Pradhan Mantri Surakshit Matritva Abhiyan (PMSMA)

3. **When was the HBYC program first implemented?**
   a. 2015–16
   b. 2016–17
   c. 2017–18
   d. 2018–19

4. **What is one of the key components of the HBYC program?**
   a. Providing free vaccinations for all age groups
   b. Conducting home visits to monitor growth, development, and nutrition of young children
   c. Distributing free textbooks to children
   d. Organizing community sports events

5. **How many home visits does an ASHA (Accredited Social Health Activist) make under the HBYC program for each young child?**
   a. Three
   b. Four
   c. Five
   d. Six

6. **What financial incentive is provided to ASHAs for completing the five additional home visits?**
   a. ₹ 200
   b. ₹ 250
   c. ₹ 300
   d. ₹ 350

7. **Which department is responsible for providing technical guidance and capacity building for the HBYC program?**
   a. Ministry of Women and Child Development (MWCD)
   b. National Health Mission (NHM)
   c. National Health Systems Resource Centre (NHSRC)
   d. Ministry of Rural Development

8. **What is the main focus of counseling provided by ASHAs under the HBYC program?**
   a. Financial management
   b. Nutrition, immunization, and early childhood development
   c. Career guidance
   d. Environmental conservation

9. **The year in which HBYC program was expanded to 690 districts across all states and union territories except Goa was?**
   a. 2020–21
   b. 2021–22
   c. 2022–23
   d. 2023–24

10. What is the role of anganwadi workers (AWWs) in the HBYC program?
    a. Conducting surgeries
    b. Providing legal support
    c. Assisting ASHAs in home visits, weighing infants, and providing supplementary nutrition
    d. Organizing health insurance plans

Answers

1.	b	2.	b	3.	d	4.	b	5.	c
6.	b	7.	c	8.	b	9.	c	10.	c

CHAPTER 28

Rashtriya Bal Swasthya Karyakram

Shaili Vyas, Surendra Singh, Parul Sharma, Nilesh Thakor

Background/Need of program/Scheme	India owes to its children a life free from death, disability and despair. This means creation of such conducive environment that help the children in country to reach their fullest potential and contribute to it. Various programs have been formulated under National Health Mission which have thus contributed to the decline in child mortality in recent times, but little to no focus was placed on reducing the birth defects, diseases, developmental delays and disabilities in children, the 4Ds. With India adding a large number of children to its population every year, the fact cannot be discounted that some of these children may be suffering from birth defects, which is then often diagnosed late resulting in increased chances of adverse outcome. Moreover, prevalence of malnutrition is still a public health problem and disease of childhood like dental caries, rheumatic heart disease, reactive airway disease, etc., often go unreported. There has also been lack of attention with regards to developmental delays which are often related to poverty, poor nutrition and lack of early stimulation; conditions prevalent in most parts of the country. A concerted effort is therefore required to address these issues at the earliest stage possible, in conjunction with provision of equitable health care that includes components of early diagnosis and management. Such interventions though require careful and joint efforts from all related stakeholders. A holistic approach that advocates preventive and promotive interventions, provides unrestricted curative services along with appropriate referral linkages will go a long in reducing morbidity and mortality, and will specifically help the marginalized and disadvantaged by lowering direct costs and out-of-pocket expenses. Rashtriya Bal Swasthya Karyakram (RBSK) is a new initiative aiming to improve health outcomes in children through provision of "Child Health Screening and Early Intervention Services". The goal being catching the children suffering from birth defects, diseases, developmental delays and disabilities in children early and placing them in the continuum of care cascade for early screening along with appropriate management and referral. This will lead to prevention of untimely death, reduced malnutrition prevalence, enhanced cognitive development, and educational attainment.[1]
Implemented since	The Rashtriya Bal Swasthya Karyakram (RBSK) was launched in 2013 by the Ministry of Health and Family Welfare of the Government of India as part of the National Health Mission with the goal of assisting all children in reaching their full potential while also providing comprehensive community care.
Goal	Its main goal is to deal with all health issues in a comprehensive way, making sure that every kid gets the right care and support without putting too much financial strain on their families.
Objectives	The objective of RBSK is to improve quality of life of children by early detection of birth defects, diseases, deficiencies, development delays, and disabilities.[1]
Beneficiaries	RBSK program targets all children aged 0–6 years in rural areas and urban slums, and children aged up to 18 years who are enrolled in classes 1st to 12th grades in government and government aided schools.

Target group under child health screening and intervention services	
Categories	**Age group**
Babies born in public health facilities and at home	Birth–6 weeks
Preschoolers in urban slums and rural areas	6 weeks–6 years
Children in 1st–12th grade at government and government-aided schools	6–18 years

Components	• Child health screening • Management and referral • Tracking and follow-up
Strategies/ Deliverables under the program	**Child health screening**: All newborn and children up to 18 years of age are screened for 4Ds namely defects at birth, deficiencies, diseases and developmental delay (including disability). The aim of health screening is early identification, early treatment and appropriate referral of the affected children. At present 32 common health conditions are screened through the program (see table below)[1]

Health conditions screened under RBSK	
A. Defects at birth 1. Neural tube defect 2. Down's syndrome 3. Cleft lip and palate/cleft palate alone 4. Talipes (club foot) 5. Developmental dysplasia of the hip 6. Congenital cataract 7. Congenital deafness 8. Congenital heart diseases 9. Retinopathy of prematurity	**B. Deficiencies** 10. Anemia especially severe anemia 11. Vitamin A deficiency (Bitot spot) 12. Vitamin D deficiency (Rickets) 13. Severe acute malnutrition 14. Goiter
C. Childhood Diseases 15. Skin conditions (scabies, fungal infection and eczema) 16. Otitis media 17. Rheumatic heart disease 18. Reactive airway disease 19. Dental caries 20. Convulsive disorders	**D. Developmental delays** 21. Vision impairment 22. Hearing impairment 23. Neuromotor impairment 24. Motor delay 25. Cognitive delay 26. Language delay 27. Behavior disorder (autism) 28. Learning disorder 29. Attention deficit hyperactivity disorder 30. Congenital Hypothyroidism, Sickle cell anemia, β-thalassemia (Optional)
E. Others 31. Tuberculosis 32. Leprosy	

Health screening is done at facility level for the newborns while Accredited Social Health Activists (ASHA) undertake screening of newborn and children up to 6 weeks at home by regular visits. Besides mobile health teams at block level are responsible for screening at Anganwadi centers and government schools.

Early Management and Referral through District Early Intervention Center (DEIC): Under the program, DEIC will be established at district hospitals around the country. DEIC aims to provide referral support to children especially those aged 6 and under who have been identified with health conditions during primary screening. The goal of early intervention is to intervene early and reduce disability. Free of cost services including surgical intervention will be available to the children at DEIC. The team that will provide these services shall include pediatricians, medical officers, staff nurses, and paramedics.

Adequate referral support is a mandate for DEIC and mapping of tertiary care facilities at government institutions will be done by manager engaged specifically for RBSK program. NHM funds will be allocated for management at such facilities with rates determined by state governments in consultation with the Ministry of Health and Family Welfare.

A brief outline of the activities performed at DEIC is given below:
- Providing referral services to referred children to confirm diagnosis and treatment.
- Screening children at the "District Early Intervention Center".
- Visit all infants delivered at the district hospital, including those admitted in SNCU, postnatal, and children wards, and to test all newborns for hearing, vision, and congenital heart problems before discharge.
- Ensure that every child born sick, preterm, with low birth weight, or with any birth defect is followed up by the DEIC.

	• All referrals for developmental delays are followed and records maintained. • The DEIC Lab Technician would evaluate the children for inborn metabolic errors and other illnesses at the district level, depending on logistics and local epidemiological factors. • Ensure collaboration with other tertiary care facilities through agreed MOU. The DEIC will be the focal point of activities under RBSK, it will serve as a clearing house, and facilitate referrals. **Mobile health team:** Mobile Health Teams are formed at block level that help in screening of children below 6 years of age at Anganwadi centers and, government and government aided schools. Each block will have at least three specialized Mobile Health Teams to screen children covering all villages within the block's jurisdiction. The number of teams may vary based on the number of Anganwadi centers, remoteness of village and school enrolment. Anganwadi centers will screen children at least twice a year, while screening will be done once a year for school going children. The Mobile Health Team will have four members: two doctors (AYUSH) (one male and one female) with a bachelor's degree, one ANM/Staff Nurse, and one Pharmacist with additional skill for computer-based data management. Proper microplanning will ensure that mobile health teams perform optimally. The block will be the unit for all microplanning activities related to mobile health team. **Capacity building**: It is vital that manpower involved in Child Health Screening and Early Intervention Services are adequately trained to provide necessary information and services. Training also helps in increasing the efficiency of the program and improves performance of personnel at all levels. A 'cascading training approach' has been implemented under RBSK that aims to 'ensure free flow of skills and knowledge'. Training modules and tools will be developed in collaboration with technical support agencies and collaborative centers, and would be standardized across the program. An appropriate budget shall be provided under training overhead. Collaborative centers will be identified across different parts of the country and will coordinate, mentor, give supportive supervision, and train health workers from different cadres. **Convergence:** Under RBSK, in order to facilitate screening of children 0–6 years of age at Anganwadi centers, there is strong convergence with the Ministry of Women and Child Development whereas for screening children enrolled in government and government-aided schools, assistance of Ministry of Human Resource Development is vital. The Ministry of Social Justice and Empowerment is assisting the identified children with disabilities by sponsoring them equipment's such as hearing aids/implants. **RBSK-ECD call center:** Ministry of Health and Family Welfare (MoHFW), Early Childhood Development (ECD) initiative attempts to supplement existing initiatives by reaching out to every expectant mother and parent of every child under the age of two years via the ECD call center. These ECD Call Centers would focus on the child's first 1000 days. The ECD call center program will help parents with information and guidance on holistic nurturing of children. The knowhow offered would be credible and will help ensure the best growth of children. **Procedures and model costing for surgeries**: Public health systems cater to a large population with limited resources and therefore the government needs to build on cost-effective health interventions that provide quality care to the poor and vulnerable populations. A prerequisite of such an exercise is information regarding the nature of costs to be incurred in provision of health programs such that evidence based decisions could be taken. The National RBSK team has thus created a list of surgical procedure packages for health disorders that require interventions under the program and costing of these packages.
Activities at various level or package of services	RBSK program envisages to identify, refer and manage defects, deficiencies, diseases and developmental delays in the target group. The program focusses on early identification and early intervention in such cases. Health screening in target group is done at various levels which include: • **Facility-based screening:** This entails screening for birth abnormalities during institutional deliveries at public health institutions, particularly at specified delivery points by ANMs, Medical Officers, and Gynecologists. Health service providers at these facilities are to be trained to identify, report, and refer birth abnormalities to District Early Intervention Centers at District Hospitals. • **Community-based newborn screening (age 0–6 weeks) for birth defects at home:** During home visits for newborn care, ASHAs screens babies up to 6 weeks old for gross birth defects; both born at home and in institutions, through the use of basic tools. ASHAs also encourage caregivers of children to visit local Anganwadi centers for screening by the dedicated Mobile Health Team at specified intervals. ASHAs will specifically mobilize the children with low birth weight, underweight and children from households known to have any chronic illness (e.g., tuberculosis, HIV, hemoglobinopathy, etc.) to the mobile health teams.

	• **Anganwadi center screening:** Dedicated mobile health teams will visit anganwadi centers at least twice a year wherein they would screen preschoolers (6 weeks–6 years) for deficiencies, diseases, developmental delays including disability. The screening tool for children aged 0–6 years includes visual aids for identifying developmental deficits. Children with developmental delays will be assessed using age-appropriate tests and referred to DEIC for further management. • **Screening at government and government-aided schools:** The block will serve as a hub for screening children aged 6–18 in government and government-aided schools. Mobile Health teams will screen school children for deficiencies, illnesses, developmental delays (including disability), and adolescent health at local schools at least once annually. The method for screening includes the use of questionnaire (ideally translated into a local or regional language) and clinical examination. • **District early intervention center:** It is established at the district hospital and aims to provide referral support for children with health issues identified during screening, including confirmation of diagnosis and treatment. In addition, DEIC will also help in screening of children, ensure that all newborns delivered at the district hospital are visited and screened, maintain records, etc.
Monitoring and evaluation of program	Monitoring of the program is done at four levels. The overall responsibility for monitoring of the program at national level lies with the Child Health Division, MoHFW, Government of India. At State, District and Block levels; nodal officers are designated, who are responsible for overseeing the program (*see* below diagram). 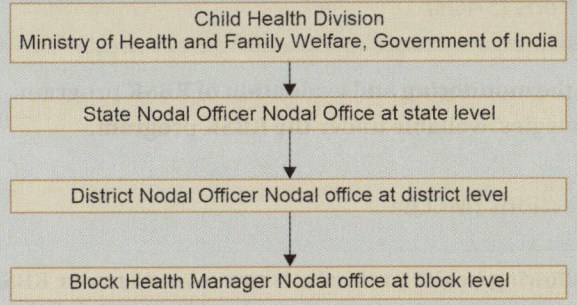 • Under RBSK, block will be the center of all activities including Child Health Screening and Early Intervention Services. • The Block Health Manager will help the CHC Medical Officer in monitoring and supervision of the program. • At the block level, it is mandatory for all healthcare stakeholders (Block Health Teams) to fill out the "Child Health Screening Card" for each child examined during the visit. • To prevent duplication and to increase the coherence in purpose, same screening card needs to be filled at all healthcare levels while examining the newborn/child, in case of any referral. These children are additionally provided unique identification numbers through the Mother and Child Tracking System (MCTS). The Mobile Block Health Teams at block level are also required to maintain a "Health Camp Register". • Birth abnormalities found by ASHAs during home visits as well as all children detected with abnormalities, need to be referred to the District Hospital/District Early Intervention Center or for further care. They can also be referred to an identified tertiary level healthcare facility. • At the district level, Early Intervention Center apart from managing the cases will also be responsible for conducting screenings, and maintaining a "DEIC Register". • A Monthly Reporting Form has been designed which needs to be filled by mobile health teams and healthcare workers posted at District Early Intervention Centers, especially from centers where deliveries also take place. Thereafter every month, the Block Health Manager, the District Nodal Officer, and the State Nodal Officer will collate and compile data from these monthly reporting format. • Compiled data would be sent on a monthly basis to the Child Health Division, Ministry of Health and Family Welfare by the State Nodal Officer. This data will be used for monitoring of the program.

Reference

1. National Health Mission, Ministry of Health and Family Welfare (MoHFW). RBSK Operational Guidelines. New Delhi: MoHFW, 2013; p. 43.

QUESTIONS

Long Answer Question (LAQ)

1. Describe in detail about the RBSK program and critically analyze its effect in lowering the child mortality in India.

Short Answer Questions (SAQs)

1. Briefly discuss the monitoring and evaluation of RBSK program.
2. Discuss the strategies available under the RBSK program.

Multiple Choice Questions (MCQs)

1. Which of the following health problems is not covered under RBSK?
   a. Rubella
   b. Vitamin A deficiency
   c. Vision impairment
   d. Developmental delay
2. Which of the following places is the hub of activity under RBSK?
   a. State
   b. District
   c. Block
   d. Anganwadi
3. All of the following are included under RBSK, *except:*
   a. Developmental delay
   b. Deficiencies
   c. Diseases
   d. Defects at 1 year of age

Answers

1. a
2. c
3. c

29 CHAPTER

Universal Immunization Programme and Mission Indradhanush

Mital Rathod, Parul Sharma, Shaili Vyas, Kajal Srivastava

Background	The Universal Immunization Programme (UIP) is one of the largest public health initiatives in the world, aimed at protecting children and pregnant women from preventable diseases through vaccination.
Need of the program/Scheme	• **Established in 1985:** The Universal Immunization Programme (UIP) was launched by the Government of India as one of the largest public health initiatives globally. • **Wide coverage:** Annually reaches over 26 million infants and 30 million pregnant women. • **Primary goals:** Aims to reduce morbidity and mortality from vaccine-preventable diseases (VPDs) such as polio, tuberculosis (TB), and measles. • **Impact and achievements:** Increased vaccine coverage, decreased VPD-related deaths, and improved overall public health. • **Ongoing challenges:** Continues to face issues with diseases like measles, TB, and pneumonia, highlighting the need for UIP's sustained efforts.
Implemented since	The UIP was launched in 1985, evolving from the Expanded Programme on Immunization (EPI) started in 1978.
Key milestones	• **1978: Expanded Programme on Immunization (EPI):** Launched with the aim to reduce morbidity, mortality, and disability from six vaccine-preventable diseases (Diphtheria, Pertussis, Tetanus, Poliomyelitis, Tuberculosis, and Measles). • **1985: Universal Immunization Programme (UIP):** EPI was renamed as UIP and expanded to cover all districts in the country. • **1995: Pulse Polio Immunization (PPI):** Launched to eradicate poliomyelitis (polio) through large-scale immunization campaigns. • **2002-2003: Introduction of Hepatitis B vaccine:** Gradual introduction of the hepatitis B vaccine in select states and subsequently expanded nationwide. • **2006: Introduction of second dose of measles vaccine:** Measles vaccination schedule was modified to include a second dose for better coverage and immunity. • **2009: Japanese Encephalitis vaccine:** Introduction of the vaccine in high-risk districts. • **2010:** Introduction of the **pentavalent vaccine (DPT+HepB+Hib)** in a phased approach. • **2014: Mission Indradhanush:** Launched to reach unvaccinated and partially vaccinated children and pregnant women in 201 high-focus districts. • **2016: Introduction of rotavirus vaccine:** Introduction of the Rotavirus vaccine to combat Rotavirus-induced diarrhea. • **2017: Pneumococcal conjugate vaccine (PCV):** Introduction of the PCV to prevent pneumococcal diseases. • **2018: Measles-Rubella (MR) vaccine campaign:** National campaign to introduce the combined MR vaccine to eliminate measles and control rubella. • **2019: Intensified Mission Indradhanush (IMI) 2.0:** Launched to cover left-out and drop-out children and pregnant women from routine immunization. • **2020: Introduction of Pneumococcal conjugate vaccine (PCV) nationwide:** Expanded nationwide to protect children against pneumonia and other pneumococcal diseases.

	- **2021: COVID-19 vaccination campaign:** Launched the largest COVID-19 vaccination drive targeting the adult population and later expanded to include adolescents. - **2022: Human Papilloma virus (HPV) vaccine introduction:** Plans to introduce the HPV vaccine for the prevention of cervical cancer.[1,2]
Goal	To achieve universal immunization coverage by providing free vaccines against VPDs to all children and pregnant women.
Targets	- Achieve and maintain 90% immunization coverage at the national level. - Reduce morbidity and mortality from VPDs.
Objectives	- To rapidly increase immunization coverage. - To improve the quality of services. - To establish a dependable cold chain system - Monitoring of performance. - To achieve self-sufficiency in vaccine production.[1]
Organogram	- **National level:** The Ministry of Health and Family Welfare (MoHFW) manages the UIP with guidance from the National Technical Advisory Group on Immunization (NTAGI). - **State level:** State Immunization Officers (SIOs) manage implementation. - **District level:** District Immunization Officers (DIOs) coordinate activities. - **Peripheral level:** Primary health centers (PHCs), community health centers (CHCs), and sub-centers deliver vaccination services.
Beneficiaries	- **Children:** All children under the age of 5 years. - **Pregnant women:** Pregnant women for tetanus and diphtheria vaccines. - **Adolescents:** Age group 10–19 years.
Components	- **Vaccines provided:** BCG, OPV, DPT, dT hepatitis B, Pentavalent, MR, Japanese Encephalitis, Rotavirus, PCV, and IPV. - **Supply chain:** Effective logistics management to ensure timely delivery and availability of vaccines. - **Cold chain management:** Maintenance of the vaccine cold chain to ensure potency.
Monitoring and Evaluation	- **Full Immunization Coverage:** Achieve and sustain 90% full immunization coverage in all districts by 2020, and work towards 100% coverage in subsequent years. - **Reducing dropouts and left-outs:** Identify and reduce the number of children and pregnant women who miss out on vaccinations through initiatives like Mission Indradhanush and Intensified Mission Indradhanush (IMI).
Strategies/ Deliverables under the program	- **Routine immunization:** Regular immunization sessions in urban and rural areas. - **Supplementary Immunization Activities (SIAs):** Special campaigns such as National Immunization Days (NIDs) for polio. - **Intensified Mission Indradhanush (IMI):** Targeting low-coverage areas to improve immunization coverage. - **Vaccine Logistics Management System (VLMS):** Monitoring vaccine stocks and distribution.

Strategies	- **Service delivery enhancement:**
	  + *Fixed, outreach, and mobile sessions:* Conducting regular immunization sessions in health facilities, community settings, and through mobile units to reach all populations, including those in hard-to-reach areas.
	  + *Integration with other health services:* Combining immunization with other maternal and child health services to ensure comprehensive care.
	- **Cold chain and logistics management:**
	  + *Strengthening cold chain infrastructure:* Upgrading and maintaining cold chain equipment to ensure the safe storage and transportation of vaccines.
	  + *Electronic vaccine intelligence network (eVIN):* Implementing eVIN for real-time monitoring of vaccine stocks and temperatures.
	- **Capacity building:**
	  + *Training of health workers:* Regular training and refresher courses for health workers on immunization practices, cold chain management, and AEFI surveillance.
	  + *Supportive supervision:* Conducting field visits and providing on-the-job training to enhance the performance and skills of health workers.

	• **Community engagement and social mobilization:**
	  ✦ *Awareness campaigns:* Running campaigns to educate the public about the importance of immunization and address vaccine hesitancy.
	  ✦ *Involvement of community leaders:* Engaging community leaders and influencers to promote immunization and increase coverage.
	• **Monitoring and evaluation:**
	  ✦ *Routine data collection and analysis:* Using HMIS and other systems to track immunization coverage, identify gaps, and take corrective actions.
	  ✦ *Periodic surveys and assessments:* Conducting surveys like NFHS and DLHS to evaluate progress and impact.
	• **Adverse Event Following Immunization (AEFI) Management:** *AEFI Surveillance:* Establishing a robust system for reporting, investigating, and managing AEFIs to ensure vaccine safety.[3]

Monitoring and Evaluation of program	• **Coverage Evaluation Surveys (CES):** Conduct periodic surveys to assess immunization coverage. • **District Level Monitoring (DLM):** Implement regular monitoring at the district level. • **Electronic Vaccine Intelligence Network (eVIN):** Provide real-time monitoring of vaccine stocks and temperatures..
Achievements of India's Universal Immunization Programme (UIP)	• Elimination of smallpox in 1977 • Elimination of polio in 2014, with the last recorded case of wild poliovirus in 2011 • Elimination of maternal and neonatal tetanus in 2015 • Successful completion of the Measles-Rubella vaccination campaign in 34 states/UTs, vaccinating 32.43 crore children as of 2024[6]

Electronic Vaccine Intelligence Network (eVIN) and Universal Vaccine Intelligence Network (uVIN): The Electronic Vaccine Intelligence Network (eVIN) and the Universal Vaccine Intelligence Network (uVIN) are digital platforms developed to enhance vaccine logistics, monitoring, and management in India which aim to ensure vaccine availability, reduced wastage, and improve immunization coverage through real-time data tracking.[4]

ELECTRONIC VACCINE INTELLIGENCE NETWORK (EVIN)

eVIN is a technology-driven initiative launched by the Ministry of Health and Family Welfare (MoHFW), Government of India, with technical support from the United Nations Development Programme (UNDP). It focuses on strengthening the supply chain of vaccines by providing real-time data on vaccine stocks, storage temperature, and distribution across the country.

Key Features of eVIN

- Real-time tracking of vaccine stocks and flows through a mobile-based application.
- Continuous temperature monitoring of vaccine storage through digital sensors.
- Data-driven decision-making for efficient vaccine distribution.
- Reduction in vaccine stock-outs and overstocking at health centers.
- Enhanced accountability and transparency in the immunization supply chain.

Impact of eVIN

- Implemented across all states and union territories in India.
- Reduced vaccine stock-outs from 30% to less than 5% in many regions.
- Improved vaccine utilization and minimized wastage.

UNIVERSAL VACCINE INTELLIGENCE NETWORK (uVIN)

uVIN is an advanced expansion of eVIN, developed to cover all vaccines beyond the Universal Immunization Programme (UIP). This includes adult vaccines, COVID-19 vaccines, and other new immunization initiatives.

Key Features of uVIN

- Covers a broader spectrum of vaccines beyond childhood immunization.
- Integrates vaccine tracking with CoWIN for enhanced COVID-19 vaccine management.

- ❖ Strengthens the digital ecosystem for immunization logistics and monitoring.
- ❖ Facilitates real-time tracking of vaccine supply across both government and private healthcare facilities.

Significance of uVIN
- ❖ Ensures seamless vaccine supply for all population groups.
- ❖ Enhances efficiency in the procurement, distribution, and monitoring of vaccines nationwide.
- ❖ Contributes to India's goal of achieving universal vaccination coverage.

Conclusion

Both eVIN and uVIN represent significant advancements in India's vaccine management infrastructure. By leveraging digital technology, these initiatives ensure the availability and quality of vaccines, ultimately strengthening the country's immunization programs.

Adverse Event Following Immunization (AEFI):[5,6]

Adverse Event Following Immunization (AEFI) refers to any unexpected health issue after vaccination, which may or may not be linked to the vaccine. It can be minor, severe, or serious, requiring proper classification and management.

Types of AEFI:
- ❖ Vaccine reaction—expected side effects (e.g., fever, swelling, and anaphylaxis).
- ❖ Immunization error-related reaction—due to mistakes in handling or giving the vaccine.
- ❖ Immunization anxiety-related reaction—fear-based response (e.g., fainting, dizziness).
- ❖ Coincidental event—unrelated health issues happening after vaccination.
- ❖ Unknown/Indeterminate—when the cause is unclear.

Brief Management

Mild cases (e.g., fever, pain) need simple treatment, such as paracetamol or cold compresses. Severe cases (e.g., anaphylaxis) need emergency care with adrenaline. Proper vaccine handling, trained staff, and AEFI tracking help reduce risks.

References

1. Ministry of Health and Family Welfare, Government of India. Ministry of Health and Family Welfare Universal Immunization Programme [Internet]. [cited 2024 Jul 18]. Available from: https://www.mohfw.gov.in/.
2. World Health Organization (WHO) India. WHO India [Internet]. [cited 2024 Jul 18]. Available from: https://www.who.int/india/health-topics/immunization.
3. National Health Portal of India. National Health Portal [Internet]. [cited 2024 Jul 18]. Available from: https://www.nhp.gov.in/.
4. UNICEF India. UNICEF India [Internet]. [cited 2024 Jul 18]. Available from: https://www.unicef.org/india/what-we-do/immunization.
5. Ministry of Health and Family Welfare, Government of India. AEFI Surveillance & Response Operational Guidelines – 2024. New Delhi: MoHFW; 2024.
6. Immunization Technical Support Unit, Ministry of Health and Family Welfare. Adverse Events Following Immunization (AEFI) Secretariat. New Delhi: ITSU; 2022.

QUESTIONS

Long Answer Question (LAQ)

1. Discuss the objectives, components and significance of UIP in India. How has introduction of newer vaccines contributed to reducing childhood morbidity and mortality?

Short Answer Questions (SAQs)

1. Discuss the importance of cold chain system in success of UIP.
2. Enlist the key challenges faced by UIP in urban slums and hard to reach rural areas.
3. Discuss the key features of eVIN and uVIN.

Multiple Choice Questions (MCQs)

1. UIP aims to provide vaccination to which age group?
   a. Adults
   b. Children under 5 years
   c. Adolescents
   d. Children and pregnant women
2. Which of following vaccine is administered at birth under UIP?
   a. DPT
   b. Hepatitis B
   c. Rotavirus
   d. Measles

Answers

1. d
2. b

CHAPTER 30

Integrated Management of Neonatal and Childhood Illnesses

Ankit Yadav, Shaili Vyas, Gneya Bhatt

Background/Need of program/Scheme	

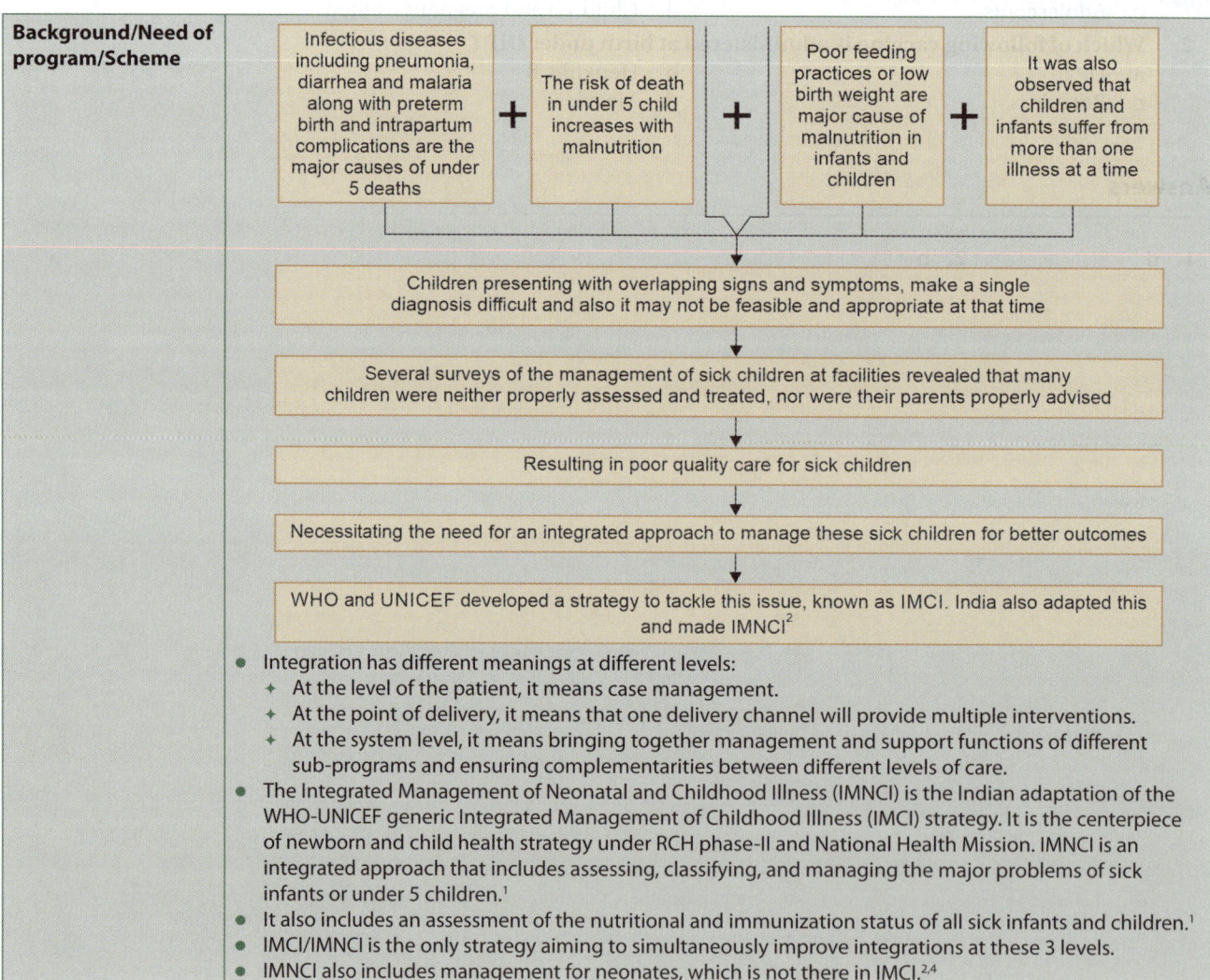

- Integration has different meanings at different levels:
  - At the level of the patient, it means case management.
  - At the point of delivery, it means that one delivery channel will provide multiple interventions.
  - At the system level, it means bringing together management and support functions of different sub-programs and ensuring complementarities between different levels of care.
- The Integrated Management of Neonatal and Childhood Illness (IMNCI) is the Indian adaptation of the WHO-UNICEF generic Integrated Management of Childhood Illness (IMCI) strategy. It is the centerpiece of newborn and child health strategy under RCH phase-II and National Health Mission. IMNCI is an integrated approach that includes assessing, classifying, and managing the major problems of sick infants or under 5 children.[1]
- It also includes an assessment of the nutritional and immunization status of all sick infants and children.[1]
- IMCI/IMNCI is the only strategy aiming to simultaneously improve integrations at these 3 levels.
- IMNCI also includes management for neonates, which is not there in IMCI.[2,4]

Chapter 30: Integrated Management of Neonatal and Childhood Illnesses

Implemented since	2003
Goal[4]	To reduce mortality, frequency and severity of illness and disability and to improve the growth and development of children

Objectives[4,6]	Implementation of IMNCI package
	• At the level of household
	• At the level of sub-center, through ANMs and
	• At the level of PHC, through medical officers, nurses, and lady health visitors (LHV).
	The objectives of training courses are:
	
	• *To train the health workers in technical skills*
	   ✦ Provide home care to young infants
	   ✦ Early referral of seriously ill children and young infants
	   ✦ Treating children with pneumonia and young infants with local bacterial infection; and
	   ✦ Treating children with dehydration by ORS solution
	
	• *To train the health worker in communication skills* Advising the mother on:
	   ✦ Keeping young infants warm
	   ✦ Feeding of infants and children
	   ✦ Development support care
	   ✦ Relieving cough by home remedies
	   ✦ Giving fluids during diarrhea
	   ✦ Observing child for danger/warning signs for follow-up and timely consultation

Beneficiaries[2,3,5]	• Sick infant up to the age of 2 months • Sick child from 2 months age to 5 years

Components[6]	The strategy includes three main components:
	1. Improvements in the case-management skills of health staff through the provision of locally-adapted IMNCI guidelines and activities to promote their use;
	2. Improvements in the overall health system for effective management of childhood illness;
	3. Improvements in family and community health care practices by:
	   • IEC campaign
	   • Promoting healthy behavior
	   • Providing counseling to caregivers and family
	   • By home visits.

Strategies/ Deliverables under the program[5]	**Introduction of color-coded chart booklets:** • Color-coded booklet has 4 columns are: 1. **Assess:** What symptoms and signs are to be checked and how to elicit them? 2. **Signs:** Summarizes the signs and symptoms present. 3. Helps in classifying each illness in the young infant or under 5 children. 4. **Identifying treatment:** Lists appropriate treatment decisions for each classification. • Assess and classify sections are organized in 3 different color codes (Pink, Yellow, Green) **Assess and classify** **Pink** — Indicate severe illness. Must be referred to a hospital or sent to doctor after giving pre-referral treatment **Yellow** — Should be treated with medicine at home. Home care advice (given) or (provided) to mother **Green** — Treated with home care without the use of medicines

158 Section III: National Health Mission

- Highlight of IMNCI (details is in Annexure):

OUT-PATIENT HEALTH FACILITY

Check for danger signs
- Convulsions
- Lethargy/unconsciousness
- Inability to drink/breastfeed
- Vomiting

↓

Assess signs and symptoms

Infant upto age of 2 months
- Check for bacterial infection/Jaundice
- Diarrhea
- Feeding problem and very low weight

Child aged 2 month to 5 years
- Cough or difficult breathing
- Diarrhea
- Fever
- Malnutrition
- Anemia

↓

Assess nutrition and immunization and potential feeding problem

↓

Check for other problems

↓

Classify conditions and identify treatment actions

Pink	Yellow	Green
Out-patient health facility • Pre-referral treatment • Advise parents • Refer child	**Treatment at OPD facility** • Give oral drugs • Advise and teach caretaker • Follow-up	**Home management** Home caretaker is counselled on how to • Give oral drugs • Treat local infections at home • Continue feeding • When to return immediately • Follow-up

- Classification and treatment are below for all conditions (sick infant up to the age of 2 months)
  - Possible bacterial Infection

Signs	Classify as	Identify treatment (urgent pre-referral treatments are in bold print)
Anyone or more of the following signs: • Fast breathing (60 or more breaths/min or more) or • Not able to feed at all or not feeding well or • Severe chest indrawing or • Movement only when stimulated or no movement at all • Convulsions or • Axillary temperature less than 35.5°C/95.9°F (or feels cold to touch) or • Axillary temperature 37.5°C/99.5°F or above (or feels hot to touch) or	Possible serious bacterial infection	• Treat to prevent low blood sugar. • Give first dose of oral amoxicillin and intramuscular gentamicin. • Advise the mother how to keep the young infant warm on the way to the hospital. • **Refer urgently** to hospital

Chapter 30: Integrated Management of Neonatal and Childhood Illnesses

Signs	Classify as	Identify treatment (Urgent pre-referral treatments are in bold print)
Anyone or more of the following signs: • Umbilicus red or draining pus or • Skin pustules	Local bacterial infection	• **Give oral amoxicillin for 5 days** • Advise the mother to give home care to the young infant • Teach the mother how to treat local infections at home • Advise the mother when to return immediately • Follow up after 2 days
• No signs of bacterial infections	Infection unlikely	• Advise the mother to give home care to the young infant

✦ Jaundice

Signs	Classify as	Identify treatment (Urgent pre-referral treatments are in bold print)
• Any jaundice in an infant aged less than 24 hours or • Yellow palms or soles	Severe jaundice	• Treat to prevent low blood sugar • Advise mother how to keep baby warm on the way to the hospital • **Refer urgently** to hospital
• Jaundice appearing after 24 hours of age and • Palms and soles not yellow	Jaundice	• Advise the mother to return immediately if the infant's palm or soles appear yellow • Advise the mother to give home care for young infants • If the infant is older than 2 weeks, refer to a hospital for assessment • Follow up after 2 days
• No jaundice	No jaundice	• Advise the mother to give home care to the young infant

✦ Diarrhea

Signs	Classify as	Identify treatment (urgent pre-referral treatments are in bold print)
Two of the following signs: • Sunken eyes • Movements only when stimulated or no movement at all • Skin pinch goes back very slowly	Severe dehydration	• **Give first dose of oral amoxicillin and intramuscular gentamicin.** • **Refer urgently to hospital** with the mother giving frequent sips of ORS on the way. • Advise the mother how to keep the young infant warm on the way to the hospital. • Advise the mother to continue breastfeeding.
Two of the following signs: • Sunken eyes • Restless, irritable • Skin pinch goes back slowly	Some dehydration	
• Not enough signs to classify as some or severe dehydration	No dehydration	• Advise mother when to return immediately • Give fluids and breastfeeds to treat diarrhea at home treatment of diarrhea at home is known as Plan A. **Plan A:** Teach the mother how to mix and give ORS. Give the mother 2 packets of ORS to use at home. Show the mother how much fluid to give in addition to the usual fluid intake: • <2 months—5 spoons after each loose stool. • 2 months up to 2 years—1/4 cup to 1/2 cup after each loose stool. • 2 years or more—1/2 cup to 1 cup after each loose stool. Tell the mother to: • Give frequent small sips from a cup. • If the infant vomits, wait 10 minutes. Then continue, but more slowly. • Continue giving extra fluid until the diarrhea stops. • Follow-up up after 2 days if no improvement

✦ Feeding problem or low weight for age

Signs	Classify as	Identify treatment (urgent pre-referral treatments are in bold print)
• Weight for age less than 3SD in infants 7–59 days old (**red on MCP card**) • Weight <1800 g in infants less than 7 days	Very low weight	• **Refer urgently to hospital** • **Warm the young infant by skin-to-skin contact if temperature less than 36.5°C/97.7°F (or feels cold to touch) while arranging referral** • **Treat to prevent low blood sugar** • Advise mother how to keep the young infant warm on the way to hospital.

• Not suckling effectively or
• Not well attached to breast or
• Receives other foods or drinks or
• Less than 8 breastfeeds in 24 hours or
• Low weight for age (weight between 1800-2500 g or weight for age **yellow on MCP card**, i.e., <-2SD) or
• Thrush (ulcers or white patches in mouth) or
• Breast or nipple problems
	Feeding problem and/or low weight	• If not well attached or not suckling effectively, teach correct positioning and attachment.
		• If breastfeeding less than 8 times in 24 hours, advise to increase frequency of breastfeeding.
		• If receiving other foods or drinks, counsel the mother about breastfeeding more, reducing other foods or drinks.
		• If not breastfeeding at all
		  ✦ Refer for breastfeeding counseling and relactation.
		  ✦ Advise mother about giving locally appropriate
		  ✦ Animal milk and teach the mother to feed with a cup and spoon
		• If low weight for age:
		  ✦ Teach the mother how to keep the young infant warm at home.
		  ✦ Advise to increase frequency of breastfeeding
		• If thrush, teach the mother to treat thrush at home.
		• If breast or nipple problem, teach the mother to treat breast or nipple problems.
		• Advise mother when to return immediately
		• Advise mother to give home care to the young infant
		• Follow-up low weight for age after 14 days
		• Follow-up any feeding problem or thrush after 2 days.

• Not low weight for age >-2SD (**green on MCP card**) and no other signs of inadequate feeding.	No feeding problem	• Praise the mother for feeding the infant well. • Advise mother when to return immediately. • Advise mother to give home care to the young infant.

- Classification and treatment is below for all conditions (from 2 month to 5 years)
  ✦ Cough or difficult breathing

Signs	Classify as	Identify treatment (urgent pre-referral treatments are in bold print)
• Oxygen saturation <90% • Chest indrawing or • General danger signs (inability to breastfeed or drink, lethargy or unconsciousness, persistent vomiting) or	Severe pneumonia or very severe disease	• **Give pre-referral dose of oral amoxicillin and IM gentamicin** • **Refer urgently to hospital**.

Chapter 30: Integrated Management of Neonatal and Childhood Illnesses

• Fast breathing respiratory rate:
   + 2–11 months ≥50/min
   + 12–59 months ≥40/min
	Pneumonia	• Advise home care for cough and cold.
		• **Give amoxicillin for 5 days**.
		• Follow-up after 2 days.

• No signs of severe pneumonia or pneumonia	No pneumonia, cough or cold	• If coughing for more than 14 days, refer for assessment. • Advise home care for cough and cold. • Follow up after 5 days, if not improving

+ Diarrhea

Signs	Classify as	Identify treatment (urgent pre-referral treatments are in bold print)
Two of the following signs: • Not able to drink or drinking poorly • Sunken eyes • Lethargic or unconscious • Skin pinch goes back very slowly	Severe dehydration	• **Refer urgently to hospital** with mother giving frequent sips of ORS on the way. • Advise the mother to continue breastfeeding

Two of the following signs:
• Sunken eyes
• Restless, irritable
• Skin pinch goes back slowly
• Drinks eagerly, thirsty
	Some dehydration	• Give fluid, zinc supplements and food for some dehydration (Plan B).
		   + The child with diarrhea of less than 14 days duration who has signs of some dehydration should be treated under your supervision with ORS for 4 hours. For this, keep the mother and child under observation, either at the health center or at the home of the child.
		   + Ask the mother to give one teaspoon of the solution to the child. This should be repeated every 1–2 minutes (An older child who can drink it in sips should be given one sip every 1–2 minutes). If the child vomits the ORS tell the mother to wait for 10 minutes and resume giving the ORS but this time more slowly than before.
		   + Breastfed babies should be continued to be given breast milk in between ORS. Any ORS which is left over after 24 hours should be thrown away. If the child wants more ORS than shown, give more.
		   + The approximate amount of ORS required (in mL) can also be calculated by multiplying the child's weight (in kg) times 75.
		• Advice when to return immediately.
		• Follow-up after 2 days if not improving.

• Not enough signs to classify as some or severe dehydration.	No dehydration	• Give fluid, zinc supplements and food to treat diarrhea at home treatment of diarrhea at home is known as Plan A.
		• Teach the mother how to mix and give ORS. Give the mother 2 packets of ORS to use at home. Show the mother how much fluid to give in addition to the usual fluid intake:
		   + <2 months—5 spoons after each loose stool.
		   + 2 months up to 2 years—1/4 cup to 1/2 cup after each loose stool.

| | | ◆ 2 years or more—1/2 cup to 1 cup after each loose stool. Tell the mother to:
• Give frequent small sips from a cup.
• If the infant vomits, wait 10 minutes. Then continue, but more slowly.
• Continue giving extra fluid until the diarrhea stops.
• Advice when to return immediately
• Follow-up after 5 days if not improving. |

◆ **Fever**

Signs	Classify as	Identify treatment (urgent pre-referral treatments are in bold print)
• Any general danger sign or • Stiff neck	Very severe febrile disease	• **Give first dose of oral amoxicillin and IM gentamicin** • **Treat the child to prevent low blood sugar** • Give one dose of paracetamol for high fever (temp. 38.5°C/101.3°F or above). • **Refer urgently to hospital**
• Positive RDT or • RDT not available and no other obvious cause of fever	Malaria/ suspected malaria	• **Give oral antimalarial as per national guidelines after making a smear** • Give one dose of paracetamol in clinic for high fever (temp. 38.5°C/101.3°F* or above). • Advise mother when to return immediately. • Follow-up after 2 days
• Negative RDT and/or other causes of fever PRESENT**	Fever- malaria unlikely	• Give one dose of paracetamol in clinic for high fever (temp. 38.5°C/101.3°F or above) • Give appropriate treatment for an identified cause of fever • Advise mother when to return immediately • Follow-up after 2 days if fever persists • If fever is present every day for more than 7 days, refer for assessment

*This cut-off is for axillary temperature
**Other causes of fever include no pneumonia: cough or cold, pneumonia, diarrhea, dysentery, skin infections, dengue, and measles

◆ **Malnutrition**

Signs	Classify as	Identify treatment (urgent pre-referral treatments are in bold print)
• MUAC <11.5 cm and/or • WFL <-3 SD score (**red color on MCP card**)* and/or • Edema of both feet	Severe acute malnutrition	• Treat the child to prevent low blood sugar. • Give **first dose of oral amoxicillin and IM gentamicin** • Refer **urgently to hospital** • Keep the child warm on the way to hospital.
• WFL <-2 SD score (yellow color on MCP card) and/or • MUAC 11.5–12.4 cm and • No edema of both feet	Moderate acute malnutrition	• Advise mother when to return immediately • Assess feeding and counsel the mother on how to feed the child • Follow-up after 30 days

Chapter 30: Integrated Management of Neonatal and Childhood Illnesses

• MUAC ≥ 12.5 cm and • WFL ≥ -2SD score and • No edema of both feet	No acute malnutrition	• If child is less than 2 years old, assess the child's feeding and counsel the mother on feeding according to the food box on the counsel the mother chart. • Advise mother when to return immediately. • If feeding problem, follow-up in 5 days.

*Look for visible severe wasting if unable to measure length/height. Classify severe acute malnutrition in the presence of visible severe wasting.

✦ Anemia

Signs	Classify as	Identify treatment (urgent pre-referral treatments are in bold print)
• Severe palmar pallor	Severe anemia	• **Refer urgently to hospital**
• Some palmar pallor	Anemia	• Give iron folic acid therapy for 14 days. • Assess the child's feeding and counsel the mother on feeding. If feeding problem, follow-up after 5 days. • Follow-up after 14 days.
• No palmar pallor	No anemia	• Give prophylactic iron folic acid if child is 6 months or older.

There are 2 types of training of manpower/personnel under IMNCI:

Type of training	Personnel to be trained	Duration	Package to be used	Place of training
Clinical skills training	Medical Officer and Pediatricians	8 days	Physicians Package	Medical college/District hospital
	Health Workers, ANMs, LHVs, Mukhya Sevikas, CDPO's and AWWs	8 days	Health Workers Package	District hospital
Supervisory skills training	Medical Officers, Pediatricians, CDPO's LHVs and Mukhya Sevikas	2 days*	Supervisory Skills package	Medical college/District hospital

*It is to be clubbed, preferably with clinical skill training. If it is not possible, then 2 days of training should be conducted within 4-6 weeks of clinical skill training.

Package of services[5]

There are 2 parts of this course/training module and services are given according to them:
1. Management of sick young infants aged up to 2 months (0 to 59 days old)
2. Management of sick children aged 2 months to 5 years (2 months to 59 months)

Young infants up to 2 months
- Assessment for General Danger Signs.
- Assess and classify young infants for possible serious bacterial infection/jaundice.
- Assess and classify for feeding problem and low birth weight.
- Assess for diarrhea.
- Assess and classify the young infant's immunization status.
- Assess the mother/caregiver's development supportive practices and counsel the mother/caregivers for practices to support child's development using MCP card.
- Assess other problems.
- Provide treatment and refer when required.
- Counsel the mother about her own health.
- Advise mother on home care to young infants.
- Correct breastfeeding problems.
- Follow up care.

	For sick child aged 2 months to 5 years • Assessment for General Danger Signs. • Assess major symptoms (Cough/Diarrhea/Fever). • Check for immunization, prophylactic vitamin A and iron-folic acid supplementation status. • Check for malnutrition and anemia. • Assess feeding if age is less than 2 years/has uncomplicated severe/moderate acute malnutrition or anemia. • Assess the mother/caregiver's development supportive practices if less than 3 years/has uncomplicated severe acute malnutrition or anemia. • Assess other problems. • Counsel for feeding and development of supportive practices. • Provide treatment and refer when required • Follow-up care

Monitoring and evaluation of program[8]	• Impact indicators for evaluating child health status:
	   ✦ NMR, IMR, U5MR
	   ✦ Prevalence of wasting, stunting and underweight
	• Coverage indicators for tracking progress:
	   ✦ Proportion of health workers who have received IMNCI training
	   ✦ Proportion of medical officers who have received IMNCI training
	   ✦ Proportion of births assisted by skilled health personnel
	   ✦ Proportion of infants less than 12 months of age with breastfeeding initiated within one hour of birth
	   ✦ Proportion of infants less than six months of age exclusively breastfed
	   ✦ Proportion of infants 6–8 months old receiving appropriate complementary feeding
	   ✦ Proportion of children 6-59 months old who have received vitamin A in the past six months
	   ✦ Proportion of children from 0 to 59 months of age who slept under insecticide-treated nets (ITNs) the previous night
	   ✦ Proportion of children from 0 to 59 months old who had suspected pneumonia in the past two weeks and were taken to an appropriate provider
	   ✦ Proportion of children from 0 to 59 months old who had suspected pneumonia in the past two weeks and received appropriate antibiotics
	   ✦ Proportion of children from 0 to 59 months old who had diarrhea in the past two weeks and were treated with oral rehydration therapy (ORT)
	   ✦ Proportion of children from 0 to 59 months old who had diarrhea in the past two weeks and were treated with an appropriate course of zinc
	   ✦ Proportion of children from 0 to 59 months old who had confirmed malaria and were treated with appropriate antimalarial drugs
	   ✦ Proportion of one-year-old children protected against neonatal tetanus through immunization of their mothers
	   ✦ Proportion of one-year-old children immunized against measles

Annexure (recording formats)[5,7]	**Management of sick young infant up to age of 2 months.** **ASK**: What are the infant's problems? Also ask whether this is initial visit or follow-up visit? **ASSESS** (Circle all signs present)

Check for possible bacterial infection/jaundice	
• Is the infant having difficulty in feeding?	

• Has the infant had convulsions?	• Count the breaths in 1 minute ____ breaths/min
	  Repeat if elevated ____ fast breathing?
	• Look for severe chest indrawing.
	• Measure axillary temperature (if not possible, feel for fever or low body temperature): Is it < 35.5°C/37.5°C (95.9°F/99.5°F) or above?
	• Look at young infant's movements.
	  If infant is sleeping, ask the mother to wake him/her
	    ✦ Does the infant move only when stimulated but then stops?
	    ✦ Does the infant not move at all?
	• Look at the umbilicus. Is it red or draining pus?
	• Look for skin pustules

	• Ask when did jaundice appeared—first 24 hrs/after 24 hrs	• Look for jaundice (yellow skin), if present. • Look at the young's infant palms and soles. Are they yellow?
	Does the young infant have diarrhea?	**Yes___ no___**

		• Look at the young infant's general condition
		Look at infant's movement
		  ✦ Does the infant move only when stimulated but then stops?
		  ✦ Does the infant not move at all?
		• Is the infant restless and irritable?
		• Look for sunken eyes.
		• Pinch the skin of the abdomen. Does it go back:
		  ✦ Very slowly (longer than 2 sec)?
		  ✦ Slowly?

	Then check for feeding problem and very low weight	

	• Has the infant breastfed in previous hour?
	If yes, how many times in 24 hours?
	_____ times
	
	• Does the infant usually receive any other foods or drinks? Yes ___ No___
	  ✦ If yes, how often? _____
	  ✦ What do you use to feed the infant? ___
		Yes_____ No_____
		• Measure weight
		  ✦ Is it less than 1800 g?
		  ✦ Is it 1800–2500 g?
		• Determine weight for age by plotting on MCP card
		  ✦ Red (< -3SD)
		  ✦ Yellow (< -2SD)
		  ✦ Green (≥ -3SD)
		• Look for ulcers or white patches in the mouth (thrush)

	Is there any indications for urgent referral Yes/No If no then ASSESS BREASTFEEDING	
	Assess breastfeeding	

	• Has the infant breastfed in previous hour?
	• If infant has not fed in the previous hour, ask the mother to put her infant to the breast. Observe the breastfeed for 4 minutes.
		• Check for attachment
		  ✦ Chin touching breast Yes_ No_
		  ✦ Mouth wide open Yes_ No_
		  ✦ Lower lip turned outward Yes_ No_
		  ✦ More areola above than below the mouth
		                                Yes_ No_
		• Is the infant able to attach?
		  ✦ No attachment at all
		  ✦ Not well attached
		  ✦ Good attachment
		• Is the infant suckling effectively (that is, slow deep sucks, sometimes pausing)?
		  ✦ Not suckling at all
		  ✦ Not suckling effectively
		  ✦ Suckling effectively
		• Does the mother have pain while breastfeeding?
		If yes, then look for:
		  ✦ Flat or inverted or sore nipples.

Check the young infant's immunization status (Circle immunizations needed today) Birth BCG OPV-0 HEP-0 6 Weeks PENTA-1 OPV-1 Rotavirus-1 fIPV-1 PCV-1 Return for next immunization on: Date_____	
Assess caregiver's practices to support child's development	
ASK: • How do you play with your baby? • How do you talk to your baby? • How do you get your baby smile?	• Look how does caregiver show he/she is aware of child's movement • Look how does caregiver comfort the child and show love
Assess other problems	
Advice given to mother for home care • Immediately after birth, baby should be put on the mother's abdomen for skin-to-skin contact. • Initiate breastfeeding within one hour of birth. • Breastfeed day and night as often as your baby wants, at least 8 times in 24 hours. Frequent feeding produces more milk. • If your baby is small (low birth weight), feed him or her at least every 2-3 hours. Wake the baby for feeding after 3 hours, if she or he does not wake self. • Breastfeed as often as your child wants. Look for signs of hunger, such as beginning to fuss, sucking fingers, or moving lips. • **DO NOT** give other foods or fluids. Breast milk is all your baby needs. • Make sure the young infant always stays warm. In cool weather, cover the infant's head and feet and dress the infant with extra clothing.	
• Advise mother to wash hands with soap and water after defecation and after cleaning the bottom of the baby. • Do not apply anything on the cord and keep the umbilical cord dry.	
Advise the mother to return immediately if the young infant has any of these danger signs: • Not able to drink or breastfeed • Becomes sicker • Develops a fever or feels cold to touch • Fast breathing • Difficult breathing • Yellow palms and soles (if infant have jaundice) • Blood in stool	

Chapter 30: Integrated Management of Neonatal and Childhood Illnesses

			• Counsel mother about feeding • Counsel mother about development supportive practices • Advice mother when to return immediately • Give any immunization needed today • Counsel mother about her own health • When the mother has to return for follow up
	Management of the sick child age 2 months upto 5 years **ASK:** What are the child's problems? Also ask if this is initial visit or follow up visit? **ASSESS**		
	Check for general danger signs		
	• Not able to drink or breastfeed • Vomiting everything • Has had convulsions • Lethargic or unconscious		
	Does the child have cough or difficult breathing?		**Yes__ No__**
	• For how long? _____ days • Count the breaths in 1 minute _____ breaths/min Fast breathing?		• Look for chest indrawing • Oxygen saturation <90%/>90%
	Does the child have diarrhea?		**Yes__No__**

	• For how long? _____ days
	• Is there blood in the stool? Yes/No
			• Look at the child's general condition. Is the child:
			  + Lethargic or unconscious?
			  + Restless and irritable?
			• Look for sunken eyes
			• Offer the child fluid. Is the child:
			  + Not able to drink or drinking poorly?
			  + Drinking eagerly, thirsty?
			• Pinch the skin of the abdomen. Does it go back:
			  + Very slowly (longer than 2 seconds)?
			  + Slowly?

	Does the child have fever? (by history or feels hot or temperature 37.5°C or above) Yes___ No___ Is it *Plasmodium falciparum* predominant area? Yes/No		
	• For how long? _____ days • If more than 7 days, has fever been present every day?		• Look or feel for neck stiffness • Look for any other form of fever
	Then check for malnutrition	**Weight___Kg**	**Length/Height__cm**

	• If child is 6 month or older, measure MUAC____cm		• Determine weight for height/length SD score by plotting on MCP card
			  + Red (< -3SD)
			  + Yellow (< -2SD)
			  + Green (≥ -2SD)
			• Look for edema of both feet
			• Look for visible severe wasting

	Then check for anemia		• Look for palmer pallor
			  + Severe palmar pallor
			  + Some palmer pallor
			  + No pallor

	• If child is 6 month or older, measure MUAC____cm	• Determine weight for height/length SD score by plotting on MCP card ✦ Red (< -3SD) ✦ Yellow (< -2SD) ✦ Green (≥ -2SD) • Look for edema of both feet • Look for visible severe wasting
	Then check for anemia	• Look for palmer pallor ✦ Severe palmar pallor ✦ Some palmer pallor ✦ No pallor

	Check the child's immunization <prophylactic vitamin A and iron-folic status (Circle immunization and vitamin A or IFA supplements needed today)
	BCG PENTA-1 PENTA-2 PENTA-3 MR-1 MR-2
	OPV-0 OPV-1 OPV-2 OPV-3 VIT A+IFA OPV-Booster
	HEP-0 Rota-1 Rota-2 Rota-3 JE-1 JE-2
	    PCV-1 PCV-2 PCV-Booster DPT-Booster-1 DPT-Booster-2
	    fIPV-1 fIPV-2 fIPV-3 Deworming
	Return for next immunization or vitamin A or IFA supplements	

	Assess child's feeding	

	• Do you breastfeed your child? Yes __ No __
	    If yes, how many times in 24 hours? ____ times
	    Do you breastfeed during the night? Yes __ No __
	• Does the child take any other food or fluids? Yes __ No __
	    If yes, what foods or fluids? _____
	• How many times per day? _____ What do you use to feed the child and how? _____
	• How large are the servings?
	• Does the child receive his own serving? _____ Who feeds the child and how? _____
	• During the illness, has the child feeding changed? Yes____ No____
	    If yes, how?	

	Assess caregiver's practice to support child's development	
	ASK How do you play with your baby? How do you talk to your baby? How do you get your baby smile?	• Look how does caregiver show he/she is aware of child's movement • Look how does caregiver comfort the child and show love?
	Assess others problem	
		Remember to refer any child who has a general danger sign and/or another severe classification
		• **Counsel mother about feeding** • **Counsel mother about development supportive practices** • **Advice mother when to return immediately** • **Give any immunization needed today** • **Counsel mother about her own health** • **When the mother has to return for follow up**

References

1. Ministry of Health and Family Welfare, Government of India. Integrated Management of Neonatal and Childhood Illness (IMNCI) [Internet]. [cited 2024 Jul 18]. Available from: https://nhm.gov.in/index4.php?lang=1&level=0&linkid=493&lid=759
2. Ministry of Health and Family Welfare, Government of India. Module 1: Introduction [Internet]. [cited 2024 Jul 18]. Available from: https://main.mohfw.gov.in/sites/default/files/7091371954Mod%201%20INTRODUCTION%20R.pdf
3. Ministry of Health and Family Welfare, Government of India. IMNCI Chart Booklet [Internet]. [cited 2024 Jul 18]. Available from: https://nhm.gov.in/images/pdf/programmes/child-health/guidelines/imnci_chart_booklet.pdf

4. Ministry of Health and Family Welfare, Government of India. Reproductive and Child Health (RCH) - IMNCI [Internet]. [cited 2024 Jul 18]. Available from: https://main.mohfw.gov.in/sites/default/files/209730261RCH%20IMNC.pdf
5. Ministry of Health and Family Welfare, Government of India. IMNCI Participants Module for Health Workers 2023 [Internet]. [cited 2024 Jul 18]. Available from: https://nhm.gov.in/images/pdf/programmes/child-health/guidelines/IMNCI-Module-2023-For-health-worker/IMNCI-Participants-Module-Health-Workers-2023.pdf
6. Park K. Park's Textbook of Preventive and Social Medicine, 27th ed. Jabalpur: Banarsidas Bhanot; 2023.
7. Ministry of Health and Family Welfare, Government of India. IMNCI Facilitator Guide for Health Worker 2023 [Internet]. Available from: https://nhm.gov.in/images/pdf/programmes/child-health/guidelines/IMNCI-Module-2023-For-health-worker/IMNCI-Facilitator-Guide-Health-Worker-2023.pdf
8. World Health Organization. Package of Interventions for Family Planning, Safe Abortion Care, Maternal, Newborn and Child Health. 2010 [cited 2024 Jul 20]. Available from: https://iris.who.int/bitstream/handle/10665/206920/9789290615361_package8_eng.pdf?sequence=1

QUESTIONS

Long Answer Questions (LAQs)

1. Describe the IMNCI strategy implemented in India, its components, and how it differs from the WHO-UNICEF IMCI strategy?
2. Discuss the objectives and the role of health workers in the IMNCI framework.

Short Answer Questions (SAQs)

1. Explain the classification and treatment approach for a sick infant with possible serious bacterial infection under IMNCI.
2. What are the components of IMNCI program?

Multiple Choice Questions (MCQs)

1. What does the color-coded booklet used in the IMNCI strategy signify?
   a. Different levels of urgency for treating sick children
   b. The nutritional status of children
   c. The type of medication required
   d. The age group of the children being treated
2. Which of the following signs would classify an infant as having severe jaundice under IMNCI?
   a. Jaundice appearing after 24 hours of age
   b. Yellow palms or soles
   c. Temperature above 37.5°C
   d. Sunken eyes
3. What is the most appropriate for a child classified with "severe acute malnutrition" under IMNCI?
   a. Provide home care and follow up after 14 days
   b. Administer a dose of oral amoxicillin and IM gentamicin and refer urgently to a hospital
   c. Provide zinc supplements and monitor at home
   d. Advise on increasing breastfeeding/feeding frequency

Answers

1. a   2. b   3. b

CHAPTER 31

Social Awareness and Action to Neutralize Pneumonia Successfully

Pallavi Singh, Rohit Katre, Parth Thakkar, Sushant Khanduri, Hetal Rathod

Need of program/Scheme	As per cause of death statistics 2015-17, office of the registrar general and census commissioner, India Childhood pneumonia continues to be the topmost infectious killer among under-five children, contributing to 16.2 percent of under-five deaths in India.[1] As per SRS 2020 under-five mortality is 32 per 1000 live birth and goal of NHP 2017 is to reduce U5M to 23 par 1000 live births by 2025. To achieve this target pneumonia mortality in children needs to be reduce lees than 3 per 1000 live births. **SAANS Campaign:** SAANS stands for **"Social Awareness and Actions to Neutralize Pneumonia Successfully"**. It is an initiative launched in 2019 in order to accelerate actions for reducing deaths due to childhood Pneumonia.[2] The initiative focuses on early detection, prompt treatment, strengthening health systems, and community awareness to achieve a significant action in pneumonia-related deaths.[3]
Implemented since	Launched in November 2019 under NHM. Expanded nationwide across all states and UTs.
Goal	To intensify action for reducing mortality due to childhood Pneumonia in India to less than 3 per thousand live births by 2025.
Objectives	• Adoption and adherence to National Childhood Pneumonia Management guidelines 2019. • Create awareness and mobilize community for Pneumonia Protection, Prevention and Treatment. • Early identification and management of under-five children to detect suspected pneumonia cases. • Strengthen facility-level management for cases of severe-pneumonia.
Objectives (Target-oriented)	• Reduce pneumonia deaths by at least 50% by 2025 through early detection and effective case management. • Ensure 90% of children under five receive complete immunization against pneumonia-preventable diseases (PCV, measles, Hib, pertussis). • Increase exclusive breastfeeding rates to 70% to improve immunity and reduce pneumonia risk. • Ensure availability of amoxicillin dispersible tablets and oxygen therapy at 100% of PHCs and CHCs by 2025. • Train at least 80% of ASHAs and ANMs in pneumonia identification and community-based treatment. • Achieve 90% household awareness on pneumonia symptoms and early care-seeking behaviors.[4]
Beneficiaries	Children under five years of age.
Components	• Assess • Classify • Pre-referral dose and refer • Management if referral not possible • Follow up
Strategies/Deliverables under the program	1. **Community awareness and behavior change communication:** Mass media campaigns through television, radio, and digital platforms to educate parents. Promotion of exclusive breastfeeding (0–6 months) and appropriate complementary feeding (after six months). Handwashing and sanitation awareness campaigns to prevent respiratory infections.

	2. **Early diagnosis and prompt treatment:** ASHAs and ANMs trained to identify pneumonia symptoms and refer cases. Availability of amoxicillin dispersible tablets at all PHCs and CHCs. Pulse oximeter-based screening at primary healthcare levels. Referral mechanisms for severe pneumonia cases to higher health facilities. 3. **Strengthening health systems and capacity building:** 100% of PHCs and CHCs equipped with pulse oximeters and oxygen concentrators. Skill-based training for doctors and nurses on pneumonia case management. Integration of pneumonia management with IMNCI (Integrated Management of Neonatal and Childhood Illnesses). 4. **Ensuring vaccine coverage:** Universal coverage of Pneumococcal Conjugate Vaccine (PCV) by 2025. Strengthening routine immunization (Measles, DPT, Hib) to cover 90% of eligible children. Mission Indradhanush expansion for vaccine coverage in high-burden districts. 5. **Intersectoral collaboration:** Partnership with ICDS, Panchayati Raj Institutions, NGOs, and private healthcare providers. Village Health and Nutrition Days (VHNDs) used for pneumonia screening and awareness activities. Integration of pneumonia awareness with Poshan Abhiyan for improved child nutrition.

Activities at various level or package of services	• To mobilize people to protect children from pneumonia, and train health personnel and other stakeholders to provide prioritized treatment to control the disease.
	• A child suffering from pneumonia will be treated with a **pre-referral dose of antibiotic amoxicillin** by Accredited Social Health Activist (ASHA) workers.
	• **Pulse oximeter** (device to monitor oxygen saturation) will be used at the Health and Wellness Centre for identification of low oxygen levels in the blood of child and if required, the child can be treated by the use of oxygen cylinders.
	• A **mass awareness campaign** will be launched about the **effective solutions for pneumonia prevention** like breastfeeding, age-appropriate complementary feeding and immunization, etc.
	• **Steps taken by India:**
	   ✦ The government aims to achieve a **target** of **reducing pneumonia deaths** among children to **less than three per 1,000 live births by 2025**.
	   ✦ In 2014, India launched **'Integrated Action Plan for Prevention and Control of Pneumonia and Diarrhea (IAPPD)'** to undertake collaborative efforts towards prevention of diarrhea and Pneumonia related under-five deaths.
	• **Community level:** Home visits by ASHAs and anganwadi workers for pneumonia detection and referral. Counseling sessions on nutrition, hygiene, and immunization at the village level. community health meetings and IEC material distribution.
	• **Primary healthcare level (PHCs, CHCs, UPHCs):** Routine pneumonia screening and pulse oximetry assessment. Amoxicillin and oxygen therapy available at all facilities. Training of healthcare workers on pneumonia management.
	• **Secondary and tertiary healthcare level (District and referral hospitals):** Advanced care for severe pneumonia cases. Availability of pediatric ICUs with ventilators and critical care support. Referral and follow-up mechanisms for discharged patients. Monitoring and evaluation of the program real-time data collection via Health Management Information System (HMIS) to track pneumonia cases and treatment outcomes. Periodic surveys (NFHS, NHFS) to assess impact on pneumonia mortality and immunization rates. ASHA and ANM performance evaluation based on case detection and treatment adherence. Quarterly review meetings at district and state levels to identify gaps and implement corrective measures.[3]

Monitoring and evaluation of program	• Health Management Information System • Supportive supervision (reporting format available from reference) • Analysis of under-five mortality and morbidity data

Key elements of the Protect-Prevent-treat (PPT) approach for pneumonia	1. **Protect (by establishing good health practices)**
	   a. Exclusive breastfeeding for 6 months
	   b. Adequate nutrition/complimentary feeding
	   c. Safe Drinking Water
	   d. Hygiene practices (Frequent handwashing, Respiratory Hygiene)
	   e. Reducing household air pollution

	2. **Prevent** (becoming ill from pneumonia and diarrhea)
	   a. Vaccination (Pertussis, Measles, Hib, PCV, Rotavirus)
	   b. Vitamin A supplementation
	   c. Health education about pneumonia risk factors, symptoms, and preventive measures
	3. **Treat**
	   a. Early identification and prompt treatment
	   b. Oxygen therapy
	   c. Case management at Community and Health Facility
	   d. Continued feeding

References

1. Cause of Death Statistics 2015-17, Office of the Registrar General and Census Commissioner, India.
2. SAANS. Available at: https://nhm.gov.in/index1.php?lang=1&level=1&sublinkid=1438&lid=790
3. Ministry of Health and Family Welfare, Government of India. SAANS Campaign Guidance Note [Internet]. New Delhi: National Health Mission; 2019 [cited 2025 Feb 22]. Available from: https://nhm.gov.in/index1.php?lang=1&level=1&lid=790&sublinkid=1438
4. Ministry of Health and Family Welfare, Government of India. Childhood Pneumonia Management Guidelines [Internet]. New Delhi: National Health Mission; 2019 [cited 2025 Feb 22]. Available from: https://nhm.gov.in/index1.php?lang=1&level=1&lid=790&sublinkid=1438

QUESTIONS

Long Answer Questions (LAQs)

1. What is Pneumonia? How do you classify it? Write in brief about Social Awareness and Actions to Neutralize Pneumonia Successfully (SAANS).
2. Explain the need for the SAANS campaign. How does pneumonia contribute to under-five mortality, and what interventions are being implemented?
3. Discuss in detail the various strategies adopted under the SAANS campaign, including community awareness, early diagnosis, vaccination, and health system strengthening.

Short Answer Questions (SAQs)

1. How is social awareness important for Pneumonia control?
2. What does SAANS stand for?
3. Why was the SAANS campaign launched?
4. What are the primary goals of the SAANS campaign?
5. Name any two key strategies of the SAANS campaign.
6. How does the campaign plan to reduce pneumonia-related mortality?

Multiple Choice Questions (MCQs)

1. All are the signs of severe pneumonia as per IMNCI, *except*:
   a. Lethargy
   b. Chest in drawing
   c. Oxygen saturation is less than 90%
   d. Only fast breathing

Chapter 31: Social Awareness and Action to Neutralize Pneumonia Successfully

2. SAAS initiative is for:
   a. To reduce the mortality due to childhood pneumonia
   b. To reduce the mortality due to infant pneumonia
   c. To reduce the mortality due to childhood upper respiratory tract infection (URTI)
   d. To reduce the mortality due to infant URTI
3. What is the tagline of SAAS initiative?
   a. Bachpan Sahi, Joh Pneumonia Nahi
   b. Pneumonia Nahi, Toh Bachpan Sahi
   c. URTI Nahi, Toh Bachpan Sahi
   d. Bachpan Sahi, Toh URTI Nahi
4. Total ____ no. of primary doses of PCV vaccine is given up to 1 year of age.
   a. 2
   b. 3
   c. 1
   d. 0
5. SAAS initiative was launched in ____.
   a. 2020
   b. 2021
   c. 2018
   d. 2019
6. What is the primary goal of the SAANS campaign?
   a. Reduce pneumonia mortality to <3 per 1,000 live births by 2025
   b. Reduce tuberculosis cases by 50%
   c. Increase childhood vaccination by 20%
   d. Improve maternal mortality rates
7. Which vaccine is specifically targeted in the SAANS campaign to prevent pneumonia?
   a. Rotavirus vaccine
   b. Pneumococcal Conjugate Vaccine (PCV)
   c. Bacillus Calmette-Guérin (BCG) vaccine
   d. Polio vaccine

Answers

1. d
2. a
3. b
4. a
5. d
6. a
7. b

CHAPTER 32

MusQan: Ensuring Child-friendly Services in Government Health Facilities

Surabhi Mishra, Niharika Verma

NEED OF THE INITIATIVE

The Government of India (GoI) strives to equitably provide quality universal health care to all children. The National Health Mission (NHM) has mandated providing quality pediatric care services through government health facilities. In the past decade, the NHM has made a concerted push to improve children's survival by increasing access to institutional care at government health facilities. Taking cognizance of the importance of quality and safety aspects in child care, the GoI has launched several initiatives, namely Facility-based Newborn Care [Special Newborn Care Unit (SNCU), Mother Newborn Care Unit (MNCU)], Home-based Care for Newborns and Young Child, and National Quality Assurance Standards (NQAS) for different levels of health facilities. As a step further in addressing all social, nutritional, and quality aspects while providing child-friendly care in government health facilities, the NHM launched a novel initiative in 2021 branded 'MusQan' for children aged between 0 and 12 years at the selected departments illustrated in **Table 32.1**.[1]

TABLE 32.1: Departments selected under the MusQan initiative at the government health facilities.[1]

District hospitals (DH)	Sub-DH	FRU-CHCs	All other LaQshya-certified facilities, medical colleges
• Pediatric OPD and ward • SNCU • NRC	• Pediatric OPD + Ward • SNCU/NBSU	• Pediatric OPD • NBSU/SNCU (if available)	• Pediatric OPD + Ward • SNCU • NRC

CHC: community health center, FRU: first referral unit; NBSU: newborn stabilization unit; NRC: nutrition rehabilitation center; OPD: out-patient department; SNCU: special newborn care unit

QoC is an important pillar of universal health coverage. For pediatric services at health facilities, the QoC is seen through the prism of the Donabedian model. Using the same model, the structure of the QoC approach adopted under the MusQan initiative has been depicted in **Figure 32.1**.

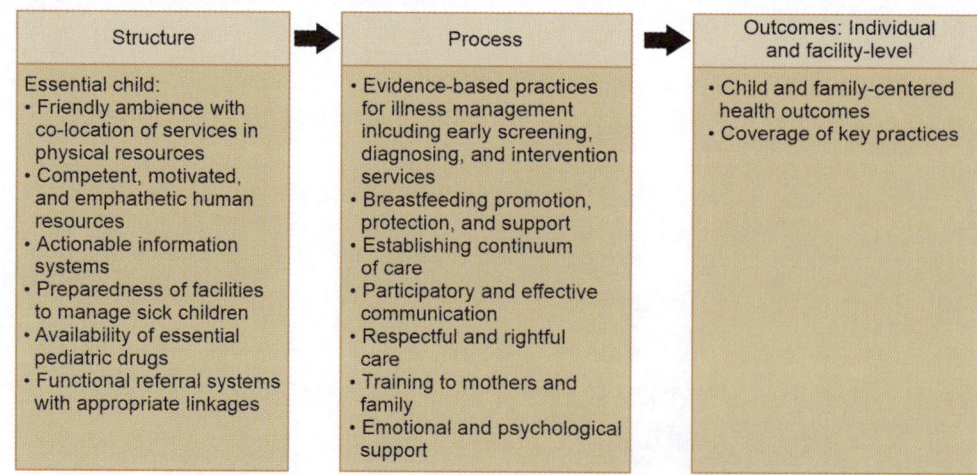

Fig. 32.1: Structure to advance quality of provisioned pediatric care under the MusQan scheme.

Goals

To ensure quality child-friendly services are provided in government health facilities to bring down preventable childhood mortality and morbidity for those aged below 12 years.

Objectives

- To provide quality child-friendly services to the pediatric age group (0–12 years) at government health facilities as per NQAS norms in a humane and supportive environment.
- To promote compliance with evidence-based guidelines and standard treatment protocols and
- To enhance the satisfaction of mothers and families seeking child healthcare.

Organogram

Under NHM, States and Union Territories (UTs) have created an institutional outline for quality initiatives. Under the territory of the National Quality Assurance Programme, the Central Quality Supervisory Committee (CQSC) implements quality initiatives at the central level. At the state and district levels, there are State and District Quality Assurance Committees (SQA-C and DQA-C) with an execution arm, namely the SQA and DQA Units (SQA-U and DQA-U). At the government health facility and department levels, there are Quality Teams and Circles, respectively. These committees, units, teams/circles also assist in implementing other quality initiatives, namely NQAS, Kayakalp, LaQshya, etc., by working at all levels in alliance with or equivalent to the Child Health Division. **(Fig. 32.2)**.

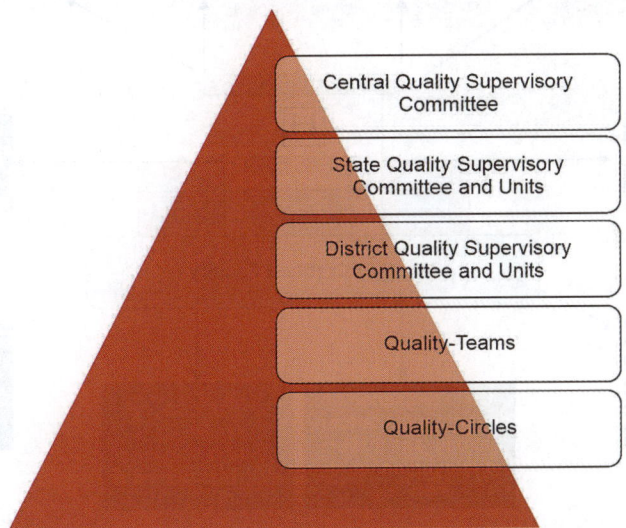

Fig. 32.2: Institutional framework under the MusQan scheme.

Beneficiaries

Paediatric age group (0–12 years) availing child care services at the government health facilities.

Strategies

- **Reinforce Clinical Protocols and Management Processes by:**
  - **Compliance with policies and standard treatment guidelines/protocols**, such as Facility-Based Newborn Care Guidelines, Pediatric Care Guidelines, and the Mother Absolute Affection program will be envisaged.
  - **By supporting early screening, diagnosis, and intervention services** at established pediatric in-patient and outpatient departments (IPD and OPD), services including emergency triage services, newborn care units [(Special Newborn Care Units (SNCUs), Newborn Stabilization Unit (NBSUs) and dedicated District Early Intervention Centers (DEIC) provide a standard level of mandated care for high-risk children.

- **Enhancing competency and skill of the healthcare professionals, including paramedical staff,** by performing periodic evaluations and providing refresher training, if required.
- **Providing facilities promoting, protecting, and supporting breastfeeding (breastfeeding corners) and nutritional counseling.**
❖ **Renovating a Government Health Facility to a Child-Friendly 'MusQan Certified' Facility** by incorporating:
  - **Dedicated childcare services near maternal health departments** (labor/delivery rooms, maternal operation theaters, recovery room complex, and postnatal ward, etc.)
  - **A visually appealing ambiance** at all pediatric IPD and OPD departments by painting the walls using soothing colors/themes in the background, sing illuminating linen, creating an exclusive pediatric zone with age-appropriate toys, games, etc.
  - **Availability and accessibility to all essential pediatric drugs** as per the Indian Public Health Standards norms for community health centers (CHC)/ sub-district hospitals (DH), DH **(Fig. 32.3)**.
❖ **Establishing two-way referral criteria and functional linkages** for follow-up services.
❖ **Providing family-centric, respectful, and dignified care** to the sick newborn/child.

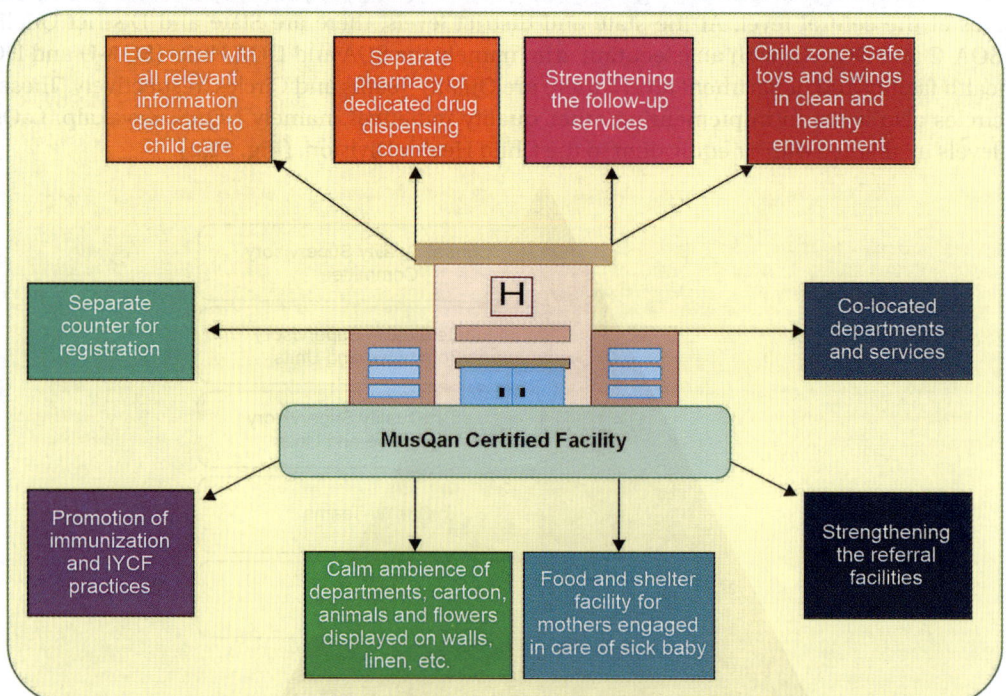

Fig. 32.3: Strategies for renovating a government health facility to a MusQan certified facility.[1]

Monitoring and Evaluation

To make newborn and childcare services friendly through the MusQan initiative, the certified facilities will undertake the following rapid improvement (RI) events:

Each event will last for a couple of months. The progress will be meticulously supported and validated by the state and district-level teams **(Fig. 32.4)**.

Norms for Certification

When the facility has achieved at least ≥70% in NQAS assessment tools, it can apply for state and national-level certification.[2-4]

> **Box 32.1: Rapid improvement events.**
> - Emergency triage assessment and treatment with referral mechanism
> - Kangaroo mother care and development support care
> - Infection prevention
> - Record keeping
> - Clinical protocols
> - Respectful and participatory care

❖ ≥70% as per NQAS protocols of Paediatric OPD, Ward, SNCU/NBSU, and NRC
❖ ≥75 % Facility-level indicators
❖ 80% Patient satisfaction

The MusQan initiative is associated with a baseline of 21 key performance indicators (KPIs) that need monthly measurements. Additionally, three other indicators are measured for updating at least biannually. All these indicators are examined periodically at state, district, and facility levels, as required. The MusQan-certified facilities must warrant that at least three-fourths of these KPIs meet their targets. Those achieving the NQAS certification must be assessed annually to assure sustenance and further facility improvement.

Incentivization

Each department at DH and first referral unit-CHCs are provided incentives of ₹ three and two lakhs, respectively, to accomplish national certification and compliance with facility-level targets. A quarter of this amount is used for staff incentivization. Remaining three-fourths for branding activities, such as signages and logos display, etc. The certificate is valid for three consecutive years depending on the state submitting the surveillance report to the National Health Systems Resource Centers and Child Health division under NHM ascertaining the sustenance status or further improvements required, if any.

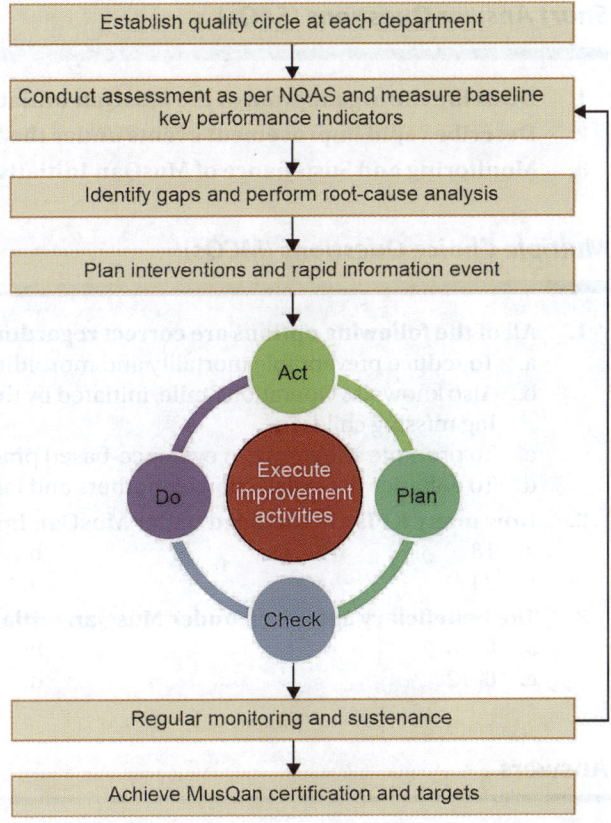

Fig. 32.4: Regular monitoring and sustenance under the MusQan initiative.[1]

References

1. Government of India. National Health Mission, MusQan – Ensuring Child-Friendly Services in Public Health Facilities. New Delhi, India: Ministry of Health & Family Welfare, New Concept Information Systems; 2021. ISBN: 978-93-82655-27-5
2. Government of India. National Health Mission, MusQan—Ensuring Child-Friendly Services in Public Health Facilities. National Quality Assurance Standards and Assessment Tools for Community Health Centres. New Delhi, India: Ministry of Health & Family Welfare, New Concept Information Systems; 2021.
3. Government of India. National Health Mission, MusQan—Ensuring Child-Friendly Services in Public Health Facilities. Road Map for MusQan Certification. New Delhi, India: Ministry of Health & Family Welfare, New Concept Information Systems; 2021.
4. Government of India. National Health Mission, Measurement System—An initiative to improve the quality of child health services. New Delhi, India: Ministry of Health & Family Welfare, New Concept Information Systems; 2021.

QUESTIONS

Long Answer Question (LAQ)

1. What are the goals, objectives, and strategies adopted under the MusQan initiative?

Short Answer Questions (SAQs)

1. Describe the organogram of the MusQan initiative.
2. Describe rapid improvement events under the MusQan initiative.
3. Monitoring and Sustenance of MusQan Initiative.

Multiple Choice Questions (MCQs)

1. All of the following options are correct regarding the MusQan initiative, *except*:
    a. To reduce preventable mortality and morbidity of children below 12 years of age
    b. Also known as Operation Smile, initiated by the Ministry of Home Affairs, focuses on rescuing and rehabilitating missing children
    c. To promote adherence to evidence-based practices and standard treatment guidelines/protocols and
    d. To enhance the satisfaction of mothers and families seeking child healthcare.
2. How many KPIs are included under MusQan initiative?
    a. 18 b. 15
    c. 24 d. 21
3. The beneficiary age group under MusQan initiative is:
    a. 0–18 b. 5–18
    c. 0–12 d. 1–12

Answers

1. b 2. d 3. c

iv. A: Adolescent Health

CHAPTER 33

Rashtriya Kishor Swasthya Karyakram

Surendra Singh, Shaili Vyas, Kajal Srivastava, Nilesh Thakor

Background/Need of program/Scheme	• **Adolescent population in India:** India has the largest adolescent population in the world, with 253 million adolescents. Ensuring their optimal growth, development, and health is essential for the country's future.
	• **Transition to adulthood:** Adolescents go through major physical, emotional, and social changes. During this period, they are vulnerable to various preventable and treatable health problems that need timely attention.
	• **Importance for sustainable development:** Adolescents are critical for achieving national development goals. Addressing the social and behavioral factors that affect their health is important to help them reach their full potential.
	• **RKSK focus areas:** The program extends beyond just **sexual and reproductive health**. It now covers:
	  ✦ **Non-communicable diseases (NCDs)**
	  ✦ **Nutrition**
	  ✦ **Injuries and violence** (including **gender-based violence**)
	  ✦ **Mental health**
	  ✦ **Substance abuse**
	• **Adolescent participation:** The program emphasizes **equity, gender inclusion**, and **adolescent participation**, recognizing adolescents as key contributors to national progress.
	• **Promotion over treatment:** There's a shift from clinic-based treatment to **preventive and promotional strategies**. The focus is on reaching adolescents in their **homes, communities, and schools**, rather than waiting for them to seek care at clinics.
	• **Key interventions:**
	  ✦ **Community-based outreach** through counselors
	  ✦ **Facility-based counseling** for adolescents
	  ✦ **Social and Behavior Change Communication (SBCC)** to promote healthy behaviors
	  ✦ Setting up **Adolescent Friendly Health Clinics (AFHCs)** at all levels of healthcare.[1]

Implemented since	The Rashtriya Kishor Swasthya Karyakram (RKSK) was introduced by the Ministry of Health and Family Welfare on January 7, 2014. The initiative aims to engage 253 million adolescents across all demographics, including both genders, rural and urban areas, and both in-school and out-of-school youth. Special attention is given to underserved and marginalized groups within this population.
Vision	All adolescents in India are able to realize their full potential by making informed and responsible decisions related to their health and well-being
Goal	The goal of the Rashtriya Kishor Swasthya Karyakram (RKSK) is to improve the health and well-being of adolescents across India. Specifically, RKSK aims to: • **Enhance adolescent health:** Provide comprehensive health services addressing physical, mental, and emotional health needs. • **Promote holistic development:** Support adolescents' growth and development through a focus on nutrition, education, and social well-being. • **Address key health issues:** Tackle critical issues such as sexual and reproductive health, non-communicable diseases, injuries, violence (including gender-based violence), mental health, and substance abuse.

	- **Increase access and equity:** Ensure that health services are accessible to all adolescents, particularly those from marginalized and underserved communities. - **Empower adolescents:** Foster greater autonomy and decision-making abilities among adolescents regarding their health and well-being. - **Strengthen community and parental involvement:** Engage communities and parents in supporting adolescent health and development. - **Implement preventive and promotional strategies:** Shift focus from clinic-based care to community-based prevention and health promotion initiatives.
Targets	To ensure the comprehensive development of adolescents, the Ministry of Health and Family Welfare launched Rashtriya Kishor Swasthya Karyakram (RKSK) on January 7, 2014. The program aims to reach out to 253 million adolescents, including both genders, from rural and urban areas, and those who are married or unmarried, as well as in-school and out-of-school youths. Special emphasis is placed on marginalized and underserved groups. RKSK broadens the scope of adolescent health beyond just sexual and reproductive health. It now addresses: - **Nutrition** - **Injuries and violence** (including gender-based violence) - **Non-communicable diseases** - **Mental health** - **Substance abuse** The program adopts a health promotion approach, shifting from traditional clinic-based services to preventive and promotional strategies. This involves engaging adolescents in their own environments—schools, families, and communities.
Objectives	- **Enhance information availability:** Expand the reach and accessibility of accurate and comprehensive information on adolescent health to educate and inform adolescents, their families, and communities. - **Improve access to services:** Boost the availability and use of high-quality counseling and health services specifically designed for adolescents, ensuring they can easily access the support they need. - **Foster collaborative partnerships:** Develop and strengthen multi-sectoral and intradepartmental partnerships to establish a safe, supportive environment for adolescents, integrating efforts across different sectors. - **Target vulnerable adolescents:** Implement focused strategies to address the needs of adolescents in high-risk geographic areas, including those from tribal regions, conflict zones, migrant communities, and out-of-school populations, to mitigate health and nutrition risks.[1]

Specific objectives	- **Improve nutrition**
	    + Reduce the prevalence of malnutrition among the target group
	    + Reduce the prevalence of iron-deficiency anemia (IDA) among the target group
	- **Enable sexual and reproductive health**
	    + Improve knowledge, attitudes and behavior, in relation to sexual and reproductive health among adolescents
	    + Reduce teenage pregnancies
	    + Improve birth preparedness, complication readiness
	    + Provide early parenting support for adolescent parents
	- **Enhance mental health**
	    + Address mental health concerns of adolescents
	    + Improved knowledge and skills on mental health issues of adolescents among the health care providers
	- **Prevent injuries and violence:** Promote favorable behavior and attitudes for preventing injuries and violence (including gender-based violence) among adolescents
	- **Prevent substance misuse:** Increase adolescents' awareness of the adverse effects and consequences of substance misuse
	- **Address NCDs:** Promote behavior change in adolescents to prevent NCDs such as hypertension, stroke, cardiovascular diseases and diabetes

Chapter 33: Rashtriya Kishor Swasthya Karyakram

Organogram	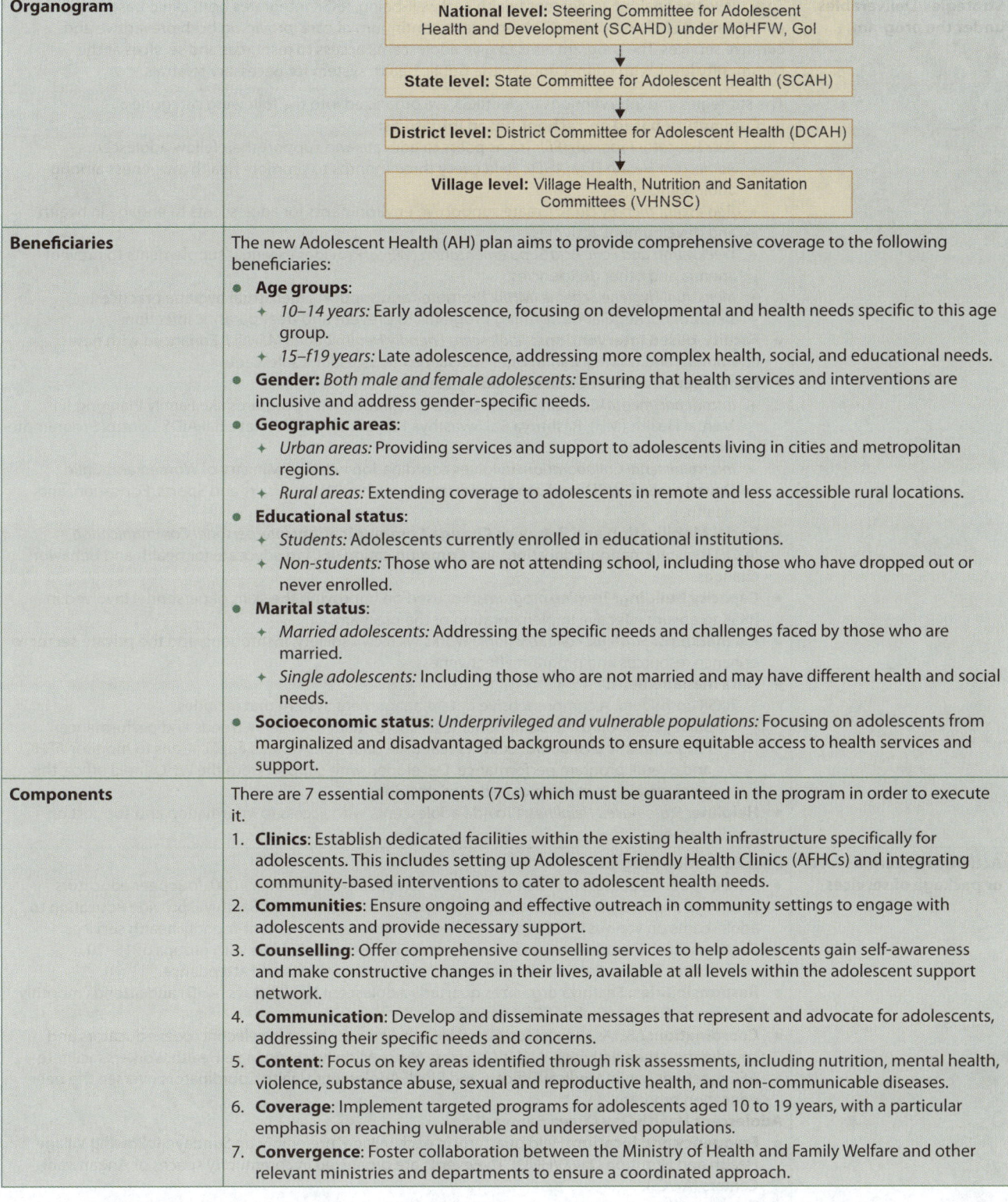
Beneficiaries	The new Adolescent Health (AH) plan aims to provide comprehensive coverage to the following beneficiaries: • **Age groups**: 　+ *10–14 years:* Early adolescence, focusing on developmental and health needs specific to this age group. 　+ *15–f19 years:* Late adolescence, addressing more complex health, social, and educational needs. • **Gender:** *Both male and female adolescents:* Ensuring that health services and interventions are inclusive and address gender-specific needs. • **Geographic areas**: 　+ *Urban areas:* Providing services and support to adolescents living in cities and metropolitan regions. 　+ *Rural areas:* Extending coverage to adolescents in remote and less accessible rural locations. • **Educational status**: 　+ *Students:* Adolescents currently enrolled in educational institutions. 　+ *Non-students:* Those who are not attending school, including those who have dropped out or never enrolled. • **Marital status**: 　+ *Married adolescents:* Addressing the specific needs and challenges faced by those who are married. 　+ *Single adolescents:* Including those who are not married and may have different health and social needs. • **Socioeconomic status**: *Underprivileged and vulnerable populations:* Focusing on adolescents from marginalized and disadvantaged backgrounds to ensure equitable access to health services and support.
Components	There are 7 essential components (7Cs) which must be guaranteed in the program in order to execute it. 1. **Clinics**: Establish dedicated facilities within the existing health infrastructure specifically for adolescents. This includes setting up Adolescent Friendly Health Clinics (AFHCs) and integrating community-based interventions to cater to adolescent health needs. 2. **Communities**: Ensure ongoing and effective outreach in community settings to engage with adolescents and provide necessary support. 3. **Counselling**: Offer comprehensive counselling services to help adolescents gain self-awareness and make constructive changes in their lives, available at all levels within the adolescent support network. 4. **Communication**: Develop and disseminate messages that represent and advocate for adolescents, addressing their specific needs and concerns. 5. **Content**: Focus on key areas identified through risk assessments, including nutrition, mental health, violence, substance abuse, sexual and reproductive health, and non-communicable diseases. 6. **Coverage**: Implement targeted programs for adolescents aged 10 to 19 years, with a particular emphasis on reaching vulnerable and underserved populations. 7. **Convergence**: Foster collaboration between the Ministry of Health and Family Welfare and other relevant ministries and departments to ensure a coordinated approach.

Strategies/Deliverables under the program	To achieve the goals of adolescent health and well-being, RKSK integrates both clinic-based and community-based approaches. This ensures a continuum of care, providing both preventive and curative services. The program aims to give adolescents access to resources and services at the community level, with connections to the public health system for necessary referrals.
	
	The strategies and interventions under RKSK are organized into the following categories:
	• **Community-based and school-based initiatives:**
	   + *Peer Educator Program (PE):* Trains peers to educate and support their fellow adolescents.
	   + *Adolescent Health Day (AHD):* Held every three months to promote health awareness among adolescents.
	   + *Adolescent friendly clubs:* Create supportive environments for adolescents to engage in health and development activities.
	   + *Weekly Iron and Folic Acid Supplementation (WIFS):* Provides essential supplements to prevent anemia and other deficiencies.
	   + *Menstrual Hygiene Scheme (MHS):* Promotes and supports menstrual hygiene practices.
	   + *Deworming:* Regular deworming programs to prevent and treat parasitic infections.
	• **Facility-based interventions:** *Adolescent Friendly Health Clinics (AFHCs):* Enhanced with new equipment and trained staff to offer specialized services for adolescents.
	• **Convergence within health and family welfare:**
	   + *Intradepartmental Coordination:* Includes integration with programs like Family Planning (FP), Mental Health (MH), Rashtriya Bal Swasthya Karyakram (RBSK), National AIDS Control Programme (NACP), and others.
	   + *Interministerial Collaboration:* Involves coordination with the Ministry of Women and Child Development (WCD) and other departments such as Youth Affairs and Sports, Education, and Health.
	• **Social Mobilization and Behavior Change Communication:** *Interpersonal Communication (IPC):* Uses Information, Education, and Communication (IEC) to advocate for health and behavior changes.
	• **Capacity building:** *Training programs:* Focused on improving the skills of personnel involved in RKSK to ensure effective implementation of the program.
	• **Partnerships:** *Strategic collaborations:* Works with civil society, institutions, and the private sector to enhance resources and program effectiveness.
	• **Data management:**
	   + *RKSK dashboard:* A comprehensive data management system that includes:
	      – *Survey dashboard:* Tracks national-level survey data to observe trends and performance.
	      – *Programmatic dashboard:* Collects real-time data from various applications to monitor AFHCs and overall program performance. Developed with support from the WHO-India office, this platform aids in making data-driven decisions.
	• **Helpline:** *State-Based Helplines:* Provide adolescents with access to information and support on various issues.

Activities at various level or package of services	**Peer Education Program** • **Role of peer educators:** In each village or area with a population of 1000, four peer educators (two boys and two girls) are selected. These peer educators, called 'Saathiya,' provide education to adolescents on various RKSK topics and help them access adolescent-friendly health services. • **Sessions:** Each Saathiya conducts weekly sessions lasting 1–2 hours with groups of 15–20 adolescents. They maintain a diary to record session summaries and attendance. • **Responsibilities:** Saathiya organizes quarterly Adolescent Health Days (AHD) and attends monthly Adolescent Friendly Club (AFC) meetings. • **Coordination:** ASHAs (Accredited Social Health Activists) assist in selecting peer educators and coordinating their activities. ANMs (Auxiliary Nurse Midwives) and Male Health Workers facilitate AFC meetings, while Medical Officers and Block Adolescent Health Coordinators oversee the peer education program. **Adolescent Health Day (Yuwa Samvad)** • **Frequency and location:** Held quarterly in each village, preferably on Sundays, following Village Health and Nutrition Day (VHND). The events are organized in community spaces or Anganwadi Centers (AWCs). • **Target audience:** All adolescents, including those aged 10-14 and 15-19, both school-going and out-of-school, as well as married adolescents.

+ *Purpose:* Reinforces adolescent health knowledge among all stakeholders, including parents and public health officials, and provides preventive and promotive health services.
+ *Coordination:* The Block Adolescent Health Coordinator manages event preparations, service delivery, and publicity.

Adolescent Friendly Club (AFC) Meetings
- *Frequency and structure:* Held monthly at the sub-center level, covering 5 villages or 5000 people. These meetings bring together Saathiya from different areas to discuss and resolve issues they face in their roles with the support of ANMs.
- *Purpose:* Provides a platform for Saathiya to address challenges and enhance their effectiveness in delivering peer education.

Adolescent Friendly Health Clinics (AFHCs)
Overview: Adolescent Friendly Health Clinics (AFHCs) are central to the Rashtriya Kishor Swasthya Karyakram (RKSK). They provide a range of services including clinical care and counseling tailored to adolescent health needs. Referrals from the Peer Education Program and Adolescent Health Days (AHD) often lead adolescents to these clinics.

Locations and staffing: AFHCs are set up at:
- Primary Health Centers (PHCs)
- Community Health Centers (CHCs)
- District Hospitals (DHs)
- Medical Colleges

They are staffed by trained professionals such as Medical Officers (MOs), Auxiliary Nurse Midwives (ANMs), and Counselors.

Key features: AFHCs are designed to be adolescent-friendly, meaning they should:
- **Equitable:** Offer services to all adolescents who need them.
- **Accessible:** Be located in places that preserve adolescents' privacy (e.g., not near obstetric wards or STI/RTI centers).
- **Acceptable:** Ensure that health providers meet adolescents' expectations.
- **Appropriate:** Provide necessary care while avoiding harmful practices.
- **Effective:** Deliver high-quality, efficient healthcare that positively impacts adolescents' health.
- **Comprehensive:** Address promotive, preventive, and curative health needs.

Services offered
- **Commodities:** Includes weekly iron and folic acid supplements (WIFS), Albendazole tablets, sanitary napkins, contraceptives, and other medicines.
- **Information and awareness:** Provided through Information, Education, and Communication (IEC) materials.
- **Counseling:** Covers topics such as diet, menstrual health, hygiene, contraceptive use, sexual health, mental health, abuse, gender violence, and prevention of non-communicable diseases.
- **Curative services:** Includes treatment for severe malnutrition, common RTIs/STIs, menstrual disorders, and non-communicable diseases.
- **Outreach services:** Conducted in schools, colleges, and communities at least twice a week by counselors.
- **Referral services:** Establishes links to secondary and tertiary care centers for further specialist care.

Adolescent Health Resource Centers (A-HRCs): AFHCs at the district level are designated as A-HRCs. These centers not only provide the full range of AFHC services but also:
- Serve as resource hubs for training healthcare professionals.
- Offer educational materials such as banners, posters, pamphlets, and audio-visual resources on adolescent health.

Benchmarks for optimal functioning: To function effectively, an AFHC should:
- Have good infrastructure.
- Be easily accessible to adolescents.
- Be well-known within the community and offer a wide range of services.
- Employ non-judgmental and competent health providers.
- Ensure privacy and confidentiality.
- Be accepted by the community and provide referral links to specialized care.

Menstrual Hygiene Scheme (MHS)[2]
Purpose: The Menstrual Hygiene Scheme (MHS) aims to ensure that adolescent girls in rural India are well-informed about menstrual hygiene. The scheme focuses on:
- **Awareness:** Educating adolescent girls about menstrual hygiene to build their self-esteem and support their broader social participation.
- **Access:** Improving availability and use of high-quality sanitary napkins in rural areas.
- **Disposal:** Promoting environmentally friendly disposal of sanitary napkins.

Key strategies:
- **Demand generation:** Using Information, Education, and Communication (IEC) efforts by Accredited Social Health Activists (ASHAs) in schools and communities to encourage the use of sanitary napkins.
- **Supply:** Ensuring a steady supply of affordable, high-quality sanitary napkins.
- **Training:** Providing ASHAs with training on menstrual hygiene, behavior change communication, and safe disposal practices.

Distribution:
- ASHAs distribute a pack of six sanitary napkins, branded as "Freedays," at a subsidized cost of ₹ 6.
- ASHAs earn ₹ 1 for each pack sold and receive one pack free each month for their own use.

Additional interventions:
- Regular sourcing and procurement of sanitary napkins.
- Ongoing training for ASHAs on menstrual hygiene and safe practices.

Weekly Iron and Folic Acid Supplementation (WIFS)[3]
The scheme aims to reduce the burden of anemia in adolescents (boys and girls). It involves supervised weekly ingestion of IFA supplementation and administration of Albendazole twice in a year (six months apart). The scheme also relies on screening of target groups, strong referral linkages, IEC and counselling.

The short-term advantage of the scheme is better human capital through nutrition; the long-term goal is to end the intergenerational cycle of anemia. The program is being carried out in both rural and urban areas of the nation.

School Health and Wellness Program
The scheme focusses on providing age-appropriate health education, and evidence-based health promotion interventions at school level.

Five components under intensification of preventive and promotive school health activities include:
1. Intensified School Health Promotion activities
2. Health Screening
3. Provision of curative and preventative services
4. Electronic Health Records
5. Upgradation of skills of emergency care

Every school shall appoint two teachers as "Health and Wellness Ambassadors" and who will receive training on how to spread knowledge about illness prevention and health promotion through engaging activities for one hour each week. Ideally, these instructors will be male and female.

The scheme is being carried out in close collaboration with the Ministry of Education.

Monitoring and evaluation of program	**Supportive supervision:** RKSK emphasizes the importance of regular monitoring through supportive supervision at multiple levels: • **Monthly reviews:** Conducted at block, district, and state levels. • **Visits:** Specific visits are made to Adolescent Friendly Health Clinics (AFHCs), Adolescent Health Days (AHDs), and Peer Education sessions to ensure quality and adherence to guidelines. **Quarterly reporting:** States are required to submit quarterly reports that include: • **Achievements:** Details on progress made towards various targets. • **Physical achievements:** Comparison of actual achievements with targets outlined in the state's Program Implementation Plan (PIP), including corresponding expenses. • **Variance analysis:** Evaluation of whether the targeted outcomes or outputs were met. If there were discrepancies, the reasons are analyzed, and corrective actions are planned. Targets may be adjusted if necessary. **Reporting format:** • Reports must be sent to the Ministry of Health and Family Welfare (MoHFW), Government of India, in specified formats. • Achievements should be expressed as percentages relative to the activities listed in the state PIP. • Reports should also include details on any corrective actions taken based on the variance analysis.

References

1. National Health Mission, Ministry of Health and Family Welfare (MoHFW). Implementation Guidelines Rashtriya Kishor Swasthya Karyakram (RKSK). New Delhi: MoHFW, 2018; p. 67.
2. National Health Mission, Ministry of Health and Family Welfare (MoHFW). Operational Guidelines Promotion of Menstrual Hygiene among Adolescent Girls (10-19 Years) in Rural Areas. New Delhi: MoHFW. p. 32.
3. National Health Mission, Ministry of Health and Family Welfare (MoHFW). Operational Framework Weekly Iron and Folic Acid Supplementation Programme for Adolescents. New Delhi: MoHFW. p. 35.

QUESTIONS

Long Answer Question (LAQ)

1. Describe adolescent health status in India and explain how RKSK is addressing this pertinent issue?

Short Answer Questions (SAQs)

1. Describe the essential components under RKSK.
2. Write short note on Adolescent Friendly Health Clinics.

Multiple Choice Questions (MCQs)

1. The specific objectives of Rashtriya Kishor Swasthya Karyakram (RKSK) includes all *except*:
    a. Enable sexual and reproductive health
    b. Prevent injuries and violence
    c. Address communicable disease conditions
    d. Improve nutrition
2. Which of the following activities is undertaken in Rashtriya Kishor Swasthya Karyakram (RKSK)?
    a. Identification of defects at birth
    b. Peer educator program
    c. Screening of communicable diseases
    d. VHSNC activities
3. Under the Friendly AFHC initiative services for adolescents should be all, *except*:
    a. Acceptable
    b. Equitable
    c. Comprehensive
    d. Complementary

Answers

1. c   2. b   3. d

CHAPTER 34

School Health Program and Menstrual Hygiene Scheme

Shaili Vyas, Pallavi Singh, Parul Sharma, Kajal Srivastava

Background/Need of program/Scheme	Integrating health and education is a crucial element of the Sustainable Development Goals (SDGs). The National Health Policy (NHP) 2017 emphasizes the importance of school health by embedding health education into the curriculum and promoting hygiene and healthy habits. Early health education and proper behavior are essential for children to lead healthy lives and achieve their full potential. Schools serve as an effective platform to educate children and adolescents about health issues, encourage healthy behaviors, establish service connections, and engage parents and communities through students. The School Health Program, part of the Health and Wellness component of the Ayushman Bharat Program, focuses on preventive and promotive health activities. These initiatives aim to integrate health education, promotion, illness prevention, and service access in a comprehensive manner at the school level. The program will address emerging social morbidities, including injuries, violence, substance misuse, risky sexual behaviors, and psychological/emotional issues. The School Health Promotion Activities under the Ayushman Bharat Programme are a collaborative effort between the Ministry of Health and Family Welfare and the Department of School Education and Literacy, Ministry of Human Resource and Development.[1]
Implemented since	The Prime Minister launched the School Health Program (SHP) under Ayushman Bharat in 2018. It is a joint initiative of both the Ministry of Health and Family Welfare and the Ministry of Human Resource Development.
Goal	The School Health Program aims to enhance students' overall health and well-being, which in turn improves their academic performance and quality of life. This goal is pursued by increasing health awareness, preventing diseases, supporting mental health, maintaining a safe and healthy environment, encouraging physical activity, promoting good nutrition, and identifying health issues early. The program seeks to instill lifelong healthy habits and foster a healthier community. The Menstrual Hygiene Scheme is designed to improve menstrual health and hygiene among adolescent girls. It provides access to affordable sanitary products, raises awareness about menstrual hygiene practices, and ensures a supportive environment. The scheme aims to reduce health risks, eliminate stigma around menstruation, and empower girls to manage their menstrual health with dignity and confidence.
Targets	• Health Education • Regular Health Screenings • Full Immunization Coverage • Mental Health Support • Promote Physical Activity • Access to Healthy Nutrition • Healthy School Environment • Parental and Community Engagement • Access to Sanitary Products • Menstrual Health Education • Safe Disposal Facilities • Address Stigma and Myths • Access to Water, Sanitation, and Hygiene (WASH) Facilities • Community and Peer Involvement

Objectives	<ul><li>To provide age-appropriate information about health and nutrition to the children in schools.</li><li>To promote healthy behaviors among the children that they will inculcate for life.</li><li>To detect and treat diseases early in children and adolescents including identification of malnourished and anemic children with appropriate referrals to PHCs and hospitals.</li><li>To promote use of safe drinking water in schools</li><li>To promote safe menstrual hygiene practices by girls</li><li>To promote yoga and meditation through Health and Wellness Ambassadors.</li><li>To encourage research on health, wellness and nutrition for children.</li></ul>
Organogram	School Health Promotion Activities under Ayushman Bharat, a collaborative initiative of the Ministry of Health and Family Welfare and the Department of School Education and Literacy, Ministry of Human Resource and Development.
Beneficiaries	School health promotion will be adopted in all government and government-aided schools nationwide.
Components	**Components of a School Health Program**[2] A comprehensive school health program encompasses various aspects to promote the physical, mental, social, and emotional well-being of students. Here are some key components: **Physical health:**<ul><li>**Nutrition:** Promoting healthy eating habits, providing nutritious meals, and addressing food insecurity.</li><li>**Physical activity:** Encouraging regular physical exercise, providing opportunities for sports and physical education.</li><li>**Health screenings:** Conducting routine health checks for vision, hearing, dental health, and other conditions.</li><li>**Health education:** Teaching students about healthy lifestyles, disease prevention, and first aid.</li></ul>**Mental health:**<ul><li>**Counselling services:** Providing counselling and mental health support for students.</li><li>**Peer support programs:** Encouraging peer support and mentoring to address emotional and social issues.</li><li>**Stress management techniques:** Teaching students relaxation techniques and coping mechanisms.</li><li>**Mental health awareness:** Promoting awareness of mental health issues and stigma reduction.</li></ul>**Social health:**<ul><li>**Character education:** Promoting positive values, social skills, and citizenship.</li><li>**Conflict resolution:** Teaching students conflict resolution skills and peaceful problem-solving.</li><li>**Peer mediation:** Training students to mediate conflicts among their peers.</li><li>**Anti-bullying programs:** Implementing programs to prevent and address bullying.</li></ul>**Emotional health:**<ul><li>**Emotional intelligence:** Teaching students to recognize and manage their emotions.</li><li>**Social-emotional learning:** Promoting social-emotional skills such as empathy, communication, and cooperation.</li><li>**Stress management:** Teaching students relaxation techniques and coping mechanisms.</li><li>**Grief counseling:** Providing support for students experiencing loss or grief.</li></ul>**Environmental health:**<ul><li>**Safe and healthy environment:** Ensuring a clean, safe, and conducive learning environment.</li><li>**Disaster preparedness:** Developing plans for emergencies and disasters.</li><li>**Environmental education:** Teaching students about environmental issues and sustainability.</li></ul>**Health services:**<ul><li>**School nurse:** Having a dedicated school nurse to provide health care services and coordinate with healthcare providers.</li><li>**First aid training:** Providing first aid training to staff and students.</li><li>**Immunization programs:** Ensuring students are up-to-date on vaccinations.</li></ul>**Community partnerships:**<ul><li>**Collaborations:** Partnering with community organizations, healthcare providers, and families to support student health.</li><li>**Advocacy:** Advocating for policies and resources that promote student health.</li></ul>

	Components of Menstrual Hygiene Scheme[3]
	The Menstrual Hygiene Scheme (MHS) typically includes the following components:
	• **Awareness and education:**
	    ◦ *Community outreach programs:* Raising awareness about menstrual hygiene, its importance, and dispelling myths and taboos associated with menstruation.
	    ◦ *Educational materials:* Providing educational materials such as booklets, pamphlets, and videos on menstrual hygiene practices.
	    ◦ *School-based programs:* Integrating menstrual hygiene education into school curricula.
	• **Access to sanitary products:**
	    ◦ *Distribution of sanitary products:* Providing free or subsidized sanitary pads or reusable menstrual products to girls and women.
	    ◦ *Vending machines:* Installing vending machines in public places, schools, and workplaces to make sanitary products easily accessible.
	    ◦ *Production and distribution:* Supporting local production and distribution of affordable sanitary products.
	• **Facilities and infrastructure:**
	    ◦ *Sanitary facilities:* Ensuring access to clean and private toilets with facilities for menstrual hygiene management in schools, workplaces, and public places.
	    ◦ *Waste management:* Providing proper facilities for the disposal of menstrual waste to prevent contamination and disease transmission.
	    ◦ *Water and sanitation:* Ensuring access to clean water and adequate sanitation facilities for menstrual hygiene.
	• **Health and hygiene promotion:**
	    ◦ *Health education:* Providing information on menstrual hygiene practices, reproductive health, and personal hygiene.
	    ◦ *Health services:* Integrating menstrual hygiene into primary healthcare services and providing related health advice.
	    ◦ *Addressing stigma and taboos:* Challenging negative social attitudes and practices related to menstruation.[4]

Activities at various level or package of services	**Package of Services under School Health**
	• **School health promotion activities:**
	    ◦ Promote healthy behavior and prevent certain diseases through age-appropriate learning.
	    ◦ Implemented by school-trained Health and Wellness Ambassadors
	• **Health screening:** The RBSK mobile health teams assess children for 30 recognized health issues to provide early detection, free treatment, and management.
	• **Provision of services:**
	    ◦ Teachers provide IFA and Albendazole tablets through WIFS and NDD programs.
	    ◦ Providing sanitary napkins
	    ◦ Vaccinating at correct age
	• **Electronic health records:** Provide electronic health records for each child
	• **Imparting skills of emergency care:** Basic first aid training for teachers
	
	Operationalization of the School Health Program
	Each school will designate two teachers, one male and one female, to serve as "Health and Wellness Ambassadors." These ambassadors will deliver health promotion and disease prevention information through engaging activities on a weekly basis. Students, acting as "Health and Wellness Messengers," will share these health lessons and contribute to improving health habits nationwide. Schools might observe Health and Wellness Day every Tuesday.
	
	Selection of Teachers as Health and Wellness Ambassadors
	It is recommended to hire proactive, self-motivated teachers with strong communication skills and the ability to engage effectively with students. Preference may be given to candidates with backgrounds in science or physical education. Health and Wellness Ambassador teachers should ideally be under the age of 45. States might recognize and reward school health promoters during campaigns as an incentive. Health and Wellness Ambassadors will be responsible for promoting health among students.

	The training module for this role will encompass topics from the MoHFW's Rashtriya Kishor Swasthya Karyakram, including improving nutrition, sexual and reproductive health, mental health, injury and violence prevention, substance abuse, non-communicable diseases, and other relevant subjects as determined in consultation with the MHRD. **Capacity Building of Health and Wellness Ambassadors** The training program will follow a cascade model, starting with national level training conducted jointly by trainers from the Ministries of Health and Education. National level master trainers will then train state level trainers (4 in no.), who will in turn train district level trainers (3 trainers/district). District level trainers will train block level trainers (3 trainers/block) who will then train teachers at the school level (2 teachers/school). The training sessions will be five days long with 30 participants per batch. Additionally, block trainers will conduct a two-day orientation for school principals. **Structure of Activities** Trained teachers and Health and Wellness Ambassadors will conduct weekly classes and complete the modules by the end of the school year as planned. Whenever possible, these sessions should be integrated into the regular schedule and taught as part of the classroom lessons. Consideration is being given to designating every Tuesday as Health and Wellness Day. Various programs, including Life Skills, AEP, Peer Instructor modules, and ASHA modules, will be adapted to provide age-appropriate content for school activities. These sessions will enhance the current health education framework. Health and Wellness Ambassadors are required to use the provided training materials. If they encounter difficulties with the lessons, they can seek assistance from the RBSK team doctor, the Block Health Coordinator, or the Medical Officer from the PHC/CHC. Schools will have a question box where students can anonymously submit their questions, ensuring unbiased queries. Health and Wellness Ambassadors will address these questions at the beginning of each meeting. Two students from each class may assist the Health and Wellness Ambassadors in running the school's health campaigns and events. These students will be known as "Health and Wellness Messengers." Peer Educators/Saathiyas from schools and communities, the Block Adolescent Health Coordinator, and ANMs will also support the outreach efforts. If available, the Block Adolescent Health Coordinator may use audiovisual tools to present various BCC materials. Teachers can also use the "Saathiya" app and helplines during discussions and meetings. Schools may occasionally hold Teen Health Days, with students selecting the themes. These events can include various activities for Adolescent Health Days, with potential involvement from parents and other stakeholders. Activities are designed to equip students with tools for managing their health and making healthy decisions. A resource kit, including an activity kit and materials such as audiovisuals, films, posters, postcards, fact sheets, and pamphlets, has been prepared to support the meetings. Teachers will receive training and awareness kits that include guides for supervising and conducting activities at schools. Additionally, schools may host events like poster-making, slogan-writing, and health quizzes. For counseling support, mobile apps, e-health/m-health tools, and other social media platforms will also be promoted.
Monitoring and evaluation of program	Monitoring and evaluation (M&E) of the School Health Program is essential to ensure its effectiveness, accountability, and continuous improvement. Monitoring involves the regular collection and analysis of data on key health indicators, such as student attendance, immunization rates, nutritional status, and the incidence of health issues, to track the program's progress against its objectives. Evaluation assesses the overall impact and outcomes of the program, determining its effectiveness in promoting health education, disease prevention, and access to healthcare services. It includes both qualitative and quantitative methods, such as surveys, focus group discussions, and health assessments. M&E helps identify gaps, challenges, and best practices, allowing for timely adjustments and evidence-based decision-making. Engaging stakeholders, including students, teachers, health workers, and parents, in the M&E process fosters transparency and community ownership, ensuring the program's sustainability and long-term success.

References

1. Operational_guidelines_on_School_Health_Programme_under_Ayushman_Bharat.pdf. Available at https://nhm.gov.in/New_Updates_2018/NHM_Components/RMNCHA/AH/guidelines
2. School Health Programme. Ministry of Health and Family Welfare. https://pmposhan.education.gov.in/Files/School%20Health%20.Programme/School_Health_Programme_B.pdf
3. Scheme for Promotion of Menstrual Hygiene. Available at: Scheme for Promotion of Menstrual Hygiene
4. Menstrual Hygiene Scheme (MHS): National Health Mission

QUESTIONS

Long Answer Question (LAQ)

1. Describe the objectives and aspects of school health services.

Short Answer Questions (SAQs)

1. Enumerate the targets under the School Health Program.
2. Explain briefly objectives and components of Menstrual Hygiene Scheme.
3. Describe the package of services provided under School Health Program.
4. Discuss monitoring and evaluation of School Health Program.

Multiple Choice Questions (MCQs)

1. In which year was the School Health Program launched in India?
   a. 2015
   b. 2017
   c. 2019
   d. 2021
2. Which of the following is *not* a component of the School Health Program?
   a. Health screenings
   b. Immunization programs
   c. Distribution of medication
   d. Mental health support
3. How do "Health and Wellness Ambassadors" contribute to the SHP?
   a. By providing basic first aid training to students
   b. By conducting weekly health promotion activities
   c. By managing electronic health records for students
   d. By coordinating with healthcare providers for referrals
4. The Menstrual Hygiene Scheme primarily focuses on:
   a. Promoting physical activity among girls
   b. Providing access to sanitary products and education
   c. Addressing childhood malnutrition
   d. Early detection of chronic diseases

Answers

1. b
2. c
3. b
4. b

35 CHAPTER

Adolescent-friendly Health Clinics

Krupal J Joshi, Krishna M Jasani, Niharika Verma

INTRODUCTION

India has the world's largest adolescent population, with approximately 253 million individuals in the 10–19 age group, constituting about 21% of the country's total population. Recognizing the distinct health and developmental challenges faced by adolescents, the Ministry of Health and Family Welfare (MoHFW) launched the Rashtriya Kishor Swasthya Karyakram (RKSK) on January 7, 2014. Initially focusing on sexual and reproductive health, RKSK has evolved to address a broader spectrum of adolescent health concerns, including nutrition, mental health, substance use, injuries, and non-communicable diseases.

Research has identified several critical barriers that hinder adolescents from accessing healthcare services:
- Limited awareness of the availability and accessibility of services.
- Social and cultural norms that act as deterrents.
- Concerns regarding the lack of privacy or confidentiality.
- Geographical and financial constraints limiting access.
- Unfriendly or unwelcoming attitudes of healthcare providers.

These challenges underscore the need for targeted interventions to improve adolescent healthcare access and delivery.[1]

Approaches to Adolescent Health Interventions

Various strategies, including family-based, school-based, community-based, and facility-based approaches, have been implemented to address adolescent health needs.

Adolescent Friendly Health Clinics (AFHCs)[2]

RKSK marks a shift from a curative to a preventive and promotive healthcare model. The initiative realigns adolescent healthcare from clinical settings to a holistic, community-based, and school-oriented approach, emphasizing health

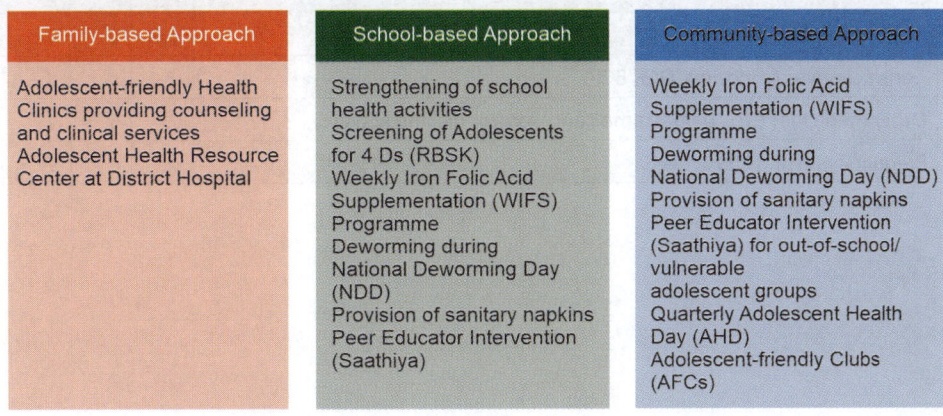

Fig. 35.1: Approaches to adolescent health interventions.

promotion and preventive care. In this context, Adolescent friendly Health Clinics (AFHCs) were introduced to offer comprehensive clinical and counseling services through the existing healthcare system.

Key Components of AFHCs

AFHCs adhere to adolescent-friendly principles:
- **Equitable:** Services are available to all adolescents in need.
- **Accessible:** Clinics are conveniently located and designed to be adolescent-friendly, avoiding placements near labor rooms, integrated counselling centers, or STI/RTI treatment centers.
- **Acceptable:** Healthcare providers are trained to ensure adolescent comfort and trust.
- **Appropriate:** Necessary care is provided while avoiding harmful or unnecessary interventions.
- **Effective:** Services demonstrate measurable improvements in adolescent health.
- **Comprehensive:** Clinics provide preventive, promotive, and curative healthcare services.

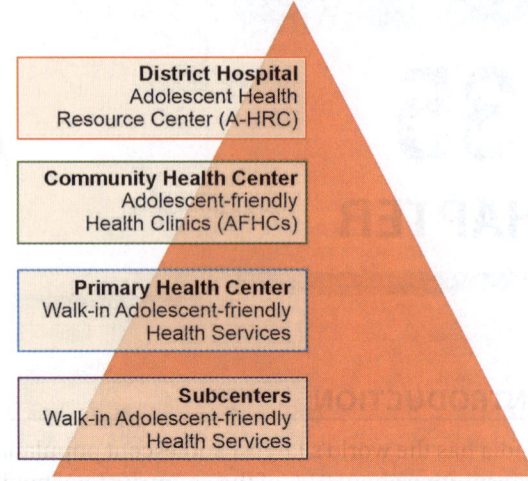

Fig. 35.2: Structure of facility-based approach.

Benchmark Criteria for AFHCs

To ensure effective service delivery, AFHCs must meet specific infrastructure and operational benchmarks:
- Clean, bright, and welcoming clinic environments
- Easily accessible locations with convenient operating hours
- Public awareness initiatives through IEC materials and clear signage
- Trained and non-judgmental healthcare providers specialized in adolescent health
- Assurance of privacy and confidentiality
- Community engagement strategies to improve service utilization
- A strong referral system linking primary and specialized care.

Package of AFHC Services

TABLE 35.1: Outlines the scope of services provided at different levels of AFHC facilities.

	Service package	DH	CHC	PHC	SC	Outreach
Information	IEC and IPC for nutrition, SRH, mental health, GBV, NCD and substance misuse	√	√	√	√	√
Commodities to be kept in AFHC	IFA/Albendazole tablets	√	√	√	√	√
	Sanitary napkin	√	√	√	√	√
	Contraceptives (condoms, OCP, ECP)	√	√	√	√	√
	Other medicines (e.g., paracetamol, anti-spasmodic and first aid)	√	√	√	√	√
	Pregnancy testing kits	√	√	√	√	√

Services to be provided in AFHC	BMI screening	√	√	√	√	√
	Hb testing	√	√	√	√	√
	RTI/STI management	√	√	√	√	√
	ANC for pregnant adolescents	√	√	√	√	√
	counseling services	√	√	√	√	√
	Management of menstrual problems	√	√	√	√	√
	Management of iron deficiency anemia	√	√	√	√	
	Screening for diabetes and hypertension	√	√	√	√	
	Management of common adolescent health problems	√	√	√	√	
	HIV testing and counseling	√	√			
	Management of physical violence and sexual abuse	√	√			
	Linkages with de-addiction centres and referrals	√	√			
	Treatment by specialists	√	√			
	Referral	√	√	√	√	√

Role of Counselors in AFHCs

Counselors are integral to the effective functioning of AFHCs, contributing significantly to their success through the following responsibilities:
* Delivering accurate information, educational resources, and counseling services on a wide range of adolescent health concerns.
* Facilitating referrals to specialized healthcare facilities, including integrated counseling and testing centers (ICTCs), De-addiction centers, and non-communicable disease (NCD) clinics, to ensure comprehensive care.
* Organizing and implementing outreach initiatives in educational institutions, youth organizations, and community spaces at least twice weekly to promote health awareness.
* Raising awareness among adolescents, parents, caregivers, and key community stakeholders about the healthcare services available to them.[3]

Convergence Approach in AFHCs

Successful implementation of AFHCs requires intra-departmental and inter-ministerial convergence, along with collaborations with civil society, private sector, and academic institutions. Addressing the six thematic areas of RKSK through this multisectoral convergence ensures a holistic approach to adolescent healthcare in India.

Through these initiatives, AFHCs ensure holistic adolescent healthcare delivery, empowering young individuals to lead healthier lives with enhanced access to medical, psychological, and social support services.

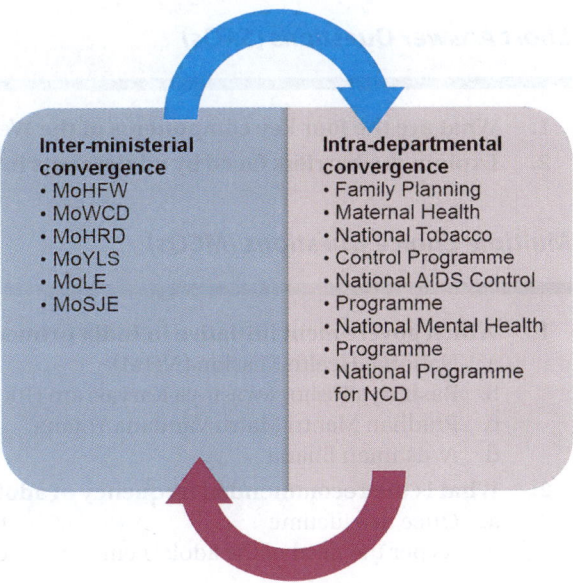

Reporting Mechanism for AFHCs

Adolescent-friendly Health Clinics (AFHCs) are required to submit monthly consolidated reports to their respective districts by the 5th of the following month. These reports must be prepared using the standardized Facility Level Consolidated

Monthly Format. The data for these reports are compiled from the Service Delivery Registers and Outreach Service Delivery Registers maintained at the AFHCs.

To facilitate effective monitoring and evaluation, a structured monthly reporting format has been established for assessment at both state and district levels. The key variables included in the report are as follows:

Variables	Boys	Girls	Total
No. of adolescents (10–19 years) registered in AFHC			
No. of adolescents (10–19 years) received clinical services			
No. of adolescents (10–19 years) received counselling services			

References

1. Implementation guidelines Rashtriya Kishor Swasthya Karyakram (RKSK) 2018. Ministry of Health & Family welfare, Government of India. Available on: https://nhm.gov.in/New_Updates_2018/NHM_Components/RMNCHA/AH/guidelines/Implementation_Guidelines_Rashtriya_Kishor_Swasthya_Karyakram(RKSK)_2018.pdf
2. Guidelines for implementation of RKSK, Adolescent Health Division, Ministry of Health and Family Welfare, Government of India. Available on: https://nhm.gov.in/images/pdf/programmes/RKSK/RKSK_Implementation_Guideline_05.03.2015.pdf
3. Guidelines for Operationalizing Model Adolescent Friendly Health Clinics (M-AFHC). Ministry of Health and Family Welfare, Government of India. Available on: https://nhm.hp.gov.in/storage/app/media/uploaded-files/M-AFHC%20guidelines.pdf

QUESTIONS

Long Answer Question (LAQ)

1. Discuss the significance of Adolescent-friendly Health Clinics (AFHCs) in improving adolescent healthcare in India. Highlight their key principles, operational benchmarks, and the role of counselors in ensuring effective service delivery.

Short Answer Questions (SAQs)

1. What are the four key components of the Weekly Iron and Folic Acid Supplementation (WIFS) Programme
2. Explain the barriers faced by adolescents in accessing healthcare services.

Multiple Choice Questions (MCQs)

1. Which government initiative in India primarily supports the establishment of AFHCs?
    a. National Health Mission (NHM)
    b. Rashtriya Kishor Swasthya Karyakram (RKSK)
    c. Pradhan Mantri Matru Vandana Yojana
    d. Ayushman Bharat
2. What is the recommended frequency of adolescent health counseling sessions under the AFHC model?
    a. Once in a lifetime
    b. Once every five years
    c. As per the need of the adolescent
    d. Only during school health check-ups

3. **Under the WIFS Programme, how often is Albendazole administered?**
   a. Monthly
   b. Weekly
   c. Biannually
   d. Annually
4. **Which of the following is not a key principle of AFHCs?**
   a. Equity
   b. Accessibility
   c. Profitability
   d. Comprehensiveness

Answers

1. b
2. c
3. c
4. c

CHAPTER 36

Peer Education Program

Krupal J Joshi, Krishna M Jasani, NIharika Verma

NEED OF THE PROGRAM

In order to cover the out of school adolescents along with the school going adolescents, the Peer Education (PE) Program engages adolescents through trained Peer Educators (Saathiyas), who facilitate discussions on RKSK's thematic areas.

Eligibility Criteria for Saathiyas

A Saathiya must meet the following criteria:
- Be between 15 and 19 years of age.
- Share similar social and demographic characteristics with the community they serve.
- Be willing to dedicate volunteer time.
- Possess strong communication skills.
- Demonstrate leadership qualities.
- Exhibit motivation and commitment to the role.

Components

To ensure maximum outreach to out-of-school adolescents, two Peer Educators—one male and one female—are designated per village, per 1,000 population, or per ASHA habitation. The selection of these educators is facilitated by the Accredited Social Health Activist (ASHA) in collaboration with the Village Health Sanitation and Nutrition Committee (VHSNC). ASHAs receive a nominal incentive of ₹ 100 for every successful selection of a Saathiya, with this incentive being disbursed biennially.[1]

Activities[2]

Weekly Sessions

Each Saathiya takes responsibility for forming a group of 15–20 adolescents within their community. These groups, composed of either boys or girls, participate in structured weekly interactive sessions lasting between one and two hours. The sessions are conducted using specially designed Peer Education (PE) kits to ensure an engaging and informative experience for participants.

Saathiyas are required to maintain a diary documenting session summaries and participant numbers. At the end of each month, they prepare a consolidated report detailing the number of sessions conducted and average attendance rates. As a non-monetary incentive, Saathiyas receive ₹ 50 per month.

Adolescent Health Day

AHD is conducted quarterly at the village level at anganwadi centers or other accessible public place, ensuring easy participation for adolescents and all stakeholders. There is a block adolescent health coordinator who coordinates the AHD. ASHAs actively engage with parents and families of adolescents to raise awareness about adolescents' unique needs.

Adolescent-friendly Club Meetings

In addition to Adolescent Health Day, monthly Adolescent-friendly Club (AFC) meetings are conducted at the subcenter level under the supervision of the ANM. Each AFC covers a population of approximately 5,000 individuals across five villages and consists of 10–20 Saathiyas. These meetings provide a platform for Saathiyas from different villages to convene and address challenges encountered during their weekly sessions, with guidance and support from the ANM.

This structured approach ensures the effective delivery of peer education, fostering adolescent health and well-being within the community.

References

1. Peer Education Program. RMNCAH+N, Adolescent Health, National Health Mission, Ministry of Health and Family Welfare, Government of India. Available on: https://nhm.gov.in/index1.php?lang=1&level=3&sublinkid=1249&lid=493
2. Peer Educator Reference Book. Rashtriya Kishor Swasthya Karyakram, National Health Mission, Ministry of Health and Family Welfare, Government of India. Available on: https://www.nhm.gov.in/images/pdf/programmes/RKSK/PE_Training_Manual/PE-Reference-book_FAQ_old.pdf

QUESTIONS

Long Answer Question (LAQ)

1. Discuss the need for Peer Education Program. What are the eligibility criteria for a Saathiya? Detail the activities conducted under this program.

Short Answer Questions (SAQs)

1. How is Adolescent Health Day organized? What is the role of block adolescent health coordinator and ASHA in its implementation?
2. Describe the role of Saathiya in Peer Education Program.

Multiple Choice Questions (MCQs)

1. Who facilitates the selection of peer educators (Saathiyas)?
    a. Anganwadi workers
    b. Accredited social health activists (ASHAs)
    c. District health officers
    d. School teachers
2. What is the age range for peer educators (Saathiyas) under the peer education program?
    a. 10–15 years
    b. 15–19 years
    c. 20–25 years
    d. Above 25 years

3. **What is the role of peer educators (Saathiyas)?**
   a. To provide financial support to adolescents
   b. To facilitate discussions on adolescent health issues
   c. To distribute iron supplements to all adolescents
   d. To provide medical treatments at AFHCs

Answers

1. b
2. b
3. b

CHAPTER 37

Scheme for Adolescent Girls

Krupal J Joshi, Krishna M Jasani, NIharika Verma

INTRODUCTION

SAG, introduced in 2010, initially focused on improving the nutritional and educational status of out-of-school adolescent girls aged 11–14 years. The scheme aimed to enhance their health and nutritional status by providing nutritional support, life skills training, and access to public services, while also encouraging their return to formal education. Following the implementation of the Right to Education (RTE) Act, the program's focus has shifted to girls aged 14–18 in Aspirational Districts and the North Eastern States.[1]

In light of this, the Scheme has been redesigned and incorporated into the broader Saksham Anganwadi and Poshan 2.0 initiative. The updated framework now specifically addresses the needs of adolescent girls aged 14–18 years, with a primary focus on regions, such as Aspirational Districts and the North Eastern States. The revised scheme emphasizes a comprehensive approach to their development, encompassing health, nutrition, education, and overall well-being.

In addition, the Government of India launched the **Kanya Shiksha Pravesh Utsav** campaign on March 7, 2022, under the **Beti Bachao Beti Padhao** initiative. This initiative is strategically designed to facilitate the re-enrollment of all out-of-school adolescent girls aged 11–14 years into formal education. The campaign aligns with the Right to Education (RTE) Act's objectives, aiming to bridge educational gaps and promote equitable access to learning opportunities for adolescent girls across the nation.

Objectives

The objectives of the revised SAG framework follow a life-cycle approach, aiming to mitigate malnutrition's intergenerational impact by targeting adolescent girls in identified regions.

Interventions under the Scheme[2]

The intervention is categorized into two components: **Nutritional Support** and **Non-Nutritional Interventions**, as outlined below:

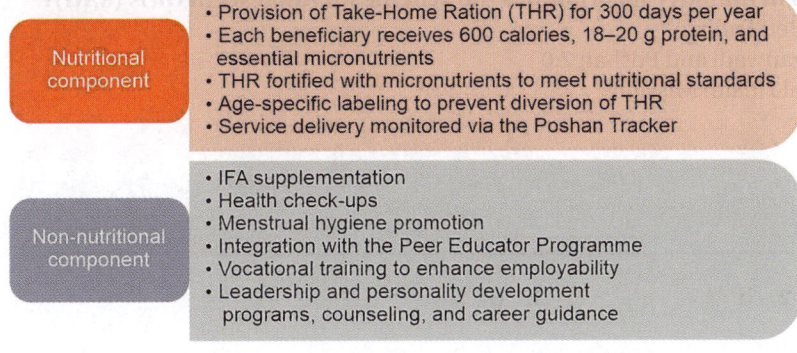

References

1. Mission Saksham Anganwadi and Poshan 2.0 scheme guidelines August 2022. Ministry of Women and Child Development, Government of India. Available on: https://wcd.delhi.gov.in/sites/default/files/WCD/generic_multiple_files/final_saksham_anganwadi_and_mission.pdf
2. Press Information Bureau, Scheme for Adolescent Girls, Ministry of women and child development Press release. (Release ID: 1811388) Available on: https://pib.gov.in/PressReleasePage.aspx?PRID=1811388

QUESTIONS

Long Answer Question (LAQ)

1. What are the objectives and interventions under Scheme for Adolescent Girls?

Short Answer Questions (SAQs)

1. What is Kanya Shiksha Pravesh Utsav campaign? Discuss the activities undertaken under the campaign.
2. Describe in detail Saksham Anganwadi and Poshan 2.0 initiative.

Multiple Choice Questions (MCQs)

1. Under the Scheme for Adolescent Girls (SAG), which group is primarily targeted for intervention?
   a. Adolescent boys aged 13–19 years
   b. All children below 10 years
   c. Out-of-school adolescent girls aged 11–18 years
   d. Only pregnant adolescents
2. What is the primary aim of the Kanya Shiksha Pravesh Utsav campaign?
   a. To provide financial aid to adolescent girls
   b. To ensure the re-enrollment of out-of-school adolescent girls into formal education
   c. To offer vocational training for unemployed women
   d. To provide free healthcare for adolescent boys
3. Which government initiative incorporates the Scheme for Adolescent Girls (SAG)?
   a. Beti Bachao Beti Padhao
   b. Saksham Anganwadi and Poshan 2.0
   c. National Rural Health Mission
   d. Digital India

Answers

1. c
2. b
3. b

CHAPTER 38

Weekly Iron Folic Acid Supplementation Program and National Deworming Day

Bhautik Modi, Akhil Dhanesh Goel

RATIONALE

Anemia is a major public health issue affecting pregnant women, children and also adolescents. In iron deficiency is the leading cause of anemia in India, making it one of the most prevalent nutritional disorders in the country.[1]

NFHS-5 data reveal that more than 59% of girls from 15 to 19 years of age and 31% of boys from 15 to 19 years of age are anaemic. Adolescent girls are particularly at risk because of rapid physical growth and loss of blood during menstruation.[2]

To address the anemia among adolescent boys and girls, the MoHFW has introduced the Weekly Iron and Folic Acid Supplementation (WIFS) program in the year 2006).[3]

Objective

Reduce the prevalence of anemia in the adolescent population (10–19 years boys and girls).

Strategies under the Program

Under the WIFS Programme for adolescents, IFA supplements are provided free of charge on a weekly basis to the designated target groups in categories A and B. Additionally, biannual administration of Albendazole tablets for deworming. This program includes the following key components:

- **Weekly Iron and Folic Acid Supplementation (WIFS):** Each adolescent receives an IFA tablet containing 100 mg of elemental iron and 500 μg of folic acid once a week.[3]
- **Anemia screening and referral:** All adolescents are screened for anemia, and those identified are referred to healthcare facilities for further management.
- **Biannual deworming:** A 400 mg dose of Albendazole is given every six months to control worm infestations.
- **Nutrition and hygiene awareness:** Counseling and education are provided to improve dietary habits and promote preventive measures against intestinal worm infections.

Beneficiaries

Two groups in both rural and urban areas:
A. Adolescent boys and girls enrolled in schools from grades 6 to 12.
B. Out-of-school adolescent girls.
The program also includes married adolescent girls.
The pregnant and lactating adolescent girls will receive IFA supplementation in accordance with the existing antenatal and postnatal care guidelines.

Package of Services

The WIFS Programme targets both adolescent boys and girls in schools, as well as out-of-school adolescent girls, regardless of their marital status. It follows a **fixed day approach** for distributing iron and folic acid (IFA) tablets, with Monday designated as the primary distribution day in schools and anganwadi centers. An additional day is allocated to reach those who miss their dose. To ensure adherence, the program emphasizes supervised consumption of IFA tablets.

Furthermore, the initiative encourages frontline workers, including anganwadi workers, ASHAs, and teachers, to take IFA tablets themselves, reinforcing their importance among adolescents and the broader community.

To identify adolescents with moderate or severe anemia, AWWs and teachers receive training to assess pallor by comparing the color of nail beds and tongues. However, this method serves only as an initial screening, and suspected cases are referred to a primary health center for hemoglobin testing. Those diagnosed with anemia receive appropriate treatment. Additionally, states conduct haemoglobin testing for school-going children through the School Health Programme.

Organogram

Weekly Iron and Folic Acid Supplementation Programme (WIFS): Roles and Responsibilities[3]

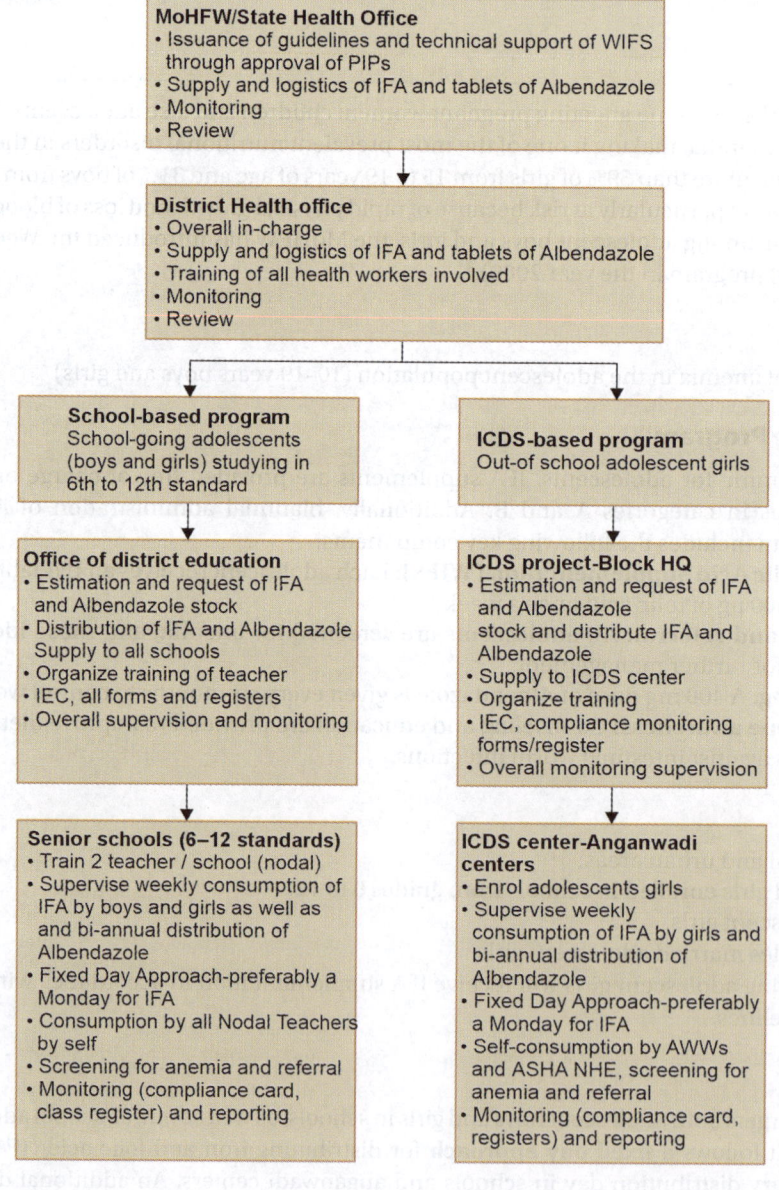

NATIONAL DEWORMING DAY

Rationale

Soil-transmitted helminth (STH. infections are widespread, impacting around 1.5 billion population, or 24% of the total population globally.[4]

Inadequate sanitation and hygiene contribute to these infections, leading to anemia and undernutrition, which negatively impact physical growth and cognitive abilities. In India, nearly 67% of children aged 6–59 months are anemic, 32% are underweight, and 35% of children under five experience stunting. Adolescents are also at high risk, with 57% of girls and 25% of boys aged 15–19 years suffering from anemia.

Severe STH infections reduce school attendance and learning capacity, affecting future economic prospects. Implementing mass deworming in schools is a cost-effective strategy that enhances health, education, and economic well-being. Research highlights that large-scale deworming programs significantly boost school participation and long-term financial stability.

In 2009, the Government of India advised state-specific mass deworming and integration with the program of vitamin A prophylaxis. Other programs, such as the National Iron Plus Initiative (NIPI) and Weekly Iron and Folic Acid Supplementation (WIFS) require deworming for children and adolescents aged 1–19 years biannual. However, many states lack effective deworming initiatives, resulting in low program coverage.

Implemented Since

The MoHFW introduced National Deworming Day (NDD) in February 10, 2015, followed by a mop-up round on February 13, 2015, to administer deworming treatment to children who missed the initial dose.[5]

The program is conducted nationwide through schools and anganwadi centers, and encouraged to involve private schools for wider coverage.

Since then, National Deworming Day is observing biannually on 10th February and on 10 August every year.

Objective

To administer age specific dose of tablet Albendazole to all children and adolescents aged 1 to 19 years, including both enrolled and non-enrolled individuals, through schools and anganwadi centers.[5]

Beneficiaries

All children between the ages of 1–19 years, including children enrolled in schools and anganwadis, as well as children who are not enrolled, are the beneficiaries of National Deworming Day.

Age	Albendazole (400 mg tablet)	Instruction
1–2 years	Half tablet	Child should chew the tablet and should consume some water if required.
2–19 years	Full tablet	For young child, with the help of a spoon the tablet should crushed and then swallow with water.

Package of Services

- Teachers to administer Albendazole tablets school-going children, while anganwadi workers (AWWs) distribute them to children under-five, out-of-school children, and adolescents.
- Children who are unwell or on medication the day do not receive the tablet. They take it after recovery or with medical advice.
- Teachers document deworming details in class registers, compile the data, and submit reports to the principal. Similarly, AWWs record information in enrollment registers and report it through anganwadi reporting forms. ASHAs, present at the anganwadi center (AWC), maintain separate records for non-enrolled children and submit them to the auxiliary nurse midwife (ANM) for incentive claims.
- Children stay in school or the AWC for at least two hours after taking the tablet to monitor potential side effects and ensure prompt medical attention if needed.

❖ Principals and AWWs compile and report the total number of dewormed children in the prescribed format. ANMs collect reports from schools and AWCs as per the given timeline.

Adverse Event Management System

Any side effect or adverse events are handled according to protocol, and the Adverse Event Management Reporting Form should be filled properly.

Emergency helpline numbers and contact details of the nearest Medical Officer at the primary health center (MO-PHC) and ANM shall be prominently displayed at the entrance for quick reference by the schools and anganwadi centers.

The Medical Officer at the PHC ensures the availability of essential medicines listed in the Adverse Event Management Protocol.

The MO-PHC shall also ensure that referral services remain fully operational to handle emergencies.

Monitoring and Supervision

Monitoring and supervision play a crucial role in ensuring the effective implementation of National Deworming Day (NDD) and assessing its impact. The key guidelines for monitoring and supervision are as follows:

❖ Teams designated by the MoHFW conduct random inspections at schools and anganwadi centers to oversee NDD activities.
❖ State, district, and block-level teams assign officials for on-ground monitoring during both NDD and the Mop-Up Day (MUD), with dedicated funds allocated for this purpose.
❖ Mobile health teams under RBSK and AYUSH doctors at the block level oversee implementation, ensuring that at least four schools or anganwadi centers are visited.
❖ The district nodal officer for deworming coordinates all monitoring and supervision efforts within the district.
❖ All collected monitoring data is submitted to the state health department's nodal officer for compilation, entry, and analysis.

References

1. Anaemia. Available on: https://www.who.int/news-room/fact-sheets/detail/anaemia#:~:text=Iron%20deficiency%2C%20 primarily%20due%20to,haemoglobin%20and%2For%20erythrocyte%20production. Last accessed on 25th January, 2025
2. NFHS 5. Available on: https://mohfw.gov.in/sites/default/files/NFHS-5_Phase-II_0.pdf . Last accessed on 2nd February, 2025
3. Operational Framework: WIFS For Adolescents. Available on: https://nhm.gov.in/images/pdf/programmes/wifs/operational-framework wifs/operational_framework_wifs.pdf Last accessed on 10th February, 2025
4. Soil-transmitted helminth infections. Available on: https://www.who.int/news-room/fact-sheets/detail/soil-transmitted-helminth-infections. Last accessed on 28th January, 2025
5. Operational Guidelines of National Deworming Day. Available on. https://nhm.gov.in/images/pdf/NDD/Guidelines/NDD_Operational_Guidelines.pdf. Last accessed on 2nd February, 2025

QUESTIONS

Long Answer Question (LAQ)

1. Write the prevalence of anemia as per NFHS-5 in India and describe the Weekly Iron Folic Acid Supplementation (WIFS) Programme in terms of objective, strategies, beneficiaries and packages of services.

Chapter 38: Weekly Iron Folic Acid Supplementation Program and National Deworming Day

Short Answer Questions (SAQs)

1. Write the interventions under the Weekly Iron Folic Acid Supplementation (WIFS) Programme to prevent anemia.
2. Enumerate the beneficiaries under the Weekly Iron Folic Acid Supplementation (WIFS) Programme.
3. Enumerate the beneficiaries under the National Deworming Day.
4. Write the rationale of the Weekly Iron Folic Acid Supplementation (WIFS) Programme.
5. Write the rationale of the National Deworming Day.

Multiple Choice Questions (MCQs)

1. National Deworming Day is celebrated on _____ every year.
   a. 1st February
   b. 10th February
   c. 1st March
   d. 10th March
2. Beneficiaries of Weekly Iron Folic Acid program are, all *except*:
   a. Adolescent girls from schools from grades 6 to 12
   b. Adolescent boys from schools from grades 6 to 12
   c. Out-of-school adolescent girls
   d. Out-of-school adolescent boys
3. Dose of Albendazole tablet for children aged 1–2 years is:
   a. 200 mg
   b. 300 mg
   c. 400 mg
   d. 500 mg
4. Dose of Albendazole tablet for children aged 2–19 years is:
   a. 200 mg
   b. 300 mg
   c. 400 mg
   d. 500 mg
5. Under Weekly Iron and Folic Acid Supplementation (WIFS) Programme, each adolescent receives:
   a. An IFA tablet containing 60 mg of elemental iron and 500 µg of folic acid every week
   b. An IFA tablet containing 60 mg of elemental iron and 100 µg of folic acid every week
   c. An IFA tablet containing 500 mg of elemental iron and 100 µg of folic acid every week
   d. An IFA tablet containing 100 mg of elemental iron and 500 µg of folic acid every week
6. Which type of prevention is Iron and Folic Acid Supplementation under WIFS?
   a. Health promotion
   b. Specific protection
   c. Primordial prevention
   d. Secondary prevention

Answers

1. b   2. d   3. a   4. c   5. d
6. b

v. N: Nutrition

CHAPTER 39

Anemia Mukt Bharat

Akhil Dhanesh Goel, Suseendar S, Manoj Kumar Gupta, Pankaj Bhardwaj, Mallika Vasantbhai Chavada

Background

Reducing prevalence of anemia is a key objective of the Poshan Abhiyaan initiative, which was launched in March 2018. In alignment with the targets set by Poshan Abhiyaan and the National Nutrition Strategy of NITI Aayog, the Anemia Mukt Bharat (AMB) strategy aims to decrease the prevalence of anemia by 3 percentage points annually among children, adolescents, and women of reproductive age (15–49 years) from 2018–2022. The Government of India has also committed to the World Health Assembly to achieve 50% reduction of anemia among women of reproductive age by 2025. This strategy is designed to improve overall health outcomes and effectively tackle the widespread issue of anemia in India. The primary objective of this initiative is to reduce the prevalence of anemia among different population groups through a lifecycle approach. This comprehensive strategy addresses anemia from infancy through adolescence, pregnancy, and into adulthood, aiming to improve overall health, cognitive development, and productivity of the Indian population.

Anemia poses a significant public health challenge in India, affecting children, adolescents, pregnant women, and women of reproductive age. It is primarily caused by iron deficiency but can also result from other nutritional deficiencies, infections, and chronic diseases. The manifestations of anemia vary by its severity and range from fatigue, weakness, dizziness and drowsiness to impaired cognitive development of children, lowered immunity, and decreased work productivity. Anemia during pregnancy is associated with postpartum hemorrhage, neural tube defects, low birth weight, premature births, stillbirths, and maternal deaths. The morbidity and mortality risks associated with anemia call for an urgent need to design an effective strategy to address this public health problem. The decline in anemia prevalence will, in turn, contribute to improved maternal and child survival rates and better health outcomes for other population groups.[1]

The prevalence of anemia in India has been documented extensively through national surveys. **Table 39.1** highlights the changes in anemia prevalence among various age groups from NFHS-3 (2006), NFHS-4 (2016), and NFHS-5 (2019–21).

TABLE 39.1: Prevalence of anemia based on findings from NFHS.

Age group	NFHS-3 (2006)	NFHS-4 (2016)	NFHS-5 (2019–21)
Children 6–59 months	69.0	58.0	67.1
Adolescent girls 15–19 years	56.0	54.0	59.1
Adolescent boys 15–19 years	30.0	29.0	31.1
Women of reproductive age	55.0	53.0	57.0
Pregnant women	55.0	50.0	52.2
Lactating women	63.0	58.0	67.1
Men 15–49 years	–	–	25.0

Despite some progress observed between NFHS-3 (2006) and NFHS-4 (2016), the overall decline in anemia prevalence has been modest, underscoring the necessity for intensified efforts. For example, anemia prevalence in children aged 6–59 months decreased from 69% in 2006 to 58% in 2016 but remains significantly high at 67.1% in 2021. Similarly, anemia in adolescent girls saw a minor decline from 56% to 54% between 2006 and 2016, and then an increase to 59.1% in 2021, indicating persistent challenges. **The data from NFHS-5 shows that anemia continues to be a critical public health**

Chapter 39: Anemia Mukt Bharat

	issue in India. The high prevalence rates among children, adolescents, and women indicate significant nutritional deficits and the need for comprehensive interventions. **The slight improvements observed between NFHS-3 and NFHS-4 have not been sustained or sufficiently impactful, demonstrating that existing measures need to be reinforced and expanded.**
Need of the program/ Scheme	Anemia remains a significant public health issue in India, affecting all age groups and contributing to adverse health outcomes. The AMB program addresses this by providing comprehensive prevention and treatment strategies to reduce the burden of anemia across the population.
Implemented since	The Anemia Mukt Bharat program has been operational since 2018. It was introduced in response to the high prevalence of anemia and its detrimental effects on public health and socioeconomic development. The program builds on the existing National Iron Plus Initiative (NIPI) and other anemia control measures, integrating them into a cohesive framework under Poshan Abhiyaan.
Goal	The overarching goal of the Anemia Mukt Bharat program is to reduce the prevalence of anemia across all age groups in India. This reduction is expected to lead to significant improvements in health outcomes, educational performance, and economic productivity.
Targets	The specific targets of the AMB program include: • Reducing anemia prevalence by one-third among children aged 6–59 months, school-aged children, adolescents, pregnant women, and women of reproductive age by 2022. • Ensuring at least 90% of the identified anemic population receives appropriate treatment and follow-up. • Increasing awareness and knowledge about anemia prevention and management through community engagement and mass mobilization activities.
Objectives	The objectives of the Anemia Mukt Bharat program are multifaceted and designed to address the issue of anemia from multiple angles. They include:[1] • Providing routine iron and folic acid (IFA) supplementation to vulnerable groups to prevent anemia. • Strengthening the capacity of healthcare facilities to test for and treat anemia effectively. • Promoting dietary diversification and the consumption of iron-rich, protein-rich, and vitamin C-rich foods. • Encouraging the fortification of staple foods with iron and other essential micronutrients. • Enhancing health and nutrition-related behaviors through targeted counseling and mass media campaigns. The AMB program adopts the **6 × 6 × 6 strategy** to address anemia comprehensively. This strategy focuses on **six target beneficiaries, six interventions, and six institutional mechanisms**. The six target beneficiaries are children aged 6–59 months, children aged 5–9 years, adolescents aged 10–19 years, pregnant women, lactating women, and women of reproductive age. **Approximately 450 million beneficiaries, nearly 50% of the country's population, will be reached through this strategy**. Six interventions under AMB strategy: 1. **Prophylactic iron and folic acid supplementation:** The key intervention of AMB program is to emphasize on routine IFA supplementation to prevent anemia across various age groups. The **Table 39.2** outlines the prophylactic dose and regimen for IFA supplementation:

TABLE 39.2: Prophylactic dose and regimen for IFA supplementation.

Age group	Dose and regime
Children 6–59 months	Biweekly 1 mL Iron and Folic Acid syrup (20 mg Iron + 100 µg Folic Acid)
Children 5–9 years	Weekly 1 Iron and Folic Acid tablet—pink color tablet (45 mg Iron + 400 µg Folic Acid)
School-going adolescents 10–19 years	Weekly 1 Iron and Folic Acid tablet—blue color Tablet (60 mg Iron + 500 µg Folic Acid)
Women of reproductive Age 20–49 years	Weekly 1 Iron and Folic Acid tablet—red color tablet (60 mg Iron + 500 µg Folic Acid)
Pregnant women and lactating mothers	Daily 1 Iron and Folic Acid tablet —red color tablet from the fourth month of pregnancy, continued throughout pregnancy and for ISO days postpartum (60 mg Iron + 500 µg Folic Acid)

The initiative includes the use of a distinct blue IFA tablet to differentiate it from the red IFA tablet provided to pregnant and lactating women.

Deworming: Under the National Deworming Day Programme, mass deworming is done biannually to prevent Soil-transmitted Helminths (STH) infections that can contribute to anemia. The **Table 39.3** outlines the dose and regimen for deworming across various age groups:

TABLE 39.3: Dose and regimen for deworming across various age groups.

Age group	Dose and regime
Children 12–59 months	Biannual dose of 400 mg albendazole (1/2: tablet for children 12–24 months and 1 tablet for children 24–59 months)
Children 5–9 years	Biannual dose of 400 mg albendazole (1 tablet)
School-going adolescents 10–19 years	Biannual dose of 400 mg albendazole (1 tablet)
Out-of-school adolescents 10–19 years	Biannual dose of 400 mg albendazole (1 tablet)
Women of reproductive age 20–49 years	Biannual dose of 400 mg albendazole (1 tablet)
Pregnant women	One dose of 400 mg albendazole (1 tablet) after the first trimester, preferably during the second trimester

2. **Intensified behavior change communication campaign:** Promoting four key behaviors improving compliance to IFA supplementation and deworming, appropriate infant and young child feeding practices, increasing the intake of iron-rich foods, and ensuring delayed cord clamping after delivery.
3. **Testing and treatment:** Using digital methods for anemia detection and providing point-of-care treatment, with more emphasis on pregnant women and school-going adolescents.
4. **Mandatory provision of iron and folic acid fortified foods:** Ensuring that public health programs include fortified foods as per prescribed and notified by the Food Safety and Standard Authority of India (FSSAI, 2016).
5. **Addressing non-nutritional causes of anemia:** Emphasize on awareness, screening and treatment for non-nutritional causes of anemia with special focus on malaria, haemoglobinopathies and fluorosis especially in endemic pockets.

The AMB strategy is implemented in all villages, blocks, and districts across India using existing delivery platforms, such as the National Iron Plus Initiative (NIPI) and Weekly Iron Folic Acid Supplementation (WIFS) program. In order to ensure accountability and effective implementation of the Anemia Mukt Bharat strategy, six institutional mechanisms are set-up at national, state and district levels, which are described below.

	Six Institutional Mechanisms The institutional mechanisms under the AMB strategy include: 1. **Intra-ministerial coordination:** Ensuring collaboration within the Ministry of Health and Family Welfare. 2. **National Anemia Mukt Bharat unit:** A dedicated unit to oversee and coordinate the AMB program. It supports and monitors the states for effective strategy implementation. 3. **National center of excellence and advanced research on anemia control (AIIMS Delhi):** NCEAR-A is an institutional mechanism envisions to develop and provide technical support to the Ministry of Health and Family Welfare, Government of India. It assists in making policy and guidelines. It also does periodic program review and check its proper implementation. It also helps for capacity building of work force by conducting training. 4. **Convergence with other ministries:** Collaborating with other government ministries to ensure comprehensive implementation of the AMB strategy. 5. **Strengthening supply chain and logistics:** Ensuring the availability and distribution of necessary supplies and supplements. So, Strengthening the procurement and supply chain mechanisms are key to effective implementation of these programs. 6. **Anemia Mukt Bharat Dashboard and Digital Portal:** A one-stop shop for anemia-related information, monitoring, and reporting. 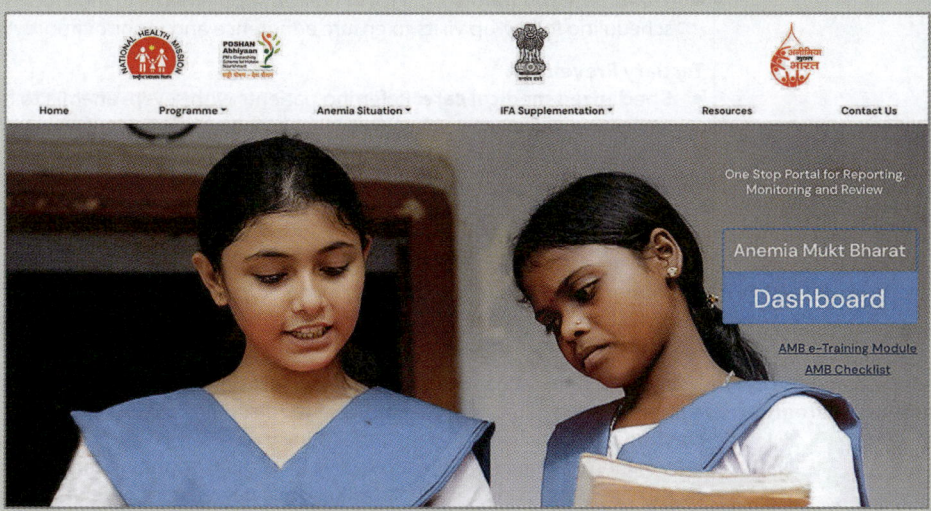
Organogram	The implementation of the Anemia Mukt Bharat program follows a structured hierarchy that includes national, state, district, and block-level officials. At the national level, the Ministry of Health and Family Welfare oversees the program, with state health departments coordinating efforts within their jurisdictions. District health officials, supported by block-level health workers, implement the program on the ground. Frontline workers, such as Accredited Social Health Activists (ASHAs), Auxiliary Nurse Midwives (ANMs), and Anganwadi Workers (AWWs) play a crucial role in delivering services and mobilizing communities. **Service delivery platforms for testing and treatment of anemia** The AMB strategy will be implemented in all villages, blocks, and districts across India using existing delivery platforms, such as the National Iron Plus Initiative (NIPI) and Weekly Iron Folic Acid Supplementation (WIFS) program. The Anemia Mukt Bharat program utilizes a comprehensive strategy to screen and treat anemia across different age groups. For children aged 6–59 months, screenings are conducted by ANMs at VHNDs, subcenters, or session sites, RSBK teams at anganwadi centers or schools, and medical officers at health facilities, with scheduled screenings and opportunistic assessments. Children aged 5–9 years are screened annually by RSBK teams in both in-school and out-of-school settings, with additional opportunistic screenings. School-going adolescents (10–19 years) are screened annually by RSBK teams within school premises. Pregnant women registered for antenatal care are tested for anemia at every ANC contact by health service providers, including those under the PMSMA initiative, using digital hemoglobinometers. This multi-tiered approach ensures early detection and timely treatment of anemia, addressing a significant public health challenge in India.

Examples of activities at various levels or package of services	**Primary Prevention**
	• **Prophylactic iron and folic acid supplementation:** Routine distribution of iron and folic acid tablets to school-going children and adolescents every week.
	• **Dietary diversification:** Promoting the inclusion of iron-rich foods, such as spinach, lentils, and citrus fruits in daily diets through community cooking demonstrations.
	• **Food fortification:** Collaborating with food manufacturers to fortify commonly consumed items, such as wheat flour and rice with iron and folic acid.
	• **Behavior change communication (BCC):** Conducting awareness campaigns in schools and communities to encourage practices, such as delayed cord clamping during childbirth and proper handwashing.
	• **Deworming:** Organizing biannual deworming drives in schools and community centers to administer albendazole tablets to children and adolescents.
	
	Secondary Prevention
	• **Screening and early diagnosis:** Conducting anemia screening camps in schools using digital hemoglobinometers to quickly identify children with low hemoglobin levels.
	• **Health check-ups:** Routine antenatal check-ups for pregnant women at health centers to monitor their hemoglobin levels and provide timely interventions.
	• **Treatment and follow-up:** Providing iron supplements to individuals diagnosed with anemia and scheduling follow-up visits to ensure adherence and monitor improvement.
	
	Tertiary Prevention
	• **Specialized medical care:** Referring patients with severe anemia to hospitals for comprehensive evaluation and management, including blood transfusions, if necessary.
	• **Management of underlying conditions:** Treating underlying causes of anemia, such as chronic infections or genetic disorders, such as thalassemia through specialized care.
	• **Rehabilitation and support**
	  ✦ **Example:** Offering nutritional rehabilitation programs for severely malnourished children diagnosed with anemia.
	• **Monitoring and long-term follow-up**
	  ✦ **Example:** Regular monitoring of patients with chronic anemia through follow-up visits by community health workers to manage their condition effectively.

Monitoring and evaluation of program	Monitoring and evaluation of the Anemia Mukt Bharat program can be achieved through a comprehensive framework that includes regular data collection and reporting via the **Jan Andolan Dashboard** of Poshan Abhiyan (under Ministry of Women and Child Development) and routine health information systems. Periodic surveys, such as the **National Family Health Survey (NFHS)** and annual health surveys provide critical data on anemia prevalence. Supervision by district and block level officials, along with feedback from community health workers and beneficiaries, ensures adherence to protocols and identifies areas for improvement.

Reference

1. Ministry of Health & Family Welfare. Anemia Mukt Bharat. Intensified National Iron Plus Initiative (I-NIPI): Operational Guidelines for Programme Managers. New Delhi: MoHFW, Government of India; April 2018. [Accessed on August 23, 2023]. Available on: https://nhm.hp.gov.in/storage/app/media/Anemia-Mukt-Bharat-Operational-Guidelines-FINAL.pdf

QUESTIONS

Long Answer Question (LAQ)

1. A 22-year-old female with 6-month amenorrhea has come for antenatal check-up when her hemoglobin was found to be 7 g%.
   a. Discuss the management of anemia in this female.
   b. Construct a district level health promotion strategy for anemia prevention and management.

Short Answer Questions (SAQs)

1. Describe the 6 × 6 × 6 strategy.
2. Describe the dietary interventions for anemia.

Multiple Choice Questions (MCQs)

1. **Anemia Mukt Bharat program addresses all below mentioned non-nutritional causes of anemia in endemic pockets, *except*:**
    a. Malaria
    b. Hemoglobinopathies
    c. Fluorosis
    d. Dengue

2. **All are correct statements under Anemia Mukt Bharat program for deworming, *except*:**

a.	Children 5–9 years	Biannual dose of 400 mg albendazole ((½ tablet)
b.	School-going adolescents 10–19 years	Biannual dose of 400 mg albendazole (1 tablet)
c.	Women of reproductive age 20–49 years	Biannual dose of 400 mg albendazole (1 tablet)
d.	Pregnant women	One dose of 400 mg albendazole (1 tablet) after the first trimester, preferably during the second trimester

3. **All are correct statements under Anemia Mukt Bharat program for anemia prophylaxis, *except*:**

a.	Children 6–59 months	Biweekly, 1 mL Iron and Folic Acid syrup (20 mg Iron + 100 µg Folic Acid)
b.	Adolescents 10–19 years	Weekly, 1 Iron and Folic Acid tablet (60 mg Iron + 500 µg Folic Acid)
c.	Women of reproductive age 20–49 years	Weekly, 1 Iron and Folic Acid tablet (60 mg Iron + 500 µg Folic Acid)
d.	Pregnant women	Biweekly, 1 Iron and Folic Acid tablet—from the fourth month of pregnancy

4. **Under Anemia Mukt Bharat program for prophylaxis of anemia in pregnant women**
    1. Iron and Folic acid tablet should be started from the fourth month of pregnancy
    2. Iron and Folic acid tablet should be continued throughout pregnancy and for 180 days postpartum
    Which of the above statements is/are correct?
    a. 1 only
    b. 2 only
    c. Both 1 and 2
    d. Neither 1 nor 2

5. **Consider the following statements regarding the Anemia Mukt Bharat strategy:**
    1. It provides prophylactic calcium supplementation for preschool children.
    2. It runs a campaign for delayed cord clamping at childbirth.
    3. It integrates deworming for children and adolescents.
    4. It addresses non-nutritional causes of anemia.
    Which of the above statements is/are correct?
    a. Only one
    b. Only two
    c. Only three
    d. All four

6. **All are primary intervention under the Anemia Mukt Bharat strategy, *except*:**
    a. Providing calcium supplements
    b. Prophylactic Iron and Folic Acid supplementation
    c. Deworming
    d. Behavior change communication

7. **What is the target reduction in anemia prevalence annually as per the Anemia Mukt Bharat initiative?**
    a. 1 percentage point
    b. 2 percentage points
    c. 3 percentage points
    d. 5 percentage points

8. Which group is NOT a target beneficiary of the Anemia Mukt Bharat program?
   a. Pregnant women
   b. Lactating mothers
   c. Elderly women
   d. Adolescent girls
9. The Anemia Mukt Bharat strategy was launched in which year?
   a. 2015
   b. 2016
   c. 2018
   d. 2020
10. Which institutional mechanism is not the part of the Anemia Mukt Bharat strategy?
    a. National Health Mission
    b. National Anemia Mukt Bharat Unit
    c. National Center of Excellence and Advanced Research on Anemia Control
    d. Strengthening supply chain and logistics

Answers

| 1. d | 2. a | 3. d | 4. c | 5. c |
| 6. a | 7. c | 8. c | 9. c | 10. a |

CHAPTER 40

National Nutrition Mission: POSHAN 2.0

Janki Bartwal, Shaili Vyas, Akash Krishali, Priti Solanki

Background/ Need of program/ Scheme[1]	The need for National Nutrition Mission (NNM) is reflected in the data of the NFHS 4 (2015–16) report: • The proportion of children under five years of age who were stunted (height-for-age), wasted (weight-for-height), severely wasted (weight-for-height), underweight (weight-for-age) was 38.4%, 21.0%, 7.5%, and 35.8% respectively. • The prevalence of anemia among children aged 6–59 months (<11 g/dL), non-pregnant women aged 15–49 years (<12 g/dL), pregnant women aged 15–49 years (<11 g/dL) and all women aged 15–49 years was 58.6%, 53.2%, 50.4%, and 53.1% respectively.
Implemented since[2-4]	The proposal for setting up the National Nutrition Mission was approved in the cabinet in December 2017. On 8th March 2018, the Hon'ble Prime Minister of India launched the proposed NNM as the POSHAN (Prime Minister's Overarching Scheme for Holistic Nourishment) Abhiyaan from Jhunjhunu district, Rajasthan. This is a flagship program of the Ministry of Women and Child Development (MWCD), and it strives to reduce stunting, undernutrition, low birth weight in children, and anemia in adolescent girls, pregnant women, lactating mothers, and children.
Goal[3]	The goals of NNM were to achieve improvement in the nutritional status of children from 0–6 years, adolescent girls, pregnant women, and lactating mothers in a time-bound manner during the next three years beginning 2017–18 with fixed targets as follows: | Objectives	Targets
Prevent and reduce stunting in children (0–6 years)	↓ by 6% @ 2% per annum
Prevent and reduce undernutrition in children (0–6 years)	↓ by 6% @ 2% per annum
Reduce the prevalence of anemia among children (6–59 months)	↓ by 9% @ 3% per annum
Reduce the prevalence of anemia among women and adolescent girls in the age group of 15–49 years anemia among Women	↓ by 9% @ 3% per annum
Reduce low birth weight (LBW)	↓ by 6% @ 2% per annum | The Government of India approved "Saksham Anganwadi and Poshan 2.0," referred to as **Poshan 2.0** during the 15th Finance Commission period, i.e., from 2021–2022 to 2025–26. It is a strategic shift in mission mode to develop practices that nurture health, wellness, and immunity from malnutrition. The Anganwadi Services Scheme for Adolescent Girls, and Poshan Abhiyaan have been re-aligned under Poshan 2.0 to maximize nutritional outcomes.
Vision[4]	It seeks to address the challenging situation of malnutrition among children up to the age of 6 years, adolescent girls (14–18 years), and pregnant and lactating women.
Objectives[4]	• To contribute to the human capital development of the country. • Address challenges of malnutrition. • Promote nutrition awareness and good eating habits for sustainable health and well-being. • Address nutrition-related deficiencies through key strategies.

Components[4]	- **Nutrition support for poshan:** It is provided through the Supplementary Nutrition Programme (SNP) for children of the age group of six months to six years, pregnant women and lactating mothers (PWLM); and adolescent girls in the age group of 14 to 18 years in Aspirational Districts and North Eastern Region (NER).
- **Early childhood care and education (ECCE) for 3–6 years:** It will cover provision for preschool learning material for the cognitive, emotional, social, and intellectual development of the child; development of muscular coordination and basic motor skills; aesthetic appreciation, independence, and creativity; good healthy habits; training and skilling needs to make all preschoolers school ready and for seamless integration of children in the age group of 5–6 years in Grade-I.
- **Anganwadi infrastructure including modern, upgraded saksham anganwadi:**
- States/UTs shall permit funding of anganwadi infrastructure, e.g., toilets, rainwater harvesting system, water purifier/installation of RO machine, etc., or any aspect of anganwadi activity, such as ECCE material with smart learning aids, audio-visual aids, child-friendly learning equipment and artwork (educational painting, practice board for children, information board), furniture, cooking utensils, kitchen infrastructure, storage facility, Poshan Vatikas (kitchen garden and nutri-gardens to bridge the dietary diversity gap by providing different vegetables, fruits, medicinal herbs round the year), etc.
- States/UTs shall co-locate those Anganwadi Centers (AWCs) running on rent and without sufficient infrastructure to nearby Government Primary Schools.
- States shall consider running mobile AWCs for beneficiaries in urban slum areas as an alternative to a brick-and-mortar AWC due to the non-availability of permanent buildings and the ceiling on the number of AWCs.
- Mini-anganwadi which fulfils the criteria of population norms of main AWC shall be upgraded to full-fledged anganwadi. In the case of tribal areas or difficult areas (such as Left Wing Extremism (LWE) districts, high altitude areas, etc.) the mini-anganwadi can be upgraded based on justification given by states.
- The Ministry of Women and Child Development (MWCD) shall consider non-operational AWCs as surrendered from the states/UTs which have failed to operationalize these AWCs and re-allocate these centers to states/UTs which require additional AWCs.
- **Poshan abhiyaan:**
- **Community mobilization and behavioral change:** It focuses on converting the agenda of improving nutrition into a Jan Andolan through the involvement of Panchayati Raj Institutions/Villages Organizations/SHGs/volunteers, etc., and ensuring wide public participation.
- **Community-based events (CBEs):** To be held twice every month by each AWC. Under it, Annaprasan Diwas, Suposan Diwas (specifically focused on orienting husbands), celebrating coming of age and getting ready for preschool at AWC, etc., are covered.
- **Jan andolan:** The month of September is celebrated as Rashtriya Poshan Maah across the country. Similarly, in/around March, Poshan Pakhwada is celebrated.
- **Incentives and awards:** Provision of incentives for 'Kuposhan Mukt Villages' will be distributed away to qualified villages/panchayats ₹ 1 lac each. About 100 awards have been provisioned annually for AWWs ₹ 50,000/- each and 50 awards annually for AWHs ₹ 40,000/- each.
- **Technology:** To empower the frontline functionaries, i.e., anganwadi workers and lady supervisors by providing them with smartphones, enabling real-time monitoring and tracking of all AWCs, AWWs, and beneficiaries on the defined indicators. 'POSHAN tracker', introduced in the year 2021 to monitor the progress of mission POSHAN 2.0, helps in the dynamic identification of stunting, wasting, and undernutrition in children and last mile tracking of nutrition service delivery. Similarly, each AWC is provisioned to be equipped with Growth Monitoring Devices (GMDs) comprising of stadiometer, infantometer, and weighing scale for infant and mother and child.
- **Best practices:** Best practices/innovations in poshan, which have won the PM's award are shared with all the states/UTs.
- **Convergence with ministries/departments/organizations:** MeiTY (for development of ICT systems), NeGD (National e-Governance Division), MyGov, MoHFW, Ministry of Education, etc.

Anganwadi Services Scheme

Package of services:
- Supplementary nutrition
- Preschool nonformal education
- Nutrition and health education

- Immunization
- Health check-up
- Referral services

Supplementary nutrition: It shall be provided at anganwadi center (AWC) during working hours. It shall be served for a minimum of 300 days in a calendar year, i.e., on an average of 25 days in a month with respect to morning snacks, Hot Cooked Meals (HCM), and Take-Home Ration (THR).

Only the beneficiaries registered at the AWC are entitled to receive it. If any beneficiary is registered at another AWC, he/she can still get the benefits of supplementary nutrition at AWC at a different location through the migration facility, which is available in POSHAN tracker.

Categories	Nutritional norms (per beneficiary per day)		Cost norms (rates-per day per beneficiary)
	Calories (kcal)	Protein (gram)	In rupees
Children (6 months–6 years)	500	12–15	8.00
Severe malnourished children (6 months–6 years)	800	20–25	12.00
Pregnant women and nursing mothers	600	18–20	9.50
Adolescent girls (14–18 years)	600	18–20	9.50

Growth measurement: Measurement of length/height and weight is essential for all children to obtain their status as normal, underweight, stunted, severe acute malnutrition, or moderate acute malnutrition. Length/Height and weight of the children from six months to six years will be measured every month.

Health services:
- **IFA prophylaxis:**
  - *Six months to five-year-old child:* IFA syrup one mL twice a week
  - *During pregnancy and post-pregnancy:* IFA tablet daily
- **De-worming:**
  - *12 months to five-year-old child:* Albendazole tablet once in six months
  - *Pregnant women:* One Albendazole tablet during the second trimester
- **Vitamin A supplementation:** Nine months to five-year-old child: Vitamin A syrup bi-annually
- **Diarrhea management:** ORS, zinc supplementation

Referral services:
- Severely malnourished (SAM) to be referred to hospital or nutrition rehabilitation center
- Care of sick children

Immunization: For pregnant women two doses of tetanus toxoid and all vaccines for children under the National Immunization schedule

Scheme for Adolescent Girls

Objective: It aims at providing nutritional support to adolescent girls in the age group of 14 to 18 years in the identified areas of the country to improve their health and nutritional status under the nutrition component and providing them IFA supplementation, health check-up, and referral service, nutrition and health education and skilling, etc., under the non-nutrition component of the scheme.

Coverage:
Adolescent girls in the age group (14–18 years) in aspirational districts of states including Assam and North-Eastern states shall be covered under the scheme for adolescent girls.

Eligibility:
The beneficiaries of the scheme will be adolescent girls in the age group of 14–18 years who will be identified by the states concerned. All beneficiaries will require an Aadhaar number to avail the benefits under the scheme.

Activities proposed under convergence	Service provider	Platform for convergence activity	Outcomes
Ministry of Health and Family Welfare (MoHFW)			
Convergence under non-nutrition component: • Iron and folic acid supplementation • Health check-up and referral service • Nutrition and health education • Ensure promotion of menstrual hygiene among adolescent girls • Ensure active participation of AGs to deal with issues and needs of adolescents and the services available through the peer educator program	Public health infrastructure by Asha and ANM	AWCs/ adolescent friendly health clinics (AFHCs)	• Focused approach towards addressing not only the nutritional needs of the AGs but also on the holistic development of the AGs • AGs shall be included as Kishori Volunteers to work with AWWs to mobilize the local AGs to meet their nutritional and health needs and to generate awareness on family planning and anemia
Ministry of Skill Development and Entrepreneurship (MSDE)			
Providing skill training to AGs	NSDC and State Skill Development Missions (SSDMs) of the states	AWCs/Training Centers formed Under Pradhan Mantri Kaushal Vikas Yojana	• Generation of livelihood opportunities for AGs trained under the scheme • AGs shall be included as Kishori Volunteers to work with AWWs to mobilize the local AGs to meet their nutritional and health needs and to generate awareness on family planning and anemia
Ministry of education			
Providing skill training to AGs	Vocational trainers in schools	Government schools	• Generation of livelihood opportunities for AGs based on district needs/ requirements and in the service sector • AGs to enrol in open schooling
Ministry of Youth Affairs and Sports (MoYAS)			
• Youth leadership and personality development training • Development and empowerment of adolescents (Life skills education, counseling, career guidance, etc.)	Organizations involved under the scheme of National Programme for Youth and Adolescent Development (NPYAD) wherein financial assistance is provided to government/ non-government organizations to take up activities for youth and adolescent development	AWCs/Platform utilized by organizations finalized by MoYAS in each financial year	Providing an opportunity for holistic development of adolescents for the realization of their fullest potential and to develop leadership qualities and personality development

References

1. National Family Health Survey 4 (2015-16). Available from https://rchiips.org/nfhs/factsheet_NFHS-4.shtml
2. ICDS Final Guidelines 2021. Available from https://wcd.nic.in/acts/icds-final-guidelines-2021.pdf
3. Administrative Guidelines for implementation of National Nutrition Mission. Available from https://wcd.nic.in/sites/default/files/Administrative_Guidelines_NNM-26022018.pdf
4. Saksham Anganwadi and Poshan 2.0 scheme guidelines. Available from https://wcd.nic.in/acts/guidelines-mission-saksham-anganwadi-and-poshan2.0.pdf

QUESTIONS

Long Answer Question (LAQ)

1. Write in detail about PM Poshan.

Short Answer Questions (SAQs)

1. Write in brief about components of PM Poshan.
2. Write in brief about beneficiaries of PM Poshan.

Multiple Choice Questions (MCQs)

1. **Following ministry is primarily responsible for Poshan Abhiyan:**
   a. Ministry of Health and Family Welfare
   b. Ministry of Rural Development
   c. Ministry of Women and Child Development
   d. Ministry of Social Justice and Empowerment
2. **National Nutrition Mission was launched on:**
   a. August 15, 2018
   b. March 8, 2018
   c. January 26, 2018
   d. July 1, 2018
3. **Community-based event, such as Suposhan Diwas is to be celebrated at AWC on:**
   a. In the month of September
   b. In/around March
   c. First week of August
   d. Twice every month
4. **The state can consider running mobile anganwadi center in which of the following scenario?**
   a. Ceiling on the total number of fixed anganwadis
   b. Non-availability of permanent infrastructure
   c. Urban slum area
   d. All of the above
   e. Only A and C

5. **Awards given under Poshan Abhiyan are:**
   a. Total 50 awards per year for anganwadi helpers
   b. ₹ 40,000 per year for anganwadi worker
   c. ₹ 10 lakhs per year for each village for 'Kuposhan-Mukt Village'
   d. ₹ 25,000 per year for Poshan panchayat
6. **Mission Poshan 2.0 focuses mainly on following beneficiaries and outcome:**
   a. Children aged 3–6 years for early formal skill-based education
   b. Adolescent girls aged 11–14 years for menstrual hygiene
   c. Pregnant women for prevention of low birth weight
   d. All of the above
7. **In the following service delivery component, along with anganwadi, health department will also get involved:**
   a. Weight measurement of infant
   b. IFA administration to the pregnant women
   c. Counseling on breastfeeding to the mothers
   d. Providing supplementary nutrition to the adolescent girls
8. **True about supplementary nutrition:**
   a. Registered beneficiaries can avail it from any anganwadi as per his/her wish
   b. It is given throughout the year with minimum of 28 days in any month
   c. Beneficiary has to be transferred through Poshan tracker to other anaganwadi in case of migration
   d. The menu of Take Home Ration is kept the same for all the states to maintain uniformity
9. **Under Mission 2.0, Poshan Vatika refers to:**
   a. Kitchen garden
   b. AWC supplying hot cooked meals
   c. Mother groups at the village level
   d. Centers of forest and agriculture departments
10. **True about Poshan tracker:**
    a. It helps in maintaining real time data of nutrition-related indicators of AWC beneficiaries
    b. It can be used to monitor any AWC and its staff activities pertaining to nutrition
    c. It provides feedback to the program managers for intervention
    d. All of the above
    e. Only 1 & 2 are correct

Answers

1. c	2. b	3. d	4. d	5. a
6. c	7. b	8. c	9. a	10. d

CHAPTER 41

Mothers' Absolute Affection

Rudresh Negi, Shaili Vyas, Nilesh Thakor

Background/Need of program/Scheme	Breastfeeding remains an accessible, acceptable, convenient and cost-effective intervention which benefits both the mother and the child and has a long-term impact on reducing the under-5 mortality and morbidity. It is an effective weapon which conforms with the life cycle approach and the continuum of care envisaged in the RMNCAH + N Programme. However, exclusive and timely breastfeeding rates were inadequate in the country prior to the operationalization of this program. Also, there were some myths and misconceptions regarding breastfeeding practices prevalent in the community. Thus, the program was launched with the intention of promoting breastfeeding and providing counseling to support breastfeeding.
Implemented since	5th August 2016
Goal	To revitalize efforts towards promotion, protection and support of breastfeeding practices through health systems to achieve higher breastfeeding rates[1]
Targets	It targets: • All states and union territories (UTs) • Around 3.9 crore pregnant and lactating mothers • 8.8 lakh ASHAs • 1.5 lakhs sub-centers • 17,000 birthing facilities/delivery points
Objectives	• Build an enabling environment for breastfeeding through awareness generation activities, targeting pregnant and lactating mothers, family members and society in order to promote optimal breastfeeding practices. Breastfeeding to be positioned as an important intervention for child survival and development. • Reinforce lactation support services at public health facilities through trained healthcare providers and through skilled community health workers. • To incentivize and recognize those health facilities that show high rates of breastfeeding along with processes in place for lactation management[1]
Organogram	• Coordination committee at state level • District as nucleus of implementation
Beneficiaries	Mainly pregnant and lactating mothers
Components[2]	**Awareness Generation (B1):** Building an enabling environment and demand generation through Mass media and Mid-media **Community level interventions (B2):** Capacity building of community health workers - ASHAs, AWWs and ANMs on breastfeeding* and Community diagoue—by ASHAs through mother' meetings; and lactation support and interpersonal communication - by skilled ANMs at VHNDs/sub-centers **Health facility strengthening (B3):** Capacity building of auxiliary nurse midwives (ANMs)/nurses doctors on lactation support and managment at facilities and Role reinforcement on breastfeeding—at all delivery points **Monitoring (B4):** Monitoring and Awards/Recognition

Fig. 41.1: Main four components and subcomponents of Mothers Absolute Affection (MAA) program.
* Anganwadi workers (AWWs) should be supporting ASHA/ANM for breastfeeding.

Strategies/ Deliverables under the program	• **Creating an enabling environment for breastfeeding** ✦ *Awareness campaigns:* Use mass media (TV, radio, SMS) and mid-media (folk performances, nukkad natak, exhibitions) to promote optimal breastfeeding practices. ✦ *Intersectoral convergence:* Coordinate advocacy with private sectors, other ministries, and development partners. • **Community-level activities** ✦ *ASHA worker training:* Single-day orientation sessions to prepare ASHAs as the primary source of information on breastfeeding. ✦ *Mothers' meetings:* Regular meetings with ASHA workers to educate and support mothers regarding breastfeeding and complementary nutrition. ✦ *Routine support:* Reinforce ASHA activities focused on breastfeeding promotion and management. ✦ *ANM capacity building:* Four-day IYCF training for ANMs to strengthen breastfeeding support at sub-centers and Village Health and Nutrition Days (VHNDs). • **Strengthening healthcare provider capacities** ✦ *Reinforcing roles:* One-day orientation for ANMs, nurses, and medical officers emphasizing breastfeeding counseling and IMS Act compliance. ✦ *Facility improvements:* Establish dedicated breastfeeding spaces, adopt BFHI guidelines, and provide IEC material in health facilities. ✦ *Training master trainers:* Capacity-building initiatives led by pediatric and community medicine departments in medical colleges. ✦ *National resource center:* Develop a resource center for supporting training and monitoring. • **Recognition and awards** ✦ *Facility awards:* State-level recognition and awards for healthcare facilities demonstrating high breastfeeding rates. ✦ *District-level recognition:* Cash awards and certificates for high-performing facilities at the district level.
Activities at various level or package of services	• **Enabling environment and demand generation** ✦ *Mass media:* Broadcasts via TV, radio, SMS, etc., promoting breastfeeding. ✦ *Community engagement:* Folk performances, street plays, exhibitions for awareness. ✦ *Intersectoral collaboration:* Advocacy with private sectors and partners. • **Community-level activities** ✦ *ASHA sensitization:* Single-day training as key breastfeeding supporters. ✦ *Mother's meetings:* Regular ASHA-led sessions to promote and manage breastfeeding. ✦ *ANM training:* Four-day IYCF training for consistent breastfeeding support. • **Healthcare provider capacity building** ✦ *Orientation sessions:* One-day refreshers for ANMs, nurses, and MOs on breastfeeding. ✦ *Advanced training:* Building master trainers for enhanced breastfeeding counseling. ✦ *Facility support:* Dedicated breastfeeding spaces and educational displays. • **Recognition and awards** ✦ *Facility awards:* Recognition for high breastfeeding rates. ✦ *District awards:* Cash prizes and certificates for outstanding performance.
Monitoring and evaluation of program	• All ASHAs to submit monitoring plans monthly to ANM • ANM to submit complied reports to Block Medical Officer • Block reports compiled and submitted to district official • District and states to submit reports detailing trainings, monitoring and visits on monthly basis Detailed statewide evaluation to be conducted post 1 year of implementation **Key monitoring indicators-** • Number and % of ASHAs for whom sensitization on IYCF was conducted in block meetings. • Number of districts conducted launch of MAA program. • Number of Mothers' meetings held. • Number and % of pregnant and lactating mothers who attended mother's meetings. • Number and % of ASHAs having IYCF info kit. • Number and % of ASHAs provided incentive for mothers' meetings. • Number and % of ANMs for whom one day sensitization was undertaken. • Number and % of ANMs and nurses trained on 4-day trainings. • Number and % of delivery points, where healthcare providers have been oriented using one day sensitization module. • Number of facilities received MAA awards (at state level).

References

1. Health Minister launches MAA programme to promote breastfeeding [Internet]. [cited 2024 Aug 20]. Available from: https://pib.gov.in/newsite/PrintRelease.aspx?relid=148531
2. Operational_Guidelines.pdf [Internet]. [cited 2024 Aug 20]. Available from: https://nhm.gov.in/MAA/Operational_Guidelines.pdf

QUESTIONS

Long Answer Question (LAQ)

1. What are the objectives of MAA program? Mention in detail the components considered in it.

Short Answer Questions (SAQs)

1. Enumerate the monitoring indicators of MAA program.
2. Critically analyze the achievements and shortcomings of MAA program.

Multiple Choice Questions (MCQs)

1. When was the MAA program launched?
   a. 2005
   b. 2016
   c. 2020
   d. 2024
2. What is the main target level for implementing the MAA program?
   a. State
   b. Division
   c. District
   d. Block
3. What is the primary goal of the MAA program?
   a. To improve maternal nutrition
   b. To increase institutional deliveries
   c. To promote, protect, and support breastfeeding
   d. To reduce maternal mortality
4. Which of the following is a key strategy in creating an enabling environment for breastfeeding under the MAA program?
   a. Providing free supplements
   b. Mid-media activities like street plays and folk performances
   c. Increasing hospital infrastructure
   d. Free vaccination drives
5. How many pregnant and lactating mothers are targeted by the MAA program?
   a. 1 crore
   b. 2.5 crore
   c. 3.9 crore
   d. 5 crore
6. Which healthcare worker is primarily responsible for community-level breastfeeding support under the MAA program?
   a. ANM
   b. ASHA
   c. Medical Officer
   d. Pediatrician
7. What type of training is provided to ANMs under the MAA program?
   a. 2-day training on child health
   b. 4-day training on Infant and Young Child Feeding (IYCF)
   c. 1-week training on maternal care
   d. No specific training

8. Which of the following is a key monitoring indicator for the MAA program?
   a. Number of deliveries conducted in hospitals
   b. Number of ASHAs sensitized on IYCF
   c. Number of immunization camps held
   d. Number of schools with hygiene programs
9. What is the incentive given to district-level facilities for achieving high breastfeeding rates under MAA?
   a. Training sessions
   b. Award of ₹ 10,000 with certification
   c. Free medical supplies
   d. Additional staff
10. Which day of the month is designated for reinforcing breastfeeding counseling under the PMSMA initiative?
    a. 1st
    b. 5th
    c. 9th
    d. 15th

Answers

1. b	2. c	3. c	4. b	5. c
6. b	7. b	8. b	9. b	10. c

CHAPTER 42

Infant and Young Child Feeding

Satabdi Mitra, Pallavi Singh, Abhay Srivastava, Parul Sharma, Shaili Vyas

Background/Need of program/Scheme	Infant and Young Child Feeding (IYCF), is crucial for a child's optimal growth and development. It encompasses the practices of breastfeeding, complementary feeding, and responsive feeding, which provide essential nutrients and support a child's immune system. IYCF is particularly important during the first 1,000 days of life, as this period is critical for brain development and the establishment of lifelong health. Adequate IYCF practices can reduce malnutrition, stunting, and mortality rates, leading to healthier and more productive children and communities.
Implemented since	The World Health Organization (WHO) and the United Nations Children's Fund (UNICEF) launched the Global Strategy for Infant and Young Child Feeding (IYCF) in 2002. This strategy aimed to improve IYCF practices worldwide and reduce child malnutrition.
Goal/vision	The goal of IYCF is to improve the nutrition and health of infants and young children through the promotion of optimal feeding practices. The vision is to create a world where all infants and young children have access to adequate nutrition and care, leading to improved growth, development, and overall health.
Targets	The target of IYCF is to improve the nutritional status of infants and young children by promoting exclusive breastfeeding for the first six months and appropriate complementary feeding from six months to two years. This is especially important in developing countries where malnutrition is a significant public health issue.
Objectives[1]	• **Promoting exclusive breastfeeding:** Encouraging mothers to breastfeed their infants exclusively for the first six months of life. • **Providing appropriate complementary feeding:** Guiding mothers on the introduction of appropriate foods at six months and beyond to meet the child's nutritional needs. • **Improving infant and young child feeding practices:** Promoting responsive feeding, ensuring hygienic food preparation, and avoiding harmful feeding practices like early or excessive introduction of solid foods. • **Reducing child malnutrition:** Addressing various forms of malnutrition, including undernutrition, stunting, and wasting, through improved IYCF practices. • **Improving child health and development:** Promoting optimal growth, cognitive development, and immune function in infants and young children. • **Reducing child mortality:** Decreasing mortality rates associated with malnutrition and related diseases. • **Empowering mothers:** Supporting and empowering mothers to make informed decisions about infant and young child feeding. • **Strengthening health systems:** Enhancing the capacity of health systems to provide IYCF support and services.

Organogram	**Key components and their roles:**
	• **Health systems:**
	  ✦ Primary healthcare centers
	  ✦ Hospitals
	  ✦ Community health workers
	  ✦ Health professionals (doctors, nurses, nutritionists)
	  ✦ Responsible for providing IYCF counseling, monitoring, and support services.

	- **Communities:**
	  + Mothers and caregivers
	  + Families
	  + Community leaders
	  + Play a crucial role in implementing IYCF practices and supporting each other.
	- **Government:**
	  + Health departments
	  + Nutrition programs
	  + Policymakers
	  + Develop and implement IYCF policies, allocate resources, and ensure access to IYCF services.
	- **Non-governmental organizations (NGOs):**
	  + International and local NGOs
	  + Provide technical assistance, advocacy, and support for IYCF programs.
	- **Research and academic institutions:** Conduct research and generate evidence to inform IYCF policies and practices.

Beneficiaries	- Infants and young children - Mothers - Families and communities

Components	**Key Components of IYCF (Infant and Young Child Feeding):**
	- **Exclusive breastfeeding:**
	  + Breastfeeding as the sole source of nutrition for the first six months of life.
	  + Provides essential nutrients, antibodies, and protection against infections.
	  + Promotes optimal growth and development.
	- **Complementary feeding:**
	  + Introduction of appropriate, nutrient-dense foods in addition to breast milk from six months onwards.
	  + Gradual increase in the variety and quantity of foods to meet the child's growing needs.
	  + Focus on locally available, culturally appropriate, and safe foods.
	- **Responsive feeding:**
	  + Attending to the child's hunger cues and feeding them in a responsive and nurturing manner.
	  + Allowing the child to self-feed and explore different textures and flavors.
	  + Creating a positive feeding environment that promotes healthy eating habits.
	- **Hygiene and sanitation:**
	  + Ensuring clean hands, utensils, and food preparation practices.
	  + Providing safe drinking water and storing food properly.
	  + Preventing food contamination to reduce the risk of illness.
	- **Nutrition education and counseling:**
	  + Providing mothers and caregivers with information and support on IYCF practices.
	  + Addressing common misconceptions and challenges related to breastfeeding and complementary feeding.
	  + Empowering mothers to make informed decisions about their child's nutrition.
	- **Community support:**
	  + Creating supportive environments that promote IYCF practices.
	  + Encouraging social norms and cultural practices that support breastfeeding and appropriate feeding.
	  + Providing community-based IYCF programs and services.
	- **Health system support:**
	  + Integrating IYCF into primary healthcare services.
	  + Training healthcare providers on IYCF practices and counseling.
	  + Ensuring access to essential IYCF supplies and resources.

Strategies/ Deliverables under the program	**Strategies:** - **Community-based IYCF programs:** Implementing programs at the community level to provide education, support, and services related to IYCF. - **Health system strengthening:** Enhancing the capacity of healthcare systems to deliver IYCF services, including training healthcare providers and improving infrastructure. - **Social marketing and communication:** Raising awareness about IYCF through various channels, such as print media, radio, television, and social media.

	• **Advocacy and policy development:** Advocating for policies that support IYCF and ensuring that IYCF is integrated into national development plans. • **Research and evidence generation:** Conducting research to generate evidence on effective IYCF practices and inform program development. • **Public-private partnerships:** Collaborating with NGOs, private sector organizations, and other stakeholders to leverage resources and expertise. **Deliverables:** • **Increased breastfeeding rates:** Promoting exclusive breastfeeding for the first six months and continued breastfeeding up to two years. • **Improved complementary feeding practices:** Encouraging the timely introduction of appropriate complementary foods and promoting responsive feeding. • **Reduced child malnutrition:** Decreasing rates of undernutrition, stunting, and wasting among infants and young children. • **Improved child health and development:** Enhancing cognitive, physical, and social development outcomes. • **Empowered mothers:** Supporting mothers to make informed decisions about their child's nutrition. • **Strengthened health systems:** Building the capacity of healthcare systems to deliver IYCF services effectively. • **Increased awareness and advocacy:** Raising public awareness about the importance of IYCF and advocating for supportive policies.
Activities at various levels or package of services	**Antenatal Care:** • IYCF counseling for pregnant women • Promotion of breastfeeding intentions • Preparation for breastfeeding and infant care **Maternal and Child Health Services:** • Skilled birth attendance • Early initiation of breastfeeding within the first hour of birth • Exclusive breastfeeding promotion • Growth monitoring and promotion (GMP) • Complementary feeding counseling • Management of common childhood illnesses **Community-based IYCF Programs:** • Home visits by health workers • Mother-to-mother support groups • Community-based nutrition education • Community kitchens or food gardens **Nutrition Education and Counseling:** • Individual and group counseling sessions • Development and distribution of IYCF materials (brochures, leaflets, posters) • Use of multimedia tools (videos, audio clips) **Food Security and Nutrition:** • Food fortification programs • Food distribution programs for vulnerable populations • Nutrition-sensitive agriculture and food systems **Water, Sanitation, and Hygiene (WASH):** • Promotion of safe water, sanitation, and hygiene practices to prevent diarrheal diseases. • Provision of clean water and sanitation facilities in communities. **Health System Strengthening:** • Training of healthcare providers on IYCF • Development of IYCF guidelines and protocols • Establishment of IYCF referral systems • Integration of IYCF into primary healthcare services **Advocacy and Policy Development:** • Advocacy for IYCF policies at national and local levels • Development and implementation of IYCF-related policies and regulations

	Research and Evidence Generation: • Conducting research to inform IYCF programs and policies • Monitoring and evaluation of IYCF intervention

Monitoring and evaluation of program	Monitoring and evaluation (M&E) are essential components of IYCF programs to assess their effectiveness, identify areas for improvement, and ensure accountability. Here are the key aspects of M&E for IYCF:
	Indicators:
	• **Process indicators:** Measure the implementation of IYCF activities, such as the number of health facilities providing IYCF counseling, the percentage of mothers receiving antenatal and postnatal care, and the coverage of community-based IYCF programs.
	• **Outcome indicators:** Measure the impact of IYCF interventions on child health and nutrition, including:
	    ✦ Breastfeeding rates (exclusive breastfeeding, continued breastfeeding)
	    ✦ Complementary feeding practices (timeliness, adequacy, diversity)
	    ✦ Child growth indicators (weight, length, BMI)
	    ✦ Child morbidity and mortality rates
	    ✦ Maternal knowledge and practices related to IYCF

Reference

1. Infant and young child feeding. WHO. Available at: https://www.who.int/news-room/fact-sheets/detail/infant-and-young-child-feeding

QUESTIONS

Long Answer Question (LAQ)

1. Enumerate recommendations of Infant and Young Child Feeding (IYCF) practices. Name parameters for assessment of IYCF.

Short Answer Questions (SAQs)

1. Briefly mention recommendations of feeding of low-birth-weight babies.
2. Discuss governmental initiatives for promotion of IYCF practices.

Multiple Choice Questions (MCQs)

3. Exclusive breastfeeding is recommended up to which age:
   a. 3 months
   b. 6 months
   c. 9 months
   d. 12 months
4. In which month 'Poshan Maah' or national nutrition month is observed?
   a. July
   b. August
   c. September
   d. October

Answers

1. b   2. c

PART B

Communicable Diseases

43. National Vector Borne Disease Control Programme
44. National Tuberculosis Elimination Programme
45. National AIDS Control Programme
46. National Leprosy Eradication Programme
47. National Viral hepatitis Control Programme
48. National Rabies Control Programme
49. Endgame Strategy for Poliomyelitis
50. Integrated Disease Surveillance Programme and Integrated Health Information Platform

CHAPTER 43

National Vector Borne Disease Control Programme

Kavita Vishwakarma, Prerna Verma, Kajal Srivastava, Parul Sharma, Rudresh Negi, Veidehi

Background/Need of program/Scheme	The National Vector Disease Control Programme (NVBDCP) in India was initiated in response to the significant burden of vector-borne diseases such as malaria, dengue, chikungunya, lymphatic filariasis, kala-azar, and Japanese encephalitis. These diseases pose a major public health challenge in India, particularly in rural and remote areas.[1]
Implemented since	The NVBDCP was launched in December 2003 to address the challenges posed by vector-borne diseases and reduce their burden across the country.[2]
Objectives[2]	<ul><li>Reduce the incidence and prevalence of vector-borne diseases.</li><li>Improve the quality of diagnosis and treatment of these diseases.</li><li>Strengthen the surveillance system for early detection and response.</li><li>Enhance the capacity of health workers and communities to prevent and control vector-borne diseases.</li><li>Promote research and innovation in vector-borne disease control.</li></ul>
Organogram[2]	<ul><li>At National level—Director General Health Services (DGHS), Ministry of Health and Family Welfare (MoHFW)</li><li>At State level—Regional Offices for Health and Family Welfare, State Vector Borne Control Society</li><li>District Health Departments at the district level</li><li>Vector Control Units at the sub-district level</li></ul>
Beneficiaries	<ul><li>Population residing in areas prone to vector-borne diseases</li><li>Healthcare workers involved in vector control activities</li><li>Communities mobilized for preventive measures</li></ul>
Components[2]	<ul><li>National Kala-Azar Elimination Programme</li><li>Japanese Encephalitis Control Programme</li><li>National Filaria Control Programme</li><li>National Malaria Elimination Programme</li><li>Dengue Control Programme</li><li>Chikungunya Control Programme</li></ul>
Strategies/Deliverables under the program[2,4]	<ul><li>Integrated Vector Management</li><li>Early Diagnosis and Prompt Treatment</li><li>Surveillance and Response</li><li>Health Education and Community Mobilization</li><li>Capacity Building</li></ul>
Activities at various level or package of services[2,4]	<ul><li>Implementation of vector control measures</li><li>Surveillance and monitoring of vector-borne diseases</li><li>Training of healthcare workers and community health volunteers</li><li>Health education campaigns</li><li>Research and innovation in vector control</li></ul>
Monitoring and evaluation of program[2]	<ul><li>Regular surveillance of vector-borne diseases</li><li>Monitoring of vector control activities and their impact</li><li>Evaluation of program outcomes and effectiveness</li><li>Feedback mechanisms for continuous improvement</li></ul>

KALA-AZAR

Need of program/ Scheme	• **Disease burden:** Visceral leishmaniasis, commonly known as kala-azar, is a significant health issue in India, particularly in 54 districts of eastern states, such as Bihar, Jharkhand, West Bengal, Uttar Pradesh. The disease manifests with symptoms, such as fever, weight loss, splenomegaly, anemia and skin lesions (in cutaneous leishmaniasis). • **Impact on health:** Kala-azar primarily affects vulnerable and at-risk populations, leading to severe health complications if untreated. The emergence of Post Kala-azar Dermal Leishmaniasis (PKDL) adds to the disease burden.[2]
Implemented since	• **Launch and integration:** The Kala-Azar Control Programme was launched in 1991 and currently the program activities are implemented under the National Vector Borne Disease Control Programme (NVBDCP), which is part of the National Health Mission (NHM).[2] • **Timeline:** Kala-azar control efforts have been integrated and intensified since the early 2000s, with a focus on reducing the incidence of the disease.[2]
Goal	**Long-term goal:** To eliminate kala-azar as a public health problem, improving the health status of vulnerable groups in endemic areas.[2]
Objectives	**Primary objective:** To reduce the annual kala-azar case incidence to less than one case per 10,000 population at the block level by the end of 2023.
Organogram	• **Central level:** Led by the National Vector Borne Disease Control Programme under NHM. • **State level:** State health departments and vector-borne disease units manage implementation. • **District and block level:** Local health officials and workers, including ASHA workers, execute on-ground activities.[2]
Beneficiaries	• **Target groups:** Vulnerable populations in endemic areas, including those affected by kala-azar and PKDL. • **Specific support:** ASHA workers receive incentives for case identification (₹ 500 for kala-azar and PKDL case identification, complete treatment and follow up), and patients receive financial support for wage loss (one time wage loss incentives/compensation of ₹ 4000 to each new PKDL patient and ₹ 500 for kala-azar patient) and nutritional supplements.[2]
Components[2,4]	• Parasite elimination and disease management using rK39 rapid diagnostic kits and oral miltefosine respectively. • **Vector control:** Integrated approaches to control the sandfly population. • **Surveillance and data management:** Utilization of systems like Kala-Azar Management Information System (KAMIS) for real-time data reporting.
Strategies/Deliverables under the program[2]	• **Early diagnosis and complete case management:** Ensuring prompt identification and treatment of cases. • **Integrated vector management and vector surveillance:** Control and monitoring of the sandfly vector. • **Supervision, monitoring, surveillance, and evaluation:** Strengthening surveillance systems and evaluating program effectiveness. • **Strengthening capacity of human resources in health:** Training and capacity-building of healthcare workers. • **Advocacy, communication, and social mobilization:** Raising awareness and encouraging behavioral change. • **Program management:** Effective management and coordination of program activities.
Activities at various level or package of services[2,4]	• **Community level:** Awareness campaigns, health education, and vector control initiatives. • **Health facility level:** Diagnosis and treatment services for kala-azar and PKDL. • **Policy and coordination level:** Intersectoral collaboration and policy implementation for disease control.
Monitoring and evaluation of program[2]	• **Real-time data monitoring:** Through systems like KAMIS, transitioning to Integrated Health Information Platform (IHIP). • **Performance incentives:** Awards for achieving and sustaining elimination targets at block, district, and state levels. • **Periodic reviews:** High-level reviews by health ministers and national leaders to assess progress.

JAPANESE ENCEPHALITIS

Need of program/ Scheme	• **Public health impact:** Japanese encephalitis (JE) is a significant public health concern in India, causing severe neurological complications and high mortality rates. JE is endemic in 355 districts across 24 states/UTs, with a significant concentration of cases in northeastern states like Assam and West Bengal. The outbreaks typically occur during the monsoon and post-monsoon periods, aligning with peak mosquito breeding seasons. India reports several thousand JE cases annually, with a high impact on children and rural communities. Survivors often suffer from long-term neurological sequelae. • **Transmission and ecology:** JE is a zoonotic viral disease transmitted from animals, particularly birds and pigs, to humans via *Culex* mosquitoes. The disease can result in severe febrile illness affecting the central nervous system.[1]
Implemented since	**Historical context:** JE was first identified in India in 1952, with the first human case reported in 1955. Major outbreaks occurred in the 1970s and 1980s. JE control was included under the National Vector Borne Disease Control Programme (NVBDCP) in 2003, within the framework of the National Health Mission (NHM).[5]
Goal	**Long-term goal:** To eliminate Japanese encephalitis (JE) as a public health problem, improving the health status of vulnerable groups in endemic areas.
Objectives	• **Reduce JE incidence:** The program aims to reduce the incidence of JE through comprehensive strategies, including vaccination, vector control, and public awareness.[5] • **Protect vulnerable populations:** Focus on reducing the disease burden among children and rural populations, who are most at risk.
Organogram	• **Central level:** Managed by the NVBDCP under the NHM, with coordination from national health authorities. • **State level:** State health departments and vector-borne disease units oversee implementation and monitoring. • **District and local levels:** Local health workers, including ASHA workers, play a crucial role in community outreach, vaccination, and surveillance activities.[5]
Beneficiaries	• **Target groups:** Children, rural populations, and agricultural workers in endemic areas, with a particular focus on those under 15 years of age who are most susceptible to severe disease. • **Vaccination and treatment access:** Provision of free JE vaccination and treatment in government health facilities.[5]
Components[4,5]	• **Disease management:** Focus on the early detection and supportive treatment of JE cases, as well as differentiation from other viral encephalitis. • **Vector control measures:** Mosquito control activities in and around human habitats, especially during peak transmission seasons. • **Vaccination efforts:** Routine immunization for children and special campaigns for adult vaccination in specific districts.
Strategies/Deliverables under the program[4,5]	• **Vaccination:** Introduction and expansion of JE vaccination in endemic regions, including routine immunization for children and targeted vaccination for adults in high-risk areas. • **Vector control:** Implementation of mosquito control measures, such as larval source reduction, use of indoor residual sprays, insecticide-treated bed nets and public education on reducing mosquito breeding sites. • **Surveillance and data management:** Strengthening of diagnostic facilities and real-time data reporting to monitor and respond to outbreaks. • **Community engagement and education:** Advocacy and communication campaigns to increase public awareness and encourage preventive behaviors by use of personal protective measures and to keep piggeries away from human settlements. • **Capacity building:** Training healthcare professionals on JE case management and outbreak response.
Activities at various level or package of services	• **Community level:** Public awareness campaigns, community engagement for mosquito control, and vaccination drives. • **Healthcare facilities:** Diagnosis, treatment, and management of JE cases, along with training for healthcare providers. • **Policy and coordination:** Regular review and adaptation of strategies based on epidemiological data and emerging trends.
Monitoring and evaluation of program[5]	• **Surveillance systems:** Enhanced diagnostic and surveillance capabilities through sentinel hospitals and laboratories. • Web-based management information system • **Periodic reviews:** Ongoing assessment of program effectiveness and adaptation of strategies to ensure continued progress in JE control.

FILARIASIS

Need of program/ Scheme	Lymphatic filariasis, commonly known as elephantiasis, is a major public health problem in India, second only to malaria. It is a disabling and disfiguring disease, causing significant physical, social, and economic burden. The disease often leads to severe swelling in limbs, hydrocele, and is associated with social stigma. With millions of people at risk, particularly in endemic regions, the elimination of lymphatic filariasis is crucial for improving public health and reducing poverty.[2]
Implemented since	The National Filaria Control Programme (NFCP) was officially launched in India in 1955, following a pilot project conducted in Orissa from 1949 to 1954. The program aimed to control the spread of filariasis, particularly in urban areas, and to train personnel to manage the program operations.[2]
Goal	**Long-term goal:** To eliminate kala-azar as a public health problem, improving the health status of vulnerable groups in endemic areas.
Objectives[2]	• To delineate and map the areas endemic to filariasis. • To implement control measures in these endemic areas to reduce transmission. • To provide treatment and care for individuals affected by filariasis, including managing chronic cases of lymphedema and hydrocele. • To train healthcare workers and personnel involved in the program.
Organogram[2]	• **National level:** National Vector Borne Disease Control Programme (NVBDCP) • **State level:** State Health Departments • **District level:** District Health Offices • **Sub-district level:** Primary health centers (PHCs) and community health centers (CHCs) • **Village level:** Sub-centers and village health workers
Beneficiaries[2]	• **At-risk populations:** Individuals living in endemic areas, particularly those in poor living conditions with high exposure to mosquito bites. • **Patients with chronic disease:** Individuals suffering from chronic conditions such as lymphedema and hydrocele. • **General public:** Through reduced transmission and awareness campaigns, the entire community benefits from the program's activities.
Components[2,4]	• **Mass drug administration (MDA):** Distribution of Diethylcarbamazine (DEC) and Albendazole to at-risk populations. • **Vector control:** Implementation of measures to control the mosquito population, including environmental management and biological control. • **Health education:** Raising awareness about the disease, its transmission, and prevention measures. • **Clinical management and care:** Providing medical care for affected individuals, including surgeries for hydrocele and management of lymphedema.
Strategies/Deliverables under the program[2,4]	• **Mass drug administration (MDA):** Regular administration of anti-filarial drugs to at-risk populations. • **Anti-larval measures:** Targeting mosquito breeding sites with anti-larval agents, particularly in urban areas. • **Environmental management:** Reducing mosquito breeding sites through activities such as filling ditches, removing waste, and draining stagnant water. • **Biological control:** Using larvicidal fish to control mosquito populations. • **Clinical management:** Detection and treatment of microfilaria carriers and patients with clinical disease.
Activities at various level or package of services[2,4]	• **National level:** Policy formulation, coordination, and funding allocation. • **State level:** Program implementation, monitoring, and coordination with national guidelines. • **District level:** Local implementation, including MDA campaigns and vector control activities. • **Sub-district and village level:** Direct service delivery, including drug distribution, vector control measures, and patient care.
Monitoring and Evaluation of program	• **Regular surveillance:** Monitoring the prevalence of the disease and effectiveness of MDA campaigns. • **Reporting mechanisms:** Data collection and reporting from the field to state and national levels. • **Joint monitoring missions:** Periodic evaluations by expert teams, including field visits to assess program implementation and impact. • **Recommendations and adjustments:** Based on monitoring and evaluation findings, recommendations are made to improve program effectiveness, such as engaging medical colleges, improving intersectoral collaboration, and addressing treatment backlogs.

MALARIA

Need of program/Scheme	Malaria remains a significant public health challenge in India, causing considerable morbidity and mortality, particularly in rural and remote areas. The disease disproportionately affects economically disadvantaged communities, contributing to poverty and limiting economic growth. With a large population at risk and the emergence of drug-resistant malaria strains, comprehensive control and elimination efforts are crucial.[3]
Implemented since	India's efforts to control malaria date back to the National Malaria Control Programme initiated in 1953. This was succeeded by the National Malaria Eradication Programme (NMEP) in 1958, which aimed at eliminating the disease. Over time, the focus shifted to control rather than eradication due to challenges such as vector resistance and logistical issues. It is merged with NVBDCP in 2003.
Objectives	• To prevent the re-establishment of malaria in Category 0 districts* • To achieve pre-elimination status in low-endemic states and territories. • To move towards malaria elimination in the entire country.[3]
Organogram[3]	• **National level:** Ministry of Health and Family Welfare (MoHFW) and National Centre for Vector Borne Disease Control (NCVBDC). • **State level:** State Malaria Control Societies/Units • **District level:** District Malaria Offices/Health Departments • **Sub-district level:** Community Health Centers (CHCs), Primary Health Centers (PHCs), Health and Wellness Centers (HWCs) • **Community level:** Village Health Workers and Accredited Social Health Activists (ASHAs)
Beneficiaries	• **High-risk populations:** People living in endemic areas, particularly pregnant women, children under five, and individuals with compromised immunity. • **General population:** Through reduced transmission and access to preventive measures and treatments.
Components[3,4]	• **Diagnosis and treatment:** Providing rapid diagnostic tests (RDTs) and artemisinin-based combination therapies (ACTs). • **Vector control:** Utilizing IRS, ITNs, and other vector control methods to reduce mosquito populations. • **Monitoring and surveillance:** Tracking disease incidence and monitoring drug and insecticide resistance. • **Capacity building:** Training healthcare workers and other stakeholders involved in malaria control.
Strategies/Deliverables under the program[3,4]	• **Early diagnosis and prompt treatment (EDPT):** Ensuring access to diagnosis and treatment, particularly in high-risk areas. • **Integrated vector management (IVM):** Using a combination of vector control measures such as indoor residual spraying (IRS), insecticide-treated bed nets (ITNs), and environmental management. • **Surveillance and epidemic preparedness:** Strengthening surveillance systems to detect and respond to malaria outbreaks. • **Behavior change communication (BCC):** Educating the public about malaria prevention and treatment. • **Strengthening health systems:** Building capacity for effective program implementation and management. Promoting research and generation of strategic information.
Activities at various level or package of services[3,4]	• **National level:** Policy development, funding allocation, coordination with international partners, and setting guidelines. • **State level:** Implementation of national strategies, training, monitoring, and evaluation. • **District level:** Local implementation of vector control, distribution of diagnostics and treatments, and public health education. • **Community level:** Direct service delivery, including testing, treatment, distribution of bed nets, and public awareness campaigns.
Monitoring and evaluation of program[3]	• **Routine surveillance:** Regular data collection on malaria cases and vector populations. • **Performance monitoring:** Assessing the effectiveness of interventions like IRS and ITNs. • **Drug and insecticide resistance monitoring:** Tracking the efficacy of treatments and vector control methods. • **Independent evaluations and audits:** Periodic assessments by external agencies or experts to review program effectiveness and recommend improvements.[3]

*Note: Category-wise distribution of districts:
- Category 0 (Prevention of re-establishment phase): Districts with zero indigenous cases of malaria.
- Category 1 (Elimination phase): Districts reporting Annual Parasite Index (API) of <1 case per thousand population
- Category 2 (Pre-elimination phase): Districts having API >1 and <2 per thousand population
- Category 3 (Intensified control Phase): Districts having API more than and equal to 2 per thousand population

DENGUE AND CHIKUNGUNYA

Need of program/ Scheme	Chikungunya and dengue fever are significant public health concern in India, causing substantial morbidity and mortality. These diseases are spread by *Aedes* mosquitoes, which are widespread in urban and rural areas. Increasing urbanization, climate change, and inadequate water management have exacerbated their spread, making comprehensive control measures crucial to protect public health.[2]
Implemented since	India's formal efforts to control dengue began in the 1960s and that of chikungunya gained momentum since 2007 with the establishment of surveillance and control measures. Over the decades, these efforts have evolved, incorporating more advanced strategies and technologies like remote sensing to address the growing challenge.
Objectives[2]	• To reduce transmission and minimize outbreaks. • To decrease morbidity and mortality. • To strengthen the capacity of health systems to respond to outbreaks. • To enhance public awareness and community involvement in prevention and control.
Organogram[2]	• **National level:** Ministry of Health and Family Welfare (MoHFW) and National Centre for Vector Borne Disease Control (NCVBDC). • **State level:** State Health Departments and Vector Borne Disease Control Units • **District level:** District Health Offices and Vector Control Units • **Community level:** Primary Health Centers (PHCs), Urban Health Centers, and Community Health Workers
Beneficiaries[2]	• **General population:** Residents in dengue-endemic areas, particularly those in urban and peri-urban regions. • **High-risk groups:** Children, the elderly, and individuals with underlying health conditions who are more susceptible to severe dengue.
Components[2,4]	• **Vector control:** Implementing measures such as environmental management, larvicide, fogging, and promoting the use of mosquito repellents and bed nets. • **Surveillance:** Regular monitoring of dengue cases, vector populations, and environmental conditions conducive to mosquito breeding. • **Laboratory support:** Strengthening laboratory capacities for the diagnosis of dengue and monitoring of vector resistance to insecticides. • **Capacity building:** Training healthcare workers, vector control staff, and community volunteers in dengue control and prevention.
Strategies/Deliverables under the program[6]	• **Integrated vector management (IVM):** This involves the use of multiple strategies to control the *Aedes* mosquito population, including source reduction, chemical control, and biological control methods.[4] • **Surveillance and response:** Strengthening disease surveillance systems to detect and respond promptly to dengue cases and outbreaks. • **Case management:** Ensuring timely diagnosis and appropriate clinical management of dengue cases.[6] • **Public health education and community mobilization:** Educating communities about dengue prevention and encouraging community participation in control measures.[2]
Activities at various level or package of services	• **National level:** Policy formulation, resource allocation, guideline development, and coordination with international organizations. • **State level:** Implementation of national strategies, monitoring and evaluation, and capacity building. • **District level:** Local surveillance, vector control activities, public awareness campaigns, and clinical management of cases.[6] • **Community level:** Household and community-level interventions, including source reduction, public education, and mobilization efforts.[2]
Monitoring and evaluation of program	• **Routine surveillance:** Tracking dengue cases and vector indices to monitor trends and identify outbreak hotspots. • **Epidemiological surveys:** Conducting periodic surveys to assess the prevalence of dengue and the effectiveness of control measures. • **Vector surveillance:** Monitoring mosquito populations and insecticide resistance patterns.[4] • **Health system performance:** Evaluating the preparedness and response capacity of health facilities and community health systems. • **Public health impact assessment:** Assessing the overall impact of the program on reducing dengue incidence and improving public health outcomes.[2]

References

1. Disease Control Programme (NHM). Annual Report 2016-17.Chapter 5.Page 55-58 Available at: https://main.mohfw.gov.in/sites/default/files/5201617.pdf (Accessed: 25 July 2024).
2. Ministry of Health & Family Welfare-Government of India. Guidelines, National Center for Vector Borne Diseases Control (NCVBDC). Available at: https://ncvbdc.mohfw.gov.in/index1.php?lang=1&level=1&sublinkid=5899&lid=3686 (Accessed: 25 July 2024).
3. National strategic plan: Malaria elimination 2023-27. Available at: https://ncvbdc.mohfw.gov.in/Doc/National-Strategic-Plan-Malaria-2023-27.pdf (Accessed: 25 July 2024).
4. NVBDCP. Available at: https://nvbdcp.gov.in/Doc/Guidelines/Manual-Integrated-Vector-Management-2022.pdf (Accessed: 25 July 2024).
5. Operational guidelines (2014). Available at: https://ncvbdc.mohfw.gov.in/WriteReadData/l892s/JE-AES-Prevention-Control(NPPCJA).pdf (Accessed: 25 July 2024).
6. National Guidelines for Clinical Management of Dengue. Available at: https://ncvbdc.mohfw.gov.in/Doc/National Guidelines for Clinical Management of Dengue Fever 2023.pdf (Accessed: 25 July 2024).

QUESTIONS

Long Answer Question (LAQ)

1. Discuss the objectives, components, and strategies of the National Vector Borne Disease Control Programme (NVBDCP) in India. How has the program evolved to tackle major vector borne diseases like malaria and dengue?

Short Answer Questions (SAQs)

1. What are the key components of integrated vector management under NVBDCP?
2. What are the main strategies to reduce the incidence of Japanese encephalitis under NVBDCP?

Multiple Choice Questions (MCQs)

1. Which of the following is a component of mass drug administration strategy for filariasis?
   a. Artemisinin
   b. Diethylcarbamazine
   c. Ivermectin
   d. Hydroxychloroquine
2. Which surveillance system is used for real time monitoring of Kala-azar cases in India?
   a. NTEP
   b. HIMS
   c. KAIMS
   d. IDSP
3. Which of the following diseases is *not* addressed by the NVBDCP?
   a. Malaria
   b. Dengue
   c. Japanese encephalitis
   d. COVID-19

Answers

1. b
2. c
3. d

44 CHAPTER

National Tuberculosis Elimination Programme

Parul Sharma, Mital Rathod, Shaili Vyas, Surendra Singh, Rakhee Khanduri

Need of the program/scheme	The National Tuberculosis Elimination Programme (NTEP), previously known as the Revised National Tuberculosis Control Programme (RNTCP), is India's flagship public health initiative aimed at eradicating tuberculosis (TB) from the country. • Tuberculosis (TB) is a major public health challenge in India, which has the highest TB burden globally, with 2.64 million new cases and 450,000 deaths in 2019. • The National TB Elimination Program (NTEP) aims to control and eliminate TB, reduce mortality and morbidity, and improve patients' quality of life. • Challenges include drug-resistant TB with 124,000 MDR/RR-TB cases reported in 2019, TB-HIV co-infection, and socioeconomic impacts, such as loss of income and stigma.[1,2]
Implemented since	• The RNTCP was launched in 1997, and it was rebranded as the NTEP in 2020 to emphasize the aim of eliminating TB by 2025. • **2017:** Launch of Nikshay Poshan Yojana, providing nutritional support to TB patients. • **2018:** Launch of the National Strategic Plan (NSP) 2017-2025, focusing on a multi-pronged approach to eliminate TB. • **2019:** Introduction of newer drugs like Bedaquiline and Delamanid for drug-resistant TB (DR-TB). • **2020:** Integration of TB services with other health programs, strengthening the Primary Health Care system. • **2020:** Implementation of a web-based, patient management system called NIKSHAY for effective monitoring and tracking of TB patients. • **2021:** Introduction of newer diagnostic tools like CB-NAAT and TrueNat for rapid TB diagnosis.
Goal	The primary goal of NTEP is to achieve a TB-free India with zero deaths, disease, and poverty due to tuberculosis.
Targets	• **By 2025:** Eliminate TB, five years ahead of the global Sustainable Development Goals (SDGs) target of 2030. • Reduce TB incidence to less than 1 case per 100,000 population per year.
Objectives[1]	• Ensure early diagnosis and prompt treatment of TB. • Prevent the emergence of drug-resistant TB. • Reduce the incidence and mortality associated with TB. • Improve TB awareness and treatment adherence.

Chapter 44: National Tuberculosis Elimination Programme

Organogram[4]	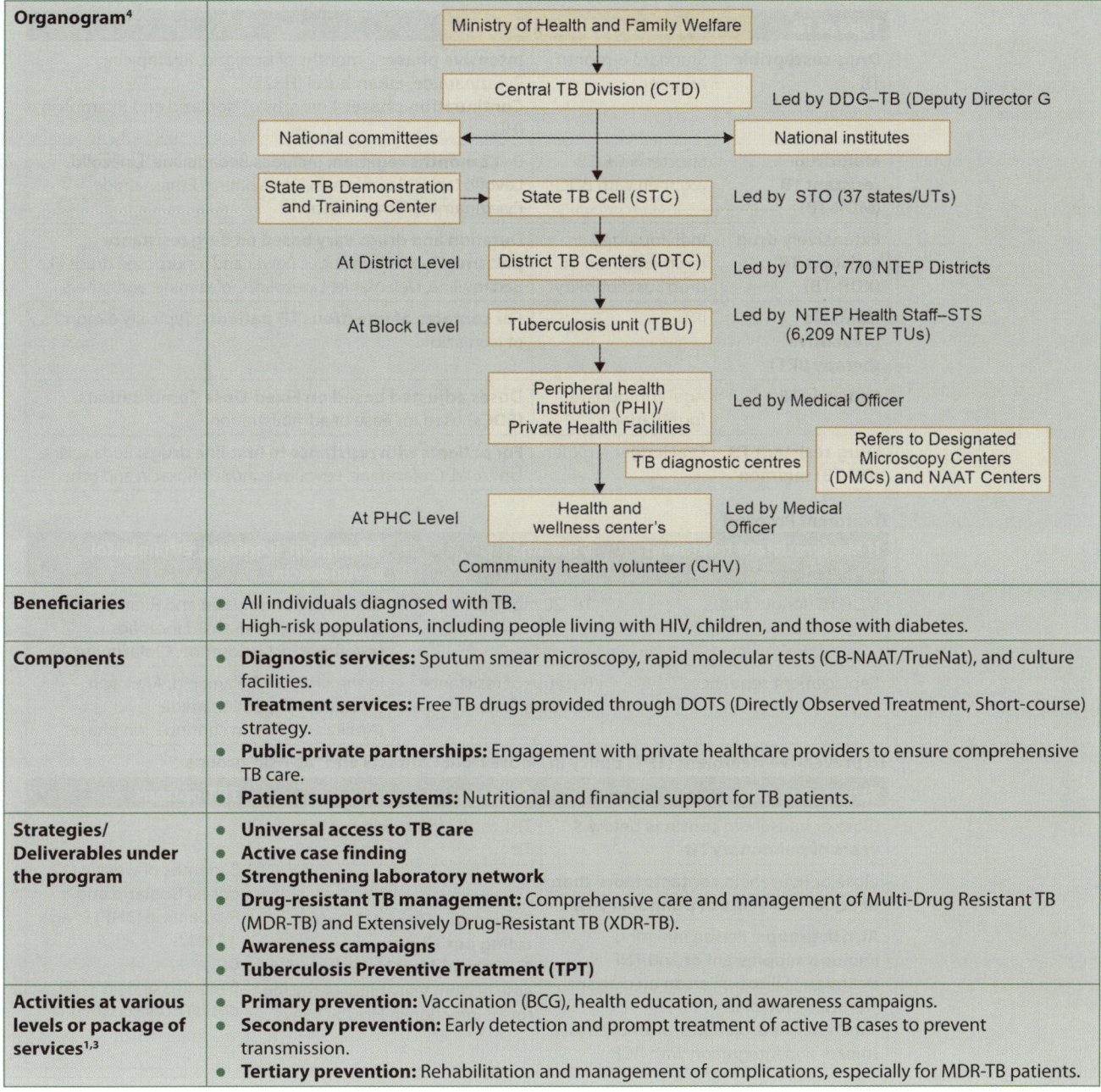
Beneficiaries	• All individuals diagnosed with TB. • High-risk populations, including people living with HIV, children, and those with diabetes.
Components	• **Diagnostic services:** Sputum smear microscopy, rapid molecular tests (CB-NAAT/TrueNat), and culture facilities. • **Treatment services:** Free TB drugs provided through DOTS (Directly Observed Treatment, Short-course) strategy. • **Public-private partnerships:** Engagement with private healthcare providers to ensure comprehensive TB care. • **Patient support systems:** Nutritional and financial support for TB patients.
Strategies/ Deliverables under the program	• **Universal access to TB care** • **Active case finding** • **Strengthening laboratory network** • **Drug-resistant TB management:** Comprehensive care and management of Multi-Drug Resistant TB (MDR-TB) and Extensively Drug-Resistant TB (XDR-TB). • **Awareness campaigns** • **Tuberculosis Preventive Treatment (TPT)**
Activities at various levels or package of services[1,3]	• **Primary prevention:** Vaccination (BCG), health education, and awareness campaigns. • **Secondary prevention:** Early detection and prompt treatment of active TB cases to prevent transmission. • **Tertiary prevention:** Rehabilitation and management of complications, especially for MDR-TB patients.

Type of TB	Treatment regimen	Details
Drug-susceptible TB	Standard 6-month regimen	**Intensive phase:** 2 months of Isoniazid, Rifampicin, Pyrazinamide, Ethambutol (HRZE) **Continuation phase:** 4 months of Isoniazid and Rifampicin (HR)
Multidrug-resistant TB (MDR-TB)	Shorter MDR-TB regimen with BDQ	**9–12 months regimen:** Includes Bedaquiline, Linezolid, Levofloxacin/Moxifloxacin, Clofazimine, Ethionamide, Pyrazinamide, Ethambutol
Extensively drug resistant-TB (XDR-TB)	Individualized regimen based on drug susceptibility	**Duration and drugs vary based on durg resistance patterns:** Typically includes newer and repurposed drugs like Bedaquiline, Delamanid, Linezolid, Clofazimine, and others
Isoniazid preventive therapy (IPT)	IPT	**For contacts of infectious TB patients:** Typically 6 months of Isoniazid
Pediatric TB	Age-appropriate formulations	**Doses adjusted based on Fixed-Dose Combinations (FDCs)** used for ease of administration
Drug-resistant TB (DR-TB) regimen	Oral longer regimen	**For patients with resistance to first-line drugs:** Bedaquiline, Linezolid, Clofazimine, Levofloxacin/Moxifloxacin and others

Treatment Protocol

H Monoresistant treatment	6 months	Rifampicin, Isoniazid, Ethambutol, Levofloxacin
MDR TB (longer oral)	18–20 months	Resistance to Isoniazid and Rifampicin: Bedaquillin (6 months), Linezolid, Levofloxacin, Cycloserine, Clofazimine.
Replacement sequence	Because of resistance or side effects	In the order…. Delamanid, Amikacin, Pyrazinamide, Ethionamide (Amikacin never in continuation phase)

TB preventive treatment (TPT) policy in House Hold Contacts and "at-risk" groups

Target population	Strategy	TPT options
Close or household **contacts below 5 years of pulmonary TB**	TPT to all after ruling out active TB	3 months of weekly (12 doses) Isoniazid and Rifapentine **(3HP)** in age >2 years or 6 months of daily (180 doses) Isoniazid **(6H)**
Close or household **contacts more than or equal to 5 years of pulmonary TB**	Testing *for TBI and TPT after **ruling out** TB disease *TPT **should not be deferred** in case of non-availability of testing for TB infection in HHC >/=5 yrs	
At-risk groups: Person initiating Immuno-suppressant or anti-TNF treatment; Silicosis; Person on dialysis; Transplant recipient Malnourished, diabetes, alcohol abuse, smoker and integration with ACF		

	TPT in HHC of DR-TB		
	Target population	Strategy	TPT options
	• Contacts of DR-TB ♦ Contact of MDR/RR-TB (FQ susceptible) or	Testing* for TBI and TPT after ruling out TB disease *TPT should not be deferred in case of non-availability of testing for TB infection in HHC >/=5 yrs	6 months of daily Levofloxacin
	♦ Contact of Isoniazid mono/poly resistant TB (R susceptible)		4R (4 months of daily Rifampicin)
	• People living with HIV (+ ART) • Adults and children >12 months • Infants <12 months with HIV in contact with active TB	TPT to all after ruling out active TB disease	1 month of daily (28 doses) Isoniazid and Rifapentine (1HP) in PLHIV age >/=13 years or 6 months of daily (180 doses) Isoniazid (6H) for age <13 years or pregnant or breastfeeding mother
	Dosage of 6H regimen		
	Regimen	Dose by age and weight band	
	6 months of daily isoniazid monotherapy (6H)	**Age 10 years and older:** 5 mg/kg/day[d] **Age <10 years:** 10 mg/kg/day (range, 7–15 mg)	
	[d]Maximum dose of H if given daily would be 300 mg/day		
Newer initiatives in NTEP	• **Fixed-dose combination (FDC):** Implemented for all ages and all types of TB. • **Isoniazid preventive therapy (IPT):** Provided for contacts of infectious TB patients. • **Drug-resistant TB (DR-TB) regimen:** Incorporation of Bedaquiline (BDQ) in treatment. • **Universal drug sensitivity testing (DST):** All sputum-positive patients are evaluated for resistance using Line Probe Assay (LPA). • **TB-mukt Gram Panchayat:** Initiative to achieve TB-free status in village councils. • **Nikshay Poshan Yojana:** Nutritional support for TB patients, providing ₹ 1000 per month. • The combination of bedaquiline (B), pretomanid (Pa), linezolid (L), and moxifloxacin (M) is a 6-month treatment regimen for multidrug-resistant (MDR) or rifampicin-resistant (RR), tuberculosis (TB). The World Health Organization (WHO) recommends this regimen for patients who have not been exposed to bedaquiline and linezolid before, or have been exposed for less than one month. • Introduction of Energy Dense Nutritional Supplementation (EDNS) for all patients with BMI <18.5. • **Pradhan Mantri TB Mukt Bharat Abhiyaan (PMTBMBA):** For a minimum of six months or a maximum of three years, the community is encouraged to adopt consented TB patients and provide them with nutritional care, nutritional supplements, further investigations, and vocational assistance. The community support person are called "Nikshay Mitra". • Scale up of TB Preventive Treatment (TPT) to other risk groups including people undergoing dialysis, living with silicosis, on immunosuppressants, organ transplant recipients, individuals with diabetes, malnutrition, smokers, alcohol-dependent individuals, healthcare workers, etc. • **Cytochrome b (Cy-Tb test):** Skin test that detects latent tuberculosis (TB) infection. It is a Third Generation Test that combines the accuracy of IGRA (interferon gamma release assay) with the case of TsTs (TVM Signaling and Transportation Systems Private Limited).		
	Details		
	Drugs	Bedaquiline, pretomanid, linezolid, and moxifloxacin	
	Treatment duration	6 months	
	Suitability	Suitable for most forms of TB, but not for extrapulmonary TB involving the central nervous system (CNS), or osteoarticular and disseminated (miliary) TB	
	Cautions	Some caution is needed when enrolling patients with CD4 counts lower than 100 cells/mm³. The safety of pretomanid during pregnancy and breastfeeding is also unclear.	
Monitoring and evaluation of the program	• **Surveillance:** Continuous monitoring of TB cases through a nationwide surveillance system (Nikshay). • **Periodic evaluations:** Regular program reviews and evaluations at the national, state, and district levels. • **Operational research:** Conducting research to identify gaps and improve program implementation.		

References

1. Ministry of Health and Family Welfare, Government of India. National TB Elimination Programme. [NTEP Official Website](https://tbcindia.gov.in)
2. World Health Organization. Global Tuberculosis Report 2023. [WHO TB Report](https://www.who.int/tb/publications/global_report/en/)
3. Central TB Division. National Strategic Plan for Tuberculosis Elimination 2017-2025. [NSP Document] (https://tbcindia.gov.in/WriteReadData/NSP%20Draft%2020.02.2017%201.pdf)
4. Organizational Structure of NTEP. Available at. https://ntep.in/mr/node/366/CP-organizational-structure-ntep

QUESTIONS

Long Answer Question (LAQ)

1. Describe the key components of NTEP. How has the transition from RNTCP to NTEP improved TB prevention and control strategies in India?

Short Answer Questions (SAQs)

1. Discuss the importance of DOTS strategy in NTEP.
2. Critically analyse Nikshay and Nikshay Poshan Yojana initiatives under NTEP.

Multiple Choice Questions (MCQs)

1. Which of the following initiatives is a part of NTEP to encourage early diagnosis and treatment adherence?
   a. Mission Indradhanush
   b. Ayushman Bharat Yojana
   c. Nikshay Poshan Yojana
   d. Pradhan Mantri Jan Aushadhi Pariyojana
2. Which strategy under NTEP focus on early case detection and treatment of TB in hard to reach areas?
   a. Active case finding
   b. DOTS
   c. National strategic plan for TB elimination
   d. ICDS
3. TPT is indicated in the following:
   a. Index TB case
   b. Contacts of TB case where active TB is ruled out
   c. Extrapulmonary TB
   d. Patients of diabetes with pulmonary TB

Answers

1. c   2. a   3. b

CHAPTER 45

National AIDS Control Programme

Shaili Vyas, Pradeep Aggarwal, Niharika Verma, Ghanshyam Ahir

Background/Need of program/Scheme	• In 1986, 10 out of 102 female sex workers were found HIV positive in Tamil Nadu. • The program was initiated to slow the spread of HIV infections, aiming to reduce the morbidity, mortality, and overall impact of AIDS in the country. • The prevalence of HIV has now come down to 0.20% (ranging from 0.17% to 0.25%) as per the HIV Estimates 2023 fact sheet[1] which was published in June 2024.

Implemented since	**Evolvement of NACP**
	• 1986: National AIDS Committee established following the detection of India's first HIV case
	• NACP Phase-I: 1992–1999
	  Major initiatives: Surveillance system to monitor the HIV epidemic, ensuring access to safe blood, and providing preventive services to high-risk populations
	• NACP Phase-II: 1999–2007
	  Major initiatives: National AIDS Prevention and Control Policy (2002), scaling up of targeted interventions for high-risk groups in states with high prevalence, National Blood Policy, National Adolescent Education Programme (NAEP), counseling, testing, and Prevention of Parent-to-Child Transmission (PPTCT) program, National Anti-Retroviral Treatment (ART) program, and State AIDS Control Societies across all states.
	• NACP Phase-III: 2007–2012
	  Major initiatives: Rapid scale-up of the service delivery facilities pan India, Providing HIV counseling and testing services to pregnant women as a vital part of antenatal care (ANC) services.
	• NACP Phase-IV: 2012–2017, extended to 2017–2021
	  Major initiatives: National HIV/AIDS toll free helpline—1097; Adoption of dual elimination of vertical transmission (of HIV & Syphilis) in NACP guidelines; Launch of NACP interventions in prisons and other closed settings
	  NACP Phase-IV Extension: 2017-21
	• National AIDS and STD Control Programme (NACP) Phase V: 2021–2026[2]
	• The NACP Phase-V builds on key initiatives such as the HIV and AIDS (Prevention and Control) Act of 2017 and its associated rules, the Test and Treat policy, Universal Viral Load Testing, Mission Sampark to restart ART for lost-to-follow up PLHIV, Community-Based Screening, the transition to a Dolutegravir-based Treatment Regimen, and active community engagement.
	• The HIV and AIDS (Prevention and Control) Act, 2017, is a central piece of legislation that protects and promotes the rights of people living with HIV. The Act prohibits the discrimination against HIV positive people including the denial, termination, discontinuation or unfair treatment with regard to Employment, Educational establishments, Health care services, Residing or renting property, Standing for public or private office and Provision of insurance.

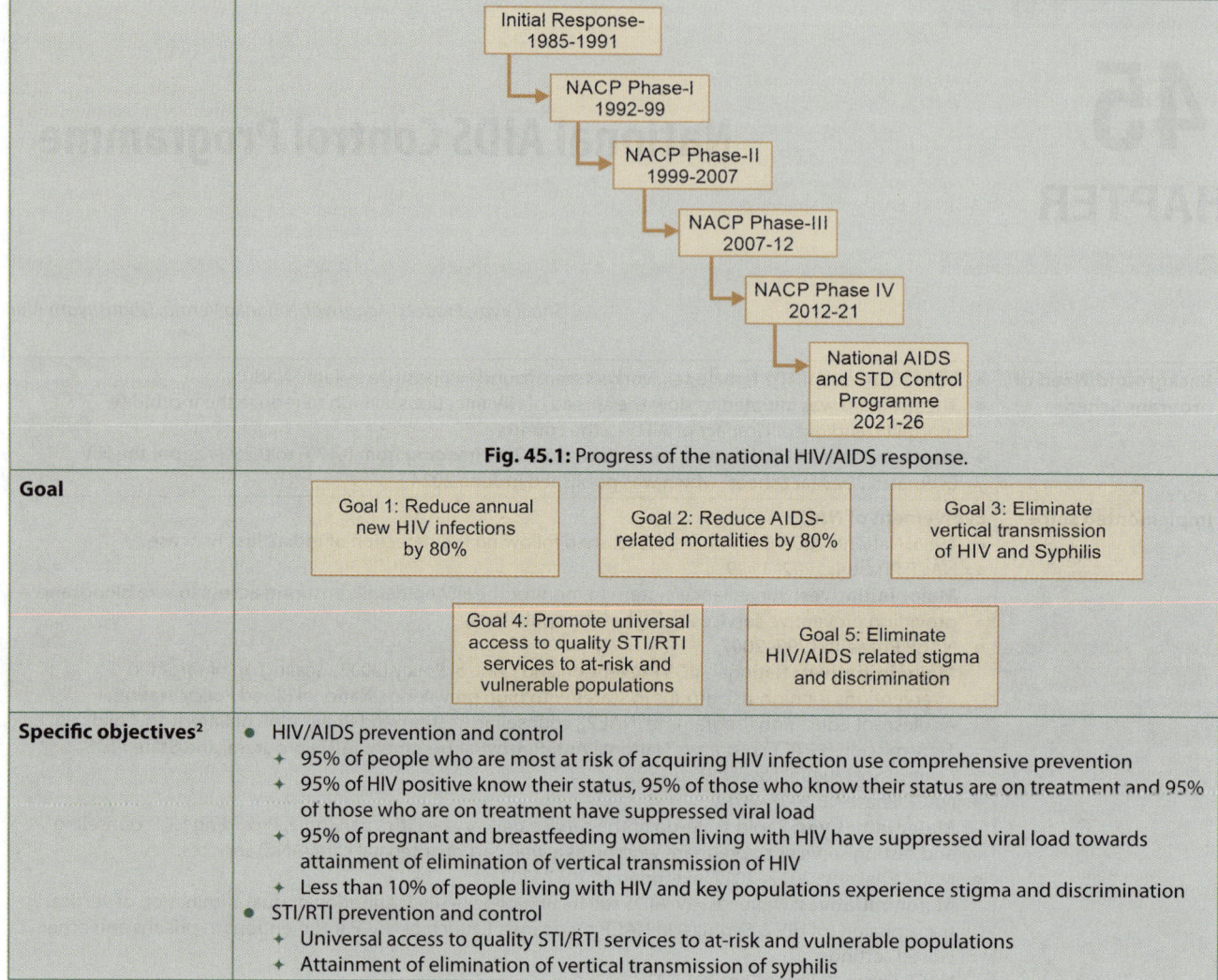

Fig. 45.1: Progress of the national HIV/AIDS response.

Goal	Goal 1: Reduce annual new HIV infections by 80% Goal 2: Reduce AIDS-related mortalities by 80% Goal 3: Eliminate vertical transmission of HIV and Syphilis Goal 4: Promote universal access to quality STI/RTI services to at-risk and vulnerable populations Goal 5: Eliminate HIV/AIDS related stigma and discrimination

Specific objectives[2]	• HIV/AIDS prevention and control
	    ✦ 95% of people who are most at risk of acquiring HIV infection use comprehensive prevention
	    ✦ 95% of HIV positive know their status, 95% of those who know their status are on treatment and 95% of those who are on treatment have suppressed viral load
	    ✦ 95% of pregnant and breastfeeding women living with HIV have suppressed viral load towards attainment of elimination of vertical transmission of HIV
	    ✦ Less than 10% of people living with HIV and key populations experience stigma and discrimination
	 • STI/RTI prevention and control
	    ✦ Universal access to quality STI/RTI services to at-risk and vulnerable populations
	    ✦ Attainment of elimination of vertical transmission of syphilis

Organogram of NACO	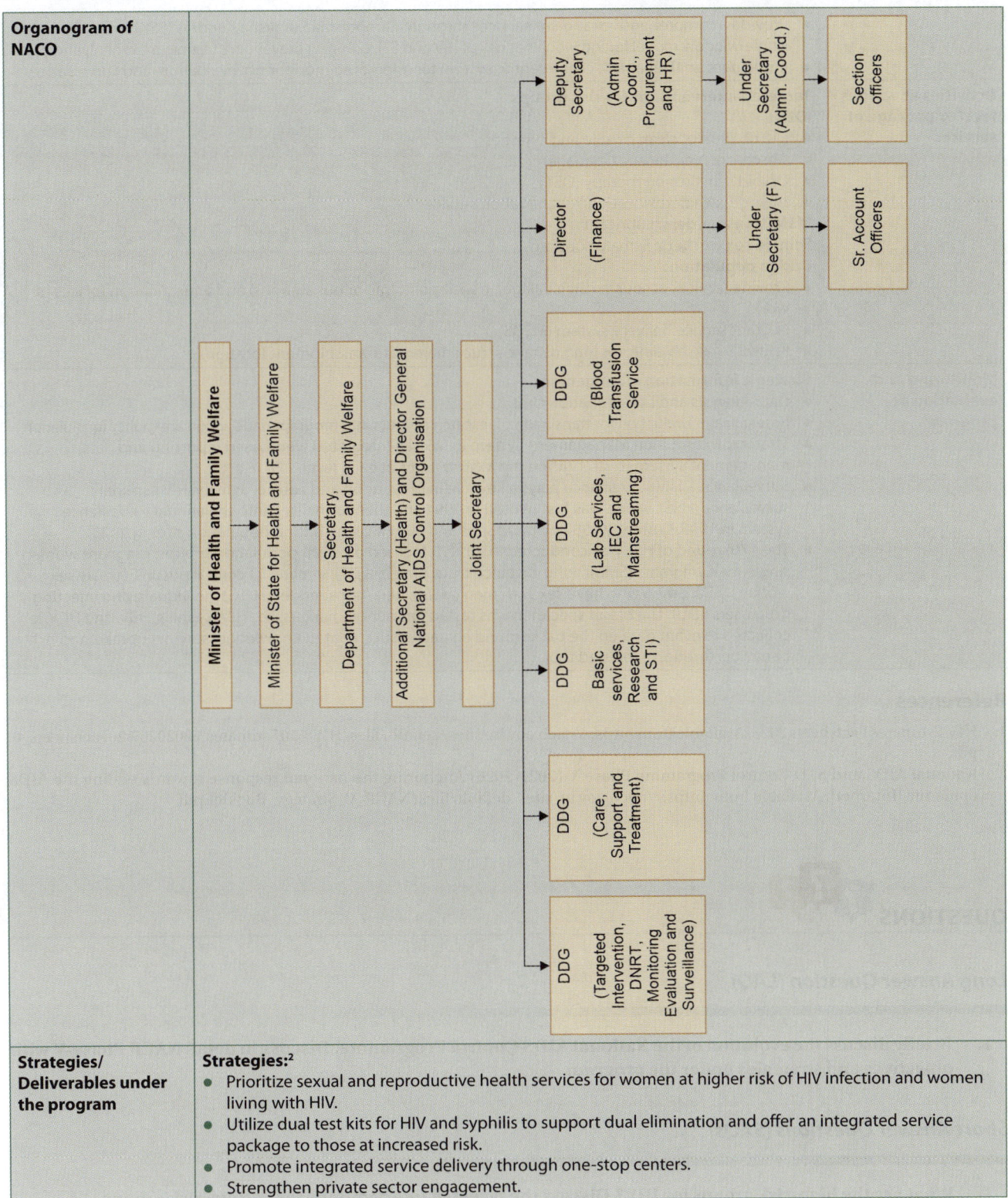	
Strategies/ Deliverables under the program	**Strategies:**[2] • Prioritize sexual and reproductive health services for women at higher risk of HIV infection and women living with HIV. • Utilize dual test kits for HIV and syphilis to support dual elimination and offer an integrated service package to those at increased risk. • Promote integrated service delivery through one-stop centers. • Strengthen private sector engagement.	

	• Provide a comprehensive range of services through "Sampoorna Suraksha Kendras (SSK)," offering a single-window model for individuals at risk of HIV and STI, covering prevention, testing, treatment, and care. • Implement an IT-enabled, client-centric system for integrated monitoring, evaluation, and surveillance.
Activities at various level or package of services	**Targeted interventions for risk groups:** **IDUs:** • Distribution of clean needle and syringes • Abscess prevention and management • Opioid substitution therapy (OST) • Linkage with detoxification/rehabilitation services **MSM/transgenders:** Lubricants **Female sex workers:** Female condom **Bridge population:** • Provide services at source (their village), transit point (rail or bus stations) and at destination (places of work) • Migrant service delivery system (MSDS) • Khushi Suraksha clinic for long distance truck drivers at transshipment locations
Monitoring and evaluation of program[2]	**Strategic information management** • Data Analysis and Dissemination Unit • Research and Evaluation for translation of research outputs into programmatic action and policy formulation • Strategic Information Management System (SIMS), an integrated web-based reporting and data management system to strengthen the M&E systems at each level. • Surveillance—HIV surveillance plays a key role in prevention and control activity. HIV sentinel surveillance (HSS), which was first piloted in 1994 and then formalized into the annual surveillance system in 1998. Currently 1557 planned sites and 600 HRG and bridge population sites in 2023. • The 17th round of HSS was conducted in 2021. It focused on eight population groups: pregnant women, single male migrants (SMM), long-distance truck drivers (LDT), inmates at central prisons, female sex workers (FSW), men who have sex with men (MSM), hijra/transgender (H/TG) individuals, and injecting drug users (IDU). The blood specimen was tested for four biomarkers, i.e., HIV, Syphilis, HBV, and HCV. It collected relevant data on the background characteristics, related knowledge, services uptake, and risk behaviors through a focused tool.

References

1. HIV Estimates Factsheets 2023. Available from https://naco.gov.in/sites/default/files/HIV%20Estimates%202023%20Factsheets_0.pdf
2. National AIDS and STD Control Programme Phase-V (2021-2026) Anchoring the national response towards ending the AIDS epidemic [Internet]. Available from: https://naco.gov.in/sites/default/files/NACP_V_Strategy_Booklet.pdf

QUESTIONS

Long Answer Question (LAQ)

1. Briefly discuss the evolution of the National AIDS Control Programme. Discuss in detail NACP Phase-V with objectives and strategies under the program.

Short Answer Questions (SAQs)

1. What are the high-risk groups for HIV? Discuss the targeted interventions for various risk groups.
2. Explain HIV Sentinel Surveillance.

Multiple Choice Questions (MCQs)

1. **High-risk groups for HIV include all, *except*:**
   a. Pregnant women
   b. Female Sex Workers
   c. Prisons inmates
   d. None of the above
2. **When was NACP launched?**
   a. 1986
   b. 1992
   c. 1990
   d. 1994
3. **In which phase of NACP was ART launched?**
   a. NACP I
   b. NACP II
   c. NACP III
   d. NACP IV
4. **What is the name of the reporting and data management system for NACP?**
   a. HIMS
   b. IHIP
   c. NIKSHAY
   d. SIMS
5. **What is the goal of NACP Phase-V?**
   a. 90% reduction in annual new HIV infections
   b. 85% reduction in annual new HIV infections
   c. 80% reduction in annual new HIV infections
   d. 95% reduction in annual new HIV infections

Answers

1. d
2. b
3. b
4. d
5. c

CHAPTER 46

National Leprosy Eradication Programme

Shweta Gangurde (Chauhan), Chaitali Borgaonkar, Parul Sharma, Kalpita Shringarpure

Background	The National Leprosy Eradication Programme (NLEP) is a centrally sponsored public health initiative which is executed under the National Health Mission (NHM) of the Ministry of Health and Family Welfare, Government of India. It aims at eliminating leprosy as a public health problem. The key NLEP focus is reduction of the incidence of leprosy, prevention of disability among affected individuals, and elimination of the disease associated stigma.[2] **History of Leprosy Program**[1] • It began as the National Leprosy Control Programme (NLCP) with the objectives to make infectious cases non-infectious and to reduce magnitude of problem. • The strategies included detection of cases of leprosy, early diagnosis and treatment with sulfone (dapsone monotherapy) and to give health education to patient, family and community.[3] • During fourth 5-year plan in 1980, the Government of India declared its resolve to "eradicate" leprosy by 2000 and made it a centrally sponsored program. In 1981, World Health Organization introduced multidrug therapy.[7] In 1983, the NLCP was renamed as Leprosy Eradication Programme. The aim of NLEP was to reduce the case load to less than 1/10,000.[2] • The program was initially localized to endemic districts but was later extended to all districts/states in 1993–1994.[9]
Need of program/ Scheme	• National Leprosy Eradication Programme came into force as the National Leprosy Control Programme in 1955. It was a centrally aided program to achieve control of leprosy. The prevalence of leprosy was 57/10,000 population in 1981, which reduced to 2.4/10,000 population in 2004.[4] • The National Health Policy 2002 set forth the goal for elimination of leprosy as a public health problem as per the World Health Organization criteria by reducing the prevalence to less than 1/10,000 population; which was achieved in December 2005. Though this was achieved at the National level, there are still few districts within the states wherein leprosy is still endemic.[5] • The major concern of the NLEP is case detection of leprosy at an early stage, provision of complete treatment, free of cost, in order to prevent occurrence of grade 2 disability (G2D) in affected persons.[6]
Vision	Leprosy-free India[2]
Mission	To provide quality leprosy services free of cost to all the sections of population, with easy accessibility, through the integrated healthcare system, including rehabilitative services after cure of the disease[1]
Description of the NLEP emblem	Symbolizes beauty and purity in lotus • Leprosy can be cured and the leprosy patient can be a useful member of the society in the form of a partially affected thumb; as depicted by a normal forefinger and the shape of house • The rising sun symbolic of hope and optimism[3]
Goals	• **Elimination of leprosy:** To maintain the elimination status at the national and sub-national levels which is defined as less than one case per 10,000 population • **Zero grade 2 disabilities (G2D):** Achieve zero cases of grade 2 disabilities among new child leprosy cases by 2025 • **Enhanced case detection:** Detect and treat all new leprosy cases annually to prevent transmission

Objectives	• **Zero disabilities among the new leprosy child cases and**
	• **Zero discrimination and stigma against persons affected by leprosy**
	1. **Reduce prevalence:** Prevalence rate less than 1/10,000 population at sub-national and district level.
	2. **Early detection and complete treatment:** Detect and treat all cases of leprosy at the earliest to prevent disability.
	3. **Disability prevention and management:** Prevent and manage disabilities among leprosy patients.
	    ✦ To reduce grade 2 disability percentage to less than 1 among new cases at national level
	    ✦ To reduce grade 2 disability cases <1 case per million population at national level.
	    ✦ Zero disabilities among new child cases.
	4. **Reduce stigma:** To have zero discrimination and stigma against persons affected by leprosy.
	5. **Strengthen surveillance:** Strengthen surveillance systems for leprosy to ensure early detection and prompt treatment.
	6. **Capacity building:** Enhance the capacity of healthcare workers and community volunteers to manage leprosy cases effectively.

Organogram	The NLEP is headed by the Deputy Director of Health Services (DGHS Leprosy) and is under the administrative control of the DGHS, Government of India. Being a centrally sponsored scheme, the NLEP strategies and plans are formulated centrally; and the program is implemented by the states/UTs.[2] 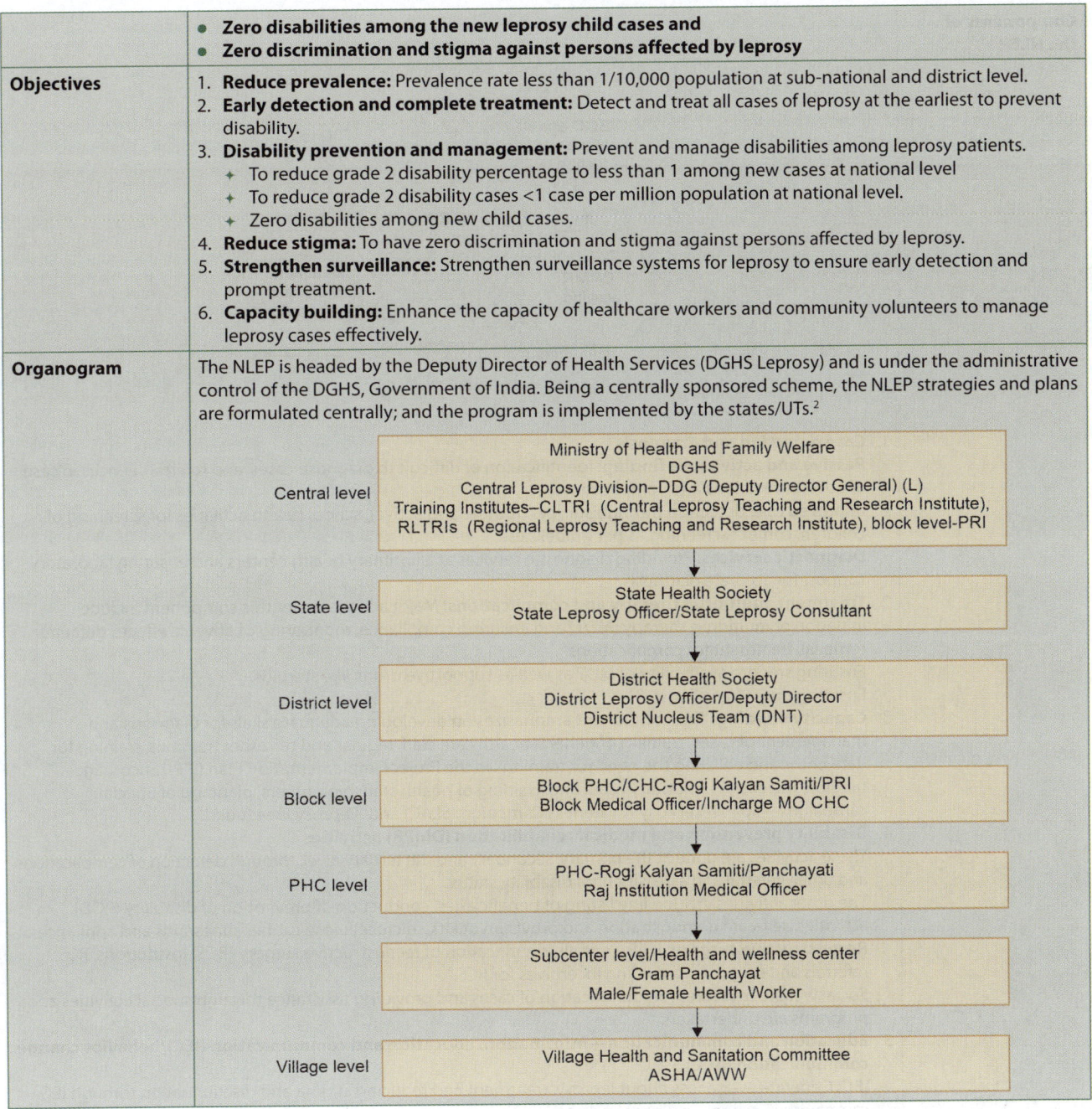

Components of the NLEP

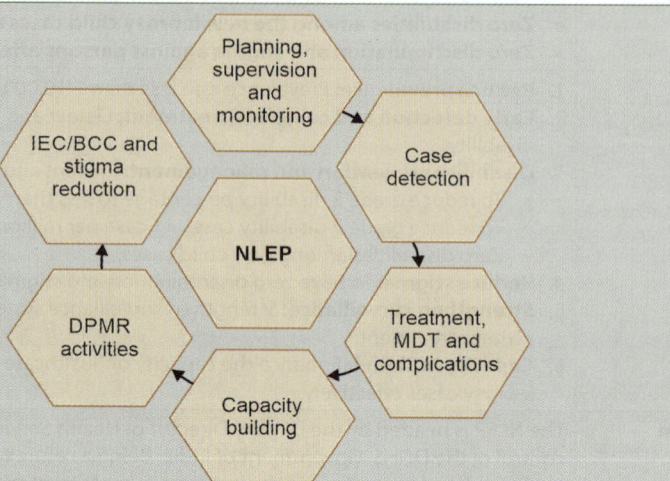

1. **Case detection and diagnosis**
   Passive and active case finding: Identification of difficult to diagnose cases, and referral services in case of adverse reactions and complications.
   Improved case detection through surveys (routine and active), school health activities for screening of children, contact screening as per guidelines.[6]
   Diagnostic services: Providing diagnostic services at all primary health centers and ensuring laboratory support for accurate diagnosis.[7]
2. **Treatment, multidrug therapy and complications:** Major actions under this component include initiation of multidrug therapy (MDT) and ensuring compliance, monitoring of adverse effects, defaulter retrieval, treatment for complications.
   Ensuring smooth availability of MDT as well as supportive drugs like steroids.
   Ensuring drugs free of cost.[10]
3. **Capacity building:** This component emphasizes on developing adequate skills for diagnosis and management of cases, training of general health care staff, regular and refresher trainings, training for data entry, and enlisting the need for trainings in the Project Implementation Plan (PIP). Encourage tangible increase in voluntary reporting, training of health staffs/volunteers, planning of Special campaigns—Sparsh Leprosy Awareness Campaign (SLAC) and "Leprosy Free India".[1,9]
4. **Disability prevention and medical rehabilitation (DMPR) activities**
   These activities are done at the primary, secondary and the tertiary level, through detection of complications and timely referral and assessment of disability status.
   The other activities include line listing of beneficiaries, conduction of prevention of disability (POD) activities, self-care demonstration and provision of kits, microcellulose rubber shoes/aids and appliances.
   Reconstructive surgery: It also entails identification of reconstructive surgery (RCS) institutions, RCS referrals and surgeries, providing incentives for RCS.[8]
   Social welfare measures for identification of cases and providing assistance through special activities and programs are undertaken.
5. **Education and communication—Information, education and communication (IEC)/behavior change communication (BCC)**
   IEC: Generate awareness about leprosy, treatment and reducing stigma and discrimination through IEC campaigns in schools, colleges and community; encouraging interpersonal communication (IPC), new strategies and methods with focus on behavior change communication.[9]
6. **Supervision and monitoring**
   Surveillance: This includes assessment of the leprosy situation in the area and the action plan, based on which surveys and field visits should be planned.
   Records and information systems: Supervision of field level healthcare workers and monitoring and evaluation of the program indicators and training needs assessment.

	Establishing a system of review meetings and feedback at all levels. Maintenance of records and reports ensuring they are complete, accurate and timely as well as implementation of NIKUSTH, a real time leprosy reporting software across India[2]

Strategies and deliverables under the program	• Decentralized integrated leprosy services through general health care system.
	   ✦ **Primary health centers:** Integrating leprosy services with general healthcare services at primary health centers to ensure accessibility.[2]
	   ✦ **Health system strengthening:** Strengthening the overall health system to provide comprehensive leprosy services, including diagnosis, treatment, and rehabilitation.[1]
	• **Early detection and complete treatment of all the new leprosy cases—community-based approach:** Utilizing a community-based approach to reach out to marginalized and underserved populations.
	• Planning of **household contact survey for early detection of cases: This is a three pronged strategy**—Leprosy case detection campaign (LCDC), focus leprosy campaign (FLC) and hard to reach areas.
	• **Capacity building of all general health services functionaries:** Through trainings and supportive supervision
	• **Involvement of ASHAs** in the detection and completion of treatment of leprosy cases on time
	• **Strengthening** of Disability Prevention and Medical Rehabilitation (DPMR) services.
	• **IEC activities** in the community to improve self-reporting to PHC and reduction of stigma.
	• **Intensive supervision and monitoring at the health and wellness centers and at primary and community health centers.** This is done by establishing village-level surveillance systems to identify new cases early and ensure prompt treatment.
	• **Regular monitoring:** Conducting regular monitoring and supervision of leprosy control activities at all levels. Intensive monitoring and supervision at health and wellness centers and at PHC/CHC.
	• **Public-private partnerships:** Integrated approach by working in collaboration with NGOs and mobilization of available resources.
	• **Undertaking research—operational research:** To identify best practices and innovations for leprosy treatment and control; including research into new diagnostic tools and treatment regime.
	• **Preventing stigma—anti-stigma campaigns and support groups:** Implementing campaigns to educate the public about leprosy and reduce the stigma and discrimination faced by affected individuals.

New strategies	Several new strategies have been devised and are under way under the NLEP such as: • The 'Sparsh Leprosy Awareness Campaign' (SLAC). This campaign was launched on Anti-Leprosy Day, i.e., 30th January in 2017 in order to reduce discrimination and stigma against persons suffering from leprosy. Gram Sabhas are organized each year in collaboration with health department with messages from the District Magistrates and Gram Sabha Pramukh (Heads of Village councils) **to reduce discrimination against persons affected with leprosy**. Pledges to reduce discrimination and felicitation of leprosy persons is done. *"Sapna" is the mascot of a common community girl, who helps spread awareness regarding leprosy through IEC messages. She can be a local school going girl who shows willingness to spread awareness. There can be many Sapnas in the village.*[9] 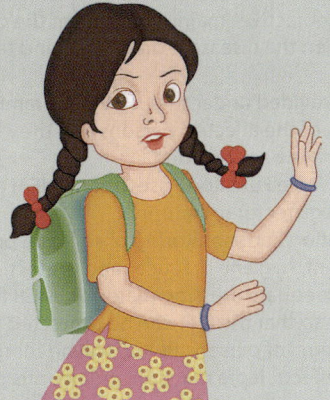 • Convergence of leprosy screening for targeting different age groups like under **RBSK** (for 0–18 yrs), **RKSK** (13–19 yrs), and CPHC—Ayushman Bharat (above 30+ years population). • Post Exposure Prophylaxis with Single Dose Rifampicin (PEP-SDR)

	<ul><li>Immunoprophylaxis through *Mycobacterium indicus pranii* (MIP) vaccine</li><li>Implementation of online reporting system ('Nikusth') for improved monitoring and supervision</li><li>Detailed investigation of grade 2 disability cases on a one-one basis</li><li>Drug resistance surveillance and modelling studies in leprosy</li><li>Active Case Detection and Regular Surveillance (ACD and RS)</li><li>District Award Scheme for achievements in NLEP</li></ul>
Package of services under the NLEP	<ul><li>**Primary prevention:** Chemoprophylaxis by single dose of rifampicin/immunoprophylaxis by *Mycobacterium indicus pranii* (MIP) vaccine to family members and contacts can give protection around 60%.</li><li>**Secondary prevention:** Early Diagnosis and Treatment through Active case detection and Regular Surveillance (ACD-RS)</li><li>**Rationale for ACDRS:** Undetected and untreated cases continue transmission and develop disability. A minimum of 6-9 months are required to develop the deformity. Despite the active case detection campaigns twice a year, grade 2 disability is being reported.</li><li>**Methodology of ACDRS:**<ul><li>Screening is done by one male and one female frontline worker identified by the Medical Officer (MO) approved by the District Leprosy Officer (DLO)</li><li>All persons above 2 years of age to be screened</li><li>Screening is done by visual examination and verbal enquiry within a span of 6 months/12 months based on endemicity of block</li></ul></li></ul>**Contact screening and tracing** The process includes activities like line listing of close contacts, screening for signs or symptoms of leprosy by trained health workers under supervision of the Community Health Officer (CHO), Health and Wellness Center Medical Officer (HWC/MO). Post Exposure Chemoprophylaxis (PEP) of a Single Dose Rifampicin (SDR) is given to eligible contacts. Incentives provided to the male and female frontline workers include ₹ 1000 per round based on having an updated screening register which is to be verified by the supervisor. Additional incentives include ₹ 250 per case detection without disability, ₹ 200 per case detection with disability, ₹ 400 for treatment completion of Paucibacillary (PB) case and ₹ 600 for treatment completion of Multibacillary case (MB). **Tertiary prevention** **Disability prevention and medical rehabilitation:** The primary objective of the NLEP is to provide comprehensive leprosy services to those persons affected by leprosy which includes (i) early detection and complete treatment of leprosy cases so that disabilities are prevented and stigma dispelled, (ii) follow up of such cases so that they do not have any complications, (iii) early identification of disabilities and deformities, if any, so that they can be managed timely. This would help mainstreaming of the cases once treated in order to help them earn their livelihood and maintain their families. The Disability Prevention and Medical Rehabilitation (DPMR) Programme is launched with a view to achieve these objectives mainly, to prevent the occurrence of any disability or deformity not already present at the time when the disease is diagnosed and to prevent the worsening of the existing disabilities and deformities.[8] The services provided under the DPMR Programme are:<ul><li>Counseling of the affected persons and their family members regarding the reason of disability and how this could have been avoided.</li><li>Thorough Nerve Function Assessment (NFA) and Eyes, Hand Feet (EHF) scoring are to be NFA card and Disability register for monitoring.</li><li>Demonstration and monitoring of self-care practices including ulcer-care, emphasis on rest, good wound management, hygiene practices and protection; and active and passive exercises.</li><li>Supply of adequate dressing materials, MCR footwear to the persons having anesthetic feet and regularly replacing it so that the feet can be protected from injuries.</li><li>Prompt referral of persons fit and willing for reconstructive surgery (RCS), complicated plantar ulcers, MDT side-effects, lepra reaction and neuritis cases not responding to steroid, pregnant and child cases developing lepra reactions and eye complications.</li></ul>

Monitoring and evaluation of the program	• **Annual case detection rate:** The case detection rate is the total number of new leprosy cases detected during the reporting year divided by the total population of the area; usually expressed as a rate per 10,000 or 100,000 population. • **Grade 2 disability rate:** The proportion of grade 2 disabled cases detected in a year amongst the new cases detected.[5] • **Prevalence rate:** The number of balance new cases under treatment as on 31st March out of the total population on 31st March into 1000.[5] **Achievements during 2021–22:** • The prevalence rate decreased to 0.41 per 10,000 population in 2020–21. • Annual new cases detection rate (ANCDR) reduced to 4.58/100000 in 2020–21. • Percentage of grade 2 disability (G2D)/visible deformity among new cases decreased from 3.05% in 2018–19 to 2.48% in 2020–21. • The G2D amongst new cases/million population decreased from 2.65/million population as on 31st March 2019 to 1.14/million population as on 31st March 2021. • Child cases percentage has reduced from 7.67% as on 31st March 2019 to 5.76% on 31st March 2021.

References

1. Kumaresan K. National Leprosy Eradication Programme (NLEP) Programmatic Management of Leprosy Public Health Specialist Gr II.
2. https://dghs.gov.in/content/1349_3_NationalLeprosyEradicationProgramme.aspx
3. https://cltri.gov.in/AboutLeprosy/NLEP_Program%20Management_DLO.pdf
4. Park K. Park's Textbook of Preventive and Social Medicine, 27th ed. Jabalpur: Banarsidas Bhanot; 2023.
5. National Leprosy Eradication Program (NLEP) Annual Report 2019-20 - Central Leprosy Division, Ministry of Health and Family Welfare, Government of India. https://naco.gov.in/sites/default/files/Annual%20Report%202019-2020%20English.pdf
6. NLEP Operational Guidelines 2019 - Central Leprosy Division, Ministry of Health and Family Welfare, Government of India. https://dghs.gov.in/WriteReadData/userfiles/file/Leprosy/2020%20Operational%20Guidelines%20for%20ACD%20and%20RS%20NLEP%20final.pdf
7. WHO Guidelines for the Diagnosis, Treatment, and Prevention of Leprosy - World Health Organization (WHO). https://www.who.int/publications/i/item/9789290226383
8. http://clinicalestablishments.gov.in/WriteReadData/516.pdf
9. National Leprosy Eradication Programme — Vikaspedia [Internet]. [cited 2024 Jul 26]. Available from: https://vikaspedia.in/health/nrhm/national-health-programmes-1/communicable-diseases/national-leprosy-eradication-programme.
10. National Leprosy Eradication Program Guidelines for Primary, Secondary and Tertiary Level Care Disability Prevention & Medical Rehabilitation; 2012.

QUESTIONS

Long Answer Question (LAQ)

1. Describe the main objectives and strategies of the National Leprosy Eradication Programme (NLEP) implemented by the Government of India. How does the program aim to achieve its goal a Leprosy Free India?

Short Answer Questions (SAQs)

1. What is the main mission of the National Leprosy Eradication Programme (NLEP)?
2. What are the primary components of the NLEP?

Multiple Choice Questions (MCQs)

1. When was the National Leprosy Control Programme renamed as the National Leprosy Eradication Programme?
   a. 1955
   b. 1981
   c. 1983
   d. 1993
2. What is the vision of the National Leprosy Eradication Programme?
   a. Leprosy-free world
   b. Leprosy-free India
   c. Leprosy-free Asia
   d. Leprosy-free districts
3. Which therapy was introduced by WHO in 1981 that played a crucial role in the NLEP?
   a. Single drug therapy (SDT)
   b. Multidrug therapy (MDT)
   c. Chemotherapy
   d. Antibiotic therapy
4. What is the main focus of IEC/BCC activities under the NLEP?
   a. Early detection of cases
   b. Ensuring compliance to treatment
   c. Generating awareness and reducing stigma
   d. Providing financial incentives to patients
5. What is the incentive for a frontline worker per round for conducting Active Case Detection and Regular Surveillance (ACD-RS)?
   a. ₹ 500
   b. ₹ 1000
   c. ₹ 1500
   d. ₹ 2000
6. Best diagnostic method for leprosy is:
   a. Droplet smear
   b. Skin smear
   c. Culture
   d. Lepromin test
7. Elimination level for leprosy is:
   a. <1/1000
   b. <1/10,000
   c. <1/100,000
   d. <10/10,000
8. Which disease is often known as a social disease?
   a. Leprosy
   b. HIV
   c. Tuberculosis
   d. Malaria
9. Strategies of leprosy eradication program include all the following *except*:
   a. Early detection and complete treatment of new leprosy cases
   b. Early diagnosis and prompt MDT, through routine and special efforts
   c. Strengthening of Disability Prevention and Medical Rehabilitation (DPMR) services
   d. Centralized services through dedicated hospitals for leprosy patients

Answers

1. c
2. b
3. b
4. c
5. b
6. c
7. b
8. a
9. d

CHAPTER 47

National Viral Hepatitis Control Programme

Ajeet Singh Bhadoria, Vineet Kumar Pathak, M Swathi Shenoy, Kavita, Kapil Gandha

Background/Need of the program	Viral hepatitis is a significant public health concern in India, contributing to considerable morbidity and mortality. Hepatitis B and C are particularly problematic, often leading to chronic liver disease, cirrhosis, and liver cancer.[1] According to the Seroprevalence of Hepatitis B and C Factsheet 2021, the national seroprevalence of hepatitis B was 0.95% (0.89–1.01). Similarly, the national seroprevalence of hepatitis C was 0.32% (0.28–0.36).[2] The prevalence of these infections, combined with low awareness and limited access to diagnosis and treatment, has underscored the need for a comprehensive public health response to prevent, diagnose, and treat hepatitis infections. The National Viral Hepatitis Control Program (NVHCP)[3] is essential to mitigate the economic burden on healthcare systems and improve the quality of life for those affected. Through the NVHCP, efforts are being made to increase awareness about hepatitis, improve screening and diagnosis, and provide affordable treatment options. In line with the Sustainable Development Goal 2030, the program envisages to achieve significant reductions in the prevalence of viral hepatitis (A, B, C, D and E) and improve the overall health outcomes for those affected.
Implemented since	The National Viral Hepatitis Control Program (NVHCP) was launched on World Hepatitis Day, July 28, 2018. The MoHFW introduced the program as part of the National Health Mission. The program is focused on providing synergistic healthcare services with the already exiting platforms and also to provide newer interventions to test and treat viral hepatitis. Through this integrated care, the program has been able to reach remote and underserved populations, ensuring that no one is left behind in the fight against viral hepatitis. The NVHCP will continue expanding its reach and impact, working towards eliminating viral hepatitis as a public health threat in India.[3]
Goal[3]	The primary goal of the NVHCP is to eliminate viral hepatitis as a significant public health threat in India by 2030, aiming for a disease-free future. This aligns with the World Health Organization's (WHO) Global Health Sector Strategy on Viral Hepatitis. By addressing these critical areas, the NVHCP aims to create a future where viral hepatitis is no longer a significant public health concern in India.
Aim[3]	• Elimination of hepatitis C by 2030 • Reduction in the infected population, morbidity and mortality associated with hepatitis B and C • Reduce the risk, morbidity and mortality due to hepatitis A and E

Targets[3]	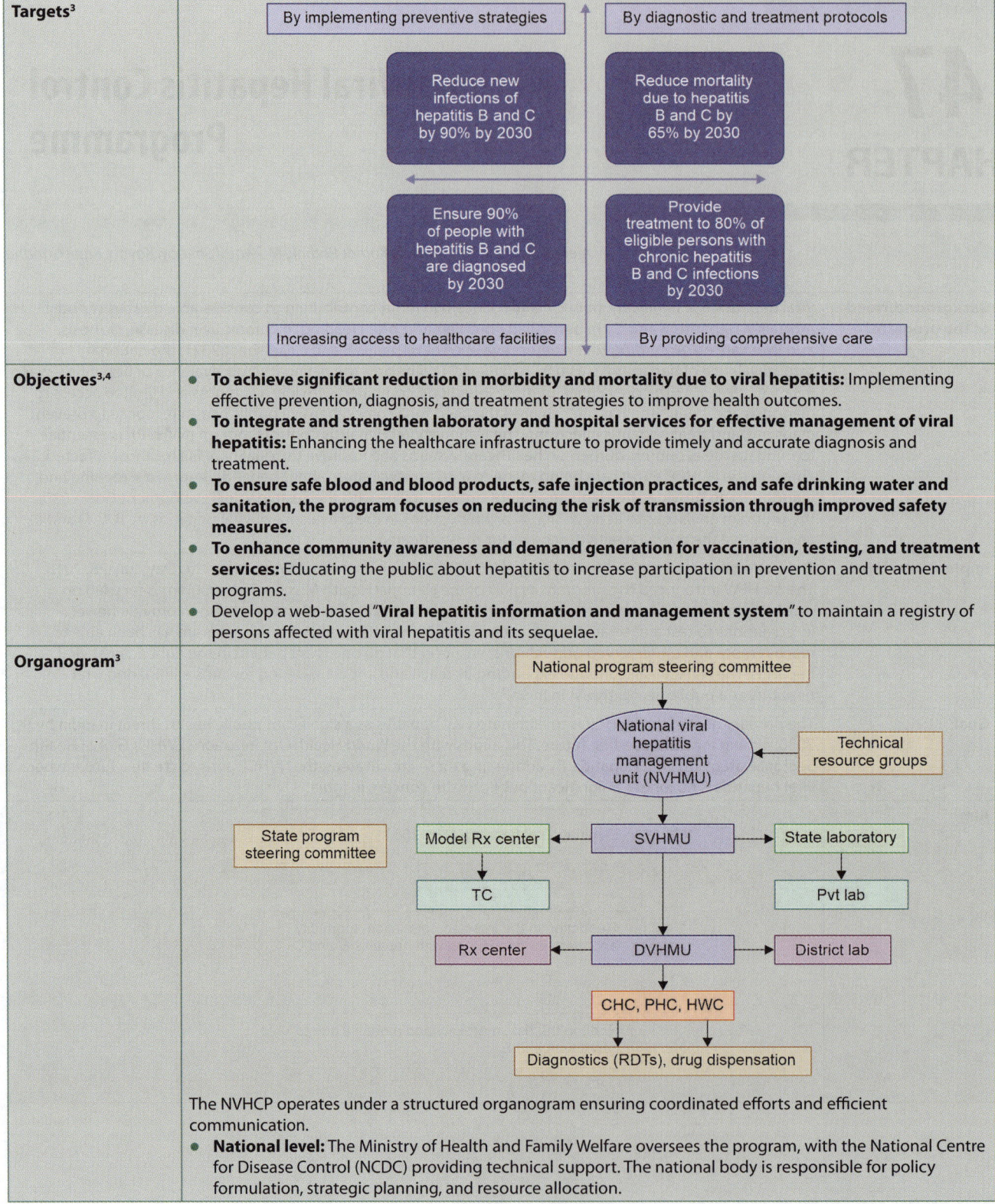
Objectives[3,4]	- **To achieve significant reduction in morbidity and mortality due to viral hepatitis:** Implementing effective prevention, diagnosis, and treatment strategies to improve health outcomes.
- **To integrate and strengthen laboratory and hospital services for effective management of viral hepatitis:** Enhancing the healthcare infrastructure to provide timely and accurate diagnosis and treatment.
- **To ensure safe blood and blood products, safe injection practices, and safe drinking water and sanitation, the program focuses on reducing the risk of transmission through improved safety measures.**
- **To enhance community awareness and demand generation for vaccination, testing, and treatment services:** Educating the public about hepatitis to increase participation in prevention and treatment programs.
- Develop a web-based "**Viral hepatitis information and management system**" to maintain a registry of persons affected with viral hepatitis and its sequelae.
Organogram[3]	The NVHCP operates under a structured organogram ensuring coordinated efforts and efficient communication.
- **National level:** The Ministry of Health and Family Welfare oversees the program, with the National Centre for Disease Control (NCDC) providing technical support. The national body is responsible for policy formulation, strategic planning, and resource allocation.

	• **State level:** State health departments implement the program with assistance from state program management units. States adapt national strategies to local contexts and ensure proper implementation and monitoring. • **District level:** District health officers manage the program with support from district program management units. Districts are responsible for operationalizing the program at the local level, conducting outreach, and ensuring service delivery. • **Primary healthcare level:** Primary health centers (PHCs) and community health centers (CHCs) deliver services directly to the community. These centers provide vaccination, screening, treatment, and community education services
Beneficiaries[3]	The beneficiaries of the NVHCP include: • **People at risk of or living with viral hepatitis:** Individuals who are either susceptible to or have contracted hepatitis B or C benefit from prevention, diagnosis, and treatment services. • **Healthcare workers exposed to infectious materials:** Medical professionals and support staff are provided with preventive measures and vaccinations to protect them from occupational exposure. • **Communities at large through enhanced public health measures and awareness campaigns:** The entire population benefits from reduced transmission risks and increased awareness of hepatitis, leading to better health outcomes and reduced healthcare costs.
Components[3,4]	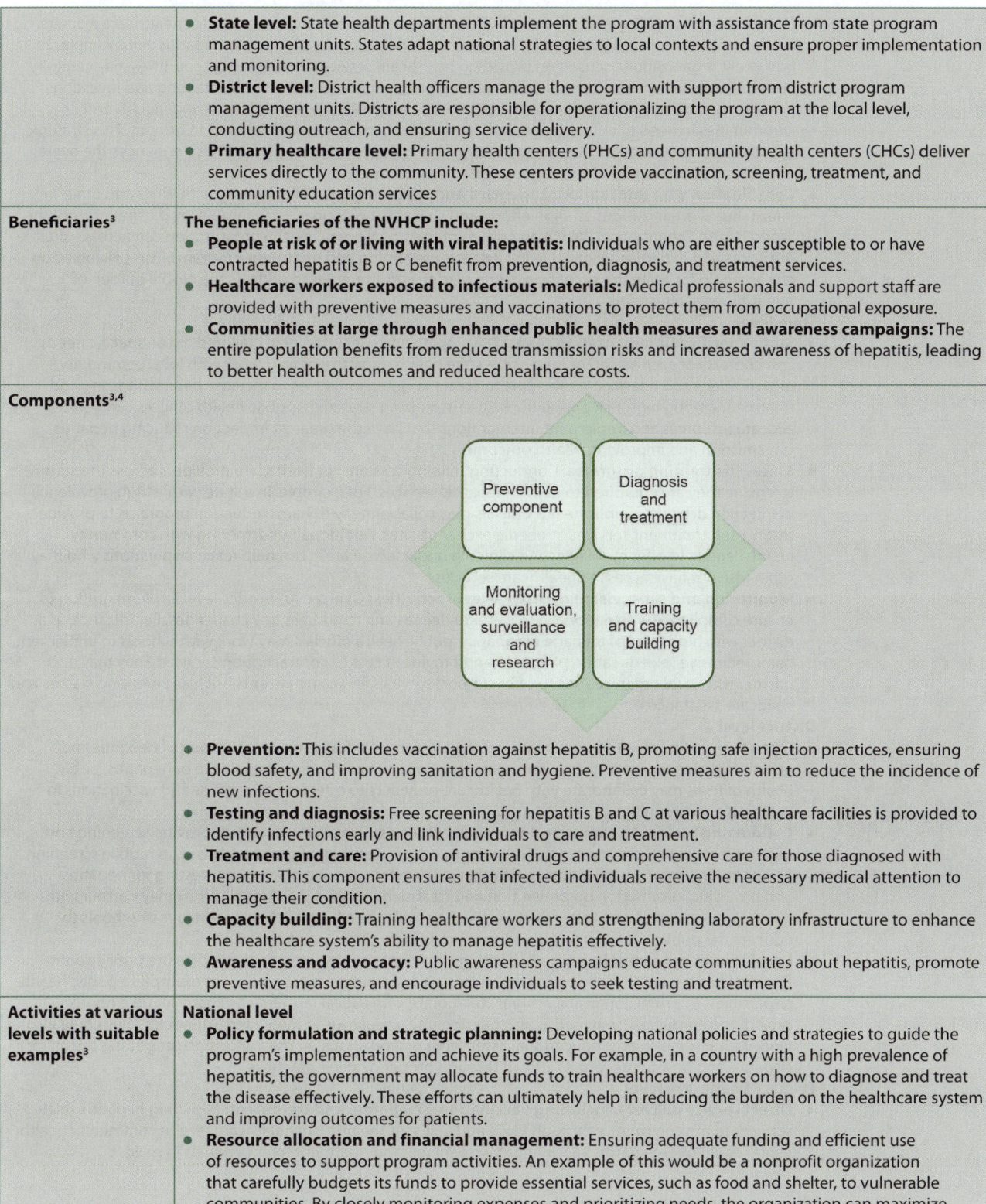 • **Prevention:** This includes vaccination against hepatitis B, promoting safe injection practices, ensuring blood safety, and improving sanitation and hygiene. Preventive measures aim to reduce the incidence of new infections. • **Testing and diagnosis:** Free screening for hepatitis B and C at various healthcare facilities is provided to identify infections early and link individuals to care and treatment. • **Treatment and care:** Provision of antiviral drugs and comprehensive care for those diagnosed with hepatitis. This component ensures that infected individuals receive the necessary medical attention to manage their condition. • **Capacity building:** Training healthcare workers and strengthening laboratory infrastructure to enhance the healthcare system's ability to manage hepatitis effectively. • **Awareness and advocacy:** Public awareness campaigns educate communities about hepatitis, promote preventive measures, and encourage individuals to seek testing and treatment.
Activities at various levels with suitable examples[3]	**National level** • **Policy formulation and strategic planning:** Developing national policies and strategies to guide the program's implementation and achieve its goals. For example, in a country with a high prevalence of hepatitis, the government may allocate funds to train healthcare workers on how to diagnose and treat the disease effectively. These efforts can ultimately help in reducing the burden on the healthcare system and improving outcomes for patients. • **Resource allocation and financial management:** Ensuring adequate funding and efficient use of resources to support program activities. An example of this would be a nonprofit organization that carefully budgets its funds to provide essential services, such as food and shelter, to vulnerable communities. By closely monitoring expenses and prioritizing needs, the organization can maximize the impact of its resources and reach more individuals in need. This strategic approach to financial management helps ensure sustainability and long-term success for the organization's mission.

- **National-level training and capacity building:** Organizing training programs for healthcare workers and administrators at the national level to enhance their capacity to manage hepatitis. For example, a non-profit organization focused on providing healthcare services in developing countries may carefully allocate funds to conduct national-level training programs. By prioritizing this training and investing in building capacity at a larger scale, the organization can effectively reach more individuals and communities in need of critical healthcare services for hepatitis prevention and treatment. This strategic approach not only ensures the sustainability of the organization's mission but also enhances the overall impact and effectiveness of its programs on a national level.
- **Coordination with international agencies and stakeholders:** Collaborating with WHO and other international organizations to align efforts and share best practices. For example, by partnering with the World Health Organization (WHO) and other international agencies, the organization can access valuable resources and expertise to improve its hepatitis prevention and treatment programs. This collaboration can also help facilitate the exchange of knowledge and strategies to address the global burden of hepatitis more effectively.

State level
- **State-specific implementation plans:** Developing and executing plans tailored to the specific needs and contexts of each state. For instance, a state health department may work with local community organizations and healthcare providers to create targeted initiatives to increase hepatitis testing and treatment among high-risk populations. By customizing strategies, public health officials can better allocate resources and implement interventions that have the greatest impact on reducing hepatitis transmission and improving health outcomes.
- **Statewide training programs:** Conducting training sessions for healthcare providers across the state to ensure they are equipped to deliver hepatitis services. For example, in a state with a high prevalence of injection drug use, public health officials may collaborate with harm reduction programs to provide testing and treatment services at needle exchange sites. Additionally, partnering with community health centers to offer mobile testing clinics in underserved areas can help reach populations who may otherwise not have access to healthcare services.
- **Monitoring and supervision of district-level activities:** Overseeing district-level implementation to ensure compliance with national and state guidelines and to address any challenges. For instance, in a district with high rates of teenage pregnancy, public health officials may work with schools to implement comprehensive sex education programs and provide access to contraception services. They may also partner with local organizations to offer support services for young parents, such as parenting classes and childcare assistance.

District level
- **District-specific action plans:** Creating detailed plans to address the local burden of hepatitis and ensure effective service delivery. For example, in a district with a high prevalence of hepatitis, public health officials may collaborate with healthcare providers to offer free screenings and vaccinations in vulnerable communities.
- **Conducting screening camps and outreach activities:** Organizing events to provide screening and raise awareness in the community. For instance, a local health department may set up mobile screening camps in rural areas where access to healthcare is limited, offering on-the-spot testing for hepatitis and providing information on prevention and treatment options. Additionally, they may partner with community organizations to conduct outreach activities at events such as health fairs or schools to educate the public about hepatitis and encourage individuals to get tested.
- **Local awareness campaigns:** Implementing communication strategies to educate the public about hepatitis and promote participation in prevention and treatment programs. For example, a public health department in a rural community might collaborate with a local farmers' market to set up a booth providing information on hepatitis and offering free screenings to interested attendees. They could also work with schools to host educational assemblies or workshops on the importance of getting tested for hepatitis and how to prevent its spread through proper hygiene practices.

Primary healthcare level
- **Direct service delivery, including vaccination, screening, and treatment:** Providing hepatitis-related services to the community through PHCs and CHCs. At the primary healthcare level, a community health center could offer hepatitis vaccinations, screenings, and treatment for individuals in need.

	• **Community engagement and education:** For example, a community health center could partner with local schools to educate students about the importance of getting vaccinated against hepatitis and provide free screenings for students. They could also collaborate with local community organizations to host workshops on hepatitis prevention and treatment options for residents.
Monitoring and evaluation[3,4]	The NVHCP has a robust monitoring and evaluation (M&E) framework to track progress and ensure accountability: • **Routine reporting:** Regular data collection and reporting from the field to state and national levels to monitor program implementation and outcomes. For example, the NVHCP could track the number of students who receive vaccinations and screenings through school partnerships to measure the impact of their education efforts. They could also analyze workshop attendance and follow-up surveys from community organizations to assess the effectiveness of their prevention and treatment programs. • **Periodic surveys:** Conducting surveys to assess program impact, coverage, and effectiveness in reducing the burden of hepatitis. For instance, the NVHCP could distribute surveys to schools participating in their vaccination program to gather data on vaccination rates and student health outcomes. They could also conduct community-wide surveys to measure awareness levels of hepatitis prevention strategies and identify areas for improvement in their education campaigns. • **Independent evaluations:** Engaging third-party evaluators for unbiased program assessments to identify strengths, weaknesses, and areas for improvement. Additionally, the NVHCP could analyze hospital data to track the number of hepatitis cases before and after implementing their program to measure its impact on disease prevalence. They could also collaborate with local health departments to monitor trends in hepatitis-related hospitalizations and inform future program strategies. • **Digital health solutions:** Utilizing electronic health records and mobile technology for real-time monitoring and data management, ensuring timely and accurate information to guide decision-making. For example, a hospital could use electronic health records to identify high-risk patients for hepatitis and provide targeted interventions to prevent transmission. Mobile technology could also be used to remotely monitor patients with chronic hepatitis, allowing for early detection of complications and timely intervention.

References

1. Ministry of Health and Family Welfare, Indian Institute of Population Sciences, Mumbai, Indian Council of Medical Research. Seroprevalence of Hepatitis B and C: Factsheet 2021.[Internet] New Delhi: Ministry of Health and Family Welfare; [cited 2024 Jul 13]. Available from: https://nvhcp.mohfw.gov.in/common_libs/Approved%20factsheet_4_10_2021.pdf
2. Mehta P, Grant LM, Reddivari AKR. Viral Hepatitis. [Updated 2024 Mar 10]. In: StatPearls [Internet]. Treasure Island (FL): StatPearls Publishing; 2024 Jan. Available from: https://www.ncbi.nlm.nih.gov/books/NBK554549
3. Ministry of Health and Family Welfare, Government of India. National Viral Hepatitis Control Program (NVHCP) [Internet]. New Delhi: Ministry of Health and Family Welfare; [cited 2024 Jul 13]. Available from: https://nvhcp.mohfw.gov.in/
4. World Health Organization - India. Combatting Hepatitis in India: Collaborative Efforts and Public Health Initiatives [Internet]. New Delhi: World Health Organization; [cited 2024 Jul 13]. Available from: https://www.who.int/india/health-topics/hepatitis

QUESTIONS

Long Answer Question (LAQ)

1. Discuss the National Viral Hepatitis Control Program (NVHCP) and its role in eliminating viral hepatitis as a public health threat in India by 2030.

Short Answer Questions (SAQs)

1. Explain the challenges in diagnosing and treating viral hepatitis in rural and underserved areas of India. Discuss the barriers to healthcare access, including infrastructure, awareness, and resource limitations.
2. Outline the role of healthcare workers in the implementation of the NVHCP at the primary healthcare level.

Multiple Choice Questions (MCQs)

1. In one boarding school, students have been eating from the same canteen. One student develop icterus, fever and pain in abdomen. Soon after those other students too had, the same complains. You are the medical officer of the boarding school. To establish the diagnosis, which test you will use?
    a. IgM for Hepatitis B
    b. IgG for Hepatitis A
    c. IgM for Hepatitis A
    d. IgG for Hepatitis B
2. The risk of transmission is highest for through needle stick injury:
    a. HBV
    b. HCV
    c. HIV
    d. All of the above
3. With which of the following types of viral hepatitis infection in pregnancy, the maternal mortality is the highest?
    a. Hepatitis A
    b. Hepatitis B
    c. Hepatitis C
    d. Hepatitis E
4. Which of the hepatitis B virus serological marker indicates the first evidence of hepatitis B infection?
    a. Anti-HBs
    b. Anti-HBc
    c. HBeAg
    d. HBsAg 264
5. Which of the following viral markers signifies the ongoing viral replication in the case of hepatitis B infection?
    a. Anti-HBs
    b. Anti-HBc
    c. HBe Ag
    d. HBs Ag
6. A person shows HBsAg$^+$, AntiHBc IgG$^+$, HBeAg$^+$, AntiHBe Ab$^-$. Diagnosis:
    a. Acute hepatitis B
    b. Vaccination
    c. Recovery from hepatitis B
    d. Chronic hepatitis B with high infectivity
7. Hepatitis B vaccine, dose schedule in adult (months):
    a. 0, 1, 2 months
    b. 2, 4, 6 months
    c. 0, 6, 12 months
    d. 0, 1, 6 months
8. During pregnancy at 37 weeks' mother found to be HBsAG positive, and then baby should receive:
    a. Hep B vaccine only
    b. Hep B vaccine + HBIG
    c. First HBIG then hep B after 1 month
    d. Only HBIG
9. A 45-day-old infant developed icterus and two days later symptoms and signs of acute liver failure appeared. Child was found to be positive for HBsAG. The mother was also HBsAG carrier. The mother's hepatitis B serological profile is likely to be:
    a. HBsAG positive only
    b. HBsAG and HBeAg positivity
    c. HBsAg and anti-HBe antibody positivity
    d. Mother infected with mutant HB V
10. A patient came in emergency with signs of dehydration and severe diarrhea. An intravenous infusion was given to correct electrolytes and fluid levels. He was discharged after 2 days. About 2 months later the patient came back with signs of jaundice and hepatitis B surface antigen was positive. He did not give history of any event, which could have led to this disease. This hepatitis infection may be labeled as:
    a. Iatrogenic
    b. Idiopathic
    c. Opportunistic
    d. Cross infection

Answers

1. c
2. a
3. d
4. d
5. c
6. d
7. d
8. b
9. b
10. a

CHAPTER 48

National Rabies Control Programme

Rohit Katre, Pallavi Singh, Manish Kumar Singh, Venu Shah

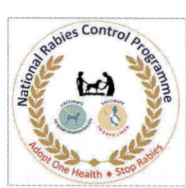

Background/Need of program/Scheme	Rabies is a significant cause of both morbidity and mortality in India, with cases reported from almost all regions except the Andaman and Nicobar Islands and Lakshadweep, highlighting the widespread nature of the disease.
Implemented since	The program was approved during the 12th Five-Year Plan by the Standing Finance Committee on October 3, 2013. It is implemented as a Central Sector Scheme under the National Health Mission.
Objectives	<ul><li>Educate healthcare professionals on rabies post-exposure prevention and the proper management of animal bites.[1]</li><li>Pushing for governments to embrace and implement the intradermal technique for pre-exposure prophylaxis for high-risk populations and post-exposure treatment for victims of animal attacks.</li><li>Strengthen the human rabies surveillance system.</li><li>Enhancement of Regional Laboratories for Rabies Diagnosis Under NRCP.</li><li>Raise community awareness through communication, advocacy, and social mobilization.</li></ul>
Organogram	**National Level**<ul><li>**National technical advisory committee on rabies**: Chaired by the DGHS, providing technical guidance and oversight.</li><li>**National Centre for Disease Control (NCDC)**: Coordinates the human health component across all states and UTs under MoHFW.</li></ul>**State Level** **State Joint Steering Committee on Rabies**: Chaired by the State Chief Secretary, overseeing program implementation and interdepartmental coordination. **District Level**<ul><li>**District Joint Steering Committee on Rabies**: Chaired by the District Magistrate/Collector, responsible for execution, monitoring, and local coordination.</li></ul>**Animal Health Component**<ul><li>**Animal Welfare Board of India (AWBI)**: Under Ministry of Environment, Forest and Climate Change responsible for pilot testing stray dog population control through sterilization and vaccination.[1]</li></ul>
Beneficiaries	<ul><li>Victims of animal bite are provided with antirabies vaccines and immunoglobulin as per their category of bite.[1]</li></ul>
Components	Activities envisaged under human health component:<ul><li>Human Health—PEP for all animal bite victims training and capacity building, strengthening surveillance of animal bites and rabies cases in human, strengthen diagnostics capacity on rabies, intersectoral coordination, information education and communication, public private partnership.[1] Activities Envisaged under Animal Health Component.[1]</li></ul>

	• Estimation of Canine Population (Dog Survey), identification of rabies risk zone, planning and implementing strategic mass dog vaccination, solid waste management (SWM), confinement and containment, community participation and Operational research, Dog Population Management (DPM), To promote responsible dog ownership.
Strategies/Deliverables under the program	• National free drug programs provide the rabies vaccine and immunoglobulin. • Surveillance, intersectoral collaboration, rabies prevention and control, and appropriate handling of animal bites. • Increasing rabies death reporting and animal bite surveillance in IDSP/IHIP portal. • Spreading knowledge about preventing rabies.
Activities at various level or package of services	**Primary Prevention** ✦ Mass vaccination of dogs. ✦ Public awareness campaigns ✦ Training and capacity building ✦ Intersectoral coordination **Secondary Prevention** ✦ Post-exposure prophylaxis (PEP) ✦ Surveillance and reporting **Other steps announced to control rabies:** • To limit the dog population, the Animal **Birth Control (Dogs) Regulations, 2023** have been proposed by the Animal Welfare Board of India (AWBI) to the appropriate authorities. • **"National Action Plan for Dog Mediated Rabies Elimination (NAPRE)** from India by 2030 was jointly announced by the Indian Ministries of Health and Family Welfare and Fisheries, Animal Husbandry and NAPRE is based on one health approach and involves many ministries. • Local bodies are involved in rabies free city initiative.
Monitoring and evaluation of program	State level Joint Steering Committee on Rabies is responsible for monitoring the collaborative activities of the State Action Plan for Rabies Elimination (SAP-RE). The committee oversees the uninterrupted supply of logistics needed for the plan's execution and ensures effective integration, cooperation, collaboration, and communication among stakeholders at all levels, following the One Health Approach.

Reference

1. National Rabies Control Program. National Center for Disease Control. Directorate General of Health Services, Ministry of Health and Family Welfare, Government of India. Available on https://rabiesfreeindia.mohfw.gov.in/

QUESTIONS

Long Answer Question (LAQ)

1. A child of age three years was brought to Primary Health Center (PHC), with a complaint of stray dog bite over his face, below the left eye. History revealed that the incidence occurred 12 hours back. Currently, there is no evidence of blood around the wound, but parents revealed that small bleeding occurred during the event. The child had a similar episode one year back also. Based on the above case scenario, write about the Epidemiological determinants of the disease which you are suspecting as a primary physician posted at this PHC. Write about the different vaccination strategy available for prevention of this disease. How are you going to manage the case?

Short Answer Questions (SAQs)

1. National Action Plan for Dog Mediated Rabies Elimination by 2030.
2. Activities under Animal Component of National Rabies Control Programme.

Multiple Choice Questions (MCQs)

1. **What is the primary aim of the National Rabies Control Programme (NRCP)?**
    a. To eliminate rabies in wild animals
    b. To control rabies in domestic animals
    c. To prevent and control rabies in humans through vaccination and awareness
    d. To promote the use of traditional medicine for rabies treatment
2. **Which committee provides overall technical guidance and oversight for the NRCP at the national level?**
    a. National Health Mission Committee
    b. National Technical Advisory Committee on Rabies
    c. Central Rabies Elimination Committee
    d. National Animal Welfare Committee
3. **Under which ministry does the National Centre for Disease Control (NCDC) operate as the nodal agency for the human health component of the NRCP?**
    a. Ministry of Environment, Forest and Climate Change
    b. Ministry of Animal Husbandry
    c. Ministry of Health and Family Welfare
    d. Ministry of Agriculture, Fisheries and Mining
4. **Which of the following is a key strategy under the NRCP for managing rabies in humans?**
    a. Mass culling of stray dogs
    b. Post-exposure prophylaxis (PEP) for animal bite victims
    c. Quarantine of rabies-infected patients
    d. Raising public awareness about rabies prevention
5. **Which agency is responsible for the Animal Health Component under the NRCP, focusing on stray dog population control?**
    a. National Institute of Virology
    b. Indian Veterinary Research Institute
    c. Animal Welfare Board of India (AWBI)
    d. National Centre for Disease Control
6. **What is the role of the State Joint Steering Committee on Rabies under the NRCP?**
    a. To develop new vaccines for rabies
    b. To oversee program implementation and coordination at the state level
    c. To manage wildlife rabies control
    d. To provide funding for rabies research
7. **Which of the following is NOT a primary prevention strategy under the NRCP?**
    a. Mass vaccination of dogs
    b. Public awareness campaigns
    c. Advanced medical care for rabies patients
    d. Animal Birth Control (ABC) programs
8. **What is the significance of post-exposure prophylaxis (PEP) in rabies control?**
    a. It provides lifelong immunity against rabies
    b. It is used to treat rabies after symptoms have appeared
    c. It prevents the development of rabies after exposure to the virus
    d. It is a primary prevention strategy used in healthy individuals

Chapter 48: National Rabies Control Programme

9. Which of the following is a component of the Animal Health Strategy under the NRCP?
   a. Surveillance of human rabies cases
   b. Mass vaccination and sterilization of stray dogs
   c. Development of rabies diagnostic kits for hospitals
   d. Quarantine of infected animals
10. The National Action Plan for Dog-Mediated Rabies Elimination (NAPRE) aims to eliminate rabies from India by which year?
    a. 2025
    b. 2030
    c. 2040
    d. 2050

Answers

1. c	2. b	3. c	4. b	5. c
6. b	7. c	8. c	9. b	10. b

CHAPTER 49

Endgame Strategy for Poliomyelitis

Hariom Kumar Solanki, Shaili Vyas, Sudeep Bhavsar

Background	In 1988, globally, there were 3,50,000 cases of poliomyelitis distributed across 125 countries.[1,2] With the background of success story of smallpox eradication in 1960 and being vaccine preventable disease, polio was eligible and suitable for eradication. However, there were two schools of thoughts, one of which was in favor of emphasizing target disease specific eradication, while the other advocated for slower but more integrated approach to public health.[2,3] **Global polio eradication initiative (GPEI):** Based on the resolution adopted in 41st World Health Assembly (WHA) in 1988 with the stated goal of global eradication of poliomyelitis, Global Polio Eradication Initiative (GPEI) came into reality. The goal was defined as:[4] • There should not be any case of clinical poliomyelitis (polio) associated with the wild poliovirus, and • Even after intensive efforts of searching, wild polioviruses should not be detected worldwide. Global Polio Eradication Initiative is led by national governments as private public partnership model with 6 partner organizations, namely World Health Organization, Rotary International, Center for Disease Control and Prevention (Atlanta, USA), United Nations Children's Fund (UNICEF), Bill and Melinda Gates Foundation and GAVI (the vaccine alliance).[5] **Polio Eradication Strategy 2022–2026: Delivering on a promise[6]** The Polio Eradication Strategy 2022–2026 reflects the kind of integrated approaches that will be required to deliver on the promise of eradication.
Goals	**Goal 1:** To permanently eradicate all poliovirus transmission in the final wild poliovirus endemic countries Pakistan and Afghanistan. **Goal 2:** To stop circulating vaccine derived poliovirus (cVDPV) transmission and prevent outbreaks in non-endemic countries.

Chapter 49: Endgame Strategy for Poliomyelitis 265

Goals

Political advocacy
- Gain and maintain access in Afghanistan through systematic advocacy with all
- Intensify advocacy with provincial governments in Pakistan

Community engagement
- Conduct multidisciplinary research into vaccine hesitancy and community mistrust
- Foster alliances with priority communities for co-design, ownership and delivery of gender-responsive program innovations

Campaigns
- Recruit, train, and appropriately support a motivated workforce that meets the needs of the community
- Introduce monitoring innovations to enable faster data feedback loops and improve quality
- Facilitate strengthening of essential immunization

Integration
- Deliver polio vaccines alongside basic public services to increase the reach of both essential and supplementary immunization, with a focus on high-risk areas
- Partner with governments, communities, and adjacent health programs to support access and reduce missed communities and zero-dose children

Surveillance
- Improve timeliness for detection from case onset to final results
- Establish pathway towards a sustainable integrated surveillance system

Enabling environment
- Increase the representation and empowerment of women at every level and across all areas of the program
- Provide targeted assistance for country programs through the GPEI hub.

Fig. 49.1: Strategic objectives and key activities for Goal 1.
*taken from Polio Eradication Strategy 2022–2026[6]

Milestones for interrupting poliovirus transmission in Afghanistan and Pakistan, 2021–2026

Afghanistan

- Intensified negotiation efforts to gain access
- Continued implementation of complementary approaches to vaccination in Inaccessible areas. High-quality delivery monitored and maintained in both accessible and inaccessible areas
- Continued long-term strengthening of immunization systems
- Rigorous review of the 2022-2026 strategy
- Beginning of the program's transition planning for certification (2024-2026)

Strategy milestones: 2021 — 2022 — 2023 — 2024 — 2025 — 2026

- Wider use of nOPV2
- Interruption of WPV1 transmission and last CVDPV2 Isolate reported
- Certify the eradication of WPV1

Pakistan
- Implement programmatic improvements:
  - Changes to frontline team management
  - New approaches for inclusive engagement for priority communities
  - Systematic, consistent dialogue with provincial leadership
- Mechanisms in place for equitable EI access and OPV co-delivery through Integrated services
- Widespread transmission limited to only core reservoirs
- Final, sporadic chains of transmission eliminated
- National and provincial governments own and are accountable for polio eradication and certification Implications
- Rigorous review of the 2022-2026 Strategy
- Beginning of the program's transition planning for certification (2024-2026)

■ Pakistan ■ Joint milestone

Fig. 49.2: Strategic objectives and key activities for Goal 2.
*taken from Polio Eradication Strategy 2022–2026[6]

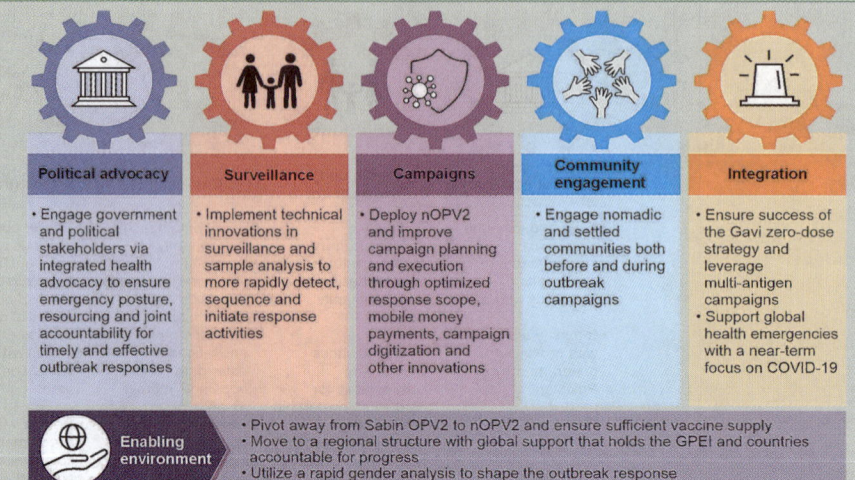

Fig. 49.3: Milestones for interrupting cVDPV transmission in outbreak and at-risk countries 2021–2030+.

(bOPV: bivalent oral polio vaccine; cVDPV: circulating vaccine derived polio virus; EI: essential immunization; IPV: inactivated polio vaccine; mOPV2: monovalent oral polio vaccine type 2;, nOPV1,3: novel oral polio vaccine types 1 & 3; nOPV2: novel oral polio vaccine type 2; OPV: oral polio vaccine; VDPV2: vaccine derived polio virus type 2; WPV1: wild poliovirus type 1)

***taken from Polio Eradication Strategy 2022-2026[6]

Global stockpile of OPV: The global stockpile of OPV is type of long-term mechanism that will ensure a supply of OPV beyond the current GPEI strategy into the post-certification period. The stockpile was established to supply OPVs in response to poliovirus outbreaks during post-certification period and once the OPV is withdrawn from essential immunization. The composition of the stockpile includes a range of monovalent, polyvalent, Sabin and Novel vaccines for all the three types of poliovirus.

Post-certification strategy

Post-certification strategy mentions about the technical functions and required standards to ensure and maintain polio free world after certification. The key goals and components of PCS are:

- **Contain the poliovirus:** Its main focus is to reduce the number of poliovirus storage and handling facilities across the world and maintain safeguards in such facilities to prevent reintroduction of poliovirus from such facilities (such as laboratories, vaccine manufacturers and research facilities, etc).
- **Protect populations:** Populations will need protection from Vaccine Derived Polio Virus (VDPVV) and vaccine associated paralytic poliomyelitis. This can be achieved by coordinated bOPV withdrawal across the world. People should also be protected against re-emergence of any poliovirus, which will be done by continuous supply and access to safe and effective vaccines.
- **Detecting and responding to polio event:** It can be achieved through maintaining sensitive sentinel surveillance systems for detecting any poliovirus promptly both in humans as well as in the environment. For this, resources in adequate capacity will be required to be made available to contain or to respond to a polio event effectively.

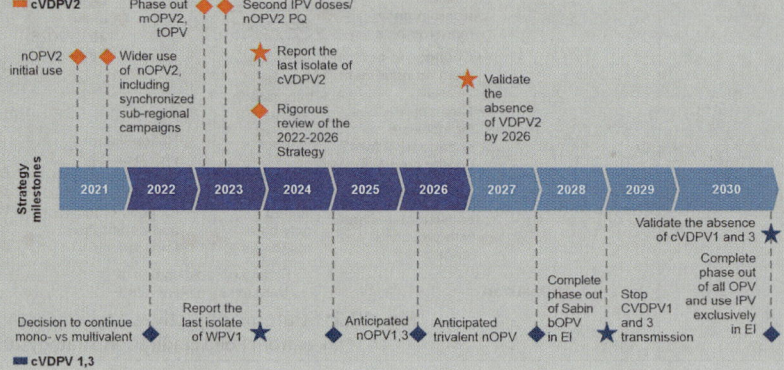

Fig. 49.4: Post-certification strategy high-level timeline.

References

1. Poliomyelitis, Detail, Fact sheets, Newsroom, Home, World Health Organization. Available at: https://www.who.int/news-room/fact-sheets/detail/poliomyelitis. Last accessed 27 July 2024
2. The Lancet Microbe. Polio eradication, elusive but achievable. Lancet Microbe. 2023 Dec;4(12):e963. doi: 10.1016/S2666-5247(23)00371-3. PMID: 38042153.
3. González-Silva M, Rabinovich NR. Some lessons for malaria from the Global Polio Eradication Initiative. Malar J. 2021 May 1;20(1):210. doi: 10.1186/s12936-021-03690-6. PMID: 33933088; PMCID: PMC8087877.
4. World Health Assembly. Global eradication of poliomyelitis by the year 2000. Resolution WHA 11.28. Geneva: World Health Organization, 1988
5. Who we are/ Global Polio Eradication Initiative. Available at: https://polioeradication.org/who-we-are/. Last accessed 27 July 2024.
6. Polio Eradication Strategy 2022–2026: Delivering on a promise. Geneva: World Health Organization; 2021. Licence: CC BY-NC-SA 3.0 IGO.

QUESTIONS

Long Answer Questions (LAQs)

1. Global Polio Eradication Initiative have been a spectacular success story in public health. Discuss critically.
2. Discuss the Polio Eradication Strategy 2022–2026 critically.

Short Answer Questions (SAQs)

1. Discuss why even after polio eradication certification, oral polio vaccine stockpile will be required to be maintained.
2. Briefly describe the key objectives and activities of Polio Eradication Strategy 2022–2026.
3. Discuss the post-certification strategy in terms of its key goals and activities.

Multiple Choice Questions (MCQs)

1. Last case of poliomyelitis due to wild poliovirus in India was detected in:
   a. Moradabad, UP
   b. Howrah, West Bengal
   c. Muzaffarpur, Bihar
   d. Garhwa, Jharkhand
2. Which of the following is NOT a partner organization in Global Polio Eradication Initiative?
   a. United Nations Children's Fund (UNICEF)
   b. Bill and Melinda Gates Foundation
   c. GAVI-the vaccine alliance
   d. United Nations Development Programme (UNDP)
3. Key pillars of Global Polio Eradication Initiative Endgame Strategy 2019–2023 include.
   a. Eradication
   b. Integration
   c. Containment and certification
   d. All of the above

4. **Post-polio eradication certification, oral polio vaccine will be required to stored for a period of about:**
   a. There will not be any need of oral polio vaccines post-certification
   b. 3–5 years
   c. 5–10 years
   d. 10–15 years

Answers

1. b　　　　2. d　　　　3. d　　　　4. d

CHAPTER 50

Integrated Disease Surveillance Programme and Integrated Health Information Platform

Neha Gawarle, Kajal Srivastava, Parul Sharma, Akash Krishali, Kinnari Gupta

Background/Need of program/Scheme	Health data in India was fragmented across various programs and departments, leading to delays in decision-making. So for early detection and rapid response to outbreaks, a robust disease surveillance system [Integrated Disease Surveillance Program (IDSP)] was launched.[1] Later, Integrated Health Information Platform (IHIP) was launched on 26th November, 2018, with the aim of providing real-time access to health data for effective public health responses and comprehensive analysis.[2]

IDSP	IHIP
Initially paper-based; now transitioning to electronic	Fully electronic and cloud-based data collection
Weekly surveillance reports	Real-time surveillance reporting
Include 12 diseases in Laboratory Confirmed (L form) and 22 diseases in Presumptive (P Form)	Covers all IDSP diseases along with other major public health concerns
No geocoding of data	All data is geocoded for precise location tracking
Takes only aggregated data	Case-based surveillance with detailed, individual-level data

Milestones[3]

National Surveillance Program for Communicable Disease (1997–1998)
↓
Integrated Disease Surveillance Project funded by World Bank (2004)
↓
IDSP became part of NRHM (2007–2008)
↓
Approved as "Integrated Disease Surveillance Programme" (2012–2017)
↓
Integrated Health Information Platform (IHIP) launched (2018)

Goals[4]
- **Surveillance:** Strengthening surveillance through integration of various departments and programs
- **Real-time data access:** Provide data for prompt decision-making.
- **Enhance disease monitoring:** Improvement in disease and outbreak through continuous disease monitoring and analysis
- **Capacity building:** Training of health workers in disease surveillance, data management, and response
- **Intersectoral coordination**

Key objective	To strengthen/maintain a decentralized laboratory-based IT-enabled disease surveillance system for epidemic-prone diseases, with the goal of monitoring disease trends and detecting and responding to outbreaks in their early stages via trained Rapid Response Teams (RRTs).[4,5]
Objectives[4,5]	- Establish surveillance units at the center, state, and district levels to integrate and decentralize monitoring activities. - Human resource development: Train State and District Surveillance Officers, Rapid Response Teams, and medical and paramedical Staff on disease surveillance principles. - Information communication technology is used to collect, compile, analyze, and disseminate data. - Strengthening public health laboratories.
Targets	- Rapid Response Team: Formation of RRT in response to outbreaks at district and state levels[1] - Timely reporting and data integration[4] - Electronic data management and advanced analysis[2] - Stakeholder engagement—including public health officials, policymakers, and community[1] - Training of health care professionals on effective use of the of the IHIP platform[5]
Organogram and components	**Flow (top to bottom):** CSU → SSU → DSU → PHC → SC Forms: L form by labs (between DSU and PHC); P form by MO (between PHC and SC); S form by ANM (below SC) **IDSP column:** - CSU: Analyze data and feedback given to state - SSU: Analyze data, reference lab, feedback to DSU - DSU: Collection of data from PHC, lab test, outbreak investigation by DRRT - PHC: Collection of data from SC, Lab test - SC: Paper based weekly reporting (18 diseases) **IHIP column:** - CSU: Analyze data and feedback given to state - SSU: Analyze data within state, reference lab, feedback to districts, identify alert (SMS/email) - DSU: Identification of early warning signs (EWS), providing descriptive epidemiological analysis, outbreak investigation by SRRT - PHC: No data collection, direct reporting - SC: Daily geocoded tablet based e-surveillance (33 diseases) S Form is for suspected case P Form is for presumptive case L Form is for laboratory surveillance. "W" form: Reporting Format for Water Quality Monitoring, filled by Health Workers and Laboratory Personnel at PHCs, CHCs, and in various other laboratories in the district. **Weekly outbreak surveillance:** - CSU, IDSP, receives disease outbreak reports from all 36 states/UTs on a weekly basis through its IDSP portal, viz., www.idsp.nic.in. Even NIL weekly reporting is mandatory. - For simple data storage and retrieval, each outbreak in the Weekly Outbreak Report is issued a unique code (outbreak ID) since 2016.
Beneficiaries	**Direct beneficiaries:**[1,4,5] - **Policy makers:** Data-driven insights for informed decision-making. - **Public health officials:** Enhanced ability to monitor and respond to health threats. - **Healthcare providers:** Access to comprehensive patient data for improved care. **Indirect beneficiaries:**[2,4] - **Patients:** Better healthcare outcomes through integrated health information. - **General population:** Reduced disease burden through early detection and response.

Strategies/Deliverables under the program[1,2,5]	**IDSP** • **Strengthen surveillance system:** Training healthcare workers on disease surveillance methods, outbreak investigation, and data management. • **Intersectoral collaboration:** Working with veterinary and animal health sectors for zoonotic disease control. • **Rapid response:** RRT is formed to ensure effective response and management of outbreaks. • **Community participation:** Creating awareness in the community regarding communicable and communicable disease and increasing awareness about early case reporting. **IHIP** • **Real-time response:** Real-time data leads to timely action by the health system, predicting outbreaks. • **Data standardization and quality control:** Implementing data quality checks and ensuring adherence to standardized reporting formats. • Building the best scientific evidence and guidelines for evidence-based decision-making.
Activities at various level or package of services[2,7,8]	**Primary prevention:** Utilizing IHIP data for identifying vulnerable populations for targeted interventions like health education and community mobilization. **Secondary prevention** • Early case identification and reporting through the IDSP surveillance network • Prompt diagnosis and treatment of cases to prevent further transmission • Utilizing surveillance data to identify clusters of cases and initiate outbreak investigations • Contact tracing and prophylaxis for high-risk individuals **Tertiary prevention** • Management of severe cases and complications • Provision of rehabilitation services to minimize long-term disability • Utilizing IDSP and IHIP data to monitor the disease burden and treatment • Development of new prevention strategies
Monitoring and evaluation of program[2,5,6,7]	**Regular monitoring:** • Monthly review meetings at all levels. • Real-time monitoring through the integrated system. **Evaluation:** • Quarterly evaluations to assess progress and address gaps. • Annual comprehensive reviews to measure impact and effectiveness. **Feedback mechanism:** • Collect feedback from healthcare workers and public health officials. • Use feedback to make continuous improvements to the program.

References

1. Outbreaks. IDSP. Available at: https://idsp.mohfw.gov.in/index4.php?lang=1&level=0&linkid=403&lid=3685
2. Disease Under Surveillance. IDSP. Available at: https://idsp.mohfw.gov.in/index1.php?lang=1&level=1&sublinkid=5985&lid=3925
3. Integrated Health Information Platform. IDSP, Ministry of health & Family Welfare. Available at: https://ihip.mohfw.gov.in/idsp/#!/mission
4. Organizational Structure. Integrated Health Information Platform. IDSP, https://ihip.mohfw.gov.in/idsp/#!/organizationalStructure
5. Overview of web-based public health surveillance system in Uttarakhand: Integrated health information platform under integrated disease surveillance programme. Available at: https://www.ijfcm.org/article-details/18749
6. Disease Under Surveillance. IDSP. Available at: https://idsp.mohfw.gov.in/showfile.php?lid=3924
7. Disease Under Surveillance. IDSP. Available at: https://idsp.mohfw.gov.in/showfile.php?lid=3923
8. https://doi.org/10.1016/j.cegh.2022.101030

QUESTIONS

Long Answer Question (LAQ)

1. What is the role of the Integrated Disease Surveillance Programme (IDSP) in India's public health system? How has the Integrated Health Information Platform (IHIP) improved disease surveillance and reporting? Discuss challenges faced in implementing these systems at different levels of healthcare.

Short Answer Questions (SAQs)

1. What is difference between IDSP and IHIP?
2. How does IDSP contribute to the early detection and prevention of outbreaks in India?

Multiple Choice Questions (MCQs)

1. What was the primary objective for the initiation of IDSP?
    a. To train healthcare workers in urban areas
    b. To increase the number of hospitals in rural areas
    c. To tackle fragmented health data and enable early diagnosis of epidemics
    d. To reduce the cost of healthcare services
2. Which form under IDSP is used by the ANM?
    a. S Form
    b. P Form
    c. L Form
    d. W Form
3. When was the integration of IDSP into the National Rural Health Mission (NRHM) done?
    a. 2004–2005
    b. 2007–2008
    c. 2012–2013
    d. 2017–2018
4. What is the main difference between IDSP and IHIP in terms of surveillance reporting?
    a. IDSP uses real-time reporting; IHIP uses weekly reports
    b. IDSP uses weekly reports; IHIP uses real-time reporting
    c. Both use weekly reporting systems
    d. Both use real-time reporting systems
5. All of the following diseases are under surveillance, *except*:
    a. Diabetes
    b. Dengue
    c. Viral hepatitis
    d. Acute gastroenteritis

Answers

1. c   2. a   3. b   4. b   5. a

PART C

Noncommunicable Diseases

51. National Programme for Prevention and Control of Noncommunicable Diseases
52. Integration of NAFLD into NP-NCD
53. National Programme for Healthcare of the Elderly
54. National Programme for Control of Blindness and Visual Impairment
55. National Programme for Prevention and Control of Deafness
56. National Mental Health Programme,
57. National Tobacco Control Programme
58. National Oral Health Programme
59. National Sickle Cell Anemia Elimination Programme
60. National Programme for Prevention and Management of Trauma and Burn Injuries (NPPMT&BI)
61. Pradhan Mantri National Dialysis Programme
62. National Programme for Palliative Care

CHAPTER 51

National Programme for Prevention and Control of Noncommunicable Diseases

Neha Gawarle, Kavita Vishwakarma, Prerna Verma, Kajal Srivastava, Nilesh Thakor

Need of program/ Scheme	Noncommunicable diseases (NCDs) have emerged as a major public health challenge in India, contributing to over 60% of total deaths. The rising prevalence of NCDs, such as cardiovascular diseases, diabetes, chronic respiratory diseases, and cancers necessitates a comprehensive approach to prevention, early diagnosis, management, and health promotion to mitigate their impact on individuals and healthcare systems.[1] Diseases under this program: • Hypertension and CVD • STEMI and other CAD/IHD • Stroke • Diabetes (type-2), Juvenile diabetes in project area • COPD • CKD • Non-alcoholic fatty liver diseases • Oral-breast-cervical cancer
Implemented since	2010-NPCDCS launched in 100 districts of 21 states ↓ 2013-14-covered all districts and came under NHM ↓ 2016-population-based screening of common NCD as a part of comprehensive primary health care ↓ 2023-NPCDCS renamed as NP-NCD included COPD, CKD, NAFLD & STEMI
Goal[1]	• To reduce premature mortality due to NCDs by 25% by 2025. • To enhance the quality of life for individuals affected by NCDs. • To strengthen the healthcare system for effective management of NCDs.
Targets[1]	2025 Targets: • Relative reduction in overall mortality from cardiovascular diseases, cancer, diabetes or chronic respiratory diseases by 25% • Reduction in alcohol use by 10% • Halt the rise in obesity and diabetes prevalence • Relative reduction in prevalence of insufficient physical activity by 10% • Relative reduction in the prevalence of raised blood pressure by 25% • Relative reduction in the mean population intake of salt less than 5 g per day by 30% • Relative reduction in the prevalence of current tobacco use by 30% • Relative reduction in the household use of solid fuel as a primary source of energy for cooking by 50% • Eligible people receiving drug therapy and counseling to prevent heart attacks and strokes by 50% • Availability and affordability of quality safe and efficacious essential medicine including generic and basic technologies in both public and private facilities by 80%

Objectives[1]	- **Prevention of NCD:** Reduce exposure to risk factors through public health interventions and policies. - **Early diagnosis:** Improve screening and diagnostic facilities for timely detection of NCDs. - **Management:** Provide effective and accessible treatment and care for individuals with NCDs. - **Capacity building:** Strengthen healthcare infrastructure and workforce for NCD management. - **Surveillance and research:** Enhance data collection, monitoring, and research to inform policy and program decisions.

Organogram and components	- **National level:** Nation NCD division
	- **Ministry of Health and Family Welfare (MoHFW),** headed by Joint secretary
	- **State level:** State NCD Cell headed by mission director (NHM)
	- **District level:** District NCD Cell headed by district nodal officer
	- **Block/PHC level:** Block health office, primary health centers, community health workers
	
	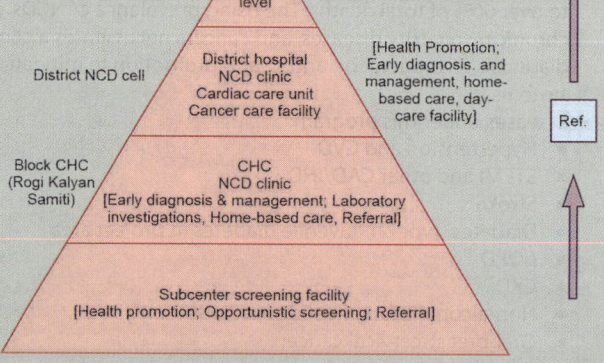
	
	Services at subcenter
	- Health promotion for behavior change
	- 'Opportunistic' screening using BP measurement and blood glucose by strip method
	- Referral of suspected cases to CHC PHC
	  Human resource—CHO, ANM, MPW-male
	PHC and CHC NCD clinic
	- Prevention and health promotion including counseling
	- Early diagnosis through clinical and laboratory investigations (Common lab investigations: Blood sugar, lipid profile, ECG, ultrasound, X-ray, etc.)
	- Management of common CVD, diabetes and stroke cases (out patient and in patients)
	- Homebased care for bed ridden chronic cases
	- Referral of difficult cases to district hospital/higher healthcare facility
	  Human resource—MO (MBBS), staff nurse, lab technician, pharmacist
	District hospital
	- Early diagnosis of diabetes, CVDs, stroke and cancer
	- Investigations: Blood sugar, lipid profile, kidney function test (KFT), liver function test (LFT), ECG, ultrasound, X-ray, etc. (if colposcopy, mammography not available, will be outsourced)
	- Medical management of cases (outpatient, inpatient and intensive care)
	- Follow-up and care of bed ridden cases
	- Day-care facility
	- Referral of difficult cases to higher healthcare facility
	- Health promotion for behavior change
	  Human resource—physician (MD), MO (MBBS), dentist, staff nurse, counselor, physiotherapist
	Tertiary center
	Comprehensive cancer care including prevention, early detection, diagnosis, treatment, minimal access surgery after care, palliative care and rehabilitation.

Chapter 51: National Programme for Prevention and Control of Noncommunicable Diseases

Beneficiaries	• General population, with a focus on individuals aged 30 and above. • High-risk groups, including those with a family history of NCDs.

Strategies/ Deliverables under the program	• **Prevention through behavior change:** To modify behavior, communication is used, with a focus on the following five messages:
	  + A greater consumption of nutritious foods
	  + A rise in physical activity from exercises, sports, etc.
	  + Steer clear of alcohol and tobacco
	  + Stress reduction
	  + Cancer warning symptoms, etc.
	• **Screening and early diagnosis:**
	  + Opportunistic screening of persons above the age of 30 years at the point of primary contact with any healthcare facility.
	  + Simple clinical examination
	  + *To identify those individuals who are at a high risk of developing NCD:*
	    – Population-based screening
	    – Estimating beneficiary and planning
	    – Methods of screening—history, BMI, BP, blood sugar, clinical breast examination
	    – Oral visual examination
	    – Visual inspection with acetic acid
	
	| *Type of NCD*
		Age of beneficiary	*Methods of screening*	*Frequency of screening*

---	---	---	---
Hypertension	30 years and above	BP apparatus	Once a year
Diabetes	30 years and above	Glucometer	Once a year
Breast cancer	30-65 years	Clinical breast examination	Once in 5 years
Oral cancer	30-65 years	Oral visual examination	Once a 5 years
Cervical cancer	30-65 years	Visual inspection with acetic acid	Once in 5 years	 • **Management:** "NCD clinic" has been established at CHC and district hospital.
Activities at various level or package of services	**Primary prevention** • Conduct awareness campaigns on healthy lifestyle choices. • Promote physical activity through community programs. • Implement tobacco and alcohol control measures. • Encourage healthy eating habits. **Secondary prevention** • Conduct regular screening camps for early detection of NCDs. • Provide risk assessment and counseling services. • Ensure timely referral and follow-up for suspected cases. **Tertiary prevention** • Provide comprehensive care and management for diagnosed NCD patients. • Establish specialized clinics for chronic disease management. • Facilitate rehabilitation and support services for patients.
Monitoring and evaluation of program	• **Data collection**: Regularly collect and analyze data on NCD prevalence, risk factors, and program impact. • **Indicators**: Track key performance indicators, such as screening rates, treatment adherence, and outcome measures. • **Feedback mechanism:** Implement a feedback system for continuous improvement of the program. • **Reporting**: Regular reporting at national, state, and district levels to ensure accountability and transparency. • **Research:** Conduct operational research to identify best practices and inform policy decisions.
Public health importance days related to NCD	World Hypertension Day – May, 17 World Heart Day – September, 29 World Stroke Day – October, 29 World Diabetes Day – November, 14 World COPD Day – November, 16 World Cancer Day—February 4

Section III: National Health Mission

Reference

1. NP-NCD Operational Guidelines.pdf [Internet]. [cited 2024 Sep 13];Available from: https://mohfw.gov.in/sites/default/files/NP-NCD%20Operational%20Guidelines.pdf

QUESTIONS

Long Answer Question (LAQ)

1. National program for control of NCDS: Describe goals, objectives, targets, strategies and monitoring of program.

Short Answer Questions (SAQs)

1. What are the various level of strategic prevention involved in NP-NCD?
2. What indicators used to evaluate the NP-NCD?

Multiple Choice Questions (MCQs)

1. World Heart Day is celebrated on:
   a. 12 September
   b. 29 September
   c. 12 October
   d. 29 October
2. For diabetes NPNC uses following as screening test:
   a. Glucometer strip
   b. Fasting blood glucose
   c. PP2Bs
   d. Glucose load test

Answers

1. b
2. a

CHAPTER 52

Integration of NAFLD into NP-NCD

Ajeet Singh Bhadoria, Vineeth Kumar Pathak, M Swathi Shenoy, Krupal Joshi

Need of the program	India is experiencing an increase in noncommunicable diseases (NCDs), which have surpassed infectious diseases as the primary cause of mortality and morbidity. Noncommunicable diseases (NCDs) currently represent more than 63% of mortality in the nation. Non-alcoholic fatty liver disease (NAFLD) has become a notable public health issue. The prevalence of NAFLD in India varies from 9% to 53%, depending on regional and demographic factors, with increased rates observed in obese or diabetic individuals.[1,2] Urbanization, changes in lifestyle, and dietary modifications have significantly contributed to the increasing prevalence of NAFLD, which shares common risk factors with other noncommunicable diseases such as cardiovascular diseases, diabetes, and hypertension.[2,3] NAFLD frequently presents without symptoms, advancing gradually and resulting in complications, such as cirrhosis and hepatocellular carcinoma (HCC) if not addressed. The integration of NAFLD management into India's broader NCD strategy is essential due to its strong link to metabolic syndrome and its potential to exacerbate healthcare burdens. The Government of India has integrated NAFLD into the National Programme for Control of Non-Communicable Diseases (NP-NCD) to enhance the comprehensive management of NCDs.[3,4]
Implemented since	The Government of India initiated the National Programme for Prevention and Control of Cancer, Diabetes, Cardiovascular Diseases, and Stroke (NPCDCS) in 2010. In response to the increasing prevalence of various conditions, including NAFLD, the program was expanded in 2023 to encompass a wider array of non-communicable diseases, resulting in the establishment of the National Programme for Control of Non-Communicable Diseases (NP-NCD).[3]
Goal	The primary goal of NP-NCD is to reduce the prevalence of NAFLD and prevent its progression to severe liver diseases through early detection, public health interventions, and effective management strategies.
Objectives	• Attain 70% screening of high-risk populations, such as individuals with diabetes, obesity, or metabolic syndrome, by the year 2030. • Achieve a 25% reduction in the progression of NAFLD to liver fibrosis, cirrhosis, and HCC through preventive care by 2025. • Enhance public awareness regarding NAFLD and associated lifestyle modifications, aiming to reach a minimum of 80% of the population by 2030.[3,4]
Organogram	The NP-NCD functions through a multi-tier system: • **National level:** The Ministry of Health and Family Welfare oversees policy formulation and strategic guidance. • **State level:** Centers of Excellence (CoEs) provide specialized care for liver diseases, conduct research, and manage complex NAFLD cases. Use of Fibroscan as diagnostic tool can be used to see fibrosis. • **District level:** District hospitals provide advanced diagnostic services for liver fibrosis detection. • **Primary level:** Primary Health Centers (PHCs) and Community Health Centers (CHCs) serve as the first point of contact, providing screening and lifestyle counseling.[3,5]
Beneficiaries	• **High-risk individuals:** Those with metabolic conditions, such as obesity, type 2 diabetes mellitus (T2DM), and dyslipidemia. • **Healthcare providers:** General practitioners, paramedics, and medical officers who will receive training on NAFLD management. • **General population:** Public health campaigns will target lifestyle changes to prevent NCDs and NAFLD.[3,4]

Components	- **Screening and diagnosis:** Early detection using non-invasive methods, such as fibrosis-4 (FIB-4) scoring and Fibroscan to assess liver health.[5]
- **Health promotion:** Community-level interventions focus on promoting healthier diets, physical activity, and alcohol abstinence.[3,5]
- **Research and surveillance:** Data collection and epidemiological studies to track the disease burden and treatment outcomes.[5,6]
Strategies/ Deliverables under the program	- **Capacity building:** Train healthcare workers, including doctors, nurses, and community health workers, to screen and manage NAFLD.[6]
- **Infrastructure strengthening:** Equip district hospitals with Fibroscan machines and other diagnostic tools.[6]
- **Referral pathways:** Establish clear referral mechanisms from primary to tertiary care, ensuring patients with advanced fibrosis receive specialized treatment.[3,6]
Activities at various levels/Package of services	**Primary Prevention** - **Health promotion campaigns:** Nationwide initiatives promoting physical activity (150 minutes of moderate-intensity exercise per week) and healthy eating habits (e.g., fiber-rich foods, reduced sugar, and fat intake).[6]
- **Tobacco and alcohol reduction:** Target smoking cessation and alcohol abstinence to mitigate liver disease risk.[5,6] **Secondary Prevention** - **Screening of high-risk individuals:** Use of FIB-4 and liver function tests (LFTs) to identify patients at risk of liver fibrosis.[5]
- **Early intervention:** Counseling and lifestyle adjustments for individuals diagnosed with simple steatosis to prevent progression to NASH or cirrhosis.[4,6] **Tertiary Prevention** - Management of advanced disease: Patients with cirrhosis or HCC are referred for specialized care at tertiary centers, including liver transplantation services where necessary.[4,6]
Monitoring and evaluation	The NP-NCD will incorporate regular monitoring systems: - **Monthly reporting:** Facilities will report screening and diagnosis data to the district and national levels.[6]
- **Performance evaluation:** Annual assessments based on indicators, such as the number of individuals screened and rates of disease progression.[6]

References

1. Duseja A, Singh SP, De A, et al. Indian National Association for Study of the Liver (INASL) Guidance Paper on Nomenclature, Diagnosis and Treatment of Nonalcoholic Fatty Liver Disease (NAFLD). J Clin Exp Hepatol. 2023 Mar-Apr;13(2):273-302.
2. Singh SP, Duseja A, Mahtab MA, Anirvan P, Acharya SK, Akbar SMF, et al. INASL-SAASL Consensus Statements on NAFLD Name Change to MAFLD. J Clin Exp Hepatol. 2023 May-Jun;13(3):518-522.
3. Ministry of Health and Family Welfare, Government of India. Final Operational Guidelines for NAFLD. 2023; Last accessed on 2025 February. Available from: https://mohfw.gov.in/sites/default/files/Operational%20Guidelines%20for%20NALFD%20Version%2020.pdf
4. Ministry of Health and Family Welfare, Government of India. Final MO Training module for NAFLD. 2023; Last accessed on: 2025 February. Available from: https://mohfw.gov.in/sites/default/files/Training%20Module%20for%20Medical%20Officers%20for%20Prevention%20and%20Control%20of%20NAFLD.pdf
5. Sarin SK, Prasad M, Ramalingam A, Kapil U. Integration of public health measures for NAFLD into India's national programme for NCDs. Lancet Gastroenterol Hepatol. 2021 Oct;6(10):777–8.
6. Musso G, Gambino R, Cassader M, Pagano G. Meta-analysis: natural history of non-alcoholic fatty liver disease (NAFLD) and diagnostic accuracy of non-invasive tests for liver disease severity. Ann Med. 2011;43(8):617–49.

QUESTIONS

Long Answer Question (LAQ)

1. Discuss the integration of non-alcoholic fatty liver disease (NAFLD) into the National Programme for Control of Non-Communicable Diseases (NP-NCD). Evaluate the challenge and future directions in the effective management of NAFLD as part of India's public health policy.

Short Answer Questions (SAQs)

1. Explain the role of lifestyle modifications in the management of non-alcoholic fatty liver disease (NAFLD).
2. Justify integration of NAFLD into NP-NCD.
3. Outline the challenges in diagnosing NAFLD at the primary healthcare level. Discuss the limitations of current diagnostic tools and the need for capacity building among healthcare professionals.

Multiple Choice Questions (MCQs)

1. Which gene polymorphism has been linked to an increased susceptibility to NAFLD?
   a. *PNPLA3*
   b. *BRCA1*
   c. *MTHFR*
   d. *HFE*
2. The expansion of NPCDCS in 2023 to include NAFLD led to the program being renamed as:
   a. National Programme for Control of Liver Diseases (NPCLD)
   b. National Programme for Prevention and Control of Metabolic Disorders (NPPMD)
   c. National Programme for Control of Non-Communicable Diseases (NP-NCD)
   d. National Liver Health Programme (NLHP)
3. What is included in India's triple burden of disease?
   a. Non-communicable diseases, communicable diseases, environmental pollution
   b. Communicable diseases, non-communicable diseases, malnutrition
   c. Infectious diseases, obesity, cardiovascular diseases
   d. Diabetes, hypertension, liver diseases
4. Which of the following diseases is NOT typically considered a communicable disease in India?
   a. Tuberculosis
   b. Malaria
   c. HIV/AIDS
   d. Nonalcoholic fatty liver disease (NAFLD)
5. The expansion of the NPCDCS in 2023 included which of the following diseases?
   a. Hypertension, obesity, diabetes
   b. Chronic kidney disease, chronic obstructive pulmonary disease, nonalcoholic fatty liver disease
   c. Tuberculosis, malaria, HIV/AIDS
   d. Dengue, hypertension, liver cirrhosis
6. What percentage of the global population is estimated to be affected by nonalcoholic fatty liver disease (NAFLD)?
   a. 10%
   b. 15%
   c. 25%
   d. 35%

7. Which of the following is a key risk factor for nonalcoholic fatty liver disease (NAFLD)?
   a. Excessive alcohol consumption
   b. Regular physical activity
   c. Low saturated fat diet
   d. Obesity
8. What is considered the gold standard for diagnosing nonalcoholic steatohepatitis (NASH) and assessing fibrosis in NAFLD patients?
   a. Ultrasound
   b. MRI scan
   c. Liver biopsy
   d. CT scan
9. Which of the following pharmacotherapies is NOT typically used in the management of NAFLD?
   a. Insulin sensitizers
   b. Statins
   c. Antioxidants
   d. Antibiotics
10. What is a significant challenge in the diagnosis of NAFLD in primary healthcare settings?
    a. Availability of general practitioners
    b. Requirement of advanced imaging techniques
    c. High prevalence of communicable diseases
    d. Lack of laboratory testing facilities

Answers

1. a	2. c	3. b	4. d	5. c
6. c	7. d	8. c	9. d	10. b

CHAPTER 53

National Programme for Healthcare of the Elderly

Abhay Srivastava, AK Srivastava, Akhil Dhanesh Goel, Margi Sheth

Background/Need of program/Scheme	• **Growing elderly population:** India's elderly population is projected to reach 300.96 million by 2051, underscoring the need for a comprehensive elderly care program. • **High prevalence of NCDs:** Noncommunicable diseases, such as heart disease, diabetes, and cancer are common among the elderly, leading to disabilities that impair daily activities. • **Inadequate health infrastructure:** India's current healthcare system is not adequately equipped to address the specific needs of the elderly, with a primary focus on maternal and child health and communicable diseases. • **Lack of geriatric specialists:** The medical education system lacks sufficient training in geriatric care, resulting in a shortage of specialists and contributing to a brain drain as professionals seek employment abroad. • **Need for a comprehensive care model:** A dedicated model of elderly care is needed, incorporating curative, promotional, preventive, and rehabilitative services to ensure healthy aging and manage chronic conditions effectively. • **Promotion of active aging:** Emphasizing active and healthy aging is crucial to enable the elderly to live dignified and fulfilling lives, which also benefits younger generations in the long term.
Implemented since	The National Programme for Health Care of the Elderly (NPHCE) has been implemented in India since 2011.[1]
Goal[1]	• Ensure accessible, affordable, and high-quality comprehensive healthcare services for the elderly. • Encourage the adoption of active and healthy aging practices. • Foster a supportive environment that embraces "A Society for All Ages."
Targets/Outcomes	• Establish 'Regional Geriatric Centers (RGCs)' in 8 Regional Medical Institutions, featuring dedicated Geriatric OPDs and 30-bed wards for elderly care, along with training and research initiatives. • Introduce 'Geriatric Medicine Post-Graduate Programs' in eight regional institutions, aiming to produce 16 specialists annually. • Implement 'Video Conferencing Units' in all eight Regional Medical Institutions for capacity building and mentoring purposes. • Set up 'District Geriatric Units' in 80–100 district hospitals, each with a dedicated geriatric OPD and a 10-bed ward. • Launch 'Geriatric Clinics/Rehabilitation Units' in community/primary health centers for domiciliary visits in selected districts. • Equip 'Sub-centers' for community outreach services and provide specialized training for public healthcare personnel in geriatric care.
Objectives[1]	• Ensure easy access to promotional, preventive, curative, and rehabilitative services for the elderly through a community-based primary healthcare approach. • Identify and address health issues in the elderly within the community, supported by a robust referral system. • Enhance the skills of medical and paramedical professionals, as well as family caregivers, to provide effective health care to the elderly.

	• Offer referral services for elderly patients through district hospitals and regional medical institutions. • Promote collaboration with the National Rural Health Mission, AYUSH, and other relevant departments, such as the Ministry of Social Justice and Empowerment.
Organogram	**National Level (National NCD Cell)** The NCD Cell constituted at the central level for planning, monitoring and implementation of the National Programme for Prevention and Control of Cancer, Diabetes, CVD and Stroke (NPCDCS) will also be responsible for PPHCE. **State Level (State NCD Cell)** Composition of Staff at State NCD Cell: • State Program Officer • Program Assistant • Finance cum Logistics Officer • Data Entry Operators **District Level (District NCD Cell)** Composition of District NCD Cell: • District Program Officer • Program Assistant • Finance cum Logistics Officer • Data Entry Operator **Facility Level** • **Regional geriatric centers (RGCs):** Act as centers of excellence, providing specialized tertiary care, training healthcare workers, and conducting research in geriatric medicine. • **District hospitals:** House dedicated geriatric wards with trained staff to offer comprehensive medical, surgical, and rehabilitative services for the elderly. • **Community health centers (CHCs) and primary health centers (PHCs):** Provide primary healthcare services with a focus on geriatric care, potentially including dedicated staff or geriatric care units. **Community Level** • **ASHAs (Accredited Social Health Activists):** Act as the link between the community and healthcare facilities, creating awareness about NPHCE services, conducting home visits, and mobilizing seniors to access care. • **Anganwadi workers:** May play a role in educating communities about healthy aging and NPHCE services, particularly in rural areas. • This is a possible structure based on the program's functionalities. The actual organizational hierarchy might vary depending on specific regions and government policies.
Beneficiaries	• Population aged 60 years and above • Frail older patients with poor functional status • Older patients with multiple medical, psychological and social problems

Components	• **National Health Mission (NHM) Integration:**
	  ✦ Provides accessible primary and secondary healthcare for the elderly through district hospitals (DHs), community health centers (CHCs), primary health centers (PHCs), and sub-centers/health and wellness centers.
	  ✦ Strengthens facilities and trains personnel to offer dedicated geriatric care, especially in remote communities.
	• **Specialized Tertiary Care (Rashtriya Varishth Jan Swasthya Yojana):**
	  ✦ Offers advanced geriatric care for complex conditions through Regional Geriatric Centers (RGCs) and National Centers for Aging (NCAs).
	  ✦ Focuses on specialized tertiary care, geriatric medicine training, and research to enhance elderly care practices.
	• **Research and data collection:**
	  ✦ Collects data on health, social well-being, and economic security of the elderly to inform program improvements and policy development.
	  ✦ Provides insights into the evolving needs of seniors to refine NPHCE services.

Chapter 53: National Programme for Healthcare of the Elderly

Strategies/Deliverables under the program[2]	NPHCE strategy emphasizes a **continuum of care**, encompassing everything from community-based primary healthcare to specialized tertiary care. **Domiciliary visit:** It ensures domiciliary care visits by trained healthcare workers. **Strengthening the Primary Care Network** • **Equipped PHCs and CHCs:** Dedicated services at PHC/CHC level including provision of machinery, equipment, training, additional human resources (CHC), IEC, etc. **Specialized Care at District Hospitals:** Establishment of special geriatric wards **Building Expertise for Advanced Care** Strengthened RGCs offer specialized tertiary care and postgraduate courses in geriatric medicine. **Educating Communities for a Supportive Environment** **IEC Campaigns:** To raise awareness about healthy aging. **Training Modules:** • Training modules have been developed for medical officers, nurses, and community health workers to deliver comprehensive geriatric care. • State-level training programs are conducted for trainers who then cascade the knowledge to healthcare workers. **NPHCE Website:** An interactive website provides information about geriatric facilities and services across India.
Activities at various level or package of services[3]	The National Programme for Health Care of the Elderly (NPHCE) offers a tiered approach to elders, with varying services provided at different levels of the healthcare system. **At Health and Wellness Center:** **Package of Services:** • Health education related to healthy aging • Domiciliary visits for attention and care to home bound/bedridden elderly persons and provide training to the family care providers in looking after the disabled elderly persons. • Arrange for suitable callipers and supportive devices from the PHC to the elderly disabled persons to make them ambulatory. • Linkage with other support groups and day care centers, etc., operational in the area. **Primary Healthcare Level (PHCs):** • **Package of services:** • Weekly geriatric clinic run by a trained Medical Officer • Health promotional activities • Conducting a routine health assessment of the elderly persons based on simple clinical examination relating to eye, ears and NCD, etc. • Provision of medicines and proper advice on chronic ailments • Referral to higher centers **Community Healthcare Level (PHCs):** • **Package of services:** • Geriatric clinic for the elderly persons twice a week. • Rehabilitation unit for physiotherapy and counseling • Domiciliary visits by the rehabilitation worker for bed ridden elderly and counseling of the family members on their home-based care. • Health promotion and prevention • Referral of difficult cases to district hospital/higher healthcare facility **District Hospital Level:** • **Package of services:** • Dedicated geriatric wards with additional resources and trained staff in geriatric care. • Comprehensive medical, surgical, and rehabilitative services for the elderly. • Management of complex health conditions requiring hospitalization. • Referral services to Regional Geriatric Centers (RGCs) for advanced care.

	Regional Geriatric Centers (RGCs):[4,5] **Package of services:** • Specialized tertiary care for complex medical and surgical conditions. • Advanced diagnostic facilities. • Rehabilitation services. • Postgraduate training programs in geriatric medicine to create a skilled workforce. • Research in geriatrics to improve best practices and identify innovative approaches. **Additional considerations:** • Capacity building initiatives, including training healthcare professionals and caregivers in geriatric care, are implemented across all levels. • Referral services ensure a seamless healthcare journey for seniors, connecting them with specialists and advanced treatment facilities when needed. • This tiered approach ensures that seniors receive appropriate care based on their needs, from preventive services at the community level to specialized care at RGCs.
Monitoring and evaluation of program	The National Programme for Health Care of the Elderly (NPHCE) recognizes the critical role of monitoring and evaluation (M&E) in ensuring program effectiveness and achieving its objectives. A robust M&E framework is vital for tracking progress towards program goals and identifying areas for improvement. **Data collection** across various NPHCE service delivery channels, including NHM facilities, RGCs, and community outreach programs, is crucial. **Periodic program evaluations,** assessing the overall impact of NPHCE interventions. This may involve conducting surveys and interviews with beneficiaries, healthcare workers, and community members to gather their experiences and perspectives. Cost-effectiveness analysis can also be employed to evaluate the program's efficiency in delivering care.

References

1. Ministry of Health and Family Welfare, Government of India. National Programme for Health Care of the Elderly (NPHCE) [Internet]. Available from: https://www.mohfw.gov.in/sites/default/files/52386925Operational%20Guidelines%20for%20NPHCE_0.pdf
2. Sharma SK, Agarwal A. Geriatric health care in India: A review of challenges and strategies. J Geriatr Care Res. 2020;8(3):120-6.
3. Nanda A, Thakur A. Strengthening geriatric health services in India: Lessons from the National Programme for Health Care of the Elderly. Indian J Public Health. 2021;65(2):231-4.
4. International Institute for Population Sciences (IIPS). Longitudinal Ageing Study in India (LASI) [Internet]. Available from: https://www.iipsindia.ac.in/content/LASI-data
5. World Health Organization. World Report on Ageing and Health [Internet]. Available from: https://www.who.int/publications/i/item/9789241565042

QUESTIONS

Long Answer Question (LAQ)

1. Discuss the strategies employed by the NPHCE to improve geriatric care in India. Include how it addresses healthcare access, capacity building, and the management of chronic diseases.

Short Answer Questions (SAQs)

1. Differentiate between the roles of the primary healthcare system and specialized geriatric units under the NPHCE.
2. Describe the key components of the NPHCE program.

Multiple Choice Questions (MCQs)

1. What is the primary focus of the national program for elderly health care in India?
   a. Maternal and child health
   b. Communicable diseases
   c. Comprehensive care for the elderly
   d. Mental health and wellness
2. By 2051, the elderly population in India is projected to reach approximately:
   a. 100 million
   b. 150 million
   c. 250 million
   d. 300 million
3. Which group is more frequently affected by immobility and home confinement after the age of 80 in India?
   a. Men in rural areas
   b. Women in rural areas
   c. Men in urban areas
   d. Women in both rural and urban areas
4. What is one of the major challenges in providing health care to the elderly in India?
   a. Lack of primary health care centers
   b. Shortage of trained geriatric specialists
   c. High prevalence of infectious diseases
   d. Low population growth
5. The concept of 'Active and Healthy Aging, in the elderly care program emphasizes:
   a. Treating only chronic diseases
   b. Promotion and prevention in health care
   c. Focusing solely on mental health
   d. Reducing the number of elderly
6. What is a significant reason why many elderly people in India do not seek medical care for their health issues?
   a. Lack of awareness
   b. High cost of treatment
   c. Perception that ill health is a normal part of aging
   d. All of the above
7. What is one of the major obstacles in providing specialized health care to the elderly in rural areas of India?
   a. Lack of interest among the elderly
   b. Limited access to specialized health services
   c. Overabundance of health care facilities
   d. Low incidence of noncommunicable diseases
8. Which elderly healthcare services are delivered at HWC-SC?
   a. Domiciliary care
   b. Health promotion services
   c. Referral services
   d. All of the above
9. Which level of health care is primarily responsible for providing basic health services to the elderly in India?
   a. Tertiary care
   b. Secondary care
   c. Primary care
   d. Quaternary care
10. What is a key characteristic of a comprehensive elderly care model?
    a. Exclusive focus on physical health
    b. Integration of health and social care services
    c. Limiting services to urban areas
    d. Providing only emergency care
11. What is the primary goal of the National Programme for Health Care of the Elderly (NPHCE)?
    a. To promote economic growth in urban areas
    b. To provide accessible, affordable, and high-quality healthcare services to the elderly
    c. To focus solely on the education of healthcare professionals
    d. To reduce the population growth rate
12. Which of the following chronic noncommunicable diseases (NCDs) is a major concern for the elderly population?
    a. Influenza
    b. Hypertension
    c. Tuberculosis
    d. Measles
13. What strategy does NPHCE employ to improve geriatric care at the community level?
    a. Eliminating all traditional healthcare practices
    b. Establishing dedicated geriatric care units within Primary Health Centers (PHCs) and Community Health Centers (CHCs)

c. Focusing solely on mental health services
d. Increasing the number of hospitals in urban areas

14. **How does the NPHCE aim to address social determinants of health for the elderly?**
    a. By focusing exclusively on medical treatments
    b. By exploring partnerships with social services organizations to combat social isolation and improve access to resources
    c. By limiting healthcare access to urban areas
    d. By providing financial support to elderly individuals only

15. **What is one expected outcome of implementing the NPHCE in India?**
    a. Decreased life expectancy among the elderly
    b. Increased rates of hospitalization among seniors
    c. Establishment of departments of geriatric medicine in 19 medical colleges
    d. Reduction in the number of caregivers available for elderly support

Answers

1. c	2. d	3. d	4. b	5. b
6. d	7. b	8. d	9. c	10. b
11. b	12. b	13. b	14. b	15. c

CHAPTER 54

National Programme for Control of Blindness and Visual Impairment

Shalki Mattas, Puneet Ohri, Rudresh Negi

Background/ Need of program/ Scheme	In India, the issue of curable and incurable blindness is creating significant social, health, and economic challenges. The primary illnesses identified as causing visual impairment and blindness in the nation include trachoma, smallpox, glaucoma, trauma to the eyes, malnourishment, and squint. It is estimated that over nine million individuals are blind and over 45 million people have vision impairment, of which five million can be cured with appropriate surgical intervention. About 2,50,000 children nationwide are blind or visually impaired, with the majority of cases being brought on by squints, traumas, and nutritional inadequacies. An estimated 14,000 preschoolers are thought to experience vision issues as a result of vitamin "A" insufficiency.[1] Beyond just how people see, vision loss and impairment affects a person's capacity, employability, income, access to healthcare and education, and more. The 2030 Agenda for Sustainable Development places a high value on vision, and since the WHO estimates that 80% of vision loss is preventable, governments must take more proactive steps to guaranteeing the health of all people's eyes.
Implemented since	The National Programme for Control of Blindness was initially implemented in India in 1976, and its 2020 target is to lower the prevalence of blindness to 0.3%. The WHO and IAPB collaborated to develop Vision 2020: The Right to Sight in 1999 with the goal of eradicating preventable blindness by 2020. With the goal of lowering the prevalence of preventable visual impairment by 25% by 2019 in comparison to the baseline prevalence in 2010, the World Health Assembly approved Universal Eye Health: Global Action Plan 2014-19 in 2013. In order to combat blindness and visual impairment, India has put in place a number of measures under its ongoing National Programme for Control of Blindness and Visual Impairment (NPCBVI).[2]
Goals	- To decrease the backlog of blindness by identifying and treating blind people at the primary, intermediate, and tertiary levels in accordance with an evaluation of the nation's total visual impairment burden. - Create and strengthen the NPCBVI's strategy for "Eye Health" and the avoidance of visual impairment by offering comprehensive eye care services and high-quality service supply. - Enhancing and upgrading RIOs to establish them as centers of excellence in a range of ophthalmology subspecialties. - Bolstering the current and creating new infrastructure and human resources to enable the provision of excellent, all-encompassing eye care in every district of the nation; - To emphasize preventive methods and raise community understanding of eye care; - Increase and expand research for prevention of blindness and visual impairment. - To ensure private practitioners' and voluntary organizations' involvement in eye care.[3]
Targets	The target under the National Health Policy (NHP) is to bring the prevalence of blindness down to 0.25% by 2025.[4]
Objectives	- **Early detection and treatment:** In order to prevent blindness, eye diseases should be recognized and treated as soon as possible. - Offering the entire range of eye care services, from prevention to recovery, is known as comprehensive eye care. - **Education and awareness:** Spreading knowledge among the general public about eye health and the value of routine eye exams. - Building capacity involves educating medical professionals about eye care and fortifying the healthcare system.[4]

Organogram	**Organization at the National Level** The Directorate General of Health Services, located in Nirman Bhawan, New Delhi, is in-charge of overseeing the National Programme for Control of Blindness (NPCBVI). A Deputy Director General (DDG) and an Additional Director General of Health Services (DGHS) support the DGHS. As the National Programme Officer, the DDG bears primary responsibility for the program's execution at the federal level. Assistant Director General and other officials support him/her. The Ministry of Health and Family Welfare (Department of Health) houses the administrative branch. Deputy Secretary and/or Under Secretary support Additional Secretary and Joint Secretary in overseeing the program. **Organization at the State Level** There are no appointed executive officers for the program in the states, in contrast to the national level. Under the general supervision of the State Health Secretary, the State Director of Health Services oversees the State Programme Officer, a Joint/Deputy Director level officer, as the accountable officer. With further assistance, a statistical assistant works alongside the State Programme Officer (NPCBVI). Implementing and overseeing the program in each of the state's districts is one of the duties of the State Programme Officer. The Director of Medical Education is the recipient of reports from Central Mobile Units assigned to the Ophthalmology Departments of the Medical Colleges. These training courses are located in the authorized medical colleges, where the Paramedical Ophthalmic Assistants (PMO/As) are trained. **Organization at the District Level** At the district level, there are two divisions of service delivery: The Chief Medical Officer (also known as the District Health Officer in certain states) oversees health programs, and the district hospital is run by a Medical Superintendent. At least one ophthalmologist is assigned to both clinical and surgical duties at each district hospital. The District Mobile Unit is connected to the district hospital wherever it is located. The operations of the eye camp are under the control of the ophthalmologist who is assigned to the Mobile Unit. The administrative head of the Community Health Centers (CHCs) and Primary Health Centers (PHCs), where the Ophthalmic Assistants are assigned, is the Chief Medical Officer/District Health Officer. **Organization at Subdistrict Level** An Ophthalmic Assistant is assigned to a block and works under the Medical Officer in-charge's general supervision. This is the final stage of the health system when an eye care specialist has been assigned. It is anticipated that more village-level implementation will be handled by health professionals and other community-based employees or volunteers. NPCBVI is a vertical health program that does not effectively reach rural and tribal populations, according to the program structure at the central, state, district, and sub-district levels. To effectively create a network in rural and tribal areas, the DBCS must expand its strategy to include additional health workers, other sectors, NGOs, and private practitioners. Health workers, health assistants, block extension educators, and other health professionals who are available in rural regions should be used for population screening, motivating the populace, and making referrals to district hospitals, eye camps, and primary health centers. Complete collaboration between the district health officer (Chief Medical Officer) and the district hospital would enable this.[5]
Beneficiaries	Patients suffering from blindness or visual impairment including the patients suffering from cataract, diabetic retinopathy {DR}, glaucoma, ocular trauma, childhood blindness, keratoplasty, squint, low vision, retinopathy of prematurity {ROP}[1]
Components	• **Free Cataract Surgery:** Giving people in need of it priority for free cataract surgery. • Comprehensive eye care involves treating diseases, such as diabetic retinopathy, glaucoma, corneal problems, and juvenile blindness in addition to cataracts. • **Population Screening:** Proactively checking for eye problems in people over 50. • **Children's Vision:** Screening and giving free eyeglasses to economically disadvantaged children with refractive problems. • Expanding eye care services to all communities in order to achieve universal coverage. • **Training for Healthcare Personnel:** Developing and improving the abilities of healthcare workers. • **Community Awareness:** Educating local populations about eye conditions. • Hospital upgrades include providing state-of-the-art facilities, ample staffing, and equipment. • Establishing vision centers with an emphasis on eye care in all primary healthcare settings. • **Mobile Eye Units:** Providing isolated communities with greater accessibility through mobile ophthalmic units.[6]

Strategies/ Deliverables under the program	Progress Report of Activities under NPCB and VI Targets and achievements during last three years				
	Year/Activity	2018-19 Achievement	2019-20 Achievement	2020-21 Achievement	2021-22* Achievement
	Cataract	66,90,830	64,33,140	35,50,765	39,56,934
	School eye screening program	8,81,929	8,56,768	1,80,723	2,52,600
	Collection of donated eyes for corneal transplantation	68,409	65,417	17,402	33,733
	Treatment/management of other eye diseases (diabetic retinopathy, glaucoma, childhood blindness, keratoplasty, etc.)	6,14,433	8,37,151	2,99,852	3,05,298
	Training of eye surgeons	125	108	32	48

*Final report for the year 2021-22 is provisional.

In order to assess the program, the "National Blindness and Visual Impairment Survey" was carried out during 2015-19 which showed reduction in the prevalence of blindness from 1% (2007) to 0.36% (2019).

A Mission Mode Cataract Surgery Campaign (Netra Jyoti Abhiyan) was begun (2022–2025) under the National Programme for Control of Blindness and Visual Impairment (NPCB and VI) with the aim of clearing the backlog of eligible cataract cases by assigning yearly targets to each State and Union Territory. A target of 75,00,000 cataract procedures was set for the FY-2022–2023; 83,44,824 cataract surgeries were performed against this aim. The goal of this campaign is to bring the rate of preventable blindness down to 0.25% by 2025.[7]

Activities at various level or package of services

Primary Eye Care Services:
Preventive and promotional vision care services are provided via comprehensive primary healthcare services provided through health and wellness centers (HWC). These include initiatives in the information, education, and communication (IEC) space to support eye donations and preventive vision care.

Secondary Eye Care Services:
- Reducing the amount of time patients must wait for cataract operations.
- **Refractive error screening and free spectacle distribution:** Through a school eye screening program, check students for refractive errors and give away free glasses to those in need. Providing older people with presbyopia (difficulty focusing on close objects) with free glasses so they can accomplish near tasks. This is a fresh project that the program has launched.
- **Visual impairment management:** All types of visual impairment, including low vision cases, are now covered by the program's expanded services. The program's emphasis has switched to the management and treatment of numerous eye disorders, including glaucoma, diabetic retinopathy, vitreoretinal diseases, corneal blindness, blindness in children.
- **Teleophthalmology network and mobile ophthalmic units:** Using a teleophthalmology network and mobile ophthalmic units to extend program reach into underserved and isolated locations.
- Enhancing the eye banking facilities and the gathering of donated eyes.

Tertiary Eye Care Services:
- Offering financial support to improve the capabilities of institutes of ophthalmology to provide specialized eye care services.
- Offering practical training to eye surgeons, enhancing their clinical and surgical expertise.
- Running information, education, and communication (IEC) campaigns.
- Conducting research and surveys in the field of eye care.[5]

Monitoring and evaluation of program

- Dashboard
- Periodic surveys
- Standard cataract surgery records[5]

References

1. Vikaspedia Domains [Internet]. Vikaspedia.in. 2020 [cited 2024 Oct 16]. Available from: https://vikaspedia.in/health/nrhm/nationalhealth-programmes-1/national-programme-for-control-of-blindness-and-visual-impairment
2. NPCBVI [Internet]. npcbvi.mohfw.gov.in. Available from: https://npcbvi.mohfw.gov.in/Home
3. REPORT: An Evaluation of the National Programme for Control of Blindness and Visual Impairment, COVID-19 Disruptions and the Way Ahead for Universal Eye Health [Internet]. IMPRI Impact and Policy Research Institute. 2022. Available from: https://www.impriindia.com/research/reports/npcbvi-eye-care-statistics/
4. Guidelines for Regional Institutes Of Ophthalmology [Internet]. [cited 2024 Oct 16]. Available from: https://npcbvi.mohfw.gov.in/writeReadData/mainlinkFile/File308.pdf
5. Update on National Programme for Control of Blindness and Visual Impairment (NPCBVI) [Internet]. pib.gov.in. Available from:https://pib.gov.in/PressReleaseIframePage.aspx?PRID=1944598
6. Blind Welfare Society. National Programme for Control of Blindness and Visual Impairment (NPCBVI): Preventing Blindness Through Comprehensive Care | Blog - Blind Welfare Society, Expanding possibilities for people with vision loss. [Internet]. Blindwelfaresociety.in. 2020 [cited 2024 Oct 16]. Available from: https://www.blindwelfaresociety.in/blogs/national-programmefor-control-of-blindness-and-visual-impairment-npcbvi-preventing-blindness-through-comprehensive-care
7. Schemes for implementation of National Programme for Control of Blindness and Visual Impairment (NPCBVI) [Internet]. 2017 [cited 2024 Oct 16]. Available from: https://daman.nic.in/nhm/documents/2019/664-22-02-2019.pdf

QUESTIONS

Long Answer Question (LAQ)

1. What are the goals of NPCB and VI? Critically analyze the implementation of this program at different levels of healthcare facilities.

Short Answer Questions (SAQs)

1. What are the key activities undertaken in NPCB and VI at secondary healthcare level?
2. Discuss the implementation of NPCB and VI at the schools.

Multiple Choice Questions (MCQs)

1. Which of the following disease is under the ambit of NPCB and VI?
   a. Cataract
   b. Tuberculosis
   c. Dengue
   d. HIV/AIDS
2. What is the target prevalence of blindness set by National Health Policy under NPCB and VI for 2025?
   a. 0.50%
   b. 0.25%
   c. 0.75%
   d. 1.0%
3. The school eye screening program under NPCB and VI focuses on:
   a. Detecting visual impairment in children
   b. Distributing free prescription glasses
   c. Eye check-ups for children from economically disadvantaged families
   d. All of the above

Answers

1. a
2. b
3. d

CHAPTER 55

National Programme for Prevention and Control of Deafness

Nitesh Kumar, Amrita Srivastava, Bhavesh Kanabar

Aspect	Details
Background/Need of program/Scheme	Hearing loss is a common sensory deficit, causing significant disability worldwide. In India, nearly 63 million people suffer from auditory impairment. The burden among school-going children is estimated at 26.4 million. This results in severe loss of productivity, both physical and economic.
Implemented since	2007 (initially as a pilot in 25 districts across 11 states/UTs)
Goal	To reduce the overall burden of hearing impairment and deafness by 25% of the current level by the end of the 12th Five Year Plan.
Targets	• Prevent avoidable hearing loss due to disease or injury • Early identification and diagnosis of ear problems causing hearing loss • Provide medical rehabilitation for persons with deafness of all age groups • Strengthen existing inter-sectoral linkages for continuity of rehabilitation program • Develop institutional capacity for ear care services by providing equipment and training personnel
Objectives	Same as targets
Organogram	• **Central level:** Central Coordination Committee • **State level:** State Health Society, State Nodal Officer • **District level:** District Health Society, District Hospital
Beneficiaries	All individuals with hearing impairment, with dedicated services for newborns to 14-year-olds. All individuals are eligible for screening.
Components	• Manpower training and development • Capacity building • Service provision • Awareness generation through IEC/BCC activities
Strategies/Deliverables under the program	• Training of healthcare workers at various levels • Strengthening infrastructure at district hospitals and other healthcare facilities • Providing screening, early diagnosis, treatment, and rehabilitation services • Conducting awareness campaigns
Activities at various level or package of services	• **Primary prevention:** IEC activities, early detection by grassroots workers • **Secondary prevention:** Ear screening camps, school ear care program • **Tertiary prevention:** Referral services, rehabilitative services, hearing aid provision
Monitoring and evaluation of program	Bottom-up approach with designated monitoring forms filled at all levels and sent to the Nodal Officer and center. Evaluates progress made by different districts, states/UTs, and the country as a whole.

NEED OF THE PROGRAM

Hearing loss is one of the most common sensory deficits in the world today. It is one of the major causes of "Years Lived with Disability" (YLD). Hearing loss accounts for 24.9 million years lived with disability (YLD) on a global scale. Health experts project that hearing impairment will become increasingly prevalent, with estimates indicating that approximately 2.5 billion individuals worldwide may experience some level of hearing loss by the year 2050. Of them, around 700 million would need hearing rehabilitation. Over a billion youth are prone to avoidable hearing loss owing to the recreational use of music aids, and over 200 million have preventable chronic infections. There is always a need for timely intervention to curb this preventable cause of deafness. The failure to act will bear insult regarding the health of the affected and would also be the reason for the financial loss. However, combining this timely intervention with public health strategies will ensure complete accessibility to all who need it.[1,2]

According to WHO, nearly 63 million people in India are suffering from an auditory impairment. As per NSSO (2001), 291 people in every one lakh population suffer from severe to profound hearing loss, of which a major share was of children between 0–14 years of life. The estimated burden among school-going children was an alarming 26.4 million.[2] This would result in a severe loss of productivity, both physical and economic.

IMPLEMENTATION OF THE PROGRAM

The program was initiated in 2007 on a pilot basis in 25 districts across 11 states/UTs. Under the 11th Five Year Plan, it was a 100% centrally sponsored scheme. The program's reach has been progressively extended in stages, now encompassing 192 districts. Plans for further expansion during the 12th Five-Year Plan period aim to incorporate an additional 200 districts by 2017. Initially 100% centrally funded, in the 12th Five Year Plan, it was decided that the center and state would have to pool in the financial resources of NRHM. Till 2013-2014, the funds were released to the State Health Societies, but from 2014-15 onwards, funds are being released through the treasury route. In 2015-16, the program was included in the health system strengthening component of the National Health Mission (NHM). Since its inception, sanctions have been given to implement the program in 595 districts. For the financial year 2022-23, the NPPCD Programme budget has been merged with strengthening the National Program Management of NRHM.[3,4]

Primary aim: The overarching goal is to reduce the overall burden of hearing impairment and deafness by a quarter of its current level by the conclusion of the 12th Five Year Plan. This will be achieved through prevention and control of major contributing factors.

SPECIFIC PROGRAM TARGETS

- Prevent hearing loss that can be avoided due to diseases or injuries.
- Facilitate early detection, assessment, and treatment of ear conditions leading to hearing impairment.
- Provide medical rehabilitation services for individuals across all age groups affected by hearing loss.
- Enhance and reinforce existing cross-sector connections to ensure continuity in rehabilitation programs for those with hearing impairments.
- Enhance institutional capacity for ear healthcare by supplying necessary equipment, materials, and training for personnel.

ORGANOGRAM[4]

Central Level

The NPPCD organization uses a top-to-bottom approach. A Central Coordination Committee is at the central level, which provides technical inputs and facilitates program implementation. The central cell supports the program division in the MoHFW and outrolls an effective management information system for efficient data collection, monitoring, and program supervision.

Chapter 55: National Programme for Prevention and Control of Deafness

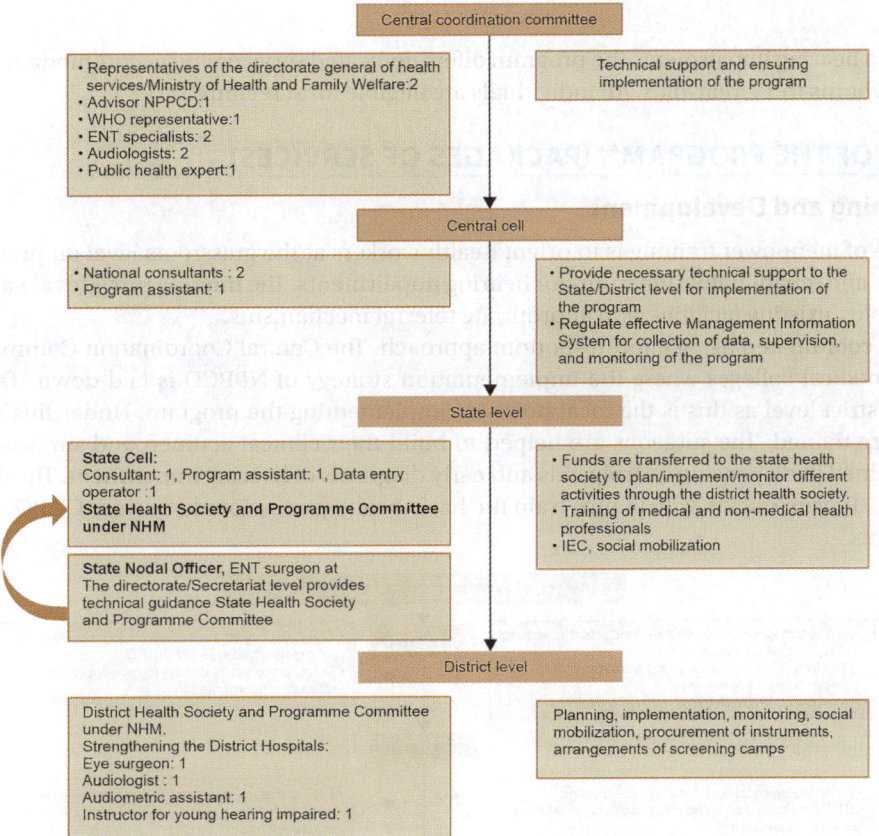

State Level

The state cell coordinates the monitoring of the program at the state and district levels. The State Health Society and Programme Committee receives the fund for program implementation at the state level and designates the fund to the District Health Society. The State Nodal Officer provides its technical guidance and ensures the optimum implementation of the program. The state society trains medical and non-medical staff in state and districts, IEC activities, and social mobilization.[4]

District Level

At the district level, the implementation of the program falls under the purview of the District Health Society.

Program execution is centered at the district level, which serves as the primary hub for implementation activities. The main focus is to provide screening, early diagnosis, treatment, and rehabilitation for hearing defects. The district hospitals (DH) are being strengthened. Each DH should ideally have:
- ENT surgeon: For clinical services and training.
- Audiologists: Providing audiological services, hearing aids, maintenance of records, and assisting in training programs.
- Audiometric assistants: Screening of hearing impairments.
- Instructor for young hearing impaired children: Providing training, therapy, and early education to impaired children.[4]

Beneficiaries

All those who have a hearing impairment. The program offers dedicated services and accommodations for the age group spanning from newborns to 14-year-olds. All individuals are eligible for screening.

COMPONENTS OF THE PROGRAM[4,5] (PACKAGES OF SERVICES)

Manpower Training and Development

The main objective of manpower training is to orient health workers at the grassroots level on prevention, promotion, early identification, and rehabilitative measures for hearing impairments. The training provides a platform to make them understand their roles, existing facilities, and appropriate referral mechanisms.

The training is coordinated using a top-to-bottom approach. The Central Coordination Committee trains the ENT specialists in the medical colleges where the implementation strategy of NPPCD is laid down. Then, a greater focus is placed on the district level as this is the focal point for implementing the program. Under this, the ENT specialists and audiologists are trained. The surgeons are helped to build their clinical acumen and surgical skills, whereas the audiologists are trained in dispensing hearing aids and early diagnosis of hearing impairment. The district-level officers train the PHC/CHC/Private doctor, who in turn train the basic health professionals, such as CDPO, ANM, AWW, school teachers, and parents.

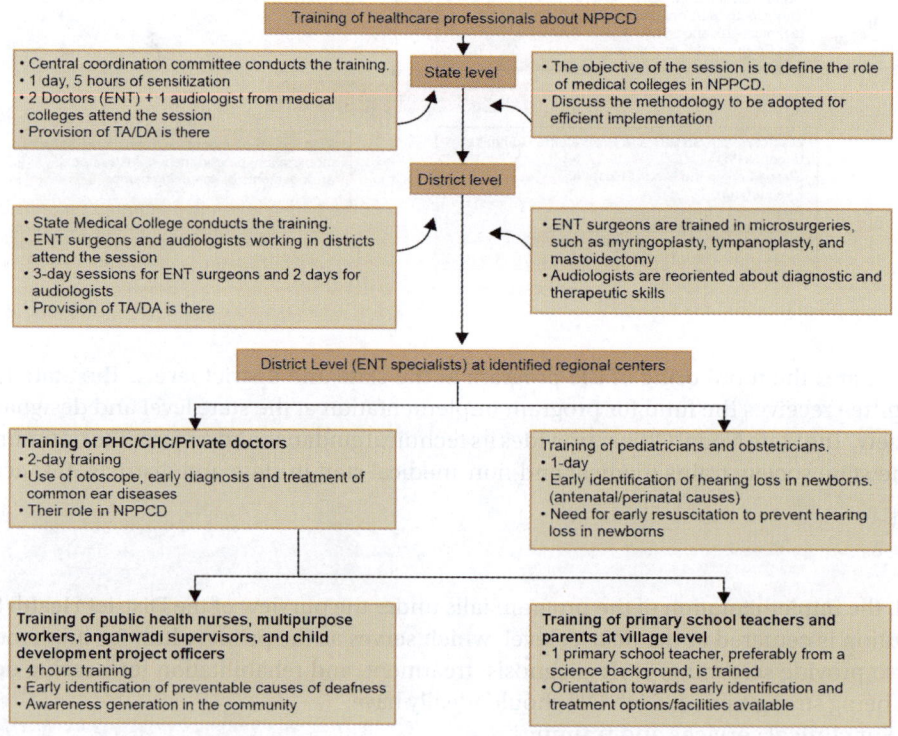

Capacity Building

The prime focus is making the district hospital a self-sustained unit. To meet program goals, the recommended staffing for each district hospital includes:
- An ENT specialist
- An audiologist
- An audiometric technician
- A hearing impairment educator

Chapter 55: National Programme for Prevention and Control of Deafness

These positions are envisioned to be filled through contractual arrangements.
This focal point implements all the preventive, promotive, and therapeutic activities.[6]

- ❖ **Service provision:**
  - The spectrum of services, viz early detection, ear screening, treatment (medical/surgical), referral and rehabilitative hearing and speech therapy are provided at different levels of health care.
  - *Early detection:* This is basically done at the grassroots level by family members, school teachers, and AWWs/ANMs by conducting house-to-house surveys. District-level gynecologists/obstetricians are responsible for the early detection of newborn deafness. A comprehensive "School Ear Care Programme" is conducted in schools in collaboration with PHCs to screen out the common causes of deafness, such as impacted wax, suppurative/serous otitis media, and otomycosis in school-going children. It is a performa-based assessment that involves both ear examination and voice testing.[7]
  - *Ear screening camps:* The screening camps for the general population are organized at CHCs/PHCs/any nearby areas in collaboration with the National Health Mission (NHM) (mainly under RBSK) and the Ministry of Social Justice and Empowerment (M/O SJ&E). The screening camps is preceded by IEC activities and are conducted by questionnaire/checklist approach. Along with the detection of hearing impairment, screening camps are also utilized to generate community awareness.
  - Ideally, each camp should have two doctors (One being an ENT specialist) and one audiologist/audiological assistant. The audiological assistant does hearing assessment by conducting tuning fork tests and informal voice tests. The ENT specialist is responsible for the referral if needed. The data pertaining to the camps is kept well-maintained.[8]
  - *Referral services:* Effective linkages are being developed from the peripheral level to the district hospital with the basic healthcare personnel at the grassroots level, such as ANM, AWW, school teachers, and family members.
  - *Rehabilitative and hearing-aid provision:* The patient requiring rehabilitative therapy is referred to an ENT specialist or audiologist at the district level. The assessment is done here, and if corrective surgery is needed, the patient is referred to State Medical College. For those whose hearing loss is not amenable to treatment and require hearing aids, the same is provided at the district level by M/O SJ&E under Assistance to Disabled Persons (ADIP) (Divyangian). The district ENT surgeon procures hearing aids and gives them only after the clearance provided by ENT specialists. For children less than 14 years, it is free, and for those over 14 years, it is provided at a subsidized rate. The hearing aids are issued as per existing norms and there is no separate budgetary allocation for it.[9]
- ❖ **Awareness generation through IEC/BCC activities**: For early identification of the hearing impaired, especially children, so that timely management of such cases is possible and to remove the stigma attached to deafness.

ACTIVITIES AT DIFFERENT LEVELS

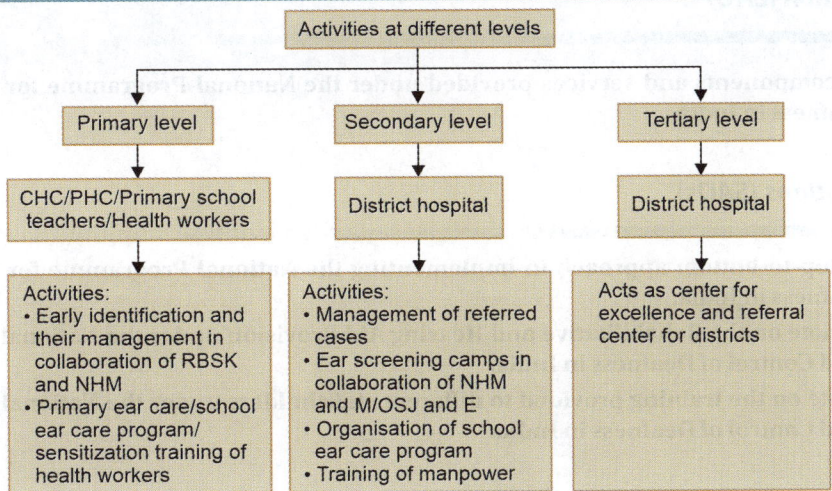

MONITORING AND EVALUATION

It is done to evaluate the progress made by different districts, states/UT, and the country as a whole. Thus, it is imperative that at all levels, the designated monitoring performance are filled properly and sent to the Nodal officer and center. Thus, a bottom-up approach is used for monitoring.

References

1. World Health Organisation. Deaf and Hearing Fact Sheet. World Health Organisation;2024. Available from: https://www.who.int/news-room/fact-sheets/detail/deafness-and-hearing-loss. [Last accessed 21st January 2025]
2. Chadha S, Kamenov K, Cieza A. The world report on hearing, 2021. Bull World Health Organ. 2021 Apr 1;99(4):242-242A. doi: 10.2471/BLT.21.285643. PMID: 33953438; PMCID: PMC8085630
3. Ministry of Health and Family Welfare, Government of India. National Programme for Prevention and Control of Deafness(NPPCD) [Internet]. Available from: https://mohfw.gov.in/?q=Major-Programmes/Non-Communicable-Diseases-Injury-Trauma/National-Programme-for-Prevention-and-Control-of-Deafness-NPPCD. [Last accessed 21st January 2025]
4. Ministry of Health and Family Welfare, Government of India. National Programme for Prevention and Control of Deafness(NPPCD).Operational Guidelines for 12th Five Year Plan[Internet]. Available from: https://mohfw.gov.in/sites/default/files/51892751619025258383.pdf [[Last accessed 21st January 2025]
5. National Health Mission, Government of India. National Programme for the Prevention and Control of Deafness (NPPCD) [Internet]. Available from:https://nhm.gov.in/index1.php?lang=1&level=2&sublinkid=1051&lid=606
6. Banerjee B. National Programme for Prevention and Control of Deafness. In: DK Taneja's Health Policies and Programmes in India.17ed.New Delhi:Jaypee Brothers Medical Publishers (P) Ltd.; 2023 . p. 547–550.
7. Ministry of Health and Family Welfare, Government of India. National Programme for Prevention and Control of Deafness(NPPCD). Guidelines for school level screening under National Program on Prevention and Control of Deafness (NPPCD)[Internet]. Available from: https://mohfw.gov.in/sites/default/files/4594720926nppcd6.pdf. [Last accessed 24th January 2025]
8. Ministry of Health and Family Welfare, Government of India. National Programme for Prevention and Control of Deafness(NPPCD). Guidelines for screening camps to be held in the districts under National Program on Prevention and Control of Deafness (NPPCD). [Internet]. Available from: https://mohfw.gov.in/sites/default/files/55594958439433520291nppcd5.pdf. [[Last accessed 24th January 2025]
9. Ministry of Health and Family Welfare, Government of India. National Programme for Prevention and Control of Deafness(NPPCD). Guidelines to prescribe BTE hearing aids under National Program on Prevention and Control of Deafness (NPPCD). [Internet]. Available from: https://mohfw.gov.in/sites/default/files/2489679489nppcd7.pdf. [[Last accessed 25th January 2025]

QUESTIONS

Long Answer Question (LAQ)

1. Describe the components and services provided under the National Programme for the Prevention and Control of Deafness in India.

Short Answer Questions (SAQs)

1. Describe the top-to-bottom approach in implementing the National Programme for the Prevention and Control of Deafness in India.
2. Write a short note on the Rehabilitative and Hearing Aid Provision under the National Programme for the Prevention and Control of Deafness in India.
3. Write short note on the training provided to different stakeholders under the National Programme for the Prevention and Control of Deafness in India.

Multiple Choice Questions (MCQs)

1. **According to the World Health Organization, how many people in India are estimated to be suffering from auditory impairment?**
    a. 25 million
    b. 43 million
    c. 63 million
    d. 83 million
2. **In which year was the National Programme for the Prevention and Control of Deafness initiated on a pilot basis?**
    a. 2005
    b. 2007
    c. 2009
    d. 2011
3. **What is the long-term objective of the National Programme for the Prevention and Control of Deafness?**
    a. To reduce the disease burden by 10% by the end of the 12th Five Year Plan
    b. To reduce the disease burden by 25% by the end of the 12th Five Year Plan
    c. To eliminate all cases of hearing impairment by 2025
    d. To provide hearing aids to all affected individuals
4. **Which of the following is NOT one of the specific program targets mentioned in the document?**
    a. Prevent avoidable hearing loss
    b. Early identification and treatment of ear problems
    c. Provide financial compensation to all hearing-impaired individuals
    d. Strengthen intersectoral linkages for rehabilitation programs
5. **At which level is the program execution primarily centered?**
    a. National level
    b. State level
    c. District level
    d. Village level
6. **Which age group is given special focus for dedicated services and accommodations under the program?**
    a. 0–14 years
    b. 15–30 years
    c. 31–50 years
    d. Above 50 years
7. **Who is responsible for the early detection of newborn deafness at the district level?**
    a. ENT specialists
    b. Audiologists
    c. Gynecologists/obstetricians
    d. Pediatricians
8. **What is the recommended number of doctors for each ear screening camp?**
    a. One doctor
    b. Two doctors (one being an ENT specialist)
    c. Three doctors
    d. Four doctors
9. **Under which scheme are hearing aids provided to those who need them?**
    a. National Health Mission (NHM)
    b. Rashtriya Bal Swasthya Karyakram (RBSK)
    c. Assistance to Disabled Persons (ADIP)
    d. Ayushman Bharat
10. **Who is responsible for training the basic health professionals, such as CDPO, ANM, AWW, and school teachers?**
    a. Central Coordination Committee
    b. State Nodal Officer
    c. District-level officers
    d. ENT specialists from medical colleges

11. What approach is used for monitoring the program's progress?
    a. Top-down approach
    b. Bottom-up approach
    c. Horizontal approach
    d. Diagonal approach
12. In which year was the NPPCD Programme included in the health system strengthening component of the National Health Mission (NHM)?
    a. 2013–14
    b. 2014–15
    c. 2015–16
    d. 2016–17

Answers

1. c	2. b	3. b	4. c	5. c
6. a	7. c	8. b	9. c	10. c
11. b	12. c			

CHAPTER 56

National Mental Health Programme

Ashish Pundir, Priya Ranjan Avinash, Parul Sharma, Bharti Koria

NATIONAL MENTAL HEALTH PROGRAMME

Background/Need of the program	Addressing burden of mental disorders and shortage of qualified professionals
Implemented since	The program was implemented in 1982.
	1996 — District Mental Health Programme included in it
	2003 — Two schemes included 'Modernization of State Mental Hospitals' 'Up-gradation of Psychiatric Wings of Medical Colleges/General Hospitals'
	2009 — Manpower development scheme became part of the program.
Objectives	• To ensure the availability and accessibility of minimum mental healthcare for all in the foreseeable future; • To encourage the application of mental health knowledge in general healthcare and in social development; • To promote community participation in the mental health service development; and • To enhance human resource in mental health subspecialties.[1]
Beneficiaries	• Person with mental health problems • Others, such as community residents, students, teachers for awareness and sensitization and counseling
Components	• District Mental Health Programme • Public-private partner model activities • Day care center • Residential/Long-term continuing care center • Community health center • Primary health center • Tertiary level activities • Mental health helpline • Support to central and state mental health authorities • Research and survey • Central IEC • Central mental health team • Mental health information system • Training/Workshops

Deliverables/ Activities under the program	**District mental health program**
	✦ Provision of mental health services: OPD, IPD, EMD services
	✦ *Outreach component:*
	  – Satellite clinic four times per month at PHC/CHC
	  – Targeted interventions:
	    ➢ Life skill education and counseling in schools
	    ➢ College counseling services
	    ➢ Workplace stress management
	    ➢ Suicide prevention services

	➢ Sensitize, engage, involve healthcare persons
	➢ Awareness camps
	➢ Community participation
	• **Public private partnership model activities:** Involve NGOs, other stakeholders for planning, implementing, training, supervision, etc.
	• **Day care center:** Rehabilitation and recovery services, such as pharmacotherapy/psychotherapy and follow-up.
	• **Residential/Long-term continuing care center:** Chronically-ill patients, not returning home, stayed at hospital are provide multidisciplinary care
	• **Community health centers:** Provision of OPD, IPD, EMD services
	Primary health centers: OPD services, counseling, case finding and mental health promotion
	• **Mental health helpline:** A country wide 24 hours dedicated helpline to provide information to public
	• **Tertiary level activities:** Manpower development schemes
	   ✦ *Scheme A (At Center of Excellence):* 10 existing mental hospitals/institutes/Medical colleges upgraded for the purpose to start/strengthen courses in psychiatry, clinical psychology, psychiatric social work and psychiatric nursing.
	   ✦ *Scheme B (PG Training Departments of Mental Health Facilities):* Provision of either starting or increasing PG courses in Government Medical College/Government Menta Hospital.
	• **Support to state and mental health authorities:** Provision of support for purchase of infrastructure and office and professional expenses.
	• **Research and survey:** Conducting research to understand regional needs, framing plan and strategies.
	• **Central IEC:** Website for information, planning, resources
	• **Central mental health team:** Team comprising consultant (Mental health), consultant (Public health), two research associates, one DEO involved in supervision, implementation of the program and support.
	• **Mental health information system:** An online data monitoring system and facilitate bilateral communication.
	• **Training/workshops:** TOTs to state and district staff who further train the field staff

Monitoring and evaluation program	Standard formats are used for recording and reporting activities, which is used by medical colleges/institutes, district, CHC and PHC.

NATIONAL MENTAL HEALTH POLICY

Framed in year	2014
Vision	To promote mental health, prevent mental illness, enable recovery from mental illness, demote stigmatization, ensure socioeconomic inclusion of mentally-ill person by providing accessible, affordable and quality health and social care to all persons through lifespan.[5]
Principles	• **Equity**: Mental health care should be provided to all irrespective of their status, area, SEC, cast. A mentally-ill person Should be provided equal rights for Job, education, participation • **Justice**: Focus on vulnerable population should be emphasized. • **Integrated care:** Services to be provided through existing healthcare system • **Evidence-based care:** Services being provided should be based on best research evidence and successful models • **Quality:** Quality should match the global standards • **Participatory and right-based approach:** Patients, care givers, community should be involved in planning, implementing, monitoring the services • **Governance and effective delivery:** Other stakeholders, such as civil society, private care provider, academic and research institution should be included for effective healthcare delivery • **Value base in all training and teaching programs:** Values, such as justice, integrity, quality, accountability and empathy included in all training forms • **Holistic approach to mental health**

Goals	<ul><li>To reduce distress, disability, exclusion morbidity and premature mortality associated with mental health problems.</li><li>To enhance the understanding of mental health in the country.</li><li>To strengthen the leadership in mental health sector at the national. state and district levels.</li></ul>
Objectives	<ul><li>To provide universal access and utilization of mental health care by mentally-ill person, vulnerable population, such as deprived sections, remote areas</li><li>To reduce prevalence and impact of risk factors associated with mental health problems.</li><li>To reduce risk and incidence of suicide</li><li>To ensure respect for rights and protection from harm of persons with mental health problems.</li><li>To reduce stigma associated with mental health problems.</li><li>To enhance availability and equitable distribution of skilled human resources for mental health.</li><li>To progressively enhance financial allocation and improve utilization for mental health promotion and care.</li><li>To recognize and address social, economic, biological and other factors related to mental health[2]</li></ul>
Strategic direction and recommendation of actions	<ul><li>**Effective governance and delivery mechanisms for mental health**<ul><li>Formulate programs, laws, allocation of budget for evidence-based mental health plans and actions.</li><li>Involvement of stakeholders</li></ul></li><li>**Promotion of mental health**<ul><li>Addressing emotional needs of the children under six years</li><li>Training anganwadi workers to impart knowledge and skills to parents of children for physical and emotional needs</li><li>Provision of life skill education to school and college going students.</li><li>Increase awareness</li><li>To work upon reducing the risk factors of women mental health</li></ul></li><li>**Prevention of mental illness, reduction of suicide and attempted suicide**<ul><li>Address stigma and discrimination</li><li>Reduce the means of suicide, such as storage of toxic pesticides.</li></ul></li><li>**Universal access to mental health services**<ul><li>Increase availability of community-based rehabilitation, short and long stay facilities and day care centers</li><li>Implement community-based programs to support family and caregivers to foster recovery of mentally-ill person</li><li>Implement program for early diagnosis, screening and treatment</li></ul></li><li>**Improved availability of adequately trained mental health human resources to address the mental health needs of the community.**<ul><li>Increase availability and training of psychiatrist, public health nurses, well trained nurses,</li><li>Increase awareness among patients and care givers</li></ul></li><li>**Community involvement for mental health and development**<ul><li>Involve patients and care givers in all welfare programs, RKS, VHSND</li><li>Inclusion of recovered person for job, education, rehabilitation</li></ul></li><li>**Research:** For implementing priority mental health research, a partnership between Center of Excellence in Mental Health, Department of Psychiatry in Medical College with NGO and Research Institution</li></ul>

NATIONAL SUICIDE PREVENTION STRATEGY[6]

Need of strategy	To address the growing concern of increasing suicide and its prevention
Framed in	2021
Aims	Decrease suicide by 10% by 2030
Implementation approach	Multisector collaboration
Goal	<ul><li>Multisectoral collaboration, institutional capacity building, reinforced leading</li><li>Enhance the capacity of health services to provide suicide prevention services.</li><li>Community involvement and support for suicide prevention, addressing stigma and discrimination</li><li>Strengthen surveillance of suicide and evidence generation.</li></ul>

Objectives	• To build an effective surveillance system for preventing suicide within three years • To establish psychiatric OPD that provide suicide prevention services, through the District Mental Health Programme in all the districts within the next five years. • To integrate mental well-being curriculum in all educational institutes within the next eight years.[3]
Strategy for first goal	• Advocate for suicide prevention and destigmatization of mental disorders amongst multiple stakeholders. • Addressing underlying psychosocial issues, such as addiction disorders. • Advocacy for provision of psychosocial care to patients with chronic and terminal illness. • Reduction in easy access to one of the most common methods of suicide • Positive media involvement for awareness
Strategy for second goal	• Build capacity for psychosocial support for persons with mental disorders and substance use disorders. • Integrate mental health service to general healthcare services. • Increasing and including qualified practitioners for care delivery • Building capacity to provide psychological first aid and psychosocial support to person who have attempted suicide and bereaved by suicide. • Helping drug abusers and addiction patients
Strategy for third goal	• Build help seeking behavior for mental health problems by removing stigma and myths associated with them. • IEC strategy for suicide prevention. • Educational club and youth club for help • Reduce workplace stressors
Strategy for fourth goal	• Strengthen self-injury/Harm data collection at the national and state level. • Strengthen suicide data collection at national and state level.

MENTAL HEALTHCARE ACT 2017[7]

Implemented year	2017
Purpose	• To provide for mental healthcare and services for persons with mental illness • To protect, promote and fulfil the rights of such persons during delivery of mental healthcare services
Provisions	
Provision of Advanced Directive	

- Person of mental illness has the right to decide his/her way of to be treated and cared
- Advanced directive would be in writing and applicable when the person with mental illness ceases to have capacity to make decision related to their treatment
- The medical officer in-charge or psychiatrist will be bound to provide treatment as per the person with mental illness advance directive.
- Advanced directive are not applicable in emergency treatment.
- In case, caregiver or relative does not want to comply to advance directive, it could be modified or nullified after submitting application to the concerned board.
- The medical Officer will not be liable to consequences of complying to advanced directive
- The Medical Officer need not be held liable for not following advanced directive if a copy of advanced directive is not given.[4]

Provision of Nominated Representative

Representative should be more than 18 years and may include relative, care giver, etc.
(If no person available to be appointed, then the director, department of social welfare as a nominated representative)
- The duties of the nominated representative would be:
  + Consider the current and past wishes, life history, values, cultural facts and best interest of mentally-ill person
  + Help him to make treatment decisions.
  + Have right to seek information on diagnosis and treatment to make right decision of mentally-ill person.

Provision for Right of Person with Mental Illness
- Right to access mental healthcare and treatment from mental health services run or funded by the appropriate government.
- Right to refuse or receive visitors and to refuse or receive and make telephone or mobile phone calls at reasonable times subject to the norms of such mental health establishment.
- Right to send and receive mail through electronic mode including through e-mail.
- Right to receive free legal services to exercise any of his rights given under this Act.
- Any person with mental illness or his nominated representative, shall have the right to complain regarding deficiencies in provision of care, treatment and services in amental health establishment
Provision of central mental health authority
The central authority comprises
- Chairperson: Secretary/additional secretary, Department of HFW
- Member ex officio: Joint secretary, Department of HFW
- Members from AYUSH, Department of Social Justice, Department of WCD, Psychiatrist, Clinical Psychologist, care givers of patients, etc.
Function of Central Mental Health Authority
- Register, maintain, compile, and publish all mental health establishments under the control of the Central Government.
- Develop quality and service provision norms, supervise, receive complaints for different types of mental health establishments under the Central Government.
- Maintain, publish, train a national register of clinical psychologists, mental health nurses and psychiatric social workers based on information provided by all State Authorities.
- Advise the Central Government on all matters relating to mental healthcare and services.
- Discharge such other functions with respect to matters relating to mental health as the Central Government may decide.
Provision of State Mental Health Authority
- **Members of the State Mental Health Authority**
- Secretary or Principal Secretary in the Department of Health of the State Government
- Joint Secretary in the Department of Health of the State Government, Director of Health Services or Medical Education
- Department of Social Welfare, Head of any of the Mental Hospitals, Head of Department of Psychiatry
- Member; one eminent psychiatrist, one psychiatric social worker, one clinical psychologist, one mental health nurse, two persons representing persons who have or have had mental illness, two persons representing care-givers, two persons representing NGOs
- **Function of State Mental Health Authority**
- Register, enlist, maintain and publish all mental health institutes except under Section 43
- State-wise ensuring quality services through monitoring, evaluation and grievance redresses
- State-wise enlist, register, train persons related to mental health, such as psychologist, mental health nurses, psychiatric social worker, etc.
Provision of responsibility of other certain agencies
- If a police officer feels a patient with mental illness ill-treated, then he will report to magistrate
- Police officer in-charge can also take responsibility of any wandering person, can take to examination by medical office and also their placement either at hospital, home or care center
Provision of decriminalization of suicide and prohibition of unmodified electroconvulsive therapy
- A mentally-ill person who have suicide attempt is decriminalized. Government will ensure rehabilitation of such person to prevent further attempts
Provision of financial punishment
- Establish a mental health facility without permission ₹ 5,000–50,000 on first contravention, ₹ 50,000–2 lakh on second contravention, ₹ 2–5 lakh on every next contravention
- Un registered practice —up to ₹ 25,000 penalty

TELE MANAS

(Tele Mental Health Assistance and Networking Across States) : Digital Component of National Mental Health Programme[2]

Background/Need of the program	It is a Digital Component of National Mental Health Program. It introduced a toll-free helpline (14416) which is available nationwide.[Available free of cost] In India , it is reported more than 11 crore suffer from mental health condition alongside treatment gap being around 80%. Hence ,this initiative was taken to bridge the treatment seeking gap for mental health conditions and improving access across India
Implementation	10th October 2022
Aim	To provide universal access to equitable, affordable, and quality mental health care through a 24 × 7 tele-mental health service
Objectives	1. **Expanding access:** To ensure anyone across India at any point of time through dedicated 24 × 7 tele-mental health facilities receive mental health services in every state and Union territory. 2. **Building a comprehensive mental health network:** In addition to counselling , to provide medical and psychosocial interventions, video consultations with specialist, e-prescriptions, follow-up care and connections to in-person services. 3. **Reaching vulnerable populations:** Providing urgent mental health care to difficult and vulnerable groups.
Beneficiaries	1. People who are finding difficult to cope up with day-to-day stressors. 2. People suffering from mental health conditions and their care givers.

Service components	1. **Tier based services**
	Tier 1 Mental Health Specialist and Trained counselors in Tele-MANAS cells(managed through 52 cells under 23 mentoring institutes and 5 regional Coordinating centers) via
	  i. **Tele-counseling:** Counsellors provide aid to individuals facing psychological distress such as family issues, relationship conflicts ,examination stress , workplace pressure and financial conflicts etc.
	  ii. **Tele-consultation:** Mental Health specialist such as psychiatrist and psychologist diagnose and manage mental health condition such as depression, anxiety, psychosis, addiction, and dementia. It also addresses urgent situation such as suicidal behavior and abrupt changes in behavior.
	Tier 2 a) Additional resources such as physical consultations and audiovisual consultations via e-Sanjeevani is provided by specialist comprises specialists from District Mental Health Programme (DMHP) facilities and medical colleges. Incase, advance treatment is indicated then TeleMANAS refers to mental health establishment for further care and evaluation.
	2. **Service for focus on mental-wellbeing and caregivers of person with mental health conditions**
	  i. Emphasis on mental well being and guidance on sleep disturbances, technology overuse, substance misuse, etc.
	  ii. Support to parents and caregivers of children and adolescents with developmental disorders such as intellectual disabilities, autism, and ADHD.

New initiatives under TeleMANAS	Launch of its mobile application for providing the following services: 1. Video consultation services 2. Mental health resources including self-care tips, stress management strategies, and tools to identify early distress signals. 3. The application provides 24 × 7 free, confidential counseling and connects users to trained mental health professionals across India. 4. Video consultations enabling to conduct history taking , clarifying concerns , and enables brief physical or Mental State Examinations (MSE). [This service is available in Karnataka, Jammu and Kashmir, and Tamil Nadu and currently being considered to be expanded across the country]

References

1. https://pib.gov.in/PressNoteDetails.aspx?NoteId=153277&ModuleId=3&reg=3&lang=1
2. https://telemanas.mohfw.gov.in/home
3. https://pib.gov.in/PressReleasePage.aspx?PRID=2063830
4. Directorate General of Health Services [Internet]. [cited 2024 Jul 16];Available from: https://dghs.gov.in/content/1350_3_NationalMentalHealthProgramme.aspx

QUESTIONS

Long Answer Questions (LAQs)

1. Mention the need of National Mental Health Programme and its beneficiaries. Describe the objectives and components of the program.
2. What are the objectives and goals of National Mental Health Policy of India? Enumerate and describe the principles, strategic direction and recommended action.
3. State the need of National Suicide Prevention Strategy and its aim, goal, objectives. Describe the strategy for achieving the goals.
4. Describe the Purpose of Mental Health Care Act. Enumerate the provision of Mental Healthcare Act 2017. Briefly describe the Provision of Mental Health Care Act 2017.

Short Answer Questions (SAQs)

1. Briefly describe the activities of different components of National Mental Health Programme.
2. Enumerate the different scheme and program incorporated into National Mental Health Programme.
3. Enumerate and briefly describe the principles of National Mental Health Policy of India.
4. Enumerate and briefly describe the strategic direction and recommended action.
5. Describe the strategy for achieving the goals.
6. As per the Mental Healthcare Act 2017, describe the Function of Central Mental Health Authority and State Mental Health Authority.
7. As per Mental Healthcare Act 2017, describe the provision of Advanced Directive.

Multiple Choice Questions (MCQs)

1. What is the primary goal of the National Mental Health Policy of India?
    a. To promote mental health
    b. To prevent mental illness
    c. To enable recovery from mental illness
    d. All of the above
2. Which principle emphasizes involving service users and caregivers in planning, development, delivery, monitoring, and evaluation of mental health services?
    a. Equity
    b. Justice
    c. Participatory and right-based approach
    d. Evidence-based care
3. What is the primary aim of the National Suicide Prevention Strategy?
    a. Reduce suicide mortality by 10% by 2030
    b. Enhance mental health services
    c. Develop community resilience
    d. Strengthen surveillance of suicide

4. **Which approach does the strategy emphasize for implementation?**
   a. Multisectoral collaboration
   b. Individual counseling
   c. Medication-based treatment
   d. Community awareness campaigns
5. **What is the primary purpose of the Mental Healthcare Act 2017?**
   a. To provide mental healthcare and services for persons with mental illness
   b. To regulate mental health professionals
   c. To promote mental health awareness
   d. To establish mental health research centers
6. **What is an Advanced Directive in the context of mental healthcare?**
   a. A legal document specifying the treatment preferences of a person with mental illness
   b. A directive issued by the Central Mental Health Authority
   c. A guideline for mental health professionals
   d. A form of emergency treatment
7. **Who can be appointed as a nominated representative for a person with mental illness?**
   a. Any relative or caregiver
   b. Only a minor person
   c. A suitable person appointed by the concerned board
   d. A medical officer
8. **What right does a person with mental illness have regarding access to mental healthcare?**
   a. Right to refuse treatment
   b. Right to receive visitors
   c. Right to access mental healthcare and treatment
   d. Right to make phone calls
9. **What is the function of the Central Mental Health Authority?**
   a. To register mental health establishments
   b. To develop quality and service provision norms
   c. To train law enforcement officials
   d. All of the above
10. **What is the penalty for executing a mental health establishment without registration?**
    a. ₹5,000 to ₹50,000 for the first contravention
    b. ₹50,000 to ₹2 lakh for the second contravention
    c. ₹2 lakh to ₹5 lakh for every subsequent contravention
    d. No penalty
11. **Which provision decriminalizes suicide attempts by mentally-ill persons?**
    a. Provision for Right of Person with Mental Illness
    b. Provision of Financial Punishment
    c. Provision of decriminalization of Suicide
    d. None of the above
12. **What is the role of the nominated representative for a person with mental illness?**
    a. To provide treatment
    b. To decide treatment preferences
    c. To support decision-making
    d. To supervise mental health establishments
13. **What is the duty of a police officer in-charge of a police station regarding mentally-ill persons?**
    a. Report ill-treatment or neglect
    b. Provide emergency treatment
    c. Arrest the person
    d. None of the above

14. **What is the purpose of prohibiting electroconvulsive therapy (ECT) without muscle relaxants and anesthesia?**
    a. To protect mental health professionals
    b. To ensure patient safety
    c. To reduce costs
    d. To improve treatment outcomes

Answers

1. d	2. c	3. a	4. a	5. a
6. a	7. a	8. c	9. d	10. c
11. c	12. c	13. a	14. b	

57 CHAPTER

National Tobacco Control Programme

Nitesh Kumar, Shaili Vyas, Akhil Dhanesh Goel, Harsha Solanki

| Background/Need of the program[1-8] | **Tobacco:** Worldwide, tobacco causes of premature death worldwide and kills half of its users. It leads to early development of cancers, cardiovascular disease, diabetes, chronic lung disease, stroke, etc. Tobacco used in smoking as well as smokeless form in India. Smoking tobacco used mainly in the form of bidi followed by cigarettes and hookah. Smokeless tobacco (tobacco chewing) includes khaini, zarda, gutkha, mishri, mava, etc.[1]
Global: Total number of tobacco users in the world has been estimated at 1.3 billion of which 80% live in low- and middle-income countries. Tobacco kills more than 8 million people each year of which more than 7 million are due to direct tobacco use while around 1.3 million are the result of non-smoking (exposed to second-hand smoke).[2,3]
India: India is the second largest tobacco producer and consumer nation and faces a dual burden of tobacco use in the form of smoking and smokeless tobacco. WHO has estimated 1.35 million (13.5 lakh) deaths occur due to tobacco use every year overall in India.
Second-hand smoke (SHS) or passive smoking is known as human carcinogens and it causes numerous health problems in infants, children and adults including more frequent and severe asthma attacks, respiratory infections, ear infections, sudden infant death syndrome, coronary heart disease, stroke, lung cancer, etc.[4,5]
Prevalence, Pattern and Trend:
Global Adult Tobacco Survey (GATS): As per the latest 2nd GATS (2016– 2017), there has been a relative decline of 17.3% of tobacco use nationwide from 34.6% reported in 2009-2010. However, still 28.6% [26.7 Crores—(42.4% men, 14.2% women)] of all adults (persons aged 15 or above) consume some or other form of tobacco in India. Overall prevalence of smoking tobacco use is 10.7% and smokeless tobacco use is 21.4% in India. Prevalence of tobacco use in rural and urban areas is 32.5% and 21.2% respectively. The prevalence of tobacco use is highest in Tripura (64.5%) followed by Mizoram (58.7%) and Manipur (55.1%) and lowest in Goa (9.7%).[6,7]
Global Youth Tobacco Survey (GYTS): GYTS is self-administered, school-based survey among 13–15 years of age. As per the latest 4th round of GYTS-4 (2019) report, tobacco usage among early adolescents is around 8.5% of (13–15 years). Highest use of any tobacco was found in Arunachal Pradesh and Mizoram (58% each) and lowest in Himachal Pradesh (1.1%).[8]
Economic burden: Estimated cost of tobacco use attributed to diseases and deaths among persons aged 35 years and older, is ₹ 1,77,341 crores (US$ 27.5 billion) in India for the year 2017-2018.
Milestones:
India has made significant progress in tobacco control since 2004 which includes implementation of the National Tobacco Control Programme (NTCP), World Health Organization Framework Convention on Tobacco Control (WHO FCTC) ratification, tobacco testing laboratories establishment, enforcement of the Cigarettes and Other Tobacco Products Act (COTPA), and the prohibitions on gutkha/smokeless tobacco and electronic nicotine delivery systems (ENDS).
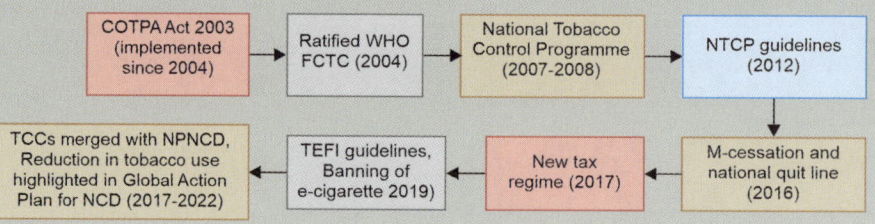 |

Chapter 57: National Tobacco Control Programme

Objectives[9]	• Awareness generation about the detrimental effects of tobacco use • Reduce production and supply of tobacco products • To ensure effective implementation of the provisions under COTPA 2003 • Help people to quit tobacco use • To facilitate implementation of strategies for prevention and control of tobacco advocated by the WHO Framework Convention of Tobacco Control (WHO-FCTC).
Organogram[9]	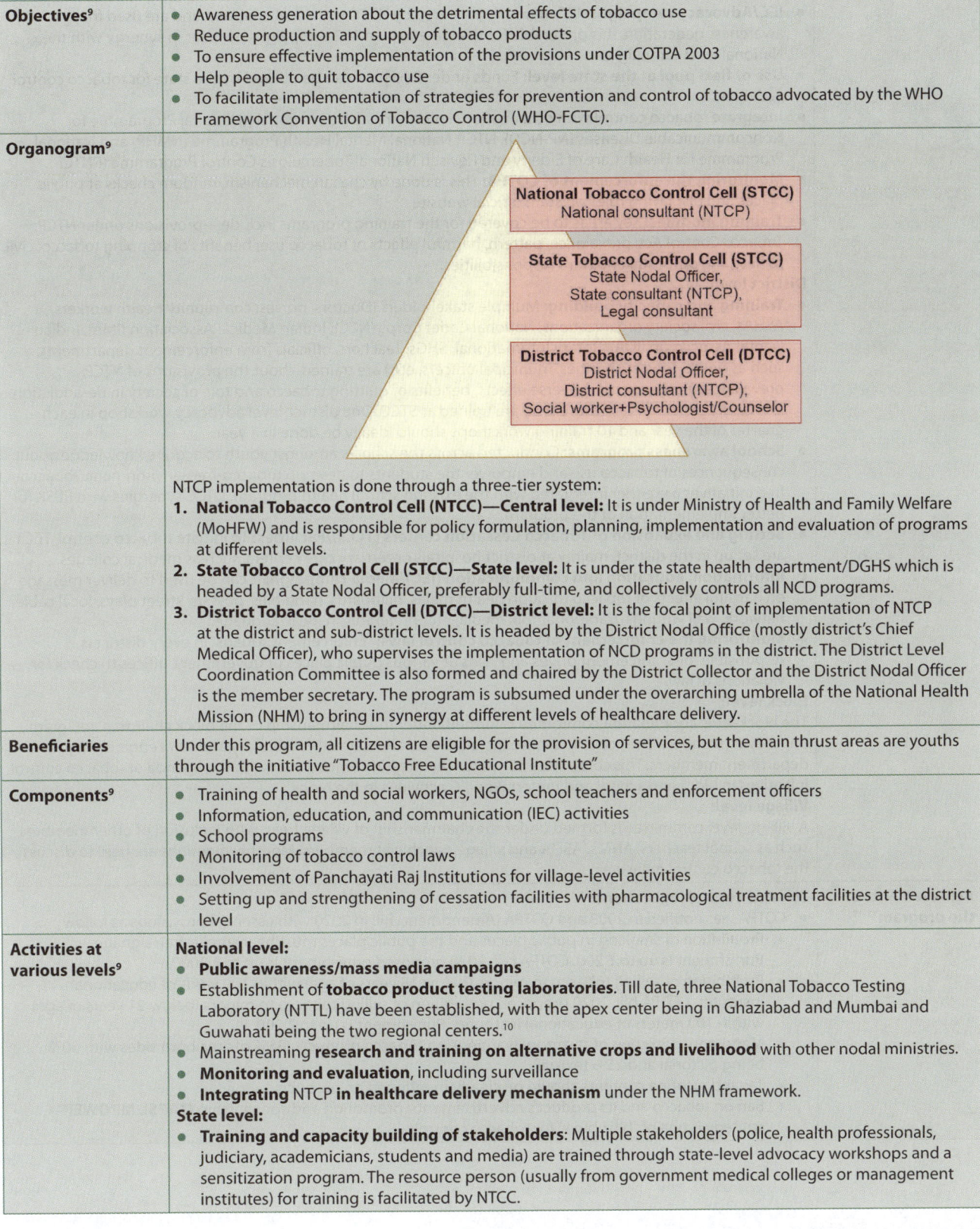 NTCP implementation is done through a three-tier system: 1. **National Tobacco Control Cell (NTCC)—Central level:** It is under Ministry of Health and Family Welfare (MoHFW) and is responsible for policy formulation, planning, implementation and evaluation of programs at different levels. 2. **State Tobacco Control Cell (STCC)—State level:** It is under the state health department/DGHS which is headed by a State Nodal Officer, preferably full-time, and collectively controls all NCD programs. 3. **District Tobacco Control Cell (DTCC)—District level:** It is the focal point of implementation of NTCP at the district and sub-district levels. It is headed by the District Nodal Office (mostly district's Chief Medical Officer), who supervises the implementation of NCD programs in the district. The District Level Coordination Committee is also formed and chaired by the District Collector and the District Nodal Officer is the member secretary. The program is subsumed under the overarching umbrella of the National Health Mission (NHM) to bring in synergy at different levels of healthcare delivery.
Beneficiaries	Under this program, all citizens are eligible for the provision of services, but the main thrust areas are youths through the initiative "Tobacco Free Educational Institute"
Components[9]	• Training of health and social workers, NGOs, school teachers and enforcement officers • Information, education, and communication (IEC) activities • School programs • Monitoring of tobacco control laws • Involvement of Panchayati Raj Institutions for village-level activities • Setting up and strengthening of cessation facilities with pharmacological treatment facilities at the district level
Activities at various levels[9]	**National level:** • **Public awareness/mass media campaigns** • Establishment of **tobacco product testing laboratories**. Till date, three National Tobacco Testing Laboratory (NTTL) have been established, with the apex center being in Ghaziabad and Mumbai and Guwahati being the two regional centers.[10] • Mainstreaming **research and training on alternative crops and livelihood** with other nodal ministries. • **Monitoring and evaluation**, including surveillance • **Integrating** NTCP **in healthcare delivery mechanism** under the NHM framework. **State level:** • **Training and capacity building of stakeholders**: Multiple stakeholders (police, health professionals, judiciary, academicians, students and media) are trained through state-level advocacy workshops and a sensitization program. The resource person (usually from government medical colleges or management institutes) for training is facilitated by NTCC.

	- **IEC/Advocacy campaigns:** IEC materials prepared by NTCC with local adaption and are used for awareness generation. It is preferable for the state to plan 1–2 campaigns per year in synergy with the National level campaigns.
- **Use of flexi pool at the state level:** Funds under flexi pool can be utilized by the state for tobacco control activities.
- **Integrate** tobacco control with other national program, such as national [(National Programme for Noncommunicable Diseases (NP-NCD), NTCP, National Mental Health Programme (NMHP) and National Programme for Health Care of Elderly and Revised National Tuberculosis Control Programme (RNTCP).
- **Monitoring the enforcement of COTPA:** This is done by challan mechanism, random checks at public places and displaying rules on state official website.
- **Training modules**: Key areas to be covered for the training programs include—provisions under NTCP; Tobacco Control Act; prevalence, pattern, harmful effects of tobacco use; benefits of stopping tobacco; civil society and other stakeholder's responsibilities.

District level:
- **Training and capacity building:** Multiple stakeholders (Doctors, nurses, community health workers, ASHAs, civil society organizations, National Cadet Corps (NCC), Indian Medical Association (IMA), Indian Dental Association (IDA), Rotary International, SHGs, Teachers, officials from enforcement departments, such as police, food authorities, municipal officers, etc.) are trained about the provisions of NTCP, prevalence of tobacco use, adverse effects, benefits of quitting tobacco and role of society in de-addiction. The resource persons are those who are trained at STCC. One district-level advocacy workshop in each quarter of the year and 10 training workshops should ideally be done in a year.
- **School awareness programs:** Conducted across the schools amongst youth to acquire knowledge about consequences of tobacco use and empower the students to develop tobacco-free-environment. Tobacco-free initiatives are either integrated with the existing school health program. DTCC synergies with RBSK for better implementation of the program.
- **Setting and expansion of Tobacco Cessation centers (TCCs)/Facilities:** To initiate tobacco control, TCCs are set up in the district, mainly at district hospitals or tertiary care centers, such as medical colleges.
- **Information, education and communication (IEC)/Media campaign:** It can be used to deliver message on harmful effects of tobacco through health melas, billboards, hand bills, posters, street plays, local cable network, wall writings, traditional/folk media, etc., preferably in local language.
- **Monitoring the enforcement of tobacco control laws:** "Enforcement squads" in every district is responsible for enforcement drives and raids at various public places or government offices to check for violations of law.

Block level:
The block-level coordination committee is formed under the chairmanship of the block chairman and gram panchayat members. The committee also includes education, health, veterinary and rural engineering department members. This committee convenes the meeting twice a year with the agenda of tobacco control initiatives in block and school and undertakes IEC activities in the block.

Village level:
A village-level committee is formed under the chairmanship of village head with inclusion of other members, such as school teachers, ANMs, ASHA and village panchayat members. Monthly meetings are held to discuss the tobacco control measures. |
| **Achievements of the program**[11-19] | **Tobacco control legislations:**[11-14]
- COTPA was notified in 2003 and COTPA (Amendment) Bill in 2020 with essential provisions as follow:
  + Prohibition of smoking in public places and the public places must bear smoke-free signage. Punishment is up to ₹ 200. COTPA bill, 2020 proposed punishment is up to ₹ 2000.
  + Prohibition of selling tobacco to minors (below 18 years of age) within 100 yards of educational institutes. COTPA bill, 2020 proposed prohibition of selling tobacco to minors (below 21 years of age) within 100 meters of educational institutes. Punishment is up to ₹ 200.
  + Mandatory depiction of statutory warnings on tobacco products (85% of area both sides with 60% being pictorial and 25% textual).
  + Tar and nicotine contents should be clearly mentioned on products.
  + Ban on tobacco and its product's advertisements, promotion and sponsorship **(TAPS)**. **MPOWER** strategy is one of "best buys" for tobacco control. |

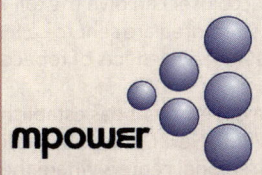

Monitor tobacco use and prevention policies
Protect people from tobacco smoke
Offer help to quit tobacco use
Warn about the dangers of tobacco
Enforce bans on tobacco advertising, promotion and sponsorship
Raise taxes on tobacco

- All tobacco products shall have legible and readable with black color font on white background textual health warning as follow:
  - Manufactured/imported/packaged on or after 1st December 2022—"TOBACCO CAUSES PAINFUL DEATH"
  - Manufactured/imported/packaged on or after 1st December 2023—"TOBACCO USERS DIE YOUNGER".
- Prevention of Food Adulteration Act, 1954 and Rules, 1955, and 1st Amendment Rules, 2004, applicable for paan masala/chewing tobacco. The ingredients are needed to be displayed.
- Cable Television Networks (Amendment) Rules, GSR 138(E), 27th February 2009: Direct advertising of tobacco products on cable television networks shall be prohibited.
- Food Safety and Standards (Packaging and Labelling) Regulations, 2011: These regulations require packages-containing food products to state name of the food, list ingredients, food additives, colors and flavors, name and complete address of the manufacturer, packager or importer, declare weight of the contents, date of packing, month and year up to which the product is best for consumption.
- Juvenile Justice (Care and Protection of Children) Act, 2015: Prohibits sale/gift of tobacco products to minors (under 18 years of age).
- Goods and Services Tax (GST) 2017: A Central Government tax that applies the highest tax slab.
- Tobacco vendor licensing requirement, 2018. States can require tobacco vendors to register with their municipal authority for a license to sell tobacco products.
- Government of India prohibited the production, manufacture, import, export, advertisement and use of electronic cigarettes.
- A film/television programs, displaying tobacco products or their use should fulfil statutory guidelines under the COTPA film and TV rules as below:
  - A strong editorial justification explaining the necessity of display of tobacco products/their use in films to the Central Board of Film Certification
  - At the beginning and middle of a film/TV program
    - An audiovisual "disclaimer" of at least 20-seconds duration on harmful effects of tobacco use
    - Minimum of 30-seconds duration of anti-tobacco health spots information
  - At the bottom of the screen during the period of display/use of tobacco products shall clearly have anti-tobacco health warning as a prominent static message.

Prohibition of Electronic Cigarettes (Production, Manufacture, Import, Export, Transport, Sale, Distribution, Storage and Advertisement) Act (2019)

Electronic Nicotine Delivery System (ENDS): Also called "e-cigs," "vapes," "e-hookahs," and "vape pens," available in the Indian market since around 2007, do not burn tobacco but use a heated liquid to deliver an aerosol-containing nicotine. Nicotine absorption from ENDS can be higher than from cigarettes and can cause acute nicotine toxicity and other respiratory, cardiovascular diseases. This is a step in the right direction to protect future generations from the perils of emerging nicotine products and a strong measure towards the Tobacco Endgame.

Key features:
- Act completely prohibits the production, manufacture, import, export, transport, sale, distribution, storage and advertisement of ENDS.
- Applicable all over India
- Futuristic: Banning not only e-cigarettes, but also heat-not-burn devices, e-hookahs and other similar devices that could be introduced in the coming years.[11,15,16]

Cessation programs:

mCessation: A text message-based mobile phone health project called mCessation was created by the MoHFW in collaboration with the WHO and the International Telecommunications Union in 2016 as part of its "Be Healthy, Be Mobile" campaign to assist tobacco users in giving up. To speak with program experts and learn how to stop using tobacco, any tobacco user can give the toll-free number **011-22901701** a missed call. Text messages that are time-specific and structured are sent to callers' mobile phones. These messages, which are sent to the person daily, center on the negative effects of tobacco use, strategies to lessen cravings, total cessation, etc.[11,17]

National Tobacco Quitline Services: The government has established a national level tobacco cessation quit line at Vallabhbhai Patel Chest Institute (VPCI), New Delhi, with a toll-free number **(1800-112-356).** These services have been extended to different regional centers where the support is provided in the regional language.[18]

Tobacco-free educational institutes (TEFI):
Seeing the menace of tobacco misuse amongst adolescents, "tobacco-free educational institute" was initiated. Various provisions included were:
- In and around the campus, there should be display of signage, such as "Tobacco Free Educational Institute", "Tobacco Free Area", and "No Tobacco Use".
- Prohibition of sale of tobacco products within 100 yards of the institute.
- Nomination of "Tobacco Monitors", who are responsible for identifying any violations of the institute's tobacco-free initiatives.
- Not to participate in any of the events sponsored by tobacco companies.

Tobacco Cessation Center (TCC):[19]
TCC is fixed premises where qualified healthcare professionals/counselors who are trained in both psychological and pharmacological interventions provide tobacco (smoke and smokeless form) cessation therapy to help patients in their attempts to quit the habit.

Objectives: To provide patient care services and community awareness.

Guidelines for patient care services:
- Within the premises of medical institution, beneficiaries should have access to tobacco cessation services.
- Offer various tobacco cessation services—behavioral and pharmacotherapy and relapse prevention.
- Services for tobacco-related medical conditions or with other existing medical conditions (tuberculosis, diabetes, hypertension, respiratory diseases, cardiovascular diseases, cancer, etc.)
- Offer Services to patient attendees/any accompanying person using tobacco.
- Integrate the TCC with prenatal care, pediatric care and adolescent care so as to provide services for vulnerable groups visiting hospital.
- Integrating TCC with AYUSH
- Establish referral services.
- Monitor effectiveness of TCC services by establishing a robust data management mechanism.

Guidelines for community awareness:
- Screening for lifestyle diseases including tobacco use, cancer screening.
- Mass community awareness activities at schools, institutions or health centers.
- Train undergraduate and postgraduate medical students, health workers and allied and healthcare professionals in organizing and conducting community-based tobacco cessation activities.
- Promote and increase visibility of the TCC through advertisements.
- Sensitize grass root health workers (ASHA/ANM/CHO) to refer tobacco users to the nearby TCC.

Coordination and collaboration: For smooth functioning of the TCC, in-charge should establish sustained coordination with concerned departments in the medical Institute to strengthen cross-referrals and also with with State Nodal Office.

Monitoring and evaluation	It is done at different levels of the program's implementation. **State level:** By strict enforcement of COTPA Act and challan mechanism, random checks at public places. **District level:** "Enforcement squads" which is responsible for monitoring and random checks at public places. **Educational institutes:** Institute will get certificate as "Tobacco-Free Educational Institutes" only after getting a self-evaluation scorecard score of 90%.
National Tobacco Control Policy: A vision for tobacco free by 2040 and beyond[20-22]	Over the past two decades, India has made significant progress in tobacco control, following a multisectoral approach. India now needs to take tobacco control to the next level of the Endgame vision by formulating a comprehensive National Tobacco Control Policy. It will be a global initiative which will serve as a roadmap for a 'Tobacco-Free India' and 'Tobacco-Free Future Generation' by 2040. The proposed policy envisages safeguarding and dissuading adolescents and youth for using any form of tobacco or use of ENDS. The NMT21C (No More Tobacco in the 21st Century) campaign and interventions for 'Tobacco-Free Future Generation' will be coordinated with GoI's ongoing efforts of implementing Tobacco-Free Educational Institution (ToFEI) guidelines.

> **Vision:** Creating a healthy, economically self-reliant and tobacco-free future for all.
> **Goal:** De-normalizing tobacco use and ensure less than 5% prevalence of tobacco use (among 15+ years population) in India by 2040.
> **Key components:**
> - Strict regulation and legislation
> - Public education and awareness campaigns
> - Support for cessation

References

1. Guidelines for Tobacco Free Educational Institution (Revised). Ministry of Health and Family Welfare, Government of India. Available from: https://ntcp.mohfw.gov.in/assets/document/TEFI-Guidelines.pdf. [Last accessed 15 July, 2024]
2. Tobacco Fact Sheet. World Health Organization; 2023. Available from https://www.who.int/news-room/fact-sheets/detail/tobacco. [Last accessed 15 July, 2024]
3. WHO global report on trends in prevalence of tobacco use 2000-2025, fourth edition. WHO, Geneva, 2021
4. Tobacco in India. World Health Organization; 2022. Available from: https://www.who.int/india/health-topics/tobacco. [Last accessed 16 July, 2024]
5. J. Kishore. National Anti-Tobacco Program. National Health Programs of India –15th edition. Century publications. New Delhi
6. GATS-2 Global Adult Tobacco Survey Fact Sheet India 2016–17. Available from: https://www. tobaccofreekids.org/assets/global/pdfs/en/GATS_ India_2016-17_FactSheet.pdf. [Last accessed 17 July, 2024]
7. Tata Institute of Social Sciences (TISS), Ministry of Health and Family Welfare, Government of India. Global Adult Tobacco Survey-2 India 2016–17. Mumbai: TISS; 2018. Available from: https://tiss. edu/view/6/mumbai-campus/school-of-healthsystems-studies/global-adult-tobacco-survey-2- india-2016-17/outcomespublications-3/. [Last accessed 17 July, 2024]
8. Ministry of Health and Family Welfare, Government of India, International Institute of Population Sciences. GYTS-4 Global Youth Tobacco Survey- Fact Sheet India. Mumbai: IIPS; 2021. Available from: https:// ntcp.nhp.gov.in/assets/document/National_Fact_Sheet_of_fourth_round_of_Global_Youth_Tobacco_ Survey_GYTS-4.pdf. [Last accessed 17 July, 2024]
9. National Tobacco Control Cell. Ministry of Health and Family Welfare, Government of India.Operational Guidelines . National Tobacco Control Programme. 2015.[Internet]. Available from: https://ntcp.mohfw.gov.in/assets/document/Guideline-manuals/Operational-Guidelines-National-Tobacco-Control-Programme.pdf [last access 25th January 2025]
10. Ministry of Health and Family Welfare ,Government of India. Operational Guidelines for National Tobacco testing laboratories.2019. [Internet].Available from: https://ncdc.mohfw.gov.in/wp-content/uploads/2024/05/3-Operational-Guidelines-for-NTTL.pdf [last access 25th January 2025].
11. Ministry of Health and Family Welfare, Government of India. Report on Tobacco Control in India 2022 .[Internet].2024. Available from: https://ntcp.mohfw.gov.in/assets/document/surveys-reports-publications/Report%20on%20Tobacco%20Control%20in%20India%202022_22%20April%202024.pdf. [Last accessed 24th Jan 2025]
12. National Health Mission. (2021). The Cigarettes and Other Tobacco Products (Prohibition of Advertisement and Regulation of Trade and Commerce, Production, Supply and Distribution) Act, 2003 and Related Rules. Available from: https://nhm.gov.in/index4.php?lang=1andlevel=0andlinkid=459andlid=692. [Last accessed 17 July, 2024]
13. The Cigarettes and Other Tobacco Products (Prohibition of Advertisement and Regulation of Trade and Commerce, Production, Supply and Distribution) Act, 2003. https://ntcp.mohfw.gov.in/assets/document/Acts-Rules-Regulations/COTPA-2003-English-Version.pdf. [Last accessed 17 July, 2024]
14. The Cigarettes and Other Tobacco Products (Prohibition of Advertisement and Regulation of Trade and Commerce, Production, Supply and Distribution) Amendment Bill 2020.pdf. Available from https://ntcp.mohfw.gov.in/assets/document/Cigarettes%20and%20other%20Tobacco%20Products%20(Prohibition%20of%20Advertisement%20and%20Regulation%20of%20Trade%20and%20Commerce,%20Production,%20Supply%20and%20Distribution)%20Amendment%20Rules,%202023.pdf. [Last accessed 18 July, 2024]
15. Chakma JK, Kumar H, Bhargava S, Khanna T. The e-cigarettes ban in India: an important public health decision. Lancet Public Health. 2020;5(8):e426. doi: 10.1016/S2468-2667(20)30063-3.
16. The Prohibition of Electronic Cigarettes (Production, Manufacture, Import, Export, Transport, Sale, Distribution, Storage and Advertisement) Act, 2019. Available from: https://ntcp.mohfw.gov.in/assets/document/The-Prohibition-of-Electronic-Cigarettes-Production-Manufacture-Import-Export-Transport-Sale-Distribution-Storage-and-Advertisement)-Act-2019.pdf. [Last accessed 20 July 2024]
17. World Health Organisation. WHO quitting toolkit: World Health Organisation, 2021.[Internet]. Available from: https://www.who.int/publications/m/item/who-quitting-toolkit.[Last accessed 25th Jan 2025]
18. mTobaccoCessation [Internet]. Available from: https://www.who.int/campaigns/world-no-tobacco-day/2021/quitting-toolkit/text-message-support/mtobaccocessation. [Last accessed 17 July, 2024]

19. Ministry of Health and Family Welfare, Government of India. National Tobacco Control Programme.National Tobacco Quit Line Services (NTQLS) [Internet].2018. Available from: https://ntcp.mohfw.gov.in/national_tobacco_quit_line_services [Cited 2025 Jan 25]
20. Ministry of Health and Family Welfare, Government of India. Operational Guidelines for Establishing Tobacco Cessation Centers in Medical Institution.[Internet].2024. Available from:https://ntcp.mohfw.gov.in/assets/document/Guideline-manuals/Operational%20Guidelines%20for%20Establishing%20Tobacco%20Cessation%20Centres%20in%20Medical%20Institutions.pdf. [Last assessed on 24th January 2025]
21. Swasticharan L, Arora M, Sinha P, Ray C, Munish V, Shrivastava R. Report on Tobacco Control in India 2022. Volume 2. WHO. Ministry of Health and Family Welfare, Government of India, Nirman Bhawan, Maulana Azad Road New Delhi 110011, India.
22. Prof Beaglehole R, Prof Bonita R, Derek Yach, et al.A tobacco-free world: a call to action to phase out the sale of tobacco products by 2040. Lancet. 2015;385(9972):10118. Available from: https://doi.org/10.1016/S0140-6736(15)60133-7.

QUESTIONS

Long Answer Question (LAQ)

1. Trace briefly the tobacco control initiatives in India since 2004. Describe briefly the components and three tier implementation framework of the National Tobacco Control Programme.

Short Answer Questions (SAQs)

1. Write briefly on tobacco cessation initiatives in India.
2. Describe briefly the provisions under "Tobacco-free educational institutes" in India.

Multiple Choice Questions (MCQs)

1. **Estimated tobacco users in the world are:**
   a. 100 crores
   b. 130 crores
   c. 80 crores
   d. 150 crores
2. **According to Global Adult Tobacco Survey 2016-17, prevalence of smokeless tobacco use in India is:**
   a. 10.7%
   b. 21.4%
   c. 12.3%
   d. 21.3%
3. **GYTS is conducted among which age group?**
   a. 15–24 years
   b. 10–19 years
   c. 20–24 years
   d. 13–15 years
4. **All are true *except*, COTPA Act 2003:**
   a. Prohibition of smoking in public places
   b. Prohibition of selling tobacco to minors (below 18 years of age)
   c. Prohibition of selling tobacco to minors (below 21 years of age)
   d. MPOWER strategy
5. **MPOWER include all, *except*:**
   a. M-Monitor tobacco use
   b. P-Protect people from tobacco smoke
   c. E- Enforce ban on TAPS
   d. R-Raise awareness

Chapter 57: National Tobacco Control Programme

6. **National Tobacco Testing Laboratories (NTTLs), Apex center is at:**
   a. Ghaziabad and Mumbai
   b. Ghaziabad
   c. Mumbai
   d. Guwahati
7. **Prohibition of Electronic Cigarettes Act (2019) ban on:**
   a. Only e-cigarettes
   b. e-cigarettes, heat-not-burn devices, e-hookahs, e-pens
   c. e-cigarettes, vape pens, e-hookahs
   d. e-cigarettes, e-hookahs
8. **According to Global Action Plan for Prevention and Control of NCD—targets set for tobacco use prevalence by 2025 is:**
   a. 30% reduction in prevalence of current tobacco user
   b. 10% reduction in prevalence of current tobacco user among adults
   c. 30% relative reduction in prevalence of current tobacco user in persons aged 15+ years
   d. 10% relative reduction in prevalence of current tobacco user among adults

Answers

1. b
2. b
3. d
4. c
5. d
6. a
7. b
8. c

58 CHAPTER

National Oral Health Programme

Lakshay Beri, Parul Sharma, Bharti Koria

Background/ Need of program/ Scheme	• Nearly 3.5 million people across the world affected with oral disease, disorders and conditions related to it.[1] • Oral health profile has been improved for many countries, but not for India • A multicentric survey by MOHFW-WHO India in 2007-08 found prevalence of dental caries in children 12 years' age 23–71.5%, in adults 48.1–86.4% and in elderly 51.6–95.1%. As same prevalence of periodontal problems among adults was found about 15.3–77.9%[2] • Various risk factors for such conditions are tobacco use, alcohol use, poor oral hygiene, infections, etc.[3] • Considering above facts India is in much need to address the situation with broad coverage of all age groups and last end areas.
Implemented since	2014-15—initiative under Twelfth Five Year Plan 1995—National Oral Health Policy drafted with the help of Indian Dental Association was accepted as a part of National Health Policy[3]
Goal	To strengthen public health facility with respect to accessible, affordable and quality oral healthcare delivery.[3]
Objectives	• To improve determinants of oral health and to reduce disparity in oral health accessibility in rural and urban population. • To reduce morbidity from oral diseases by strengthening oral health services initially at district and subdistrict level. • To integrate oral health services with other general health services especially with other national health programs. • To encourage promotion of public private partnership models for achieving better public health goals.
Organogram	• **National Oral health Cell (NOHC):** This comprises administrative and technical personnel under the overall guidance of Deputy Director General (NCD) in DGHS (Directorate General of Health Services) and Joint Secretary (NOHP). They will be assisted by Chief Medical Officer In-Charge of NOHP and a National Consultant. Overall implementation of the program will be seen by Joint Secretary and Under Secretary. • **State Oral Health Cell (SOHC):** At the state level, State Nodal Officer would be the in charge of NOHP. This cell would work in collaboration with the State NCD Cell existing for other existing NCD programs. • **District Oral Health Cell (DOHC):** The District Oral Health Cell will be headed by an identified District Oral Health Officer. They will share manpower available with district for other existing programs for non-communicable diseases.[4]
Components (National Oral Health Policy 2021)	• Raising the **fund:** For strengthening and broadening the scope of oral health care across the country. • Provision of comprehensive **oral health care**: Promotive and preventive measures, such as promoting healthy eating habits, oral health education in pregnant women, preventing tobacco/alcohol abuse, IEC/BCC, oral health screening, tooth-brushing activities in school, dental cleaning, fluoride varnish application and pit and fissure sealant programs. • To raise adequate **infrastructure** in the three tier healthcare delivery system of the country with a special focus on rural, hard to reach and tribal areas. • To establish an **oral health-promoting environment conducive** to lead a quality life. It commits to provide appropriate preventive and promotive measures for all age groups, with a special focus on priority populations. • To promote **involvement of community leaders**, Panchayati Raj Institutions, self help groups and civil society to empower communities to take informed decisions, facilitate need-based planning, implement, monitor, and evaluate the activities.[2]

Strategies/ Deliverables under the program	• **IEC and behavior change communication (BCC):** These shall include instructions on oral hygiene, simple methods of prevention of oral problems, dietary counseling, early identification and referral, oral care for pregnant women, instructions during school program on dental caries prevention, analgesics for toothache, etc. • **Training:** General oral health training of all healthcare staff and special training of nodal officers. • **Human resources:** Hiring of dental surgeons, dental hygienists and dental assistants on contract basis. • **Logistic support:** Provision of dental chair with equipment and consumables. • **Comprehensive program management:** Involves coordination and linkages with various stakeholders.
Activities at various levels	**Tertiary level activities (central level activities)** • Designing IEC material be shared with other states. • Organizing national/regional training programs • Conduct national and regional workshops to train the paramedical health functionaries **District level activities (under the umbrella of NHM):** • Manpower support (dentist, dental hygienist and dental assistant) • Logistic supply, such as consumable and equipments • Regular IEC, training and capacity building
Monitoring and evaluation	The program shall be monitored at all the levels from district to central level, utilizing existing HR support of noncommunicable disease (NCD) cell and under the program.

References

1. World Health Organization. Oral diseases. Available from www.who.int [online] . Last accessed on 26/01/2025.
2. National Oral Health Programme, draft National Oral Health Policy 2021. MOHFW, GOI.
3. National Oral Health Programme, Annual Report 2020-21, MOHFW, GOI, Nirman Bhawan, New Delhi. [online]
4. Operational guidelines. National Oral Health Programme 2012-17. MOHFW, GOI. [online]

QUESTIONS

Long Answer Question (LAQ)

1. Describe in detail components and strategies of NOHP.

Short Answer Questions (SAQs)

1. Enumerate objectives of NOHP.
2. Describe briefly activities under NOHP.

Multiple Choice Questions (MCQs)

1. The Indian Dental Association was formed in the year:
   a. 1947
   b. 1948
   c. 1949
   d. 1950
2. The first initiative of oral health program was taken in the year:
   a. 1947
   b. 1948
   c. 1949
   d. 1995

3. Which five year plan was pioneer to National Oral Health Programme?
   a. 10th FYP
   b. 12th FYP
   c. 16th FYP
   d. 18th FYP
4. Tertiary level activities include all, *except*:
   a. Designing IEC material
   b. Training programs
   c. Workshops
   d. None of above
5. District level activities under oral health program include, *except*:
   a. Manpower support
   b. Logistic supply
   c. Regular IEC
   d. None of above
6. National Oral Health Programme directly coms under control of:
   a. Deputy director NCD
   b. Deputy director CD
   c. Secretariat HFW
   d. Commissioner HFW
7. Risk factors for oral problems includes all, *except*:
   a. Alcohol
   b. Smoking
   c. Gargling
   d. Non hygiene
8. A nationwide survey regarding oral health was done in the year:
   a. 1947
   b. 1999
   c. 2001
   d. 2007
9. Core components of National Oral Health Programme includes following:
   a. Manpower training
   b. Fund raising
   c. Logistic management
   d. All of above
10. Tooth decay is mainly caused by:
    a. Acid
    b. Fibers
    c. Calcium
    d. Fluoride

Answers

1. b	2. d	3. b	4. d	5. d
6. c	7. d	8. d	9. d	10. a

CHAPTER 59

National Sickle Cell Anemia Elimination Programme

Mansi Kala, Shaili Vyas, Pritesh Patel

Background/Need of program/Scheme	A single base pair mutation in the B globin gene is the source of sickle cell disease, a monogenetic condition. The homozygous state inheritance is the most frequent kind, although co-inheritance of HbS and HbC is more common in Africa. Clinical manifestation of sickle β thalassemia varies. Numerous thoughts and studies have been prompted by the protection against malaria in sickle cell disease sufferers. With 8.6% of the world's population being tribal, India has the highest concentration of these populations worldwide. The Sickle gene is widespread in the tribal population, with prevalence ranging from 1–40%. The condition has major financial and economic repercussions, including screening, emergency and primary care, medications, hospital stays, blood transfusions, and bone marrow transplants.[1]
Implemented since	On July 1, 2023, Prime Minister Narendra Modi announced the National Sickle Cell Anemia Elimination Mission. The mission's objectives are to identify, stop, and treat sickle cell anemia in India's tribal and high-prevalence areas. The initial focus will be on 17 states with high SCD prevalence, with plans to expand to non-tribal districts. The initiative aims to minimize redundancy and optimize resource use by integrating with National Health Mission (NHM) processes.
Goal	To eliminate sickle cell anemia as a public health problem in India before 2047.
Targets	It will target individuals from 0–40 years of age and pregnant woman
Objectives[1]	• Provision of affordable, accessible and quality care to all SCD patients. • To reduce the prevalence of SCD and sickle cell trait
Organogram	In India, the Sickle Cell Disease Programme is run at several administrative levels using a hierarchical organizational framework. Overseeing the Programme Sub-Committee are NGOs and several departments under the direction of the State Health Society. This structure is replicated at the district and block levels, where representatives from the relevant departments serve as committee chairs. Village/Urban Health Committees organize neighborhood groups for screening events and awareness initiatives at the local level.
Beneficiaries	As part of the National Health Mission, the initiative would concentrate on population-based screening, prevention, and management of sickle cell anemia in all tribal and other high-prevalence states/UTs of India, starting at age zero and extending gradually up to age forty. The goal would progressively expand to include all states and UTs, with an initial concentration on high incidence and tribal states. In three and a half years, the goal is to test, counsel, and treat seven crore individuals for sickle cell disease.
Components[1]	**Human Resources** • **Use of current human resources:** States are urged to make efficient use of current staff members in order to prevent and eradicate SCD. • **Additional provision:** States may alter responsibilities in light of local circumstances, but there will be one counselor for every two PHC/UPHC-HWCs for counseling and facilitating services. **Module Construction** • **Expert team:** The MoHFW assembled a group of specialists on SCD who created comprehensive training materials. • **Target personnel:** At Ayushman Bharat Health and Wellness Center (AB-HWC), training modules are created for primary healthcare workers, like as medical officers, community health officers, staff nurses,

	MPW/ASHA: Training Modules • Medical Officers: • Community Health Officers: • Staff Nurses: • MPW/ASHA: **Availability of Training Materials** • Copies of training materials will be provided to all states. • Digital versions will be available on the sickle cell support corner, sickle cell portal developed by MoHFW, and websites of MoHFW and NHSRC.

Strategies/
Deliverables under
the program
	Sensitization and Community Awareness: Make house calls and participate in IEC events through the media.
	Engage Influential Members of the Community: Provide support groups and therapy.
	• **Diagnosis and screening:**
	  ✦ Set up camps with MMUs in schools and other isolated locations.
	  ✦ Provide counseling and provide referrals for further evaluation and care.
	  ✦ Assist with adoption program registration.
	• **Primary healthcare level activities:**
	  ✦ Perform teleconsultations and screenings.
	  ✦ Offer guidance and preventative actions.
	  ✦ Handle emergencies and start hydroxyurea.
	• **Specialized care and capacity building:**
	  ✦ Offer prenatal screening and transfusion at tertiary facilities.
	  ✦ Create COEs in relation to bone marrow transplants.
	  ✦ Assist in developing healthcare workers' capacity.
	• **Program performance monitoring and evaluation:**
	  ✦ Establish an electronic register.
	  ✦ Make modifications and effect assessments using data.
	• **Advocacy and policy formulation:**
	  ✦ Create standards and promote the inclusion of PMJAY.
	  ✦ Encourage studies on the management of SCD.

Activities at various level or package of services	**Basic prevention:** • To avoid having a kid with a homozygous genotype, premarital and preconception counseling will be provided. • To prevent sickle cell disease in offspring, genetic counseling and testing will be implemented in areas with a high frequency. • Due to cultural and ideological disparities on genetic issues, such as human reproduction, community support and engagement will be essential. **Screening and secondary prevention:** • Early identification and treatment of sickle cell illness by screening for the sickle cell trait, which lowers mortality and enhances quality of life. • Primary, secondary, and tertiary care therapy of sickle cell disease **Tertiary prevention and screening:** • Advanced diagnosis and treatment techniques at tertiary institutions; • Management of sickle cell disease at the primary, secondary, and tertiary care levels • Integration of AYUSH • Assistance for patients • Adoption by the community
Monitoring and evaluation of program	Through dashboards, the sickle cell portal will track mission progress and offer resources at the federal, state, and local levels. Under collaboration with NITI Aayog, performance evaluation and grading will be based on predetermined metrics. • Total sick cell disease screened patients • Evaluation of screening and outreach efforts among the targeted demographics. • Amount of patients with sickle cell trait diagnosed • Finds trait carriers who might pass on the illness to their progeny. • Number of people with sickle cell illness diagnosed

Chapter 59: National Sickle Cell Anemia Elimination Programme

- Shows prevalence and verifies instances that need to be managed.
- Total number of ill individuals filed at institutions
- Monitors how patients interact with medical services.
- Count of patients getting penicillin injection for prophylaxis
- Assures infection prevention, which is essential for managing diseases.
- The quantity of patients receiving care.

Reference

1. OperationalGuidelines.pdf [Internet]. [cited 2024 Oct 7]. Available from: https://sickle.nhm.gov.in/uploads/english/OperationalGuidelines.pdf

QUESTIONS

Long Answer Question (LAQ)

1. Describe in detail about the national sickle cell anemia elimination program with specific mention of the strategies under the program.

Short Answer Questions (SAQs)

1. Explain how will you monitor the sickle cell elimination program in your region?
2. Describe the activities performed under sickle cell elimination program.

Multiple Choice Questions (MCQs)

1. India set a goal to eliminate SCD by the year:
   a. 2027
   b. 2037
   c. 2047
   d. 2057
2. Beneficiaries of National Sickle cell Anemia Elimination Mission are:
   a. 0–18 years of age
   b. 0–40 years of age
   c. 0–5 years of age
   d. 0–2 years of age
3. National Sickle cell Anemia Elimination Mission was launched in:
   a. 2021
   b. 2022
   c. 2023
   d. 2024
4. To realize the aims of National Sickle cell Anemia Elimination Mission the following platforms can be used:
   a. Anemia Mukt Bharat
   b. IMNCI
   c. IDSP
   d. NTEP

Answers

1. c
2. b
3. c
4. a

CHAPTER 60

National Programme for Prevention and Management of Trauma and Burn Injuries (NPPMT&BI)

Immanual Joshua, Vinothini J, Sanjeev Pandey, Akhil Dhanesh Goel, Rudresh Negi

Background/Need of program/Scheme	The Global Status Report on Road Safety 2018 states that in 2016, annual road traffic deaths rose to 1.35 million. Road traffic injuries are now the leading cause of death for individuals aged 5–29 and the eighth leading cause of death for all age groups. In India, road injuries are among the top four leading causes of death and health loss for people aged.[1] Many regions, especially those along major highways and in densely populated urban areas, struggle with insufficient healthcare infrastructure and a shortage of trained personnel to handle emergencies effectively.[2] To address these gaps, the goal is to reduce fatalities and improve recovery outcomes by enhancing emergency care and specialized burn management.
Implemented since	The trauma care initiative started as a pilot project during the 9th Five Year Plan (FYP) and was later expanded to a national level during the 11th and 12th FYPs. Similarly, the Burn Injury Management component was launched as a pilot during the 11th FYP and implemented nationwide during the 12th FYP. In 2017, these two components were merged into the "National Programme for Prevention and Management of Trauma and Burn Injuries".[3]
Goal	The primary goal of the NPPMT&BI is to reduce the incidence, severity, and mortality of trauma and burn injuries through a comprehensive and integrated approach that includes emergency care, injury prevention, and rehabilitation services.
Objectives	**Trauma care objectives** • Establish a network of trauma care facilities aimed at reducing preventable deaths from traffic accidents by adhering to the golden hour principle. • Develop an efficient referral and communication system between ambulances, trauma centers, and within trauma centers themselves. • Develop a National Injury Surveillance and Trauma Registry along with a Capacity Building Centre to collect, compile, analyze, and disseminate data for informed policy-making and preventive measures. • Set up trauma registry centers to ensure the provision of high-quality services. • Formulate a National Trauma System Plan. • Enhance public awareness through targeted IEC (Information, education, and communication) activities.[4] **Burn care objectives** • Set up burn units with the necessary facilities for managing and rehabilitating burn injuries in designated government medical colleges and district hospitals. • Raise awareness about burn injuries among the public, especially targeting women, children, and workers in industrial and hazardous occupations. • Create a Burn Data Registry integrated with the National Injury Surveillance Centre to collect, analyze, and use burn injury data to reduce the number of cases. • Conduct research to understand the behavioral, social, and other factors contributing to burn injuries, which will help in planning, monitoring, and evaluating effective programs. • Provide training programs on burn injury management for doctors, nurses, and paramedical staff in the identified district hospitals and government medical colleges.[5]

Chapter 60: National Programme for Prevention and Management of Trauma and Burn Injuries (NPPMT&BI)

Organogram	The NPPMT&BI is run by the Trauma and Burns Division (PMU) in the Hospital-II Section of the Ministry of Health and Family Welfare. The structure is as follows: • **National level:** The Ministry of Health and Family Welfare, overseen by the Health and Family Welfare Minister. • **State level:** State Health Departments, which handle the program's implementation in selected hospitals. • **District level:** District Hospitals, Civil Hospitals, and Medical Colleges, responsible for carrying out the program's activities locally.
Beneficiaries	• **Trauma care:** Government District Hospitals, Civil Hospitals, and Medical Colleges with 100 or more beds (or fewer in NE/hilly regions) located on or near accident-prone roads. • **Burn care:** State Government Medical Colleges with high caseloads of burn injuries.[3]
Component	The program comprises two main components: • **Trauma care:** Focused on strengthening emergency facilities, including infrastructure development (OT/ICU/wards), procurement of essential equipment, and human resource augmentation. • **Burn injury management:** Emphasizes the establishment of dedicated burn units with specialized infrastructure, equipment, and trained personnel.[3]
Strategies/Deliverables under the program	• **Infrastructure development:** Establishment and upgrading of trauma and burn care facilities in selected hospitals. • **Training and capacity building:** Training of doctors, nurses, and paramedics in emergency care techniques (BLS and ATLS). • **Public awareness:** IEC activities to educate the public on first aid and good Samaritan laws. • **Data collection and research:** Establishment of National Injury Surveillance Centers for data collection and analysis. • **Resource allocation:** Financial assistance for infrastructure, equipment, and human resources. • Funding is allocated with a 60:40 split between the Central and State Governments, with North-East and Hilly States receiving 90% from the Central Government and 10% from the State Governments, and Union Territories without legislatures receiving 100% of the funding from the Central Government.[3]

Activities at various level or package of services	• **Primary level:**
	  ✦ Basic first aid and initial treatment for both trauma and burns
	  ✦ Stabilization and immediate transportation to higher-level facilities
	  Facilities:
	  ✦ Local emergency centers providing initial care
	  Training:
	  ✦ Community-based first aid and basic life support (BLS) for responders
	• **Secondary level:**
	  ✦ Intermediate trauma and burn care at district hospitals
	  ✦ Specialized trauma and burn units for emergency treatment and stabilization
	  Facilities:
	  ✦ Trauma and burn wards in district hospitals
	  Training:
	  ✦ Advanced trauma life support (ATLS) and burn injury management training for healthcare professionals
	  ✦ Trauma technician and burn care courses
	• **Tertiary level:**
	  ✦ Comprehensive trauma and burn care including surgeries and intensive care
	  ✦ Specialized trauma and burn centers with advanced facilities
	  Facilities:
	  ✦ Regional trauma and burn centers with advanced diagnostic and treatment capabilities
	  Training and research:
	  ✦ Specialized training programs for advanced trauma and burn care
	  ✦ Trauma and burn registries for data analysis and policy formulation

	- **Quaternary level:**
	  + High-tech and comprehensive care for severe trauma and burns, including rehabilitation
	  + Premier centers with extensive resources and specialized services
	Facilities:
	  + National Trauma and Burn Care Centers with integrated services and advanced technology
	  + Regional Apex Trauma Centers with heli-ambulance services
	Training and research:
	  + Cutting-edge training and research programs
	  + Coordination with national and international agencies for continuous improvement in trauma and burn care[3]

Monitoring and evaluation of program	- **Monitoring mechanisms:** Regular field visits and inspections by the Trauma and Burns Unit to ensure compliance with program guidelines. - **Data reporting:** Hospitals are required to submit periodic reports on service delivery, infrastructure status, and patient outcomes. - **Evaluation:** Annual reviews by a Screening Committee and approval from the Hon'ble Health and Family Welfare Minister to assess the program's effectiveness and identify areas for improvement.[3,6,7]

References

1. Wang K, Li Z. Global, regional, and national burdens of road injuries from 1990 to 2021: Findings from the 2021 Global Burden of Disease Study. Injury. 2025 Mar 1;56(3):112221.
2. Kumar A. The Transformation of The Indian Healthcare System. Cureus. 15(5): e39079.
3. National programme for Prevention & Management of Trauma & Burn Injuries (NPPMT&BI) | Ministry of Health and Family Welfare | GOI [Internet]. [cited 2025 Feb 19]. Available from: https://mohfw.gov.in/?q=basicpage-6
4. Prog brief Trauma component .pdf [Internet]. [cited 2025 Feb 19]. Available from: https://mohfw.gov.in/sites/default/files/Prog%20brief%20Trauma%20component%20.pdf
5. Prog brief Burn component.pdf [Internet]. [cited 2025 Feb 19]. Available from: https://mohfw.gov.in/sites/default/files/Prog%20brief%20Burn%20component.pdf
6. Monitoring Format NPPMBI.pdf [Internet]. [cited 2025 Feb 19]. Available from: https://mohfw.gov.in/sites/default/files/Monitoring%20Format%20NPPMBI.pdf
7. Monitoring reporting format for TCF .pdf [Internet]. [cited 2025 Feb 19]. Available from: https://mohfw.gov.in/sites/default/files/Monitoring%20reporting%20format%20for%20TCF%20.pdf

QUESTIONS

Long Answer Question (LAQ)

1. Discuss the objectives and strategies of the National Programme for Prevention and Management of Trauma and Burn Injuries. How are these strategies implemented at primary, secondary and tertiary levels of care?

Short Answer Questions (SAQs)

1. Examine the role of Trauma and Burn Data Registers under the National Programme for Prevention and Management of Trauma and Burn Injuries.
2. How is effective monitoring and evaluation done in the National Programme for Prevention and Management of Trauma and Burn Injuries?

Multiple Choice Questions (MCQs)

1. **The primary goal of NPPMT&BI is:**
   a. To reduce burn injuries by 50%
   b. To reduce the incidence, severity and mortality from trauma and burn injuries
   c. To eliminate all road traffic injuries
   d. To provide universal health coverage
2. **Which of the following principle is crucial in reducing preventable deaths from trauma as per NPPMT&BI?**
   a. Silver hour
   b. Golden hour
   c. First aid principle
   d. Emergency response principle

Answers

1. b
2. b

CHAPTER 61

Pradhan Mantri National Dialysis Programme

Shweta Gangurde (Chauhan), Kajal Srivastava, Parul Sharma, Hinal Baria

Background/Need of program/Scheme	Chronic kidney disease (CKD) is a global public health concern that also poses a significant social and financial burden. It is a chronic illness where the kidneys do not function as they should. In India, an estimated 220,000 more people receive an end-stage renal disease (ESRD) diagnosis each year, necessitating 34 million dialysis sessions.[1] There are currently 4,950 dialysis centers, the most of which are in the private sector, however they are unable to meet this demand. The average session fee for a patient is ₹2,000, or approximately ₹3.4 lakhs, each year. Additionally, patients and their families usually incur large travel fees because they regularly have to travel great distances to receive dialysis services. Almost all impacted households experience extreme financial hardship as a result of this financial load.[2]
Implemented since	Following a presentation by the Secretaries Group on Health and Education, the Hon'able Prime Minister sought a mechanism to improve access to dialysis services in light of this pressing need. The Ministry of Health and Family Welfare (MoHFW) assessed various Public-Private Partnership (PPP) models for dialysis services that have been implemented in states like West Bengal, Kerala, Karnataka, Mumbai, and Delhi NCR with support from the National Health Systems Resource Centre (NHSRC). Experts from PGIMER, AIIMS, and private service providers met on February 16, 2016, to discuss the specifics of the program's implementation. In order to provide free dialysis services to the underprivileged, the Pradhan Mantri National Dialysis Programme (PMNDP) was launched on April 7, 2016, as a component of the National Health Mission (NHM). Ayushman Bharat Health Account (ABHA) IDs can be used by dialysis patients to register on the PMNDP's National PMNDP portal, which was introduced in May 2022.[3]
Goal	The One Nation-One Dialysis program was developed under NHM with the goal of facilitating dialysis services for underprivileged patients wherever in the nation, in keeping with the idea of "One Nation-One Service."
Targets	• As of December 31, 2022, the program has been deployed across all 36 States/UTs, covering 641 districts and 1350 dialysis centers, with 8871 hemodialyzer equipment. • The Government of India has directed the states and union territories to extend PMNDP coverage to every district in the nation.
Objectives	• The Pradhan Mantri National Dialysis Programme (PMNDP) aims to enhance district hospitals by offering affordable dialysis services. • To leverage the existing capacity of the private sector in the dialysis care segment, the program is implemented through public-private partnerships in several states, while others use an in-house system for service delivery. The objectives of the program are: • **Accessibility:** To ensure dialysis services are available in all districts of the country, particularly in rural and underserved areas. • **Affordability:** To reduce the financial burden on patients by providing free or highly subsidized dialysis services. • **Quality care:** To standardize and improve the quality of dialysis services provided in public health facilities. • **Capacity building:** To enhance the capacity of healthcare providers through training and infrastructure development.

Chapter 61: Pradhan Mantri National Dialysis Programme

Organogram	• **Ministry of Health and Family Welfare (MoHFW):** Overall policy formulation, funding allocation, and strategic direction. ↓ • **National Health Mission (NHM) Steering Committee:** Oversight and coordination of the program at the national level. ↓ • **State Nodal Officer:** Implementation and monitoring at the state level, coordination with districts. ↓ • **District Nodal Officer:** Operational management at the district level, ensuring service delivery.
Beneficiaries[3]	• For Below Poverty Line (BPL) economic group: 100% expenses are directly covered under NHM by the government. • For non-BPL patients: They can get treated at the district hospitals by paying the same rates as paid by the government for the BPL patient.
Components	The program has two components, namely hemodialysis (HD) services and peritoneal dialysis (PD) services.
Strategies/Deliverables under the program	• By public-private partnership mode to provide dialysis treatments in district hospitals throughout states. • The service provider should provide medical staff, dialysis machines, RO water plant infrastructure, dialyzers, and consumables. • The payer government should give district hospitals with space, drugs, power, and water, as well as cover the cost of dialysis for low-income patients.
Activities at various level or package of services[3]	• Establishing dialysis centers within district hospitals and various public health facilities is a strategic initiative aimed at enhancing access to advanced dialysis treatments. These centers are furnished with modern dialysis equipment and requisite infrastructure to ensure optimal patient care. • To ensure high standards of care, the engagement of private dialysis service providers is encouraged to oversee and manage the dialysis units and guarantees adherence to stringent care standards. • Furthermore, the implementation of regular training programs for healthcare professionals, including nephrologists, nurses, and technicians, is crucial. These programs are designed to uphold the highest standards of care through continuous professional development. • Additionally, financial assistance from the central government is secured to offset the expenses associated with the establishment of dialysis units and to facilitate the provision of free or subsidized dialysis sessions. This support is instrumental in ensuring equitable access to life-saving treatments.
Monitoring and evaluation of program	Continuous monitoring and process evaluation are necessary to assess the impact of the program at various level of care.

References

1. National Health Systems Resource Centre (NHSRC). Pradhan Mantri National Dialysis Programme (PMNDP). Available from: https://nhsrcindia.org/sites/default/files/2021-07/PMNDP.HD_.pdf
2. Lok Sabha. Pradhan Mantri National Dialysis Programme (PMNDP) - Reference Notes. Available from: https://loksabhadocs.nic.in/Refinput/New_Reference_Notes/English/PRADHAN%20MARI%20NATIONAL%20DIALYSIS%20PROGRAMME.pdf
3. Ministry of Health and Family Welfare (MoHFW). Introduction of Pradhan Mantri National Dialysis Program (PMNDP). Available from: https://pmndp.mohfw.gov.in/en/introduction-of-pradhan-mantri-national-dialysis-program-pmndp

QUESTIONS

Long Answer Question (LAQ)

1. Discuss the rationale behind the implementation of the Pradhan Mantri National Dialysis Programme under the Public-Private Partnership (PPP) model. How does this model address the challenges faced by patients with End-Stage Renal Disease (ESRD) in India?

Section III: National Health Mission

Short Answer Questions (SAQs)

1. How does the One Nation–One Dialysis initiative aim to improve access to dialysis services across India?
2. What strategies are in place under the PMNDP to ensure high standards of care in dialysis services?

Multiple Choice Questions (MCQs)

1. What is the primary public health concern addressed by the Pradhan Mantri National Dialysis Programme (PMNDP)?
   a. Chronic kidney disease (CKD)
   b. Diabetes
   c. Cancer
   d. Heart disease
2. How many new end-stage renal disease (ESRD) diagnoses are estimated to occur each year in India?
   a. 100,000
   b. 220,000
   c. 500,000
   d. 1,000,000
3. When was the Pradhan Mantri National Dialysis Programme (PMNDP) officially launched?
   a. February 16, 2016
   b. April 7, 2016
   c. December 31, 2022
   d. May 1, 2022
4. Which of the following is a key goal of the PMNDP?
   a. To increase the number of dialysis centers in private hospitals
   b. To provide free kidney transplants
   c. To ensure dialysis services are available to underprivileged patients across the nation
   d. To encourage private health insurance for dialysis patients
5. As of December 31, 2022, how many dialysis centers had been established under the PMNDP?
   a. 4950
   b. 1350
   c. 641
   d. 8871
6. Which of the following groups receive 100% coverage for dialysis expenses under the PMNDP?
   a. All citizens
   b. Middle-income families
   c. Below poverty line (BPL) patients
   d. Patients with private health insurance
7. Which of the following is NOT a key objective of the PMNDP?
   a. Accessibility of dialysis services in rural and underserved areas
   b. Affordability by reducing financial burdens
   c. Providing free kidney transplants to all patients
   d. Capacity building through training and infrastructure development
8. What is the approach used by the PMNDP to implement dialysis services in various states?
   a. Public-private partnerships (PPP)
   b. Sole government funding
   c. Private donations
   d. Crowdfunding
9. Which organization is responsible for policy formulation and strategic direction for the PMNDP?
   a. Indian Medical Association
   b. National Health Mission Steering Committee
   c. Ministry of Health and Family Welfare (MoHFW)
   d. World Health Organization
10. What is the role of the district hospitals in the PMNDP's implementation strategy?
    a. To serve as centers for specialized care only for paying patients
    b. To provide space and resources for dialysis centers, covering costs for low-income patients
    c. To recruit patients for private dialysis centers
    d. To ensure dialysis centers are run exclusively by government-employed nephrologists

Answers

1. a
2. b
3. b
4. c
5. b
6. c
7. c
8. a
9. c
10. b

CHAPTER 62

National Programme for Palliative Care

Soumya Swaroop Sahoo, Vipul Nautiyal, Rashmi Bhujade

| **Background/ Need of the program** | As a strategy to improve the quality of life for patients and their families dealing with health issues related to life-threatening illnesses, palliative care (PC) is defined by the World Health Organization (WHO) as preventing and relieving suffering through early detection, assessment, and management of pain and other issues such as psychological, spiritual, and physical issues.[1]
PC can be commenced from diagnosis and endures all through treatment till dissolution support after the death of a patient. It is predicated on the person-centered, holistic concept of chronic care within the framework of acute episodic treatment.[2]
By addressing patients' psychological needs and relieving pain and other physical symptoms, it lessens their suffering. For terminally sick patients, providing a PC is like extending years to their lives. While palliative care is less expensive than most other specialty procedures, it nevertheless has a very high cost-benefit ratio.[3] |
|---|---|

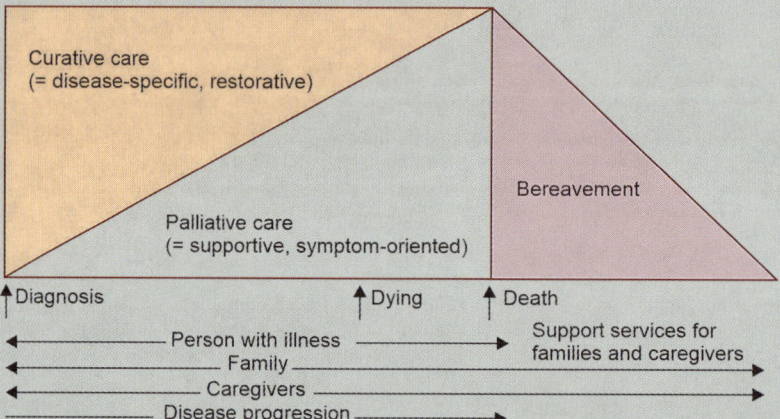

Suggested model of palliative care [adapted from the Integrated Model of Care proposed by the World Health Organization in 1990.[4]

India is now the world's most populated nation, surpassing China. Because of the significant burden of preventable chronic illnesses, people are living longer (because of advances in therapy and medicine). However, this has resulted in a sharp decline in quality of life, financial hardship for families, and strain on the healthcare system. The majority of AIDS patients experience discomfort, and about 80% of cancer patients receive their diagnosis when their disease is already advanced. Palliative care is necessary for these patients because they all have significant medical demands. The only practical course of care and treatment for these people is the management of pain as well as other symptoms. Evidence demonstrates that PC improves hospital compliance with care quality standards, promotes survival, shortens hospital and ICU stays and facilitates transitions between care environments.

The World Health Organization considers PC to be a vital part of comprehensive cancer and AIDS care.

Palliative care is not covered by public or commercial health delivery systems because medical insurance does not cover it, or does not cover it sufficiently, and because the majority of health policies do not acknowledge palliative care as a legitimate field. Less than 4% of Indians have access to PC, and most of the nation's palliative care services are concentrated in a few states, including Kerala. In community settings, India has a need for PC services ranging from 1.5 to 43.1 per 1000 people.[5,6] In India, the availability, accessibility, and affordability of palliative care services are severely limited. It is therefore imperative that PC services be given priority in accordance with our commitment to advancing toward Sustainable Development Goal 3.8 and the National Health Policy.

Chapter 62: National Programme for Palliative Care

History of palliative care in India	The WHO and the Indian Government were consulted during the 1994 formation of the Indian Association of Palliative Care (IAPC). Its initiatives focus on providing end-stage chronic medical disorders, cancer, AIDS, and other life-limiting illnesses with care that includes advocacy, palliative care capacity building, and access to pain management. IAPC introduced the Children's Palliative Care program in 2010, which targets HIV-positive children's pain management. Additionally, the IAPC has established minimal requirements for palliative care services at various levels.
	The Indian Government introduced the National Programme for Palliative Care (NPPC) in 2012. Palliative care falls within the National Health Mission's (NHM) "Mission Flexipool." The National Palliative Care Programme's implementation has not been given its own budget. However, in order to apply for funding under NHM, the states and territories may draft their submissions on PC in accordance with sample project implementation plans. The nation now has two centers of excellence that are officially WHO Collaborating Centers. The "WHO Collaborating Center for Training and Policy on Access to Pain Relief is located in Thiruvananthapuram, Kerala, while the WHO Collaborating Center for Community Participation in Palliative Care and Long-term Care is located in Kozhikode, Kerala.
Goal	The goal is to guarantee that the underprivileged have access to reasonable, high-quality pain management and palliative care as a necessary component of healthcare at all levels of the healthcare system, in accordance with community needs.
Vision	• Enabling everyone who needs it in the nation to have access to palliative care and pain management at a reasonable cost that is safe and high-quality. • To bring in the dimension of 'Long-term care principles' and 'palliative care principles' within the healthcare systems
Objectives	• **Capacity building:** To increase the ability to deliver PC services "within the National Programme for Prevention of Non-Communicable Diseases (NPNCD), National Programme for Health Care of the Elderly (NPHCE), National AIDS Control Programme (NACP), and National Health Mission (NHM)—all" of which are currently running government health programs. • **Improve access to medical and scientific use of opioids:** To maintain safeguards against misuse and diversion while improving the legal as well as regulatory framework and supporting implementation to guarantee access to the availability of opioids for medicinal and research applications • **Reinforce attitudinal switch among health professionals:** Enhance and incorporate PC and long-term care ideas into the medical, nursing, pharmacy, and social work curricula to influence the attitudes of healthcare practitioners. • **Foster behavior reshaping of Community:** To encourage societal and behavioral transformation by raising public awareness and developing knowledge and abilities in the areas of palliative care and pain management. Community-owned projects that support the current healthcare system would be encouraged as a result. • **Provision of PC in private sectors** • **Develop protocol and keep track** to guarantee progress towards the objective, create national standards for PC services, and update the program's architecture and execution on a regular basis.
Organogram	NPPC is a program that is sponsored centrally. **Funding pattern:** A 40% portion of the states' A model PIP, which is a framework of operational and financial parameters, has been allocated (10% for the NE and Hill states). The GOI: State share would be 90:10 in the Northeast and Hill states and 60:40 overall. The PIPs may be submitted by state governments for review under the National Health Mission's "Mission Flexipool."[7]
Beneficiaries	Patients with a wide range of life-limiting illnesses are among the recipients. Adults with chronic illnesses "such as cardiovascular diseases (38.5%), cancer (34%), chronic respiratory diseases (10.3%), AIDS (5.7%), and diabetes (4.6%), make up the majority of patients in need of palliative care. Chronic renal illness, chronic liver illness, rheumatoid arthritis, neurological disorders, dementia, congenital malformations, and drug-resistant tuberculosis" are among the other chronic ailments that require it. In addition, PC services are required for long-term issues brought on by neurological illnesses like cerebral palsy, blood disorders, such as thalassemia, and congenital abnormalities.
Strategies/ Deliverables under the program	• Contribute vital funds to strengthen the capability of the major health initiatives for non-communicable diseases, such as cancer, HIV/AIDS, and initiatives aimed at the senior population. • Funding for the district hospital's palliative care services and the state's palliative care cell[7]

334 Section III: National Health Mission

Activities at various level or package of services	• Contribute vital funds to strengthen the capability of the major health initiatives for noncommunicable diseases, such as cancer, HIV/AIDS, and initiatives aimed at the senior population. • Funding for the district hospital's palliative care services and the state's palliative care cell At every stage of treatment, particularly community and home-based care, efficient palliative care services are incorporated into the current healthcare system. They are tailored to fit into particular social, cultural, and economic contexts. ASHA, volunteers, community health officers (CHO), and multi-purpose health workers (MPHWs) make up the palliative care team. PC is to be provided at two levels: 1. Home and community level 2. Health system level **Home and community level:** The primary caregivers are relatives and family members. However, palliative care delivery is inadequate, especially in rural regions, due to low levels of awareness and knowledge. The caregivers and volunteers need to be trained to provide standardized home-based care. They can be enabled to care for patients in a way that is specific to their needs and limited resources by receiving basic training in nursing, infection control, bedridden patient care, and end-of-life care. Their empowered participation improves the quality of care offered. **Health system level:** This package is provided through the health and wellness center.[8] 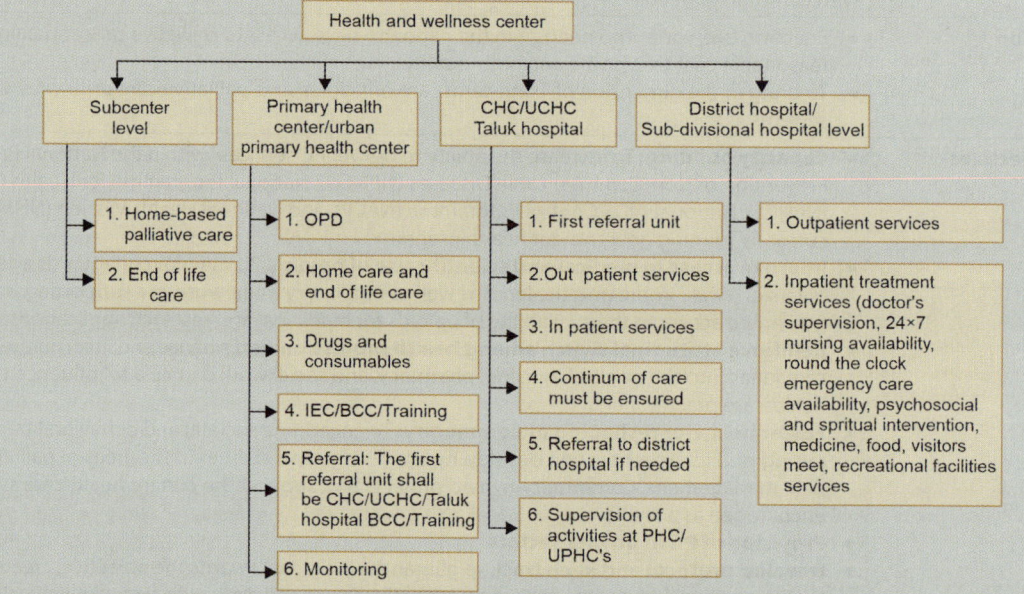
Monitoring and evaluation of program	The state and the district will report on the financial and physical progress accomplished under the various program components on a regular basis, following the format specified by the Central Division. Furthermore, the State Palliative Care Cell's program coordinator or the state program/Nodal program officer will conduct routine monitoring visits to the districts.

References

1. World Health Organization. WHO Definition of Palliative Care [Internet]. Geneva: World Health Organization; [cited 2024 Aug 05]. Available from: http://www.who.int/cancer/palliative/definition/en
2. Stjernsward J, Clark D. Palliative medicine—a global perspective. In: Doyle D, Hanks G, Cherny N, Calman K (Eds). Oxford textbook of palliative medicine. 3rd ed. Oxford: Oxford University Press; 2004. p. 1197-1224.
3. Gunderson Lutheran Health System. Transforming Healthcare: End-of-Life Care. Feb 3, 2009.
4. WHO Guide for Effective Programmes: Cancer Control - Knowledge into Action. World Health Organization. 2007. Available onlinhttps://www.who.int/cancer/ media/FINAL-PalliativeCareModule.pdf. Accessed 09 Aug 2024.
5. Chandra A, Bhatnagar S, Kumar R, Rai SK, Nongkynrih B. Estimating the Need for Palliative Care in an Urban ResettlementColony of New Delhi, North India. Indian J Palliat Care. 2022; 28:434-8.

6. Sudhakaran D, Shetty RS, Mallya SD, Bidnurmath AS, Pandey AK, Singhai P, et al. Screening for palliative care needs in the community using SPICT. Med J Armed Forces India. 2023;79:213-9.
7. Directorate General of Health Services, Ministry of Health and Family Welfare. Proposal of Strategies for Palliative Care in India (Expert group report). New Delhi: Ministry of Health and Family Welfare; November 2012. p. 23.
8. Ministry of Health and Family Welfare (MoHFW). Operational guidelines for palliative care at Health and Wellness Centres. Government of India.

QUESTIONS

Long Answer Question (LAQ)

1. What is the need of palliative care program in India? Enumerate its objectives and the provisions under the program at different levels of health system.

Short Answer Questions (SAQs)

1. Home-based palliative care.
2. Role of ASHA in national program on palliative care.

Multiple Choice Questions (MCQs)

1. What is the full form of NPPC?
    a. National Programme for Palliative care
    b. National Programme for Preventive Care
    c. Nutritional Programme for Preventive Care
    d. Nutritional Programme for Palliative Care
2. The Government of India launched The National Programme for Palliative Care (NPPC) in the year:
    a. 1949
    b. 1994
    c. 2012
    d. 2021
3. What is the primary goal of palliative care?
    a. To cure the disease
    b. To prevent the spread of disease
    c. To promote the health
    d. To improve the quality of life of patients and their families
4. Beneficiaries for NPPC are:
    a. Patients with acute illness
    b. Persons who are at risk of chronic ailment
    c. Patients with life-limiting illnesses
    d. None of the above
5. Palliative care needs to be initiated at:
    a. Terminal stage of disease
    b. Before the occurrence of disease
    c. At the time of diagnosis of chronic ailment
    d. After all curative options are exhausted

6. **Various packages of NPPC are provided through:**
   a. Schools
   b. Health and wellness centers
   c. Anganwadi centers
   d. None of the above

7. **Which one of the following is not part of the palliative care team?**
   a. Community health officer (CHO),
   b. Multi-purpose health worker (MPHW),
   c. ASHA, and volunteers
   d. Anganwadi worker

8. **Which of the following is a key component of palliative care?**
   a. Aggressive curative treatment
   b. Comprehensive pain and symptom management
   c. Routine diagnostic testing
   d. Intensive surgical interventions

9. **In the context of palliative care, what does the term " pain relief " refer to?**
   a. Physical pain only
   b. Psychological and emotional pain only
   c. Physical, emotional, social, and spiritual pain
   d. Pain that cannot be treated

10. **How can public health initiatives contribute to the development of palliative care services?**
    a. By focusing solely on curative treatments
    b. By promoting early integration of palliative care into the healthcare system
    c. By discouraging the use of palliative care in non-cancer illnesses
    d. By restricting palliative care to specialized palliative care units

11. **The National Programme for Palliative Care is part of:**
    a. The 'Mission Flexipool' under the National Health Mission (NHM)
    b. RMNCAH+N
    c. National AIDS Control Programme
    d. National Vector-borne Disease Control Programme

Answers

1. a
2. c
3. d
4. c
5. c
6. b
7. d
8. b
9. c
10. b
11. a

PART D

Nutrition

63. Integrated Child Development Services Scheme
64. PM-Poshan Scheme/Mid-Day Meal—Pradhan Mantri Poshan Shakti Nirman
65. National Iodine Deficiency Disorders Control Programme
66. National Programme for Prevention and Control of Fluorosis
67. Antyodaya Anna Yojana

CHAPTER 63

Integrated Child Development Services Scheme

Surendra Singh, Shaili Vyas, Hinal Baria

Background/Need of program/Scheme	Saksham Anganwadi and Poshan 2.0 (henceforth Poshan 2.0) is an Integrated Nutrition Support Programme. It aims to address the problems associated with malnutrition in children, teenage girls, pregnant women, and nursing mothers by establishing a convergent ecosystem to foster and create activities that support immunity, wellbeing, and health as well as by strategically changing the nutrition content and delivery. The themes of Poshan 2.0 will include Maternal Nutrition, AYUSH-Promoted Wellness, and Infant and Young Child Feeding Norms. Convergence, governance, and capacity-building will serve as its three pillars. The reason for Mission Poshan 2.0 is related to the difficulties encountered with the existing supplementary feeding program. Nutrition policies have remained stable over the years and have been slow to evolve towards a more integrated approach to food security. Past attempts to improve food quality and distribution has been ineffective. ICDS Anganwadi services have focused on ensuring adequate caloric intake, neglecting the quality and diversity of diets, and changing behavior towards better nutrition. The focus of the current program has been primarily on caloric intake rather than balanced micronutrient-deficient diets in take-home rations (THR) and hot cooked meals (HCM). Traditional knowledge in food practices was not used. Program execution and implementation have been affected by the lack of effective participation of beneficiaries and local stakeholders, highlighting low community ownership or participation in local anganwadi activities. One of the main challenges is poor enforcement and the lack of tracking. Poshan 2.0 key strategies include developing good eating habits for long-term health and well-being, raising nutrition awareness, and developing corrective measures to address deficiencies in nutrition. It also includes developing green eco-systems, such as Poshan Vatikas and strategies for communication. The goals of Mission Poshan 2.0 include increasing the use of millets in the diet, diversifying the diet, and fortifying food. Through the use of wholesome regional foods to close dietary gaps, nutrition awareness initiatives under Poshan 2.0 seek to promote long-term health and wellbeing. Consumption of micronutrient-rich foods, such as dark green leafy vegetables, lentils, and fruits high in vitamin C, is encouraged by dietary diversification within the anganwadi platform.[1]
Implemented since	The Government of India (GoI) is dedicated to advancing child and maternal health through various programs that focus on their holistic development. The Integrated Child Development Scheme (ICDS), launched on October 2, 1975, aims to provide pre-school education and break the cycle of starvation, illness, reduced learning capacity, and mortality.[1] In the financial year 2021–22, the GoI restructured the ICDS and POSHAN Abhiyaan (Prime Minister's Overarching Scheme for Holistic Nourishment) into Saksham Anganwadi and POSHAN 2.0. This updated scheme includes the following sub-programs: • ICDS: Anganwadi Services Scheme • Poshan Abhiyaan • Scheme for adolescent girls (SAG)
Goal	The initiative was designed to tackle the pressing issue of malnutrition among children under six, adolescent girls (ages 14 to 18), pregnant women, and mothers, addressing their health, nutrition, and developmental needs. The program is aligned with the Sustainable Development Goals (SDGs), particularly SDG 2 and SDG 4, which emphasize quality education and nutrition.[2]

Objectives	Poshan 2.0 integrates the Supplementary Nutrition Programme, Scheme for Adolescent Girls, and Poshan Abhiyaan into a unified Nutrition Support Programme. Its key objectives are: • Contributing to the development of human capital in the country; • Tackling malnutrition challenges; • Promoting nutrition awareness and healthy eating habits for sustained health and wellbeing; • Addressing nutritional deficiencies through targeted strategies.[2]
Organogram	For effective implementation the scheme is organized as shown in **Flowchart 63.1**. Coordination committees at each focal point help in efficient delivery of services with the Ministry of Women and Child Development acting as the nodal department.[1] **Flowchart 63.1:** Organogram of ICDS scheme.[1] **Center** Ministry of Health and Family Welfare, GoI — Ministry of Women and Child Development, GoI **State** Director Health Service, State Coordinator — Director Social Welfare/Project Officer In-Charge ICDS **District** District Chief Medical Officer — District Social/Tribal Welfare /ICDS Program Officer **Block** Medical Officer In-Charge — Child Development Project Officer **Sector** Health Assistant Female/Lady Health Visitor — Mukhya Sevika **Subcenter** Health Worker Female/Auxiliary Nurse Midwife **Village** Health Guide/ASHA — Anganwadi Worker and Anganwadi Helper Immunization, health check-up and, referral services — Supplementary nutrition, preschool nonformal education, and nutrition and health education Administrative unit for an ICDS project is a Community Development Block in rural areas, Tribal Development Block in predominantly tribal areas and slums in urban areas. As per the norms of the scheme, a rural/urban project is to cater to a population of one lakh while a tribal project is required to cater to a population of 35,000.[1] **Funding pattern**[3] Poshan 2.0 is an ongoing centrally-sponsored program being implemented through the state governments/UT administrations based on a cost sharing ratio between the Central Government and the State Government.[3] **Anganwadi service scheme team**[1] The District Programme Officers (DPOs), Child Development Project Officers (CDPOs), supervisors, anganwadi workers, and anganwadi helpers make up the Anganwadi Service Scheme team. Anganwadi workers are female frontline honorary workers, who are chosen from the local community. She also works as a social change agent, encouraging the community to promote improved treatment of women, girls, and young children. In addition, the medical officers collaborate with the scheme functionaries to build a team that includes the Auxiliary Nurse Midwife (ANM) and Accredited Social Health Activist (ASHA) to achieve convergence of various services.[1]

Chapter 63: Integrated Child Development Services Scheme

	Anganwadi service scheme team			
	Geographical coverage	**Job title**	**Job description**	**Norm**
	Village level/community	Anganwadi helper (AWH)	Cooking, cleaning	1/1 AWW
	Village level/community	Anganwadi worker (AWW)	Service provider	1/800 population
	Sector level	Mukhya sevika	Supervisor	1/20–25 AWW
	Block/project level	Child development project officers (CDPOs)	Program manager and supervisor	All AWCs at project level
	District	District magistrate	Chairman, supervisor	All AWCs in district

	In addition, ANM, ASHA, Lady Health Visitor (LHV), Medical Officer (MO), Block Development Officer (BDO) also help in provision of services in Anganwadi Service Scheme[1]
	Staff Norms
	1 Anganwadi center: 1 Anganwadi worker
	1 Anganwadi helper
	Population norms (For setting up anganwadi center)

	Rural/Urban projects:	• 400–800 1 AWC • 800–1600 2 AWCs • 1600–2400 3 AWCs • Thereafter in multiples of 800 1AWC
	For mini AWC	• 150–400 1 mini AWC
	For tribal/Riverine/Desert, hilly and other difficult area/Project	• 300–800 1 AWC • 150–300 1 mini AWC
	Anganwadi on demand	• Where a settlement has at least 40 children under 6 years but no AWC[1]

Beneficiaries	Poshan 2.0 seeks to address the challenging situation of malnutrition among children up to the age of 6 years, adolescent girls (14–18 years) and pregnant and lactating women.[2]
Components	• Nutrition support for POSHAN through Supplementary Nutrition Programme (SNP) for children of the age group of six months to six years, pregnant women and lactating mothers (PWLM); and for adolescent girls in the age group of 14–18 years in aspirational districts and North Eastern Region (NER) • Early childhood care and education [3–6 years] and early stimulation for (0–3 years) • Anganwadi infrastructure including modern, upgraded Saksham anganwadi; and • Poshan Abhiyaan[2]
Strategies/Deliverables under the program	• Strengthening the program with clear focus on accelerating achievement of maternal and child outcomes, repositioning early child development centrally. • Developing an implementation framework with programmatic, management and institutional reforms, in mission mode. • Strengthening partnership between the central, state, panchayati raj institutions/urban local bodies and communities. • Transform the scheme into a learning organization, backed by a strong monitoring and evaluation function, accountability and transparency. • Strengthening capacity development • Improving basic Infrastructure and service delivery through anganwadi centers (AWCs), etc.[4]
Activities at various level or package of services	Package of services under ICDS The Anganwadi Services Scheme delivers a comprehensive package of services to eligible beneficiaries, which includes: • **Supplementary nutrition** • **Preschool nonformal education**

- **Nutrition and health education**
- **Immunization**
- **Health check-ups**
- **Referral services**

Of these, immunization, health check-ups, and referral services focus on health and are offered through the National Health Mission (NHM) and public health infrastructure.

Supplementary nutrition:[2]
- As one of the key elements of the anganwadi services, supplementary nutrition is distributed through a network of 14 lakh anganwadi centers across the country. This component is designed to close the gap between the Recommended Dietary Allowance (RDA) and the Average Daily Intake (ADI). Only registered beneficiaries at anganwadi centers (AWCs) are eligible to receive supplementary nutrition, which is provided during operational hours.
- The National Food Security Act (NFSA) of 2013 mandates the provision of supplementary nutrition for all pregnant and lactating women for up to six months post-childbirth, as well as for children aged six months to six years, including those suffering from malnutrition.
- Supplementary nutrition is offered for at least 300 days annually, or around 25 days each month.

Beneficiaries: This includes pregnant and lactating women, children aged 6–36 months, severely malnourished (SAM) children, and adolescents aged 14–18 years who receive Take-Home Rations (THR). Children aged 3 to 6 years benefit from hot cooked meals (HCM) and breakfast.

Nutrition: Beneficiaries receive two servings daily, consisting of Morning Snacks and Hot Cooked Meals (HCM), to encourage dietary diversity and consumption of fresh food.

Distribution: THR is distributed twice a month, ideally on the 1st and 15th of every month. For SAM children, additional nutrition is provided in the form of THR. However, THR is not to be distributed as raw rations. Where applicable, states may substitute THR with hot cooked meals. Beneficiaries, including pregnant women, lactating mothers, and children aged six months to three years, are not required to attend anganwadi centers daily for THR.

THR shall be distributed regularly to registered beneficiaries. The beneficiaries in the categories of PW & LM, Children six months to three years are not expected to visit the AWCs daily. The distribution of THR to beneficiaries shall be made twice a month, preferably on 1st and 15th of each calendar month uniformly.

The nutritional standard and cost norms for the beneficiaries under the scheme are presented in the following table:

Nutritional standards for the beneficiaries under the scheme

Categories	Supplementary food	Nutritional norms (per beneficiary per day)	
		Calories (KCAL)	Protein (G)
Children (6–36 months)	Take home ration	500	12–15
Children (3–6 years)	Morning snack and hot cooked meal	500	12–15
Severely malnourished children (6–72 months)	Take home ration	800	20–25
Pregnant women and nursing mothers	Take home ration	600	18–20
Adolescent girls (14–18 years)	Take home ration	600	18–20

Preschool Nonformal Education[1]
- Anganwadi centers provide nonformal education to children aged three to six years by creating a joyful and stimulating environment that fosters their overall development.
- The daily three-hour play-based activities are culturally relevant and use locally made materials developed by trained anganwadi workers.
- This program encourages social, emotional, cognitive, physical, and aesthetic growth through a child-centered, play-oriented approach.

Nutrition and Health Education[1]
- Nutrition, Health, and Education (NHED) form an essential part of the anganwadi worker's responsibilities.
- As part of the Behavior Change Communication (BCC) strategy, NHED aims to build the long-term capacity of women, particularly those aged 15–45, empowering them to manage their own health, nutrition, and development needs, as well as those of their children and families.

Immunization[1]
- Immunization is a critical service for pregnant women and infants, protecting children from vaccine-preventable diseases in line with the National Immunization Schedule.
- Anganwadi workers (AWWs) assist the health system by identifying and registering eligible beneficiaries, organizing immunization camps, promoting the benefits of vaccination, and conducting follow-ups.

Health Check-ups[1]
- Health services include care for children under six, antenatal care for pregnant women, and postnatal care for nursing mothers.
- AWWs, in collaboration with Primary Health Center (PHC) staff, provide regular health check-ups, monitor weight, manage malnutrition, treat diarrhea, conduct de-worming, distribute basic medications, and identify individuals at risk.

Referral Services[1]
- During health check-ups and growth monitoring, children who are ill or malnourished and in need of immediate medical attention are referred to the Primary Health Center or its subcenters.
- Anganwadi workers are trained to detect disabilities in young children, document the cases in a special register, and refer them to the medical officer for further evaluation and treatment.

Service delivery framework[1]

Services	Target group	Responsibility
Immunization*	Children below six years, pregnant and lactating mothers	MO, ANM, ASHA, AWW
Supplementary nutrition	Children (six months to six years), pregnant and lactating mothers, adolescent girls	AWW, AWH
Health checkup*	Children below 6 years, pregnant and lactating mothers	MO, ANM, ASHA
Referral service*	Children below 6 years, pregnant and lactating mothers	MO, ANM, ASHA
Preschool education	Children in the age group of 3–6 years	AWW
Nutrition and health education	Women in age group of 15–45 years	MO, ANM ASHA, AWW

*AWW assists ANM in identifying the beneficiaries/MO: Medical Officer; ANM: Auxiliary Nurse Midwife; AWW: Anganwadi Worker; AWH: Anganwadi Helper; ASHA: Accredited Social Health Activist.

Monitoring and evaluation of program[1,5,6]

Monitoring of program
Effective monitoring and supervision are essential for the successful implementation of the program. The Ministry of Women and Child Development (MoWCD) serves as the central agency responsible for overseeing the scheme's activities. Recognizing the importance of monitoring, MoWCD has introduced various initiatives to modernize the program's Management Information System (MIS). A comprehensive monitoring and evaluation system has been established to track projects via monthly progress reports (MPRs) from each project.
- The key elements of this system include MPRs submitted by anganwadi workers to the Child Development Project Officer (CDPO) through supervisors, and further to the State Government or Union Territory Administration, as well as the ICDS Control Room at MoWCD, using the updated MIS format.
- In addition to MPRs, a multi-tiered administrative framework has been created to ensure effective implementation, encompassing monitoring at all levels, from the central level down to the community level in villages.

Central Monitoring Unit	
National Mission Steering Group	National Empowered Program Committee
State Monitoring Unit	
State Mission Steering Group	State Empowered Program Committee
District Level Monitoring	
District ICDS Mission	District Level Monitoring and Review Committee (DLMRC)
Block Level Monitoring	
Block ICDS Mission Committee	Block Level Monitoring Committee (BLMC)
Village Level	
Village Health Sanitation and Nutrition Committee (VHSNC)	Anganwadi Level Monitoring and Support Committee (ALMSC)

References

1. Ministry of Women and Child Development. Government of India. Mission Saksham Anganwadi and Poshan 2.0 - Scheme Guidelines. New Delhi: MoWCD; 2022. 78 p.
2. Ministry of Women and Child Development. Integrated Child Development Services. ICDS Scheme [Internet]. [New Delhi (India): MoWCD, GoI]; 2015 [updated 2015 Aug 17; cited 2024 Jun 26]. Available from: https://wcd.nic.in/integrated-child-development-services-icds-scheme
3. Institute of Economic Growth. Evaluation of ICDS Scheme of India. New Delhi: NITI Aayog; 2020 Feb. 144 p.
4. Ministry of Women and Child Development. ICDS Mission. The Broad Framework for Implementation. New Delhi: MoWCD. 141 p.
5. Ministry of Women and Child Development. Integrated Child Development Scheme (ICDS). Manual for District- Level Functionaries. New Delhi: MoWCD; 2017. 32 p.
6. Central Monitoring Unit (CMU), National Institute of Public Cooperation and Child Development. Monitoring and Supervision of Anganwadi Centres and ICDS Projects. New Delhi: NIPCCD. 98 p.

QUESTIONS

Long Answer Question (LAQ)

1. Write in detail about Poshan 2.0.

Short Answer Questions (SAQs)

1. Write short note on Anganwadi Services Scheme.
2. Write short note on Scheme for Adolescent Girls.

Multiple Choice Questions (MCQs)

1. **What is the main goal of Saksham Anganwadi and Poshan 2.0?**
   a. Promote early childhood education
   b. Address malnutrition in children, adolescent girls, pregnant women, and lactating mothers
   c. Improve employment opportunities for women
   c. Increase access to higher education for girls

2. **Which ministry is responsible for monitoring and implementing the Integrated Child Development Scheme (ICDS)?**
   a. Ministry of Health and Family Welfare
   b. Ministry of Women and Child Development (MoWCD)
   c. Ministry of Education
   d. Ministry of Social Justice and Empowerment

3. **What are the three main pillars of Mission Poshan 2.0?**
   a. Education, Healthcare, Sanitation
   b. Maternal Nutrition, AYUSH-Promoted Wellness, Infant and Young Child Feeding Norms
   c. Convergence, Governance, Capacity-Building
   d. Economic Development, Social Welfare, Employment

4. **Which age group of children is covered under the nonformal preschool education component of ICDS?**
   a. 0–3 years
   b. 3–6 years
   c. 6–10 years
   d. 10–14 years

5. **What is the purpose of Take-Home Ration (THR) in the ICDS program?**
   a. To provide raw food ingredients
   b. To bridge the gap between Recommended Dietary Allowance (RDA) and actual intake
   c. To improve sanitation in households
   d. To promote vaccination

6. **How many days per year is supplementary nutrition provided under ICDS?**
   a. 200 days
   b. 250 days
   c. 300 days
   d. 365 days

7. **Which population norm is required for setting up an anganwadi center (AWC) in rural/urban projects?**
   a. 200–500 people
   b. 400–800 people
   c. 800–1200 people
   d. 1200–1600 people

8. **What is the role of the anganwadi worker in the ICDS scheme?**
   a. Supervising anganwadi helpers
   b. Monitoring and promoting nutrition and health education
   c. Providing legal aid to women
   d. Managing school enrollments

9. **Which group is NOT a target of the ICDS program under Poshan 2.0?**
   a. Adolescent girls aged 14–18
   b. Children under 6 years of age
   c. Elderly individuals over 60 years of age
   d. Pregnant and lactating mothers

10. **Who assists the anganwadi worker in identifying beneficiaries for immunization and health services?**
    a. District Magistrate
    b. Auxiliary Nurse Midwife (ANM)
    c. Accredited Social Health Activist (ASHA)
    d. Both B and C

Answers

1. b
2. b
3. c
4. b
5. b
6. c
7. b
8. b
9. c
10. d

CHAPTER 64

PM—Poshan Scheme/Mid-Day Meal—Pradhan Mantri Poshan Shakti Nirman

Janki Bartwal, Shaili Vyas, Priti Solanki

Background/Need of the program	Pradhan Mantri Poshan Shakti Nirman (PM Poshan)' was approved by the Government of India for providing one hot cooked meal in government and government—aided schools from 2021–22 to 2025–26. This is the Centrally Sponsored Scheme.[1] This was before known as 'National Programme for Mid-Day Meal in Schools' popularly known as Mid-Day Meal Scheme. The scheme is being enforced by the Ministry of Education. Under the scheme, there is provision of hot cooked meal to children of preschools or Bal Vatika (before class I) and children studying in classes I to VIII. It is being implemented across the country covering all the eligible children without any discrimination of gender and social class. **Rationale:**<ul><li>**Preventing classroom hunger:** Children from weaker sections of the society who come to school without having breakfast or some children even if they had a meal in the morning feel hungry by afternoon and are not able to concentrate in class. It will be helping those family who cannot afford lunch box and hence could prevent "classroom hunger".</li><li>**Promoting school participation:** More children will enroll in the schools as well as enhancement of attendance in the school.</li><li>**Facilitating healthy growth of children:** School meals can also act as a regular source of "supplementary nutrition" for children and facilitate their healthy growth.</li><li>**Intrinsic educational value:** It can be used as an opportunity to inculcate good habits among children, such as washing one's hands before and after eating and to educate them about the importance of clean water, good hygiene, etc.</li><li>**Fostering social equality:** School children from all the different social background will sit together to eat the meal.</li><li>**Enhancing gender equity:** Help in removing the social barriers for girls to attend the school. Gives employment to women as cook.</li><li>**Psychological benefits:** It will facilitate overall cognitive, emotional and social development.</li></ul>
Objectives[1]	The objectives of the scheme are to address two of the pressing problems for majority of children in India, viz. hunger and education by:<ul><li>Improving the nutritional status of children studying in Bal Vatika and classes I—VIII in government and government-aided schools and Special Training Centers (STCs).</li><li>Encouraging poor children, belonging to disadvantaged sections, to attend school more regularly and help them concentrate on classroom activities.</li><li>Providing nutritional support to children of elementary stage in drought affected areas during summer vacation and during disaster times.</li></ul>
Beneficiaries under scheme	<ul><li>All children enrolled and studying in government and government-aided schools are entitled for one hot cooked meal on all schools' days.<ul><li>Bal Vatika (i.e., just before class I)</li><li>Class I-V</li><li>Class VI-VIII</li></ul></li><li>All children enrolled in classes I-V under National Child Labour Project (NCLP) schools of Ministry of Labour and Employment, Government of India.</li></ul>

Components of the scheme[1]	• **Food grains:** Cost is borne entirely by Central Government. Rice @ ₹ 3 per kg, wheat @ ₹ 2 per kg and coarse grain @ ₹ 1 per kg is provided to states/UT. The norms under the scheme are as follows:

S. No.	Items	Primary	Upper primary
A. Nutrition norms per child per day			
1.	Calorie	450 kcal	700 kcal
2.	Protein	12 g	20 g
B. Food norms per child per day			
1.	Food grains	100 g	150 g
2.	Pulses	20 g	30 g
3.	Vegetables	50 g	75 g
4.	Oil and fat	5 g	7.5 g
5.	Salt and condiments	As per need	As per need

- **Material cost:** Covers expenditure on pulses, vegetables, cooking oils, condiments, fuel, etc.
- **Honorarium to cook-cum-helpers:** A minimum honorarium of ₹ 1000 per month is paid. The states are free to give over and above the prescribed minimum from their own resources. 1 cook-cum-helper for 25 students, 2 cook-cum-helpers for 26–100 students and thereafter 1 additional for every 100 students.
- **Transportation assistance:** It is as per public distribution system rate prevailing in the particular state/UTs for foodgrain transportation from Food Corporation of India godown to school doorsteps. It is limited to a maximum of ₹ 1500 per metric tonne for states/UTs except in North Eastern Region and, there Himalayan states, and two UTs.
- **Management, monitoring and evaluation:** It comprise of 3% cost of food grains, cooking cost, honorarium cost to cook-cum-helper and transport assistance. About 90% fund released to states/UTs and 10% as national component. About 50% fund is earmarked at school level expenditure and remaining 50% at block, district and state level.
- **Kitchen-cum-stores:** For 100 students, 20 sqm area of kitchen cum stores may be constructed and an additional 4 sqm may be added for every addition of up to 100.
- **Kitchen devices:** Gas stoves, storage containers, utensils for cooking and serving with replacement every five years.
- **Repair of kitchen-cum-stores:** ₹ 10,000 for repair of every kitchen cum stores constructed 10 years ago.
- **Innovation and flexibility:** About 5% of the aggregate cost of food grains, cooking cost, honorarium cost to cook-cum-helper and transport assistance.
- **Meals during summer vacation:** There is also a provision of meals during summer vacation in drought affected areas and during closure of schools in disaster affected areas.

Menu under scheme: It consists of varied, locally available and culturally acceptable food items. Food from each food group will be selected providing varied nutrients and children will also not get bored. Inclusion of green leafy vegetables, whole legumes and millets, etc., in the diet will ensure reduction in the prevalence of anemia, providing good source of protein, vitamins and minerals and other micronutrients respectively. Involvement of parents and children while preparing the menu.

Convergence with other development programs: Convergence with Ministry of Health and Family Welfare, Ministry of Rural Development and Panchayati Raj, Ministry of Women and Child Development, Ministry of Agriculture, etc., for kitchen cum store, kitchen devices, school nutrition gardens, social audit, hand washing facilities, drinking water, dining halls, supplementary nutrition, etc.

School health component: Health check-ups under Rashtriya Bal Swasthya Karyakaram, with referral to nearest primary health center, micronutrients, such as Iron Folic acid tablets are provided weekly and deworming is done biannually in convergence with MoHFW.

Reference

1. Pradhan Mantri Poshan Shakti Nirman Guidelines. Available from https://pmposhan.education.gov.in

QUESTIONS

Long Answer Question (LAQ)

1. Write in detail about PM Poshan.

Short Answer Questions (SAQs)

1. Write in brief about components of PM Poshan.
2. Write in brief about beneficiaries of PM Poshan.

Multiple Choice Questions (MCQs)

1. **Nodal Ministry for Implementation of PM Poshan:**
    a. Ministry of Health and Family Welfare
    b. Ministry of Education
    c. Ministry of Women and Child Development
    d. Ministry of Rural Development
2. **Correct full form of PM Poshan:**
    a. Pradhan Mantri Poshan Shakti Nirman
    b. Prime Minister Poshan Shakti Nirman
    c. Pradhan Mantri Poshan Abhiyan
    d. Prime Minister Poshan Abhiyan

Answers

1. b
2. a

65 CHAPTER

National Iodine Deficiency Disorders Control Programme

Vinod chayal, Jyotsana, Bharti Koria

Background/Need of program	Iodine is an essential micronutrient that is required at 100–150 µg daily for normal growth and development of human beings.[1] National Goitre Control Programme was launched in India in 1962. In august 1992, it was further renamed as the National Iodine Deficiency Disorders Control Programme with a broad view to cover a wide spectrum of iodine deficiency disorders (IDD), such as mental and physical retardation, deaf-mutism, cretinism, stillbirths, abortion, etc.[2] Most of the districts of India are endemic to Iodine deficiency disorders.[3]
Goals	• To bring down the prevalence of iodine deficiency disorders (IDD) below 5% in the entire country. • To ensure 100% consumption of adequately iodized salt (15 ppm) at the household level.
Target	To reach the target of more than 90% household-level coverage of adequately iodized salt of universal salt iodization.
Objectives	• Regular surveys to assess the magnitude of iodine deficiency disorders in various districts. • Supply of iodized salt in place of common salt. • Resurveys to assess iodine deficiency disorders and the impact of iodized salt every five years in the districts. • Laboratory monitoring of iodized salt and urinary iodine excretion. Health education and publicity.
Components	• Establishment of IDD control cell • Establishment of IDD monitoring labs • Idd survey/resurvey • Production and distribution of 52 lakh mt of iodized salt • Lab testing of iodized salt and urinary iodine excretion • Qualitative iodized salt testing at the community level • Health education and publicity • Training programs • Monitoring and evaluation Financial assistance is being provided to states/UTs for conducting financial surveys to assess the magnitude of goiter and other IDD.
Beneficiaries	People of all ages, both sexes and people of different socioeconomic statuses, particularly pregnant women and young children.
Organogram	National level → Ministry of Health and Family Welfare (Nodal Ministry) ↓ Central level → Central Nutrition and IDD Cell (DGHS) ↓ State level → State/UT IDD Cell (State Health Directorate)

Important activities carried out at the central IDD cell of DGHS are as follows[2]	The IEEC's salt commissioner maintains close liaison with the Ministry of Industry/Transport, providing technical guidance to states/UTs. They conduct independent IDD surveys, conduct training for state health personnel, and collect data for effective advice. The commissioner oversees iodized salt quality control at production, distribution, and consumer levels, coordinating with the Ministry of Railways. They manage IEC activities and financial aspects of state IDD cells.
Responsibilities of the state IDD cell	The IEC is responsible for coordinating with wholesalers and retailers to check iodine levels of iodized salt, distributing it through open markets and public systems, monitoring consumption, conducting IDD surveys, training medical staff, and disseminating information through various channels, including salt testing kits for iodine awareness.
Prevention[3]	**Primary prevention:** • The main strategy for the control and prevention of IDDS is universal salt iodization. Potassium iodate is the most commonly used agent for iodization of salt. Iodization is done at a dose of 30 ppm at the production level and 15 ppm at the consumer level. • Screening of beneficiaries through IDD surveys at the district level. • Daily consumption of the recommended amount of iodized salt in the diet. • Consumption of iodine-rich food and avoid goitrogenic food items. • In high-risk areas that have delays in the accessibility of iodized salt, iodized oil can be given to women and children. It is available in the form of oral drops and intramuscular (IM) injections. A single IM injection can provide protection to a pregnant female for up to one year postpartum. However, oral drops have to be repeated every six months to one year. • Monitoring of iodine levels in different salt samples. • Health education and awareness regarding the consumption of iodized salt in the diet. **Secondary prevention:** • Early diagnosis through estimation of serum levels of t3, t4 and tsh, urine iodine excretion, and heel prick test in neonates for congenital hypothyroidism. • Treatment can be medical or surgical depending on the severity of the disease. **Tertiary prevention:** Disability limitation and rehabilitation of the physically- and mentally-retarded children through psychological support.
Monitoring and evaluation[2]	The chairmanship of the DGHS has been established to assess the implementation status, monitoring and evaluation of the program. IDD monitoring laboratories in each state has been set up with a view to effectively monitoring the quality of iodated salt and the content of iodine in urine samples. There are three levels of laboratory monitoring of NIDDCP: 1. At the primary level, the estimation of the iodine content of salt by the titration method is being done. 2. At secondary level monitoring, the estimation of urinary iodine excretion for the bio-availability of iodine is being done. 3. At the tertiary level of laboratory monitoring, neonatal scanning for thyroid-stimulating hormones is used.

References

1. World Health Organization. Assessment of iodine deficiency disorders and monitoring their elimination. Geneva: World Health Organization; 2007.
2. Directorate General of Health Services, Ministry of Health and Family Welfare, Government of India. Revised Policy Guidelines on National Iodine Deficiency Disorders Control Programme. [Internet]. New Delhi: Ministry of Health and Family Welfare, Government of India; 2006 [cited 2024 Sept 24]. Available from: https://nhm.gov.in/images/pdf/programmes/ndcp/niddcp/revised_guidelines.pdf
3. Pandav CS, Yadav K, Srivastava R, Pandav R, Karmakar MG. Iodine deficiency disorders (IDD) control in India. Indian J Med Res. 2013;138:418–33.

QUESTIONS

Long Answer Question (LAQ)

1. Briefly describe the National Iodine Deficiency Disorders Control Programme. Discuss the preventive strategies adopted and activities at various levels of prevention in detail.

Short Answer Questions (SAQs)

1. What are iodine deficiency disorders? How will you prevent them?
2. Illustrate the organogram of National Iodine Deficiency Disorders Control Programme.
3. Explain briefly about the aims, objectives, targets of the National Iodine Deficiency Disorders Control Programme.

Multiple Choice Questions (MCQs)

1. Iodine content in iodated salt at manufacturing and distribution level is as follows:
   a. 30 ppm and 15 ppm
   b. 15 ppm and 30 ppm
   c. 15 ppm and 20 ppm
   d. 30 ppm and 20 ppm
2. Average daily requirement of iodine of an adult per day is:
   a. 50–100 µg
   b. 100–150 µg
   c. 250–300 µg
   d. 300–500 µg
3. Amount of financial assistance per district provided to State/UT IDD control cells for conducting surveys for assessing the magnitude of goiter and other IDD is:
   a. 50,000
   b. 40,000
   c. 30,000
   d. 25,000
4. Which is the Nodal Ministry of NIDDCP?
   a. Ministry of Health and Family Welfare
   b. Ministry of Woman and Child Development
   c. Ministry of Health Nutrition and Indigenous Medicine
   d. Ministry of Education

Answers

1. a   2. b   3. d   4. a

CHAPTER 66

National Programme for Prevention and Control of Fluorosis

Pankaj Bhardwaj, Nitin Kumar Joshi, Akhil Dhanesh Goel, Jaydeep Ghevaria

Background/Need of program	Fluorosis is resulting from prolonged exposure to high levels of fluoride, typically through drinking water, food products, or industrial emis manifests primarily in three forms—dental fluorosis, skeletal fluorosis, and non-skeletal fluorosis, each with distinct but severe implications for individual and public health. Groundwater contamination is the primary driver of fluorosis in India, with fluoride levels often exceeding the World Health Organization's suggested limit of 1.5 mg/L, reaching as high as 30 mg/L in some areas.[1] Dental fluorosis is often the first visible sign of fluoride overexposure, particularly in children. It occurs when excessive fluoride intake disrupts the normal development of tooth enamel, leading to discoloration and pitting of the teeth.[2] Skeletal fluorosis, resulting from chronic fluoride ingestion over many years, is a more severe and debilitating condition. In its early stages, it may be asymptomatic or present with joint stiffness and Advanced skeletal fluorosis is irreversible, and treatment focuses on managing symptoms and preventing further exposure. Non-skeletal fluorosis affects various soft tissues and organs. Chronic fluoride exposure has been linked to gastrointestinal issues, neurological symptoms, and adverse effects on the endocrine system.[3] The Bureau of Indian Standards (BIS) sets the desirable limit of fluoride in drinking water at 1 ppm (1 mg per Liter). High fluoride levels have been reported in 230 districts across 19 states as of April 2014 (data from the Ministry of Drinking Water and Sanitation).[4] Reducing fluoride intake from these sources is crucial for improving health and preventing fluorosis, which can be achieved through awareness programs.[5] To address fluorosis, the Indian Government has implemented the National Programme for Prevention and Control of Fluorosis (NPPCF).
Implementation	The National Programme for Prevention and Control of Fluorosis (NPPCF) was launched by the Government of India during the 11th Five Year Plan in 2008–09. The initial implementation covered 100 endemic districts across 17 states/UTs, six districts were selected from each of the six zones of the country based on information collected from the Ministry of Drinking Water and Sanitation. The districts included: • **Southern zone:** Nellore (Andhra Pradesh) and Dharampuri (Tamil Nadu) • **Western zone:** Jamnagar (Gujarat) • **Northern zone:** Nagaur (Rajasthan) • **Eastern zone:** Nayagarh (Odisha) • **Central zone:** Ujjain (Madhya Pradesh) During the 12th Five Year Plan, an additional 95 districts were included, expanding the program's reach.[6]
Goals, targets, and objectives	The primary goal of NPPCF is to mitigate the health effects of fluorosis and prevent further exposure to high levels of fluoride in drinking water, thereby reducing the incidence of fluorosis related morbidities in the affected population. The objectives are as follows: • **Baseline survey data:** Collect, assess, and utilize baseline survey data on fluorosis from the Ministry of Drinking Water and Sanitation to guide program activities. • **Comprehensive management:** Implement comprehensive management strategies for fluorosis in the selected areas. • **Capacity building:** Build capacity at various levels of the healthcare delivery system for the prevention, diagnosis, and management of fluorosis cases.[5,6]

Organogram	The National Programme for Prevention and Control of Fluorosis (NPPCF) in India follows a structured approach involving various sectors and professionals. At the central level, the Ministry of Health and Family Welfare (MoHFW) provides overall policy direction, planning, and funding for the NPPCF. Under the MoHFW, the Directorate General of Health Services (DGHS) implements the NPPCF at the national level and coordinates with state governments. Key roles within the DGHS include the Director (Public Health), who oversees the implementation and monitoring of NPPCF, the Programme Manager (NPPCF), who manages day-to-day operations and liaises with states to ensure adherence to program guidelines, and Technical Experts/Consultants who provide technical support, conduct research, and offer recommendations for program improvement. Under the program, no regular posts are sanctioned at either the central or district levels. Coordination at the central level is managed by the Adviser Nutrition/In-charge of Nutrition and IDD within the Directorate General of Health Services. At the state level, coordination is overseen by the State Nodal Officer, and at the district level by the District Nodal Officer. The program employs contractual staff, including one National Consultant and one Data Entry Operator (DEO) at the national level, and one District Consultant, one Lab Technician, and three Field Investigators (for six months) at the district level.[5,6]
Beneficiaries	The beneficiaries of the NPPCF include populations living in areas with high fluoride content in groundwater. Specifically, individuals affected by fluorosis, which may manifest as dental, skeletal, or non-skeletal forms.
Components	The key components of the NPPCF include: • **Community diagnosis:** Through surveys and mapping. • **Capacity building:** Of healthcare professionals and laboratory technicians. • **IEC (information, education, communication)** • **Treatment and rehabilitation:** For fluorosis-affected individuals.[5,6]
Strategies/ Deliverables under the program	The NPPCF adopts a multifaceted strategy, including: • **Early diagnosis and treatment:** Through community surveys and health check-ups. • **Safe drinking water supply:** Promoting the use of low-fluoride water sources. • **Health education and awareness:** Utilizing IEC strategies to inform communities. • **Capacity building:** Training for medical and paramedical staff on fluorosis management. • **Intersectoral coordination:** Collaborating with various sectors to ensure comprehensive program implementation.[5,6]
Activities at various levels/Package of services	Details of activities proposed under NPPCF at various levels is mentioned in **Table 66.1**.

TABLE 66.1: Activities proposed under NPPCF at various levels.

S. No.	Level	Activities
1.	Community (Village)	• Assess the entire endemic village and identify persons with fluorosis for provisional diagnosis. • Awareness-cum-Training Programme for Medical Officers of PHC/CHC and district hospitals, paramedical workers, ICDS workers, PRI functionaries, and teachers about symptoms and prevention of fluorosis. • Line listing and color-coding of water sources for safe drinking, intervention activities for prevention, and referral system for surgeries. • Introduce behavioral changes through IEC approaches. • Promote intersectoral cooperation for prevention and control of fluorosis, emphasizing safe water sources. • Implement selected interventions for prevention, health promotion, safe water supply, and monitor impact. • Record fluorosis prevalence and manage non-skeletal fluorosis through interventions.
2.	Community Health Centers (CHCs)/FRU	• Implement similar activities for CHC staff and block level functionaries. • Conduct training programs for clinical examination and management of fluorosis cases for Medical Officers and health personnel. • Organize Training-cum-Awareness Programmes for BDC, ICDS staff, and block level functionaries. • Conduct diagnostic tests for urine fluoride levels and skeletal fluorosis, if facilities are available. • Monitor village/PHC level activities. • Facilitate referrals.

Monitoring and evaluation of the program	S. No.	Level	Activities
	3.	District	• Implement similar activities as CHC level at district level. • Develop fluorosis mapping using water fluoride estimation data and dental fluorosis surveys in school children. • Develop and implement detailed training programs for Medical Officers and health personnel for comprehensive management of fluorosis. • Organize training-cum-awareness programs for DDC, ICDS, and education personnel. • Establish diagnostic support for dental, skeletal, and non-skeletal fluorosis. • Provide basic medical, surgical, and rehabilitative activities for diagnosed cases. • Monitor and refer difficult cases to nearby medical college hospitals. • Designate the CMO as the Nodal Officer for NPPCF.
	4.	State	• Plan and execute program activities, monitor, conduct mid-term evaluation, and report to the Center (GOI) through the State Nodal Officer. • Manage receipt and disbursement of funds. • Process utilization certificates and submit physical progress reports to the Center (GOI). • Assist central team in follow-up activities. • Regularly monitor district progress.
	5.	Center	• Develop, plan, and implement the program through states/UTs. • Manage and release funds to states/UTs. • Conduct supervision, monitoring, and impact assessment. • Review performance.

Monitoring and evaluation are critical aspects of NPPCF. This involves:
- **Regular reporting:** From district and state levels to the central level.
- **Impact assessment:** Evaluating the effectiveness of interventions through health surveys and feedback mechanisms.
- **Supervision:** Continuous oversight by central and state health authorities to ensure adherence to program guidelines and achievement of objectives.[5,6]

References

1. Kashyap SJ, Sankannavar R, Madhu GM. Fluoride sources, toxicity and fluorosis management techniques – A brief review. 2021; 2, 100033.
2. Bose S, Yashoda R, Puranik MP. A review on defluoridation in India. International Journal of Applied Dental Sciences. 2018; 4(3), 167–71.
3. Shen L, Feng C, Xia S, Wei Y, Zhang H, Zhao D, et al. Progressive Research in the Molecular Mechanisms of Chronic Fluorosis. IntechOpen, 2019.
4. Khyalia P, Duhan SS, Laura JS, Nandal M. A comprehensive analysis of fluoride contamination in groundwater of rural area with special focus on India. Elsevier BV, 2024; (pp. 201–212).
5. Directorate General of Health Services, Ministry of Health & Family Welfare, Government of India. National program for prevention and control of fluorosis (NPPCF) revised guidelines (2014).https://mohfw.gov.in/sites/default/files/5698574563321459874546.pdf Accessed on 03 Feb 2025.
6. Government of India. (n.d.). Indexl :: National Health Mission. National Programme for Prevention & Control of Flurosis (NPPCF). https://nhm.gov.in/indexl.php?lang=l&level=3&sublinkid= 1055.Accessed on 03 Feb 2025.

QUESTIONS

Long Answer Question (LAQ)

1. Discuss the need for the National Programme for Prevention and Control of Fluorosis (NPPCF) in India, highlighting the health, economic, and social impacts of fluorosis.

Short Answer Questions (SAQs)

1. What are the primary objectives of the NPPCF?
2. Write a short note on monitoring, and evaluation of NPPCF.

Multiple Choice Questions (MCQs)

1. What is the primary source of fluoride exposure leading to fluorosis in India?
   a. Agricultural crops
   b. Industrial emissions
   c. Groundwater contamination
   d. Air pollution
2. Which form of fluorosis is characterized by the calcification of ligaments and immobility of joints?
   a. Dental fluorosis
   b. Skeletal fluorosis
   c. Non-skeletal fluorosis
   d. Neurological fluorosis
3. What is the suggested limit for fluoride in drinking water set by the World Health Organization (WHO)?
   a. 0.5 mg/L
   b. 1.0 mg/L
   c. 1.5 mg/L
   d. 2.0 mg/L
4. Which of the following is NOT a component of the NPPCF?
   a. Community diagnosis
   b. Capacity building
   c. Industrial emission regulation
   d. IEC (Information, education, communication)
5. What is the primary goal of the NPPCF?
   a. To eliminate all fluoride sources in India
   b. To mitigate the health effects of fluorosis and prevent further exposure
   c. To provide universal dental care
   d. To replace groundwater with surface water
6. Which level of NPPCF activities involves developing fluorosis mapping using water fluoride estimation data?
   a. Community level
   b. Primary health centers (PHCs)
   c. District level
   d. State level
7. What is the role of the State Nodal Officer under the NPPCF?
   a. Manage the receipt and disbursement of funds
   b. Conduct fluorosis diagnosis at the community level
   c. Oversee fluoride removal in water treatment plants
   d. Organize national awareness campaigns
8. Which of the following is a key strategy of the NPPCF?
   a. Increasing fluoride levels in drinking water
   b. Early diagnosis and treatment through community surveys
   c. Promoting fluoride-rich diets
   d. Industrial fluoridation of water

Answers

1. c
2. b
3. c
4. c
5. b
6. c
7. a
8. b

CHAPTER 67

Antyodaya Anna Yojana

Rudresh Negi, Parul Sharma, Hathila, Parul Katara

Background/ Need of program/ Scheme	In post-Independent India, poverty and food dependency were substantial and increased with intermittent periods of draughts, famines and wars. This led to the establishment of the public distribution system in 1960s to combat critical food shortages with focus on urban areas. With the advent of green revolution, it was expanded to tribal areas and areas with high incidence of poverty. This was further revised to "revamped" Public distribution system (PDS) in 1992, and officially converted from universal to targeted public distribution system (TPDS) in 1997. The National Sample Survey (NSS) revealed that around 5% of the population in India sleeps 'without two square meals a day.' Thus, to make TDPS more focused and targeted towards this population, Antyodaya Anna Yojana was launched for the provision of food security to the poorest of the poor population.[3,5]
Implementation	AAY was initially launched for one crore poorest of the poor families in December 2000. It has been expanded three times since its launch as 1st expansion on 5th June, 2003; 2nd expansion on 3rd August, 2004 and 3rd expansion on 12th May 2005, increasing the number of families in each expansion by 50 lakh.[5]
Goal	• To reduce hunger among the poorest segments of the Below Poverty Line (BPL) population. • To provide food security to poorest segment from the Below Poverty Line families.[7]
Organogram	It is operated under the Ministry of Consumer Affairs, Food and Public Distribution with the joint responsibility of Central Government and State/Union Territory (UT) Governments

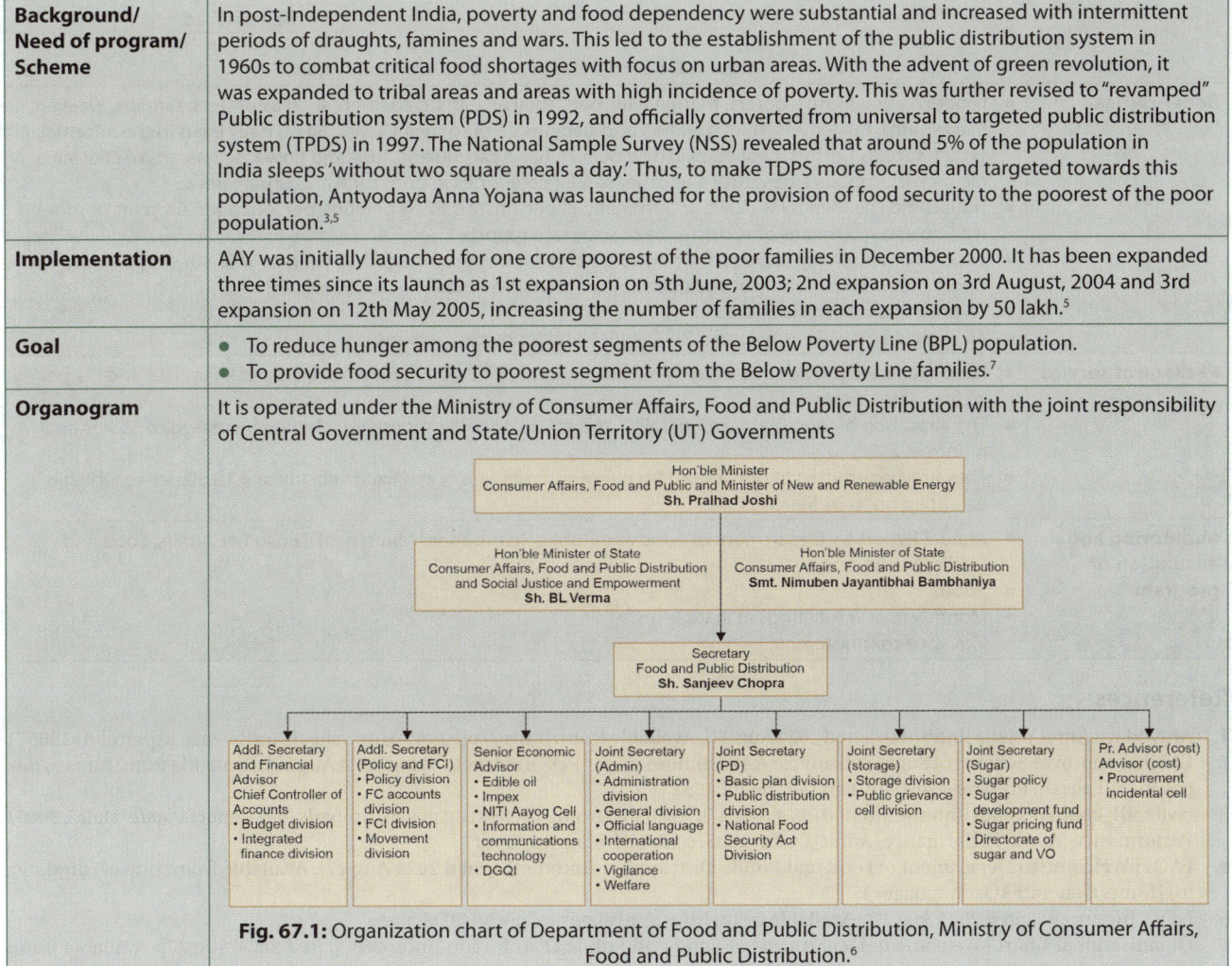

Fig. 67.1: Organization chart of Department of Food and Public Distribution, Ministry of Consumer Affairs, Food and Public Distribution.[6]

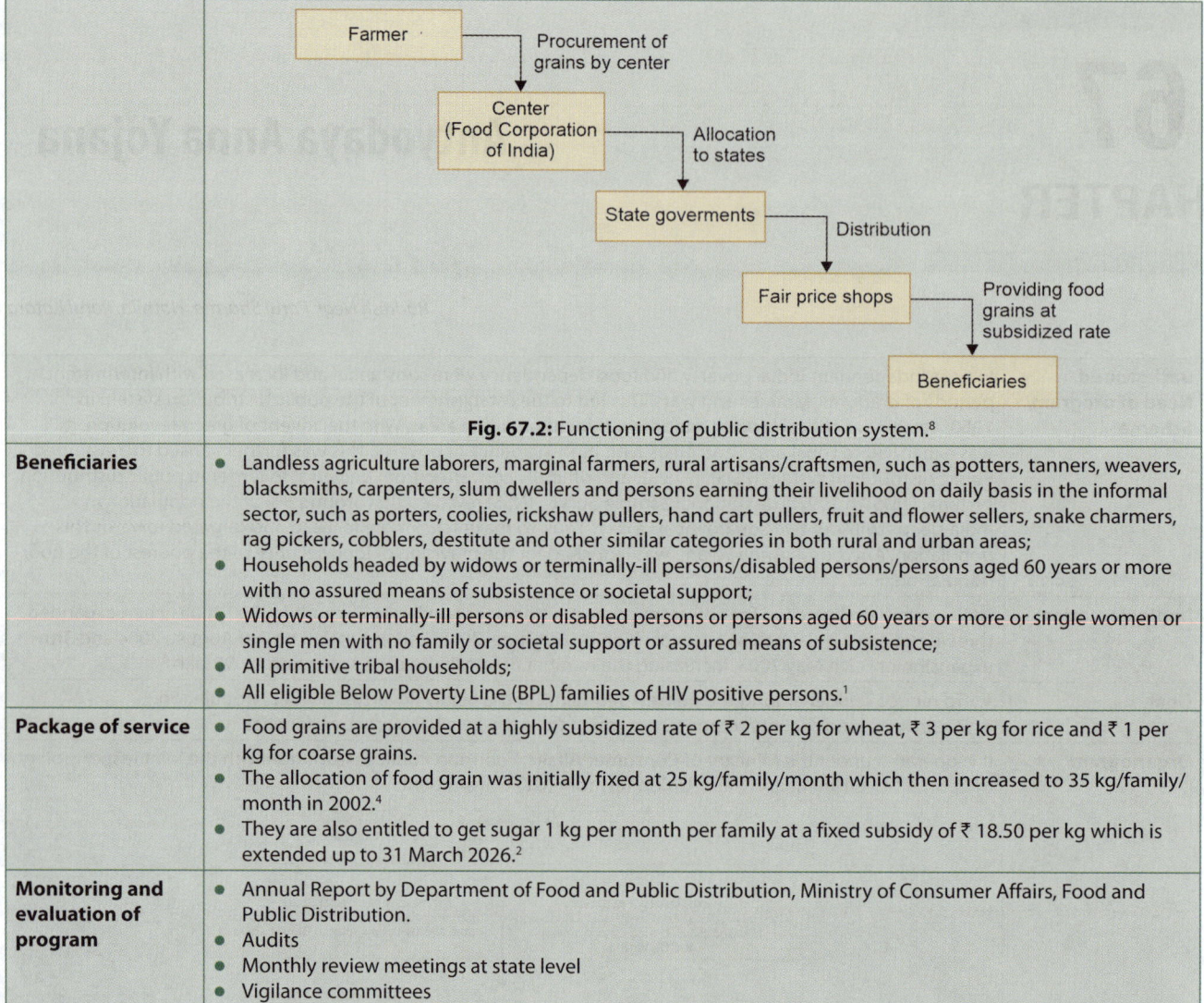

Fig. 67.2: Functioning of public distribution system.[8]

Beneficiaries	• Landless agriculture laborers, marginal farmers, rural artisans/craftsmen, such as potters, tanners, weavers, blacksmiths, carpenters, slum dwellers and persons earning their livelihood on daily basis in the informal sector, such as porters, coolies, rickshaw pullers, hand cart pullers, fruit and flower sellers, snake charmers, rag pickers, cobblers, destitute and other similar categories in both rural and urban areas; • Households headed by widows or terminally-ill persons/disabled persons/persons aged 60 years or more with no assured means of subsistence or societal support; • Widows or terminally-ill persons or disabled persons or persons aged 60 years or more or single women or single men with no family or societal support or assured means of subsistence; • All primitive tribal households; • All eligible Below Poverty Line (BPL) families of HIV positive persons.[1]
Package of service	• Food grains are provided at a highly subsidized rate of ₹ 2 per kg for wheat, ₹ 3 per kg for rice and ₹ 1 per kg for coarse grains. • The allocation of food grain was initially fixed at 25 kg/family/month which then increased to 35 kg/family/month in 2002.[4] • They are also entitled to get sugar 1 kg per month per family at a fixed subsidy of ₹ 18.50 per kg which is extended up to 31 March 2026.[2]
Monitoring and evaluation of program	• Annual Report by Department of Food and Public Distribution, Ministry of Consumer Affairs, Food and Public Distribution. • Audits • Monthly review meetings at state level • Vigilance committees

References

1. Antyodaya Anna Yojana [Internet]. [cited 2024 Aug 27]. Available from: https://pib.gov.in/newsite/PrintRelease.aspx?relid=186571
2. Cabinet approves Scheme of Sugar Subsidy for AAY Families under PDS [Internet]. [cited 2024 Aug 27]. Available from: https://pib.gov.in/pib.gov.in/Pressreleaseshare.aspx?PRID=2001052
3. civilvolII_chapter_5.pdf [Internet]. [cited 2024 Aug 27]. Available from: https://cag.gov.in/uploads/old_reports/state/Delhi/2005/Performance_Audit/Performance_Audit_Delhi_2005/civilvolII_chapter_5.pdf
4. FAQs | Welcome to Department of Food and Public Distribution [Internet]. [cited 2024 Aug 27]. Available from: https://dfpd.nic.in/Home/GeneralFAQs?language=1
5. NFSA [Internet]. [cited 2024 Aug 27]. Available from: https://nfsa.gov.in/portal/PDS_page
6. Organisational Chart | Welcome to Department of Food and Public Distribution [Internet]. [cited 2024 Aug 27]. Available from: https://dfpd.gov.in/Home/OrganisationalChart?language=1
7. Public Distribution System (PDS) [Internet]. PMF IAS. 2024 [cited 2024 Aug 27]. Available from: https://www.pmfias.com/public-distribution-system-pds/
8. Reports | Welcome to Department of Food and Public Distribution [Internet]. [cited 2024 Aug 27]. Available from: https://dfpd.nic.in/Home/DocumentReport?language=1

QUESTIONS

Long Answer Question (LAQ)

1. Mention the beneficiaries and benefits provided under Antyodaya Anna Yojana. Describe the evolution of this scheme.

Short Answer Questions (SAQs)

1. What are the monitoring and evaluation mechanisms for Antyodaya Anna Yojana?
2. Critically analyze Antyodaya Anna Yojana using the SWOT analysis technique.
3. Enlist the beneficiaries of Antyodaya Anna Yojana.

Multiple Choice Questions (MCQs)

1. In which year, the Antyodaya Anna Yojana was launched to provide highly subsidized food to millions of the poorest families?
   a. 1966
   b. 1972
   c. 1997
   d. 2000
2. All are eligible for Antyodaya Anna Yojana, *except*:
   a. All primitive tribal households
   b. All eligible Below Poverty Line (BPL) families of HIV positive persons.
   c. Households headed by widows
   d. Above Poverty Line (BPL) families of HIV positive persons.
3. Allotted food grains per family per month under Antyodaya Anna Yojana currently is:
   a. 25 kg
   b. 35 kg
   c. 45 kg
   d. 55 kg
4. Antyodaya Anna Yojana is implemented under which Ministry?
   a. Ministry of Health and Family Welfare
   b. Ministry of Women and Child Development
   c. Ministry of Home Affairs
   d. Ministry of Consumer Affairs, Food and Public Distribution.
5. Antyodaya Anna Yojana was launched to help the:
   a. Children under six years of age
   b. Women in the rural area
   c. Poorest of poor
   d. Social workers
6. Antyodaya Anna Yojana is linked with:
   a. Public distribution system
   b. Mid-day meal
   c. Special Nutrition Programme
   d. None of the above

Answers

1. d
2. d
3. b
4. d
5. c
6. a

PART E

Digital Health Initiatives

68. National Digital Health Mission (NDHM)/Ayushman Bharat Digital Mission(ABDM)
69. eSanjeevani—National Telemedicine Service
70. e-Health Initiatives in India

CHAPTER 68

National Digital Health Mission (NDHM)/ Ayushman Bharat Digital Mission (ABDM)

Sharon Baisil, Abhay Srivastava, Akhil Dhanesh Goel

INTRODUCTION

The Ayushman Bharat Digital Mission (ABDM), which was rebranded as the National Digital Health Mission (NDHM) in 2021, is a transformative initiative initiated by the Government of India to establish a unified digital health ecosystem throughout the nation. This mission addresses the historical challenges of India's healthcare system, such as fragmented health data, limited interoperability among stakeholders, and inequitable access to quality care, especially in rural and underserved areas.[1]

A seamless and efficient healthcare delivery system that promotes universal health coverage is the objective of ABDM, which is achieved through the utilization of digital technologies. The COVID-19 pandemic further highlighted the urgent need for scalable digital solutions, which accelerated the adoption of digital health infrastructure under ABDM. The mission strives to align with the National Health Policy (NHP) 2017 and the Sustainable Development Goals (SDGs) to ensure efficient, accessible, inclusive, affordable, timely, and safe healthcare for all.[2]

NEED OF THE PROGRAMME/SCHEME

India's healthcare system has long faced numerous challenges, necessitating a comprehensive digital transformation. These challenges include:
- **Fragmented health data:** The traditional paper-based system leads to a lack of continuity in patient care and difficulties in data sharing between healthcare providers. This fragmentation hinders a holistic view of patient health, leading to inefficiencies and errors.
- **Limited interoperability:** The absence of standardized systems prevents seamless data exchange among various healthcare stakeholders, such as providers, insurers, and patients. This lack of interoperability results in fragmented care and difficulties in accessing patient records.
- **Inequitable access to care:** Significant disparities exist in access to quality healthcare, particularly in rural and underserved regions. These disparities are further exacerbated by a lack of infrastructure and healthcare professionals.
- **Data-driven decision-making:** There is a critical need to support public health surveillance, research, and policy formulation with robust data. The current paper based systems and lack of interoperability makes this difficult.

ABDM is designed to address these gaps by creating an integrated digital health infrastructure that ensures every citizen has access to quality healthcare services. The mission aims to replace paper-based records with longitudinal Electronic Health Records (EHRs), enable seamless data exchange, bridge urban-rural disparities through telemedicine and digital health infrastructure, and support data-driven decision-making.[1]

IMPLEMENTATION TIMELINE

The implementation of ABDM has progressed through several key milestones:
- **2020:** The National Digital Health Mission (NDHM) was proposed, along with the release of the Health Data Management Policy (HDM Policy) to ensure privacy and consent-based data sharing.
- **August 15, 2020:** The National Digital Health Mission was officially launched.

- **September 27, 2021:** NDHM was formally relaunched as the Ayushman Bharat Digital Mission (ABDM).
- **2021:** Nationwide rollout of Ayushman Bharat Health Account (ABHA) IDs was initiated.
- **2023:** Integration of telemedicine services (e-Sanjeevani) and vaccination digitization via the U-WIN portal was implemented.
- **2024–2025:** Expansion to 73 crore ABHA IDs and the development of AI-driven health platforms in collaboration with IIT Kanpur are planned.
- The mission is envisioned to be fully implemented across the country over the next few years, transforming the landscape of healthcare delivery in India.

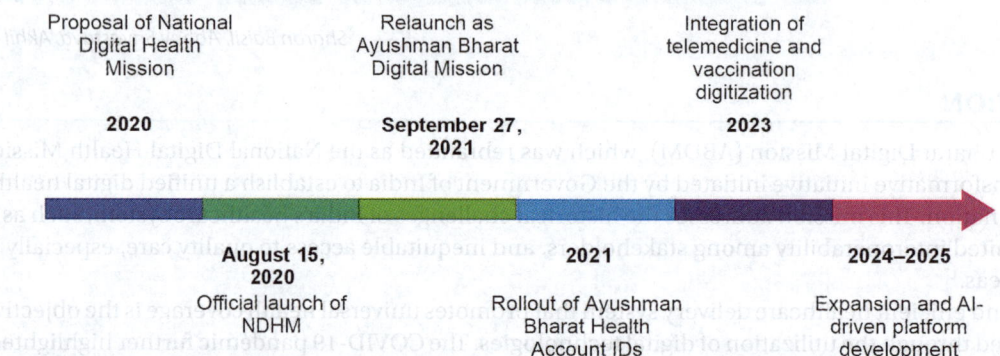

Key Milestones in the Ayushman Bharat Digital Mission

The National Health Authority (NHA), the apex body responsible for the implementation of Ayushman Bharat Pradhan Mantri Jan Arogya Yojana (AB-PMJAY), is implementing ABDM. The mission is being rolled out in a phased manner, with pilot projects conducted in several states and union territories to test and refine the digital health infrastructure.[1,3]

GOAL

The primary goal of ABDM is to establish a national digital health ecosystem that facilitates universal health coverage in a safe, effective, affordable, accessible, and expeditious manner. The process entails the establishment of cutting-edge digital health systems, the management of central digital health data, and the facilitation of seamless data exchange between healthcare providers and patients. Improving health outcomes, reducing healthcare costs, and empowering citizens to make informed decisions about their health are the objectives of the mission. In addition, ABDM encourages the adoption of open standards by all stakeholders in the digital health ecosystem, thereby promoting interoperability and innovation.

TARGETS

ABDM has set several key targets to achieve its vision of a digitally empowered healthcare system:
- **ABHA registrations:** Creation of 73 crore ABHA IDs by January 2025, with 49.15% of beneficiaries being women.
- **Healthcare provider integration:** Registration of over 5 lakh healthcare professionals and over 2 lakh Ayushman Arogya Mandirs for primary care.

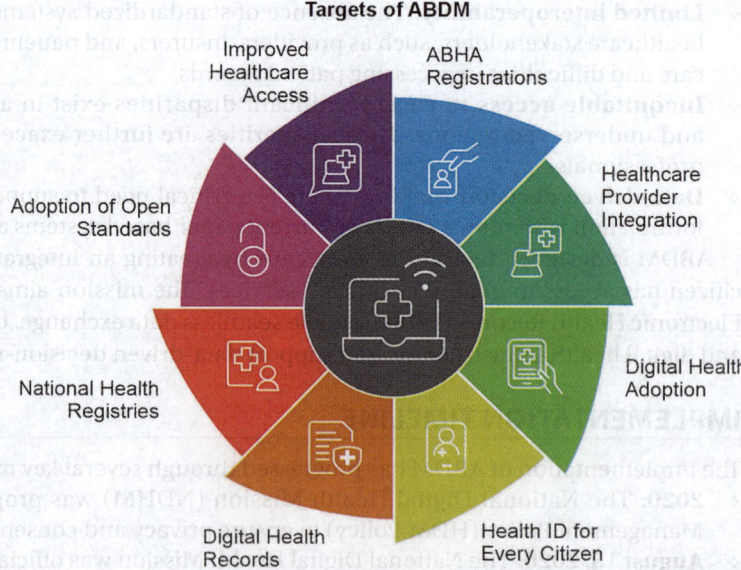

- ❖ **Digital health adoption:** 100% digitization of vaccination records via U-WIN, with 27.77 crore vaccine doses recorded by 2024.
- ❖ **Health ID for every citizen:** Providing every Indian citizen with a unique Health ID, which will serve as a repository of all health-related information.
- ❖ **Digital health records:** Enabling access to personal health records through a digital platform, allowing patients to share their health information with healthcare providers securely.
- ❖ **National health registries:** Creating and maintaining national and regional registries of clinical establishments, healthcare professionals, and health workers.
- ❖ **Adoption of open standards:** Enforcing the adoption of open standards by all stakeholders to ensure interoperability and seamless data exchange.
- ❖ **Improved healthcare access:** Enhancing access to healthcare services, especially in remote and underserved areas, through telemedicine and other digital health solutions.

OBJECTIVES

To achieve its overarching goal and targets, ABDM has several specific objectives:
- ❖ Establish a federated architecture for Electronic Health Records (EHRs), Health Facility Registries (HFR), and Healthcare Professional Registries (HPR).
- ❖ Implement FHIR R4 standards for health data exchange.
- ❖ Provide assisted ABHA registration for low-resource settings.
- ❖ Foster health-tech startups through the ABDM Sandbox and Digital Health Incentive Scheme (DHIS).
- ❖ Enforce the Health Data Management Policy for consent-based data governance.
- ❖ Develop and oversee the infrastructure necessary for the seamless exchange of the fundamental digital health data.
- ❖ Facilitate the development of a wide range of digital health systems that encompass the sector, from disease management to wellness, by encouraging the adoption of open standards by all actors in the National Digital Health Ecosystem.
- ❖ Develop an electronic health record system that adheres to international standards and is readily accessible to service providers and citizens on the basis of citizen consent.
- ❖ Establish a unified source of information regarding clinical establishments, healthcare professionals, health workers, and pharmacies, national and regional registries should be established.

ORGANOGRAM

The institutional framework of ABDM operates at different levels:
- ❖ **Ministry of Health and Family Welfare (MoHFW):** Responsible for policy formulation and overall supervision of ABDM. MoHFW provides guidance to the National Health Authority for implementation and works towards the legal and regulatory framework for NDHM. Additionally the ministry issues necessary directions for adoption of NDHM by all health related initiatives across the country.
- ❖ **National Health Authority (NHA):** Leads the implementation of ABDM and coordinates with various stakeholders. NHA proposes policy support, develops models for self-financing, and manages the day-to-day operations of ABDM.
- ❖ **Ministry of Electronics and Information Technology (MeitY):** MeitY works with MoHFW for legal and regulatory framework for NDHM and provides guidance on the technological framework. MeitY will play a key role in providing guidance on proper technological framework, leveraging digital services in proper fashion, and adopting emerging technologies.
- ❖ **State health agencies:** Responsible for onboarding facilities, healthcare professionals, and conducting Information, Education, and Communication (IEC) activities at the state level.
- ❖ **Technical partners:** Institutions like IIT Kanpur (for AI platforms) and the WHO's Global Initiative on Digital Health (GIDH).
- ❖ **Mission steering group:** Oversees and guides the mission, with the chairpersonship of the Hon'ble Minister of Health and Family Welfare.
- ❖ **Empowered committee:** Takes necessary policy-level decisions and supervises the roll-out of the mission, chaired by the Secretary of Health and Family Welfare.

- **Board of directors:** Provides administrative leadership, develops policy direction, and creates models for self-financing and sustainability.
- **CEO:** Implements policies and decisions approved by the Board of Governors.
- **Operations:** Coordinates with the Ministry of Health and Family Welfare (MoHFW) and the States/UTs, engages with the private sector, and resolves technical and operational issues.

BENEFICIARIES

ABDM benefits a wide range of stakeholders in the healthcare ecosystem:
- **Citizens:** Access to portable health records, teleconsultations, and preventive care. They can access their health records with just a few clicks, reduce the need for repeated diagnostic tests, and have centralized access to healthcare services.
- **Healthcare providers:** Streamlined workflows through e-Hospital and e-Sanjeevani, better access to patient information, and enhanced decision-making capabilities.
- **Healthcare facilities:** Streamlined processes, improved data management, and enhanced coordination with other facilities.
- **Policymakers:** Real-time data for resource allocation, outbreak response, and better monitoring and evaluation of health programs.
- **Government:** Improved policy-making and progress towards achieving Sustainable Development Goals (SDGs) related to health.
- **Researchers:** Benefit from the availability of aggregated information to evaluate the effectiveness of various programs and interventions.[1]

KEY COMPONENTS

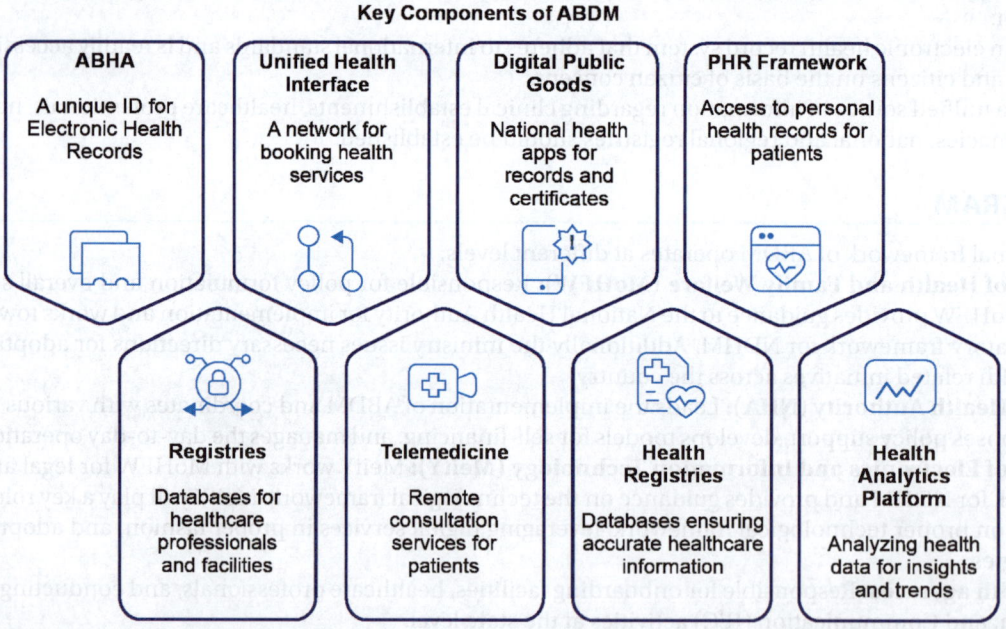

Key Components of ABDM

- **ABHA** — A unique ID for Electronic Health Records
- **Unified Health Interface** — A network for booking health services
- **Digital Public Goods** — National health apps for records and certificates
- **PHR Framework** — Access to personal health records for patients
- **Registries** — Databases for healthcare professionals and facilities
- **Telemedicine** — Remote consultation services for patients
- **Health Registries** — Databases ensuring accurate healthcare information
- **Health Analytics Platform** — Analyzing health data for insights and trends

ABDM comprises several key components:
- **ABHA (Ayushman Bharat Health Account):** A 14-digit unique ID for Electronic Health Records (EHRs), linked to Aadhaar or mobile numbers. This ID will serve as a repository of all health-related information, with a goal of creating 73 crore ABHA IDs by 2025. Uttar Pradesh and Maharashtra are leading in registrations.
- **Registries:**
  - **Healthcare Professionals Registry (HPR):** A verified database of doctors and other healthcare professionals.

- **Health Facility Registry (HFR):** A comprehensive registry of public and private healthcare facilities, mapped for standardized care.
- **Unified Health Interface (UHI):** An open network for booking appointments, lab services, and e-pharmacies.
- **Telemedicine:**
  - **e-Sanjeevani:** Provides teleconsultation services, including 17.6 lakh tele-mental health consultations via TeleMANAS.
- **Digital public goods:**
  - **Aarogya setu:** Expanded as a national health app for lab reports and vaccination certificates.
  - **U-WIN portal:** Digitized immunization records for 7.43 crore beneficiaries.
- **National health electronic registries:** Comprehensive databases of healthcare facilities and healthcare professionals, ensuring accurate and updated information.
- **Federated personal health records (PHR) framework:** Secures the availability of health data for medical research by enabling patients and healthcare providers to readily access healthcare reports and data.
- **National health analytics platform:** Enables the analysis of aggregated and anonymized health data, thereby facilitating research, policy-making, and the acquisition of insights into healthcare trends and patterns.
- **Additional horizontal components:** These include the Unique Digital Health ID, health data dictionaries, payment gateways, and supply chain management for pharmaceuticals.[2]

STRATEGIES AND DELIVERABLES

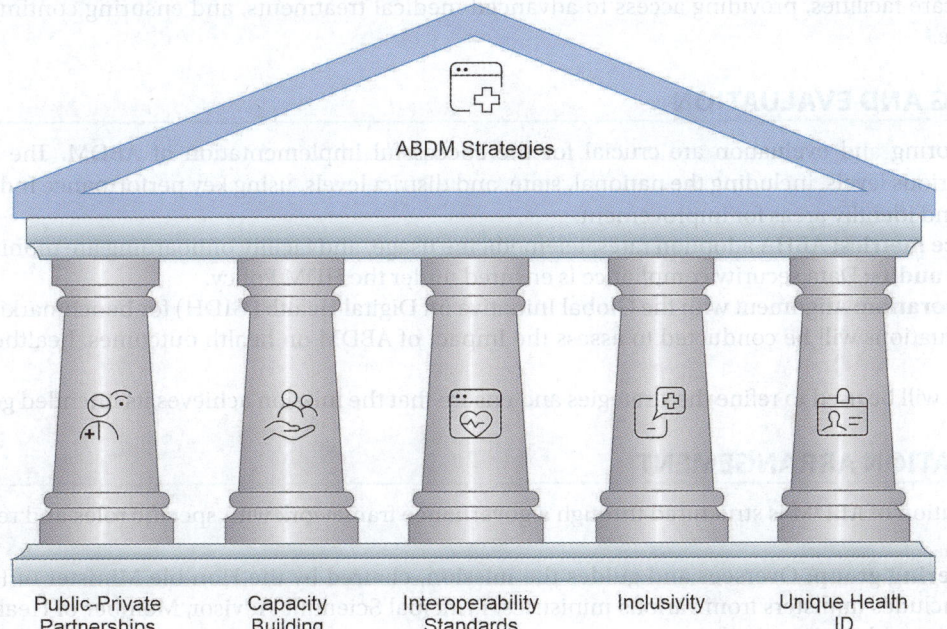

ABDM employs several strategies to achieve its objectives and deliver tangible outcomes:
- **Public-private partnerships:** The Digital Health Incentive Scheme (DHIS) incentivizes hospitals to adopt EHRs.
- **Capacity building:** Training modules for healthcare workers on ABDM tools are provided.
- **Interoperability standards:** FHIR-based APIs are implemented for EHR integration.
- **Inclusivity:** Multilingual apps and offline ABHA registration are available for better accessibility.
- **Development of a unique health ID:** Each citizen will be assigned a unique health ID that serves as a repository for all health-related data.
- **Establishing health data consent managers:** These will be associated with the unique health IDs of the patients and will facilitate the seamless exchange of health records between the patient and the doctor.

- **Providing healthcare services via a mobile app and website:** Healthcare services will be accessible via an official website and mobile application.
- **Enabling digital doctors:** Healthcare professionals can act as digital doctors, providing prescriptions remotely with free digital signatures.

ACTIVITIES ACROSS PREVENTION LEVELS

ABDM focuses on providing a continuum of care across primary, secondary, and tertiary levels of healthcare:
- **Primary prevention:**
  - Health education is disseminated through Aarogya Setu and community health workers.
  - Vaccination drives are enhanced through U-WIN's SMS alerts and QR-based certificates, improving coverage. Promoting health and wellness through digital platforms, providing information on healthy lifestyles, and facilitating early detection of diseases.
- **Secondary prevention:**
  - Early diagnosis through screening for noncommunicable diseases (NCDs) at Ayushman Arogya Mandirs.
  - Teleconsultations via e-Sanjeevani OPD reduce referral delays. Enabling timely access to diagnostic services and specialist consultations through telemedicine, and ensuring efficient management of chronic diseases.
- **Tertiary prevention:**
  - EHRs for continuity of care enable post-treatment follow-ups.
  - AI-driven care includes federated learning platforms for predictive analytics. Facilitating seamless referrals to tertiary care facilities, providing access to advanced medical treatments, and ensuring continuity of care after discharge.[4]

MONITORING AND EVALUATION

Effective monitoring and evaluation are crucial for the successful implementation of ABDM. The mission will be monitored at various levels, including the national, state, and district levels, using key performance indicators (KPIs) to track progress and identify areas for improvement.
- **Performance metrics:** ABHA adoption rates, telemedicine usage, and facility onboarding are monitored.
- **Third-party audits:** Data security compliance is ensured under the HDM Policy.
- **WHO collaboration:** Alignment with the Global Initiative on Digital Health (GIDH) for benchmarking.
- Regular evaluations will be conducted to assess the impact of ABDM on health outcomes, healthcare access, and efficiency.
- The findings will be used to refine the strategies and ensure that the mission achieves its intended goals.

IMPLEMENTATION ARRANGEMENT

The implementation of ABDM is structured through a governance framework with specific roles and responsibilities at various levels:
- **Mission steering group:** Oversees and guides the mission, chaired by the Hon'ble Minister of Health & Family Welfare. It includes ministers from various ministries, Principal Scientific Advisor, Member of Health (NITI Aayog) and Secretaries of the ministries.[5]
- **Empowered committee:** Takes policy-level decisions and supervises the roll-out of the mission, chaired by the Secretary of Health & Family Welfare. It includes the CEO of NITI Aayog and Secretaries from various ministries and organizations.
- **Ministry of Health and Family Welfare (MoHFW):** Provides overall supervision and guidance, along with working towards the legal and regulatory framework for NDHM.
- **Ministry of Electronics and Information Technology (MeitY):** Provides guidance on the proper technological framework and emerging technologies.
- **National Health Authority (NHA):** Leads the implementation and coordinates with various stakeholders.

The mission is implemented in a phased manner, following the approach of 'Think Big, Start Small, Scale Fast':

❖ **Phase 1:** Pilot in selected Union Territories with a focus on setting up the technological platforms and building capacity of the stakeholders for the use of Federated Health ID, PHR, and Registries. It includes field testing of the product in selected public and private institutions.
❖ **Phase 2:** Expansion of the pilot to additional states and expansion of the service bouquet. This phase includes onboarding of the States and the State governments setting up a dedicated team for NDHM implementation. It includes the integration of existing systems, such as eHospital, eSanjeevani, eSushrut, and Digilocker.[6]
❖ **Phase 3:** Nationwide roll-out, operationalizing and converging with all health schemes across India, along with promotion, on-boarding and acceptance of NDHM across the country.

The implementation is based on the Agile India Enterprise Architecture (Agile IndEA) Framework, emphasizing a minimalist approach, a federated architecture model, and API-based access.

Security and privacy are crucial aspects of the implementation. The security architecture is based on the principle of "Zero Trust Architecture". Various policies like Health IDs, Data Sharing, Security, and Privacy policies are enforced. The legal and regulatory requirements are aligned with the Personal Data Protection Bill, 2019, and other relevant acts. Informed consent is ensured for collecting, storing, using, and sharing health data.[7]

Active stakeholder engagement is ensured through continuous inputs during conceptualization, development, and roll-out. An agile procurement strategy is used to achieve the timely implementation of the mission. A Government Community Cloud or Virtual Private Cloud infrastructure is adopted to host data building blocks. Secure Health Networks are established for sensitive data access.

A dedicated team is working to achieve the mission's objectives. This includes a core project management team, development and management teams in various verticals, and leveraging existing teams working on PM-JAY.

CONCLUSION

The Ayushman Bharat Digital Mission (ABDM) represents a paradigm shift in India's healthcare delivery, emphasizing equity, innovation, and interoperability. By establishing a nationwide, comprehensive, and integrated digital health ecosystem, ABDM will make a substantial contribution to the attainment of the National Health Policy 2017 and the Sustainable Development Goals (SDGs) in the health sector. Despite challenges like digital literacy and funding sustainability, ABDM's success in registering a large number of citizens and pioneering AI-driven tools positions India as a global leader in digital health. Understanding ABDM's framework is critical for postgraduates to navigate future public health innovations. The mission is designed to ensure that healthcare becomes more effective, accessible, and affordable to all, promoting a healthier India.

REFERENCES

1. Ministry of Health and Family Welfare, Government of India. National Digital Health Blueprint [Internet]. New Delhi: Ministry of Health and Family Welfare; 2019 [cited 2025 Feb 09]. Available from: https://ndhm.gov.in
2. National Health Authority, Government of India. Ayushman Bharat Digital Mission [Internet]. New Delhi: National Health Authority; 2021 [cited 2025 Feb 09]. Available from: https://www.nha.gov.in
3. Ministry of Electronics and Information Technology, Government of India. Digital India [Internet]. New Delhi: Ministry of Electronics and Information Technology; 2015 [cited 2025 Feb 09]. Available from: https://www.digitalindia.gov.in
4. Government of India. National Health Policy 2017 [Internet]. New Delhi: Ministry of Health and Family Welfare; 2017 [cited 2025 Feb 09]. Available from: https://www.mohfw.gov.in
5. NITI Aayog. Strategy for New India @75: Building an Inclusive and Sustainable Future [Internet]. New Delhi: NITI Aayog; 2018 [cited 2025 Feb 09]. Available from: https://niti.gov.in
6. Indian Council of Medical Research. ICMR Guidelines for Digital Health Research [Internet]. New Delhi: ICMR; 2021 [cited 2025 Feb 09]. Available from: https://www.icmr.gov.in
7. Ministry of Health and Family Welfare, Government of India. Guidelines for the Use of Digital Technologies in Healthcare [Internet]. New Delhi: Ministry of Health and Family Welfare; 2020 [cited 2025 Feb 09]. Available from: https://www.mohfw.gov.in

QUESTIONS

Long Answer Question (LAQ)

1. Critically assess the Ayushman Bharat Digital Mission (ABDM)'s potential to revolutionize India's healthcare by analysing its objectives, components, and implementation strategies while evaluating the challenges it faces, and propose mitigation measures.

Short Answer Questions (SAQs)

1. Explain the significance of a federated architecture for health data management as proposed by ABDM. Discuss how it differs from centralized systems and its implications for data privacy and security, referring to the relevant sources.
2. Outline the key components of the ABDM ecosystem, and explain how they interrelate and contribute to the mission's objectives.

Multiple Choice Questions (MCQs)

1. What is the primary goal of the Ayushman Bharat Digital Mission (ABDM)?
   a. To promote the use of paper-based health records
   b. To create a national digital health ecosystem supporting universal health coverage
   c. To limit access to health services in rural areas
   d. To focus on tertiary care alone
2. Which of the following is a key component of ABDM that provides a unique 14-digit ID for citizens' health records?
   a. Health Facility Registry (HFR)
   b. Unified Health Interface (UHI)
   c. Ayushman Bharat Health Account (ABHA)
   d. Health Professionals Registry (HPR)
3. According to the sources, what standards are being implemented by ABDM to enable health data exchange?
   a. ISO 9001
   b. FHIR R4
   c. ICD-10
   d. SNOMED CT
4. Which body is primarily responsible for the implementation and coordination of ABDM with the states?
   a. Ministry of Health and Family Welfare (MoHFW)
   b. National Health Authority (NHA)
   c. State Health Agencies
   d. Technical Partners
5. What is the U-WIN portal primarily used for under the ABDM?
   a. To digitize immunization records
   b. To book appointments for telemedicine
   c. To register healthcare professionals
   d. To access personal health records

Chapter 68: National Digital Health Mission (NDHM)/Ayushman Bharat Digital Mission (ABDM)

6. **What is a key objective of ABDM concerning equity in healthcare?**
   a. Providing digital services exclusively in urban areas
   b. Restricting access to assisted ABHA registration in low-resource settings
   c. Providing assisted ABHA registration for low-resource settings
   d. Prioritizing private healthcare providers

7. **What does the term HIP stand for in the context of ABDM?**
   a. Health Insurance Provider
   b. Health Information Provider
   c. Healthcare Infrastructure Platform
   d. Health Innovation Program

8. **Which of the following is NOT a primary focus of the National Digital Health Mission (NDHM) as described in the sources?**
   a. Creating a national health ID for all citizens
   b. Creating national health registries
   c. Enabling access to personal health records through digital platforms
   d. Promoting traditional paper-based health records

9. **What is the role of the Health Claims Platform (HCP) within NDHM?**
   a. To provide teleconsultation services to patients
   b. To manage the national health registries
   c. To facilitate the submission and processing of e-claims for health insurance
   d. To act as a mobile app for citizens to access health services

10. **What does NDHM aim to ensure regarding access to health data?**
    a. Healthcare providers have direct access to all patient records.
    b. Data is publicly available and accessible to everyone without consent
    c. Patients have complete control over their records and can share with consent
    d. The Government has centralized control over all patient data.

Answers

1. b	2. c	3. b	4. b	5. a
6. c	7. b	8. d	9. c	10. c

CHAPTER 69

eSanjeevani—National Telemedicine Service

Amit Sachdeva, Rivu Basu

INTRODUCTION: BRIDGING THE HEALTHCARE DIVIDE

eSanjeevani, India's national telemedicine initiative, is transforming healthcare accessibility, particularly for remote and underserved regions. Launched in 2019 by the Ministry of Health and Family Welfare, this cloud-based telemedicine platform provides digital consultations, ensuring medical expertise reaches even the most isolated areas.[1,2]

THE EVOLUTION OF eSANJEEVANI: A DIGITAL LEAP IN HEALTHCARE

India's healthcare system has long struggled with geographic and economic disparities. While urban centers have access to specialists, rural populations often lack even basic medical care. The government's Digital India, Ayushman Bharat, and National Health Policy initiatives sought to bridge this gap. The COVID-19 pandemic accelerated the adoption of telemedicine, leading to the rapid expansion of eSanjeevani.[3-5]

Developed by the Center for Development of Advanced Computing (C-DAC), Mohali, eSanjeevani ensures secure, scalable, and free teleconsultations for millions of Indians. Unlike private telemedicine platforms that cater primarily to urban populations, eSanjeevani focuses on public healthcare and equity, ensuring that healthcare is universally accessible.[6-8]

KEY FEATURES OF eSANJEEVANI[3,6,7]

- **Scalability**: Handles millions of consultations nationwide.
- **Dual-mode functionality**: Supports Doctor-to-Doctor (AB-HWC) and Patient-to-Doctor (OPD) models.
- **Cloud-based and mobile-friendly**: Accessible via desktops, tablets, and smartphones.
- **Multilingual support**: Ensures inclusivity across linguistic and cultural barriers.
- **Integration with Ayushman Bharat**: Enhances coordination between primary, secondary, and tertiary healthcare services.
- **Electronic health records (EHRs)**: Enables digital prescriptions and patient history tracking.

TWO MODELS OF eSANJEEVANI: EXPANDING ACCESS TO HEALTHCARE[1,4,7]

1. eSanjeevani AB-HWC: Strengthening Primary Healthcare

Designed to connect rural patients with specialists, this model operates on a **Hub-and-Spoke Model**:
- **Hubs**: Specialists at medical colleges and district hospitals provide virtual consultations.
- **Spokes**: Health and Wellness Centers (HWCs) in rural areas facilitate patient-doctor interactions.

Impact
- Reduces patient travel and costs.
- Empowers primary healthcare providers with expert guidance.
- Enhances chronic disease management.

Case Study

Himachal Pradesh: In a remote Himalayan village, a patient experiencing chest pain consulted a cardiologist through eSanjeevani AB-HWC. The diagnosis and treatment recommendations helped prevent a potential cardiac emergency without requiring travel to a distant hospital.

2. eSanjeevani OPD: Bringing Healthcare to Homes

This model enables individuals to consult doctors remotely via smartphones, tablets, or computers, eliminating long waiting hours and reducing infection risks.

Key Benefits

- Enables remote chronic disease management.
- Provides virtual mental health consultations.
- Reduces hospital overcrowding.
- Facilitates quick and seamless e-prescriptions.

Case Study

A Working Mother in Delhi: A corporate professional, juggling work and childcare, used eSanjeevani OPD for a pediatric consultation instead of taking time off work. She received an e-prescription instantly, avoiding unnecessary hospital visits.

SPECIALIZED HEALTHCARE SERVICES VIA eSANJEEVANI

1. Chronic Disease Management

eSanjeevani ensures continuous care for hypertension, diabetes, cardiovascular diseases, and cancer.

Impact

- Enables remote monitoring of blood pressure and glucose levels.
- Provides personalized treatment adjustments.
- Facilitates virtual tumor board meetings for cancer care.

Case Study

Jharkhand: A lung cancer patient received expert consultation from AIIMS Delhi without leaving her village, improving her treatment outcomes significantly.

2. Maternal and Child Healthcare

- Facilitates prenatal and postnatal consultations.
- Ensures pediatric care for early disease detection.
- Supports nutrition and vaccination programs.

Case Study

Odisha: A pregnant woman at risk of preeclampsia received timely remote intervention, saving her and her baby's life.

3. Emergency and Critical Care

- Enables tele-stroke networks for rapid intervention.
- Supports real-time teleradiology and telepathology.

Case Study

Madhya Pradesh: A stroke patient received life-saving remote guidance from a neurologist, preventing permanent disability.

4. Mental Health Services

- Provides confidential therapy and psychiatric consultations.
- Addresses stigma-related barriers to mental health treatment.
- Supports crisis intervention and suicide prevention.

Case Study

Bihar: A rural student battling depression and anxiety received virtual counseling from NIMHANS psychiatrists, helping her regain mental well-being.

THE IMPACT OF eSANJEEVANI: A PARADIGM SHIFT

1. Accuracy and Reliability

- 74% diagnostic concordance with in-person consultations proves telemedicine's effectiveness.
- EHR integration improves long-term patient tracking and care.

2. Cost Savings for Patients

- Eliminates travel costs and lost wages.
- Saves an average of USD 25 per consultation.

3. Reducing Travel Burden

- Reduces patient travel by 18 km on average.
- Makes healthcare more accessible for the elderly and disabled.

4. A Global Benchmark

With over 130 million consultations, eSanjeevani is the world's largest government-led telemedicine initiative, offering a model for other developing nations.

5. COVID-19: A Critical Lifeline

- Provided uninterrupted medical care during lockdowns.
- Shifted non-critical consultations online, reducing hospital burden.
- Increased access to mental health services.

CHALLENGES AND FUTURE DIRECTIONS

1. Expanding Digital Infrastructure

- **Challenge:** Limited internet access in rural areas.
- **Solution:** Broadband expansion, satellite internet, and telehealth kiosks.

2. Training Healthcare Workers

- **Challenge:** Skill gaps among Community Health Officers (CHOs) and primary care providers.
- **Solution:** Nationwide telemedicine training programs and AI-assisted decision support.

3. Strengthening Data Security

- **Challenge:** Cybersecurity risks and patient privacy concerns.
- **Solution:** Implement end-to-end encryption, blockchain-based health records, and multi-factor authentication.

4. AI and IoT Integration

- **Challenge:** Limited use of smart healthcare technology.
- **Solution:** AI-powered diagnostics, IoT-based health monitoring, and predictive analytics for disease outbreaks.

5. Global Expansion
- ❖ **Challenge:** Adapting eSanjeevani for diverse healthcare systems.
- ❖ **Solution:** International collaborations, affordable cloud-based deployment, and localized telemedicine models.

CONCLUSION: eSANJEEVANI—A BLUEPRINT FOR THE FUTURE

eSanjeevani is more than just a telemedicine platform—it is a healthcare revolution. By making quality medical consultations accessible to every Indian, regardless of location or financial status, it is setting a precedent for digital healthcare globally. As AI, IoT, and data analytics further evolve, eSanjeevani is poised to lead the future of smart, inclusive, and equitable healthcare, ensuring that no patient is left behind.

eSanjeevani: A Revolution in Digital Healthcare—Key Highlights

Category	Key iInsights
Introduction	eSanjeevani is India's national telemedicine platform, bridging healthcare gaps, ensuring universal access to specialists, and transforming rural and urban healthcare.
Core technology	A cloud-based, AI-integrated telemedicine system handling millions of users daily with seamless connectivity across all health levels.
Service models	• **eSanjeevani AB-HWC:** Doctor-to-doctor teleconsultations, connecting rural HWCs to specialists via a Hub-and-Spoke model. • **eSanjeevani OPD:** Patient-to-doctor teleconsultations, enabling home-based virtual care.
Hub-and-spoke model	• **Hub:** Medical colleges and district hospitals house specialists • **Spoke:** Health and Wellness Centers (HWCs) in remote areas connect patients to experts.
Key benefits	• Specialist access for underserved areas. • **Reduced travel and costs:** Saves an average of 18 km per patient trip. • **Enhanced diagnosis and treatment:** 74% diagnostic accuracy matches in-person care. • **Continuity of care:** Chronic disease management for diabetes, hypertension, cancer, and mental health. • **Digital inclusivity:** Free e-prescriptions, tele-pathology, and radiology analysis. • **COVID-19 lifeline:** Ensured uninterrupted healthcare during lockdowns.
Clinical applications	• **Chronic disease management:** Virtual follow-ups for hypertension, diabetes, and cancer patients. • **Maternal and child health:** Remote pregnancy monitoring, pediatric care, and immunization counseling. • **Emergency and critical care:** Tele-stroke interventions and AI-assisted diagnostics. • **Mental health support:** Accessible therapy and counseling, reducing stigma.
Economic impact	• **Cost savings:** Each consultation saves $25 in travel and medical expenses. • **Travel reduction:** Average 18 km saved per patient visit. • **Scalability:** 130M+ consultations completed, making it the world's largest government telemedicine project.
Challenges and solutions	• **Digital divide:** Expand broadband and satellite internet in rural India. • **Healthcare workforce training:** Train CHOs and frontline workers for telemedicine. • **Data security risks:** Implement AI-driven encryption and multi-factor authentication. • **AI and IoT integration needed:** Use AI diagnostics, wearables, and real-time monitoring. • **Global expansion:** Adapt eSanjeevani for developing nations facing similar healthcare challenges.
Future prospects	• **AI-powered telehealth:** Integration of machine learning for predictive analytics. • **5G-enabled rural expansion:** Faster, real-time specialist consultations. • **Blockchain-based health records:** Secure, portable patient history tracking. • **Global replication:** A model for low-cost, high-impact telemedicine worldwide.
Conclusion	eSanjeevani is not just a telemedicine service—it is India's healthcare revolution. With AI-driven advancements, workforce training, and continued government support, it is paving the way for universal digital healthcare, setting a global benchmark in telemedicine.

References

1. Ministry of Health and Family Welfare, Government of India. eSanjeevani - National Telemedicine Service [Internet]. Available from: https://esanjeevani.mohfw.gov.in/#/
2. Digital India Programme, Government of India. eSanjeevani - A Digital Healthcare Initiative [Internet]. Available from: https://www.digitalindia.gov.in/initiative/esanjeevani/
3. National Portal of India. eSanjeevani Programme – Online OPD [Internet]. Available from: https://www.india.gov.in/esanjeevani-programme-online-opd
4. Department of Medical, Health & Family Welfare, Rajasthan Government. User Guide for Citizens – eSanjeevani [Internet]. Available from: https://rajswasthya.nic.in/PDF/eSanjeevani/USER%20GUIDE%20CITIZENS.pdf
5. Board of Governors, Medical Council of India. Telemedicine Practice Guidelines [Internet]. Available from: https://esanjeevani.mohfw.gov.in/assets/guidelines/Telemedicine_Practice_Guidelines.pdf
6. India.gov.in – National Government Services Portal. eSanjeevani - National Telemedicine Service [Internet]. Available from: https://services.india.gov.in/service/detail/esanjeevani-national-telemedicine-service
7. India Stack. eSanjeevani - Revolutionizing Digital Healthcare [Internet]. Available from: https://www.indiastack.global/esanjeevani/
8. Centre for Development of Advanced Computing (C-DAC), India. eSanjeevani - National Telemedicine Service [Internet]. Available from: https://www.cdac.in/index.aspx?id=product_details&productId=eSanjeevaniNationalTelemedicineService

QUESTIONS

Long Answer Question (LAQ)

1. eSanjeevani is considered a revolutionary step in India's healthcare system. Explain how it operates through its two service models, AB-HWC and OPD, and discuss its impact on healthcare accessibility. Highlight its role in chronic disease management, maternal care, emergency healthcare, and mental health support. What economic benefits does it offer, and what challenges must be addressed to ensure its long-term success?

Short Answer Questions (SAQs)

1. What are the key features of eSanjeevani, and how does it enhance healthcare accessibility in rural India?
2. Describe the hub-and-spoke model in eSanjeevani AB-HWC. How does it connect rural patients to specialists?
3. How has eSanjeevani helped reduce healthcare costs and travel time for patients? Provide specific data or examples.
4. Discuss the role of eSanjeevani during the COVID-19 pandemic. How did it help maintain uninterrupted healthcare services?
5. What are the primary challenges in implementing eSanjeevani, and what steps can be taken to overcome them?
6. How can Artificial Intelligence (AI) and wearable health devices improve the efficiency of eSanjeevani in the future?

Multiple Choice Questions (MCQs)

1. What are the two primary service models of eSanjeevani?
   a. Tele-Stroke Network & e-Pharmacy
   b. eSanjeevani AB-HWC & eSanjeevani OPD
   c. AI-Powered Diagnostics & Virtual Health Assistants
   d. Rural Healthcare Mission & Urban Health Drive

Chapter 69: eSanjeevani—National Telemedicine Service

2. **How does the Hub-and-Spoke model in eSanjeevani AB-HWC function?**
   a. Patients directly consult specialists at home without any intermediary
   b. It connects local Health & Wellness Centers (HWCs) to specialists at tertiary hospitals
   c. It operates as a hospital-based referral system for in-person consultations
   d. It provides AI-generated prescriptions without human intervention
3. **Which of the following is NOT a key benefit of eSanjeevani?**
   a. Reducing patient travel distance and associated costs
   b. Providing instant online consultations with AI-generated diagnosis
   c. Ensuring access to specialist care in rural areas through telemedicine
   d. Offering mental health support via virtual consultations
4. **During the COVID-19 pandemic, how did eSanjeevani contribute to healthcare accessibility?**
   a. It replaced all physical hospital visits with virtual consultations
   b. It provided uninterrupted access to doctors, reducing hospital crowding and exposure risks
   c. It was only used for COVID-19 patients and not for general medical concerns
   d. It acted as a vaccine registration portal rather than a telemedicine service
5. **Which of the following is a major challenge faced by eSanjeevani in its implementation?**
   a. Excessive patient engagement due to its overwhelming popularity
   b. The lack of doctors willing to participate in teleconsultations
   c. Limited internet connectivity in rural areas, requiring satellite-based expansion
   d. Government policies restricting telemedicine use in public health

Answers

| 1. b | 2. b | 3. b | 4. b | 5. c |

CHAPTER 70

e-Health Initiatives in India

Shaili Vyas, Niharika Verma, Sharon Baisil

Background	According to WHO, e-Health is defined as "the cost-effective and secure use of information and communications technologies in support of health and health-related fields, including health-care services, health surveillance, health literature, and health education, knowledge and research." "It encompasses multiple interventions, including telehealth, telemedicine, mobile health (mHealth), electronic medical or health records (eMR/eHR), big data, wearables, and even artificial intelligence." India is currently experiencing a significant rural-to-urban migration which is driven by various factors, including inadequate healthcare infrastructure. The existing healthcare facilities are insufficient to meet the demands of the rural population, resulting in a substantial gap between healthcare needs and service availability. e-Health initiatives by Government of India have emerged as a promising solution due to their accessibility and affordability, even in the most remote regions of the country. The integration of Information and Communication Technology (ICT) in healthcare delivery presents a valuable opportunity for resource-limited settings to optimize healthcare services and enhance overall public health outcomes.
Goal	To improve the efficiency and effectiveness of public healthcare system in the country
Initiatives	
National health portal[1,2]	• NHP was launched on 14th November, 2014. It acts a single point IT-enabled gateway to the authentic health-related information and government health programs and services to citizens and stakeholders in "6 languages: Hindi, English, Tamil, Gujarati, Bengali, and Punjabi." • "Center for Health Informatics (CHI)" has been established by the "National Institute of Health and Family and Welfare (NIHFW)" to manage NHP related activities. • There are different sections on NHP Portal along with useful links and screen-shots. • The portal handles many health initiatives like "mCessation, Mera Aspataal, MyHealthRecord, Pradhan Mantri Surakshit Matritva Abhiyaan (PMSMA), etc". • NHP voice-based web portal has also been launched. It provides the information to the users through 24 × 7 toll-free number 1800-180-1104. It allows users to interact with the app in their preferred language for receiving the authentic information.
Mera Aspataal (my hospital)[3]	• It is an initiative for receiving feedback from the patients for the services utilized at the hospital which is obtained through multiple channels such as "Short Message Service (SMS), Outbound Dialling (OBD) mobile application and web portal. These services are designed to be user-friendly". • The patient can submit the feedback for the hospitals visited in the last 7 days in seven different languages either on mobile app or a web portal. • The aim of Mera Aspataal initiative is to assist the government in making informed decisions to enhance the quality of healthcare services in the public facilities, thereby improving the patient experience and establishing a patient-centred and accountable health system.
India fights dengue[4]	• It is a mobile application which was launched on 7th April, 2016. • The 'India Fights Dengue' Mobile App provides information about dengue, ways of preventing and controlling it, its symptoms, checking the availability of hospitals and blood banks, and other related information.
No more tension mobile app[5]	• It is stress management mobile application which has been launched to helps users to manage stress. • The primary objective of 'No More Tension' mobile application is to educate the users about stress, including its definition, effects, symptoms and management strategies. • The application enables the users to assess their stress levels and provide evidence-based techniques for stress reductions like meditation and yoga.

"Mother and child tracking system (MCTS)/ reproductive child health (RCH) application"[6]	• MCTS is an individual-based tracking system designed to ensure the timely delivery of antenatal, postnatal and delivery services, as well as the systematic tracking of children to ensure complete immunization. • It has been implemented nationwide across all the States and Union Territories with the objective of improving Infant Mortality Rate, Maternal Mortality Rate, minimizing morbidity and enhancing service delivery. The system provides alerts to health service providers regrading due services list, identifies service delivery gaps and disseminates targeted health promotion messages to beneficiaries. • Reproductive and Child Health (RCH) is an enhanced version of MCTS that captures comprehensive data on "all RCH related services including family planning, maternal health, Child health and immunization". The application provides for early identification and continuous tracking of the beneficiaries throughout the reproductive lifecycle.
Kilkari[7]	• The Kilkari is a mobile-based public health initiative designed to support maternal and child health by disseminating critical information through Interactive Voice Response (IVR) technology. • Launched on January 15, 2016, as part of India's Digital India initiative, the program delivers "free, weekly, time-sensitive 72 audio messages on pregnancy, childbirth, and neonatal care to women registered in the Reproductive and Child Health (RCH) portal". • Currently operational in 20 States and Union Territories, the program initiates message delivery during the second trimester of pregnancy and continues until the child reaches one year of age. • Beneficiary data is systematically retrieved from the RCH portal via web-based services to ensure timely and accurate dissemination of information. • Toll free number: 1800-3010-1703
mCessation[8]	• mCessation is a mHealth strategy to encourage and support tobacco users who are willing to quit tobacco use. • In this strategy, those tobacco users who desire to quit tobacco give a missed call to Toll free number 011-22901701.
mDiabetes[9]	• It is a mobile-based initiative aimed at the prevention and management of diabetes, accessible by giving a missed call to 011-22901701. • The mDiabetes delivers text messages in "12 languages including English, Hindi, Kannada, Tamil, Malayalam, Bengali, Marathi, Gujarati, Telugu, Punjabi, Assamese, and Oriya" to promote awareness and support diabetes care. • It provides text messages twice a week for six months.

ANM OnLine (Anmol)[10]	• "ANMOL is a tablet-based application designed for the Integrated Reproductive and Child Health (RCH) Register" which enables ANMs to enter and update beneficiaries' data within their designated jurisdiction.
	• The application serves as a job aid to the ANMs by providing real-time access to essential information including due list, dashboard and guidance based on data entered etc for service delivery.
	• It also includes the multimedia educational tools such as Videos / audios on subjects like high-risk pregnancy, immunization, family planning etc. for use by ANMs.
	• **Key features:**
	  ✦ Real time data entry and updates by the ANM
	  ✦ Enhanced data accuracy and quality
	  ✦ Easily accessible training materials
	  ✦ Functionality remains unaffected even with poor Internet connectivity.

Mobile academy[11]	• Introduced in 2016, Mobile Academy is a free audio-based training program on Reproductive Maternal Neonatal and Child health, designed to refresh the knowledge of Accredited Social Health Activist (ASHA) on life-saving preventive healthcare practices. The program aims to improve the quality of ASHAs' interaction with new and expectant mothers and their families. • At present, the programme utilizes Interactive Voice Response (IVR) technology which is audio-based, making it accessible via a simple voice call, independent of mobile handset type. • The course consists of modules that equip ASHAs with the necessary skills to provide preventive care and appropriate referrals for mothers and children, through all the stages of pregnancy until the child's first two years of life. • The curriculum is organized into chapters, lessons and quizzes, with a cumulative assessment determining the pass/fail outcome. • Currently, Mobile Academy is available in "five languages: Hindi, Oriya, Assamese, Bengali and Telugu". • **Toll free number: 1800-3010-1704**

Aarogya Setu[12]	• Arogya Setu is a mobile application which was launched in April 2020 to protect the citizens during the pandemic of COVID-19. • It supports the scheduling, rescheduling, cancellation of Covid-19 vaccination appointment. It also allows users to download their vaccination certificate and request modifications in the certificate as needed. • Now, this digital application has transformed into National Health App offering a whole plethora of digital health services powered by Ayushman Bharat Digital Mission (ABDM). • Through Aarogya Setu, individuals can register for an Ayushman Bharat Health Account (Digital Health ID) and utilize it for seamless interaction with participating healthcare providers. • It also facilitates the scheduling of online medical consultations through the eSanjeevani OPD application, enabling users to book virtual doctor appointments and consult healthcare professionals remotely from their residences. • The application facilitates the secure and efficient exchange of digital health records, including laboratory reports, prescriptions, and diagnoses, from verified healthcare professionals and service providers.
e-Hospital[13]	• The e-Hospital application is a Hospital Management Information System (HMIS) designed to streamline and optimize the internal workflows and operational processes of healthcare facilities. • Implemented using a Software as a Service (SaaS) model, e-Hospital is deployed on a cloud infrastructure and is available to Central Government/State Government/Autonomous/Cooperative hospitals. **Objectives:** • To deploy e-Hospital, e-BloodBank, and ORS applications in government healthcare institutions to enhance digital healthcare management. • To offer online patient portal to deliver citizen centric healthcare services, including online appointment scheduling, online access to lab reports and real-time blood availability status. • To provide healthcare facilities with application related technical support through dedicated call center/ helpdesk.
e-BloodBank[13]	• The e-BloodBank application is a digital blood bank management system to streamline the process of blood collection, storage and distribution • It facilitates real time monitoring and coordination among blood banks, hospitals and donors, ensuring optimal resource utilization and accessibility. **Key features:** • User friendly and configurable • Simple registration process for blood transfusion center or storage unit • Real-time blood stock availability • Instant blood request functionality • Comprehensive blood donation records • Information on upcoming blood camps in nearby district
Online registration system[13]	• ORS is a key component of Digital India Initiative to enhance the patient access to healthcare services through integration with Ayushman Bharat Health Account (ABHA). • ORS functions as a nationwide digital framework that connects multiple hospitals to facilitate online appointment scheduling for OPD consultations. • By integrating with HMIS, it has digitized counter-based OPD registration process, thereby reducing manual workload and improving efficiency. • Through ORS, patients can schedule appointments with different hospital departments using their ABHA credentials.
Services e-Health assistance and teleconsultation (SeHAT)[14]	• Launched on 27th may, 2021, SeHAT is the tri-services teleconsultation service developed by the Ministry of Defence to provide telemedicine services for the entitled personnel and their families. • The SeHAT Stay-Home OPD functions as a virtual outpatient department (OPD), enabling patients to consult with healthcare professionals remotely via the internet. It supports multimodal communication, including video, audio, and text-based interactions, allowing real-time clinical consultations through smartphones, laptops, desktops, or tablets. This system ensures high-quality healthcare delivery while allowing patients to receive medical guidance without the need for physical hospital visits. **Key features:** • Secure and structured video consultations between patients and hospital-based physicians, ensuring professional medical guidance from any location. • User-friendly interface, requiring minimal effort for navigation and interaction. • Completely free-of-cost service, accessible via the official SeHAT OPD portal (https://sehatopd.gov.in) or through the SeHAT mobile applications, available on both the Google Play Store and Apple App Store.

e-RaktKosh[15]	**e-RaktKosh** is an integrated, **web-based blood bank management system** designed to automate and streamline blood bank operations across the country. Officially launched on **April 7, 2016**, the system incorporates **Aadhaar-based linkage** to enhance donor identification and record-keeping. • Key components • Biometric Donor Management System to identify, track, and regulate donors based on health status, donation history, and eligibility criteria • Blood Processing Module for essential processes, such as blood grouping, transfusion-transmitted infection (TTI) screening, antibody testing, and component separation in accordance with predefined protocols • Centralized Blood Inventory Management System maintaining a real-time database of blood stock availability across multiple blood banks • Biomedical waste management system for disposal of discarded blood and other waste generated during the process • Donor Registry Management for rare blood group donors and tracks regular donors to promote repeat donations • Automated Alert and Notification System sending real-time notifications and alerts to relevant stakeholders regarding donor eligibility, inventory updates, and other critical information

References

1. e-Health. Ministry of Health and Family Welfare, Government of India. Available at https://mohfw.gov.in/?q=Organisation/departments-health-and-family-welfare/e-Health-Telemedicine
2. Revolutionizing Healthcare: Digital Innovations in India's Health Sector. Press Information Bureau, Government of India, Ministry of Health and Family Welfare. Available at https://pib.gov.in/PressNoteDetails.aspx?NoteId=151782&ModuleId=3&reg=3&lang=1#_ftn10
3. Mera Aspataal (My Hospital). Ministry of Health and Family Welfare, Government of India. Available at https://meraaspataal.nhp.gov.in/about_us
4. India Fights Dengue, Strategy and plan of action for effective community participation for prevention and control of dengue. Ministry of Health and Family Welfare, Government of India. Available at https://ncvbdc.mohfw.gov.in/Doc/Strategy-plan-actions-ECP-Dengue.pdf
5. Shri JP Nadda launches "Healthy India Initiative" magazine and "No More Tension" Mobile Application. Press Information Bureau, Government of India, Ministry of Health and Family Welfare. Available at https://pib.gov.in/newsite/PrintRelease.aspx?relid=153444
6. Mother and Child Tracking System (MCTS). Available at: http://nrhm-mcts.nic.in/
7. Update on Kilkari Scheme. Press Information Bureau, Government of India, Ministry of Health and Family Welfare. Available at https://www.pib.gov.in/PressReleasePage.aspx?PRID=2004362
8. mCessation. National Tobacco Control Program, Ministry of Health and Family Welfare, Government of India. Available at https://ntcp.mohfw.gov.in/mcessation
9. mDiabetes. Arogya World. Available at https://arogyaworld.org/mdiabetes/
10. ANMOL User Manual Version 5.0.12. Ministry of Health and Family Welfare, Government of India. Available at https://nhmmizoram.org/upload/Anmol%205.0.12%20User%20Manual_28May2024.pdf
11. Mobile Academy. ARMMAN-Helping Mothers and Children. Available at https://armman.org/mobile-academy/
12. Aarogya Setu App. Available at: https://www.india.gov.in/content/aarogya-setu-app
13. eHospital. NAtional Information Centre. Available at: https://www.nic.in/project/ehospital/
14. Website of Services eHealth Assistance and Teleconsultation (SeHAT) Out Patient Department (OPD), Ministry of Defence. Available at; https://sehatopd.gov.in/
15. e-RaktKosh: Centralized Blood Bank Management System. Available at:https://eraktkosh.mohfw.gov.in/BLDAHIMS/bloodbank/transactions/bbpublicindex.html

QUESTIONS

Long Answer Question (LAQ)

1. What is e-Health? How does it contribute to the advancement of healthcare services in India? Comment on the information and communication technologies (ICT) initiatives for improving efficiency and effectiveness of the public healthcare system of india.

Short Answer Questions (SAQs)

1. Discuss e-Health initiatives initiated by Ministry of Health and Family Welfare to improve maternal and child health.
2. What is m-Health? Enlist the mobile health initiatives launched by Government of India.

Multiple Choice Questions (MCQs)

1. Which of the following best describes e-Health?
    a. The use of electronic devices exclusively for hospital administration
    b. The application of digital technologies to improve healthcare delivery and accessibility
    c. Method of online shopping for medicines only
    d. A system limited to storing patient records in digital format
2. All of the following are service delivery and tracking apps, *except*:
    a. Mera Aspataal
    b. MCTS
    c. Nikshay
    d. Kilkari
3. Refresher training of Ashas is conducted through:
    a. Anmol
    b. RCH portal
    c. National health portal
    d. Mobile academy

Answers

1. b 2. a 3. d

PART F

Miscellaneous

71. Ayushman Bharat Programme
72. Pradhan Mantri Bhartiya Janaushadhi Pariyojana
73. Beti Bachao Beti Padhao
74. Kayakalp
75. National Jal Jeevan Mission
76. Swachh Swasth Sarvatra (SSS) Initiative
77. Pradhan Mantri Ujjwala Yojana
78. Ujjawala Scheme for Prevention of Trafficking and Rescue, Rehabilitation and Reintegration of Victims of Trafficking
79. National Programme on Climate Change and Human Health
80. Voluntary Blood Donation Programme
81. National Organ Transplant Program
82. National Programme for Control and Treatment of Occupational Diseases
83. National Programme on Containment of Anti-Microbial Resistance (AMR)
84. Social Security Schemes for Unorganized and Organized Sectors
85. Schemes for Intellectual Disability
86. Pradhan Mantri Swasthya Suraksha Yojana (PMSSY)
87. Affordable Medicines and Reliable Implants for Treatment
88. National Action Plan for Prevention and Control of Snakebite Envenoming

CHAPTER 71

Ayushman Bharat Programme

Ritesh Singh, Parul Sharma, Nilesh Thakor

Background/Need of program/Scheme	Ayushman Bharat was introduced to address several key challenges in India's healthcare system: **Healthcare access disparities:** Many Indians, especially those in rural areas and from economically weaker sections, struggle to afford essential healthcare services. **Financial protection:** • Out-of-pocket healthcare expenses can lead to catastrophic financial burdens. Financial barriers often prevent people from getting the treatment they need. • High medical expenses can push families below the poverty line. **Lack of quality healthcare infrastructure:** Many parts of India, especially rural areas, lack adequate healthcare facilities and skilled medical professionals. **Less focus on emerging diseases:** • India faces a dual burden of communicable and non-communicable diseases. • There is a need for increased emphasis on preventive healthcare (regular check-ups, screenings, and health education) to tackle emerging health challenges.
Implemented since	The scheme has been implemented since September 2018.
Goal	• Ayushman Bharat is a flagship healthcare scheme of the Government of India, introduced as per the National Health Policy 2017. • It aims to achieve Universal Health Coverage (UHC), ensuring that everyone receives the healthcare they need without financial hardship.[1]
Targets	• **Upgrade health centers:** Transform existing Sub-Health Centers (SHCs) and Primary Health Centers (PHCs) into Health and Wellness Centers (HWCs) to ensure universal access to comprehensive primary healthcare services. • **Provide Health Coverage:** Offer health coverage and financial protection to deprived households that lack access to essential healthcare services.
Objectives	**To reduce the burden on hospitals by promoting early detection and preventive care, improving overall health outcomes.** • **Universal health coverage (UHC):** Ensure that everyone has access to quality healthcare services without financial barriers. • **Financial protection:** Protect individuals and families from catastrophic healthcare expenses. • **Enhanced healthcare access:** Improve access to healthcare services, especially for underserved and marginalized populations. • **Improved quality of care:** Focus on raising the quality standards of healthcare facilities and services. • **Promoting wellness and preventive care:** Emphasize prevention, health promotion, and early detection to reduce disease burden. • **Technology integration and transparency:** Leverage digital health technology for better service delivery, monitoring, and transparency in the healthcare system.
Organogram	**Service Delivery Levels:** **Family/household and community level:** *Roles of ASHA and MPW:* • ASHA workers and multi-purpose workers (MPWs) visit homes for: • Community mobilization to improve healthcare-seeking behavior. • Risk assessments, screening, and follow-up for primary and secondary prevention. • Counseling and creating supportive environments in families and communities.

	Follow-up support: • ASHAs ensure treatment compliance through regular home visits. • They also help organize meetings for patient support groups. **Community Platforms:** Platforms like Village Health and Nutrition Days (VHNDs), Village Health, Sanitation, and Nutrition Committees (VHSNCs), and Mahila Arogya Samities are used to engage the community. **Health and Wellness Centers (HWCs):** • **Service availability:** HWCs are open for at least six hours daily, providing general OPD services and follow-up care for chronic illnesses. • **Team member roles:** Outreach services and home visits are scheduled to ensure someone is always available at the HWC for OPD and chronic illness management. *Chronic Illness Follow-Up:* • Patient group meetings are held on fixed days for specific conditions: • Hypertension/Diabetes: Wednesday afternoons. • Elderly care: Thursday afternoons. **First referral level:** *Referral Pathways:* The referral site depends on the illness and availability of specialists. Consultations for acute illnesses are typically done by: • Medical Officers (MOs) at PHCs. • Specialists at CHCs or District Hospitals (DHs), either in person or via teleconsultation. Over time, each state aims to establish: • First Referral Units (FRUs) at the CHC level. • District Hospitals (DHs) equipped with a full range of specialist services for comprehensive referral support.
Beneficiaries	**PM-JAY (Pradhan Mantri Jan Arogya Yojana):** • Beneficiary families are identified based on the 2011 Socio-Economic Caste Census (SECC). • Selection is done using specific deprivation and occupational criteria. **Health and Wellness Centers (HWCs):** These centers are designed to benefit everyone in the community, offering services accessible to all.
Components	**Ayushman Arogya Mandir (health and wellness centers):** These centers focus on providing primary healthcare services near the community. Services include: • Maternal and child health care. • Screening and management of non-communicable diseases (NCDs). • Basic diagnostic services. **Pradhan Mantri Jan Arogya Yojana (PM-JAY):** PM-JAY provides health insurance coverage to over 65 crore people, making it the world's largest government-funded healthcare program. *Coverage includes:* • Up to ₹ 5 lakh per family per year for secondary and tertiary care hospitalization. • A wide range of medical treatments, such as surgeries, diagnostics, and medications. *Comprehensive healthcare approach:* • Ayushman Bharat moves away from segmented healthcare delivery to a comprehensive, need-based service model. • The focus is on holistic interventions covering prevention, promotion, and ambulatory care at the primary, secondary, and tertiary levels. *Continuum of care:* • The scheme integrates care across various levels through two main components: • Health and Wellness Centers (HWCs): Provide primary care services close to communities, focusing on preventive and promotive healthcare. • Pradhan Mantri Jan Arogya Yojana (PM-JAY): Offers financial protection through health insurance for secondary and tertiary care to economically weaker families.

Strategies/ Deliverables under the program	*Universal health coverage:* • Ayushman Bharat aims to provide financial protection against high healthcare costs. • The scheme covers over 14 crore vulnerable families, ensuring the poorest sections of society can access quality healthcare without financial burden. *Empowering the poor:* • The scheme gives beneficiaries the freedom to choose where they receive treatment, enhancing patient autonomy. • It encourages private hospitals to join the network, increasing the availability of quality healthcare across the country. *Focus on preventive healthcare:* • Health and Wellness Centers (HWCs) focus on promoting preventive care, like regular check-ups and screenings. • The goal is to reduce the incidence of diseases and encourage a healthier population. *Strengthening healthcare infrastructure:* • The scheme has led to investments in healthcare infrastructure, especially in rural and underserved areas. • It has driven the development of new hospitals, upgrades to existing facilities, and the deployment of more healthcare professionals to improve service delivery. *Digital Integration:* • The PM-JAY scheme operates through a digital platform for smooth and cashless transactions at empaneled hospitals. • This system ensures transparency, efficiency, and accountability in identifying beneficiaries, verifying entitlements, and delivering healthcare services.
Activities at various level or package of services	• **Pregnancy and childbirth care:** Comprehensive care during pregnancy and safe delivery. • **Neonatal and infant health care:** Health services for newborns and infants. • **Childhood and adolescent health care:** Health services focused on children and adolescents. • **Family planning and reproductive health:** Family planning, contraceptive services, and other reproductive health care. • **Communicable diseases management:** Management of communicable diseases, including services under national health programs. • **Common communicable diseases and minor illness care:** Outpatient care for simple illnesses and minor ailments. • **Noncommunicable diseases (NCDs):** Screening, prevention, control, and management of NCDs. • **Common ophthalmic and ENT care:** Basic care for eye, ear, nose, and throat problems. • **Oral health care:** Basic dental and oral health services. • **Elderly and palliative care:** Health services for the elderly and those needing palliative care. • **Emergency medical services:** Immediate medical care in emergencies. • **Mental health services:** Screening and basic management of mental health issues.
Monitoring and evaluation of program	**Responsibility and Oversight:**[2] **State and district levels:** A designated program management team is responsible for overall monitoring and supervision of Health and Wellness Centers (HWCs). **Block level:** The block nodal officer oversees the rollout of HWCs and monitors progress monthly. **IT Platform:** A digital platform generates reports on population health indicators and disease surveillance for effective monitoring at block, district, and state levels. **Indicator A—Reported to State and National Levels:** 1. Outpatient (OP) visits per capita in each district/state. 2. Hospitalization rate (per 100,000 population) in each district/state. 3. Annual primary care empanelment rate: Proportion of families registered with HWCs. 4. Three ANC Rate: Proportion of pregnant women receiving three antenatal checkups. 5. SBA-assisted delivery rate/Institutional delivery rate. 6. Perinatal mortality rate by district. 7. Under-5 mortality rate by district. 8. Full immunization rate by district.

9. Child malnutrition rate by district.
10. Exclusive breastfeeding rate at DPT3.
11. Pediatric hospitalization rate.
12. Proportion of children with diarrhea/ARI receiving appropriate treatment.
13. Cardiovascular mortality in the 15–60 years age group.
14. Accidental death rates.
15. Major surgeries per one lakh population.
16. Leprosy indicators: Annual new case detection rate, prevalence rate, new cases with Grade II disability, and treatment completion rate.
17. Tuberculosis case detection rate.
18. Annual parasite index for malaria.
19. HIV in ANC clinics/STD clinics rate.
20. Proportion of chronic NCD patients on regular follow-up/medication.
21. Average Out-of-Pocket (OOP) costs per hospitalization episode.
22. Average OOP costs for ARI/diarrhea treatment in children under five.

Indicator B-Available at the District Level:
1. OP visits per capita for each facility HMIS
2. Beds per lakh population
3. Bed Occupancy Ratio
4. Anemia in pregnancy rate
5. Hypertension in pregnancy rate
6. Full ANC rate
7. C-Section rate
8. Complicated pregnancy rate
9. Medical termination of pregnancy rate
10. Stillbirth rate
11. Weighing efficiency and low birth weight rate
12. Maternal deaths—absolute numbers per district
13. Maternal deaths by cause of death
14. Death of women in 15 to 45 year age group due to unknown causes
15. Late still births
16. Early neonatal deaths
17. Neonatal deaths
18. 0–1 Infant deaths
19. 1–4 deaths
20. Full immunization rate of each vaccine
21. Severe Acute Malnutrition (SAM), Moderately Acute Malnutrition (MAM) rates
22. Mild, moderate and severe malnutrition rates
23. Breastfeeding within first hour
24. Hospitalization specifically for: Sick newborn, pneumonia, diarrhea and dehydration.
25. Oral Rehydration Therapy (ORT) for diarrhea rate
26. Appropriate treatment for ARI rate.
27. Any notified vaccine preventable disease
28. % of population of 30 years and above screened for HT
29. % of those screened positive for HT who were examined at PHC/CHC
30. % of those who were initiated on treatment at PHC or above who are still under treatment, uninterrupted for last three months
31. % of those currently on treatment who have achieved blood pressure control
32. % of population of 30 years and above screened for DM
33. % of those screened positive for DM who were examined at PHC/CHC
34. % of those who were initiated on treatment at PHC or above who are still under treatment, uninterrupted for last three months
35. % of those currently on treatment who have achieved blood sugar control
36. % of population of 30 years and above screened for Oral Cancer
37. % of women of 30 years and above screened for Breast Cancer

	38.	% of women of 30 years and above screened for cervical cancer
	39.	% of those who were screened positive for each of the cancers that underwent biopsy at CHC/DH
	40.	% of those who underwent treatment for each of the cancers who are screened periodically

References

1. Ayushman Bharat. Comprehensive Primary Health Care through Health and Wellness Center. Operational Guidelines. NHSRC (Available on URL: https://www.nhm.gov.in/New_Updates_2018/NHM_Components/Health_System_Stregthening/Comprehensive_primary_health_care/letter/Operational_Guidelines_For_CPHC.pdf)
2. Towards Universal Health Coverage. Ayushman Bharat Health and Wellness Centres. A compendium of Health and Wellness Centres operationalization. April 2018 – November 2020. (Avaialble on URL: https://ab-hwc.nhp.gov.in/download/document/Towards_Universal_Health_Coverage_HWCO_14_12_20_for_web.pdf)

QUESTIONS

Long Answer Question (LAQ)

1. What are the strategies implemented under Ayushman Bharat scheme? How is the program evaluated?

Short Answer Questions (SAQs)

1. What are the components of Ayushman Bharat?
2. Enumerate the objectives of Ayushman Bharat Programme.

Multiple Choice Questions (MCQs)

1. Which key challenge does Ayushman Bharat primarily address in the Indian healthcare system?
   a. Reducing pollution
   b. Healthcare access disparities
   c. Economic development
   d. Industrial growth
2. What is the main goal of the Pradhan Mantri Jan Arogya Yojana (PM-JAY) under Ayushman Bharat?
   a. Provide free medication to everyone
   b. Offer health insurance coverage for secondary and tertiary care hospitalization
   c. Build new hospitals in urban areas
   d. Promote traditional medicine
3. How much health coverage is provided per family per year under PM-JAY?
   a. ₹1 lakh
   b. ₹2 lakh
   c. ₹3 lakh
   d. ₹5 lakh
4. Which census is used for identifying PM-JAY beneficiaries?
   a. 2001 Population Census
   b. 2011 Socio-Economic Caste Census (SECC)
   c. 2021 Population Census
   d. National Sample Survey
5. Which level of care does the Ayushman Bharat Programme primarily emphasize for early detection and prevention?
   a. Tertiary care
   b. Secondary care
   c. Primary care
   d. Quaternary care

6. **What is the role of ASHA workers under the Ayushman Bharat Programme at the community level?**
   a. Conduct surgeries
   b. Mobilize the community, risk assessments, and follow-up care
   c. Provide tertiary healthcare services
   d. Manage financial transactions

7. **What is the primary objective of the Health and Wellness Centers (HWCs)?**
   a. Deliver high-end surgical care
   b. Provide primary healthcare services near the community
   c. Offer only pharmaceutical services
   d. Manage large-scale emergency cases

8. **Which of the following is not a key objective of Ayushman Bharat?**
   a. Promoting preventive healthcare
   b. Enhancing healthcare access
   c. Establishing new private hospitals in urban areas
   d. Ensuring financial protection from high healthcare expenses

9. **Which digital platform is used for smooth, cashless transactions under PM-JAY?**
   a. Ayushman Bharat Portal
   b. Aarogya Setu
   c. National Health Stack
   d. UPI Health Gateway

10. **Which of the following services are offered at Health and Wellness Centers (HWCs)?**
    a. Specialized surgeries
    b. Maternal and child healthcare, screening for NCDs
    c. Ayurvedic treatments
    d. Cosmetic surgeries

Answers

1. b	2. b	3. d	4. b	5. c
6. b	7. b	8. c	9. a	10. b

CHAPTER 72

Pradhan Mantri Bhartiya Janaushadhi Pariyojana

Kartik Prajapati, Parul Sharma, Purushottam Giri, Deepika Aggarwal

Background/ Need of program/ Scheme	The majority of Indians lack access to reasonably priced medications, even though their country is one of the world's top exporters of generic medications. Compared to inpatient treatment, the overall cost of outpatient care is substantially higher. According to the National Sample Survey Organization's (NSSO) 71st Round (January–June 2014) report on health in India, the purchase of medications accounted for almost 72% of all non-hospitalized treatment expenditures in the rural sector and 68% in the urban sector. The Brookings study argues that the Out-of-Pocket Expenditure (OOPE) warrants special attention as it leads to impoverishment, with 7% of the households falling below the poverty line on account of health expenses.[1] A medicinal product under PMBJP is priced on the concept of a maximum of 50% of the average price of the top three branded medicines. Therefore, the price of Janaushadhi medicines is cheaper at least by 50% and, in certain circumstances, by 80–90% of the market price of branded medicines. The PMBJP's implementing agency, the Pharmaceuticals and Medical Devices Bureau of India (PMBI), has generated over ₹1000 crore in sales during the last financial year, which runs through February 15, 2023. This has resulted in savings for the populace of almost ₹6,000 crore.
Implemented since	It began as the Jan Aushadhi scheme in 2008 and was redesigned as the Pradhan Mantri Janaushadhi Yojana in September 2015. In order to broaden even further, it was renamed the Pradhan Mantri Bhartiya Janaushadhi Pariyojana (PMBJP).
Goal	Making quality generic medicines available at affordable prices to all.
Targets	The target established by the government is to have 25,000 Pradhan Mantri Bhartiya Janaushadhi Kendras (PMBJKs) open nationwide by March 31, 2027.
Objectives	• Ensure access to quality medicines for all sections of the population, especially the poor and deprived ones. • Create awareness about the generic medicines through education and publicity to counter the perception that quality is synonymous with the high price. • Generate employment by engaging individual entrepreneurs in opening the PMBJP kendras. • Extend coverage of quality generic medicines so as to reduce out-of-pocket expenditure on medicines and thereby redefine the unit cost of treatment per person.
Organogram	The Department of Pharmaceuticals founded the Pharmaceuticals and Medical Devices Bureau of India (PMBI), formerly the Bureau of Pharma Public Sector Undertakings of India (BPPI), on December 1, 2008, with the main goal of establishing a targeted and capable organization to carry out the Jan Aushadhi Campaign. PMBI is governed by a Chief Executive Officer (CEO) and is registered under the Societies Registration Act, 1860. The Secretary of the Department of Pharmaceuticals chairs the Governing Council, which approves policy decisions. Under the direction of the Joint Secretary of the Department, an Executive Council (EC) periodically evaluates PMBI's performance.
Beneficiaries	Qualifications for opening Pradhan Mantri Bhartiya Janaushadhi Kendra applicants must possess a D Pharma or B Pharma degree, or they must hire someone with a D Pharma or B Pharma degree and provide documentation of this at the time of application submission or final approval. Any company or non-profit applying for a PMBJK must hire people with a B Pharma or D Pharma degree and provide documentation of this at the time of application submission or final approval. Reputable NGOs and charitable groups would be the preferred agency on government hospital grounds, including medical universities, although individuals would also be qualified.[2,3]

Components	- **Low-priced medications:** Through Pradhan Mantri Bhartiya Janaushadhi Kendras (PMBJKs), the program seeks to offer high-quality generic medications at a price that is 50–90% less than that of branded ones. In terms of safety, effectiveness, and quality, these medications are on par with branded ones.[3]
- **Extensive Pradhan Mantri Bhartiya Janaushadhi** Kendra Network: According to the latest reports, the program has created more than 9,000 PMBJP Kendras throughout India. To guarantee that everyone has access to reasonably priced medications, these stores are open in a variety of cities, towns, and rural areas.
- **Accessibility of essential drugs:** The program offers more than 1,600 medications as well as more than 250 surgical and consumable supplies. Anti-diabetics, cardiovascular medications, anti-cancer medications, analgesics, antipyretics, vitamins, and more are on the list of medications.
- **Entrepreneurial incentives:** To encourage the establishment of new PMBJP Kendras, the government offers incentives, such as a one-time grant of up to ₹2.5 lakh. Extra rewards for SC/ST candidates, female entrepreneurs, and those starting businesses in underdeveloped areas. financial assistance for the purchase of furniture, printers, and PCs.[4]
- **Quality control:** Labs accredited by the National Accreditation Board for Testing and Calibration (NABL) test the medications sold through Janaushadhi Kendras. They guarantee quality and safety by adhering to the Indian Pharmacopoeia's (IP) standards.
- **Campaigns for awareness:** To inform the public about the advantages of generic medications, awareness campaigns and initiatives are conducted. These include raising awareness through social media, print media, and electronic media.
- **Transparency and E-government:** To ensure system transparency, the government uses IT-enabled services to keep an eye on pricing, supply chain management, and medication availability. Customers can also use a smartphone app to look up costs and available medications.
- **Assistance for the medical system:** By lowering patients' out-of-pocket costs and supplying medications that are necessary to treat both acute and chronic illnesses, PMBJP promotes the broader healthcare system.
- **Product range expansion:** With an emphasis on introducing more life-saving medications and lowering their cost for the average person, the PMBJP's drug selection continues to expand.[5]
- **Collaborations:** To supply medications, the government has partnered with both private businesses and public sector enterprises (PSUs). These collaborations provide a consistent and sustainable supply of necessary medications.
- **Janaushadhi suvidha sanitary napkin:** On August 27, 2019, Janaushadhi Suvidha Oxo-biodegradable Sanitary Napkins were introduced as a significant step towards guaranteeing the health security of Indian women. They will be sold at ₹1/-per pad only. All around the nation, over 10,000 PMBJP Kendras are selling Janaushadhi Suvidha napkins. As of November 30, 2023, Suvidha Napkins' total sales value was 47.87 crores.[6]
Strategies/ Deliverables under the program	- Establishing a network of stores called Jan Aushadhi Kendras to provide reasonably priced generic medications all over India.[6]
- **Providing generic medicines at reasonable prices:** Generic medications are offered at 50% to 90% less than their branded equivalents.
- **Working together with pharmaceutical manufacturers:** Assuring a consistent supply of high-quality medications requires cooperation with both public and private manufacturers.
- **Ensuring quality control:** All medications supplied undergo stringent quality testing at labs approved by the NABL.
- **Publicity and awareness campaigns:** Encouraging the use of generic medications by means of community involvement and broad media outreach.
- **Incentives for store owners:** Providing financial assistance and training to encourage the establishment of Jan Aushadhi Kendras.
- **Broadening product offering:** Increasing the selection of goods, such as essential prescription drugs for long-term illnesses.
- **Integrating with national health programs:** Working together to improve healthcare delivery through national health initiatives.
- **Digitalization and supply chain management:** Setting up a centralized system for inventory control and real-time tracking.
- **Emphasizing underserved and rural areas:** To increase access to medications, Jan Aushadhi Kendras are being established in underserved and rural areas.

	It is run by both private business owners and government organizations. • **Regular incentive:** The previous ₹2,50,000/- incentive for Kendra owners has been increased to ₹5,00,000/-, which would be awarded at 15% of monthly purchases, up to a monthly maximum of ₹15,000. • **Special incentive:** The PMBJP will receive a one-time incentive of ₹2,00,000 (in addition to regular incentives) for computers, printers, and furniture and fixtures. Kendras have been established in the northeastern states, the Himalayan regions, island territories, and underdeveloped areas designated as aspirational districts by NITI Aayog. These locations have also been opened by women entrepreneurs, Divyang, SCs, and STs. • Janaushadhi medications are 50% to 90% less expensive than branded ones found on the free market. • In order to guarantee product quality, medications are exclusively purchased from vendors who have earned World Health Organization-Good Manufacturing Practices (WHO-GMP) certification. • To guarantee the highest quality, every batch of the medication is examined at labs approved by the "National Accreditation Board for Testing and Calibration Laboratories (NABL)." • A 20% profit on each drug's MRP (excluding taxes) will be given to the operating agency.
Activities at various level Or package of services	**Primary prevention** • To ensure awareness among the masses, various media platforms, such as print, outdoor, TV, social media, etc., are being used regularly. The government is also adopting an integrated approach for spreading awareness about PMBJP with state governments. Promotion workshops are also organized across India with kendra owners, doctors, and various important dignitaries. • The product basket has also been expanded to provide a complete range of medicines for increasing footfall to the Kendras. • New medicines and nutraceuticals products, such as protein powder, malt-based food supplements, glucometers, etc., have been launched. • State health and associated government authorities have been requested on a regular basis to open Jan Aushadhi kendras in various government hospitals and associated premises by providing rent-free spaces. **Secondary prevention** The Pradhan Mantri Bhartiya Janaushadhi Pariyojana (PMBJP) plays a crucial role in secondary prevention by providing affordable access to medications that help manage chronic illnesses and prevent complications. Through over 9,000 Janaushadhi Kendras, the program offers essential medications for conditions, such as diabetes, hypertension, cardiovascular diseases, and respiratory disorders at 50–90% lower costs. This affordability encourages early and consistent treatment, which is key to stopping disease progression and avoiding severe outcomes, such as heart attacks, strokes, and kidney failure. PMBJP ensures the availability of life-saving drugs, promoting long-term treatment adherence, especially for those with lower and middle incomes. By reducing out-of-pocket healthcare expenses, the program enables more patients to access and sustain their treatments without financial hardship, thus improving health outcomes and preventing the worsening of their conditions. **Tertiary prevention** PMBJP lowers the chance of serious health crises by assisting patients in managing conditions, such as diabetes, heart disease, and cancer. Patients can easily obtain life-saving medications at Kendras nationwide, which promotes adherence to treatment plans. The initiative helps people to properly prioritize their health by reducing the financial burden related to managing chronic diseases. In the end, this continuous assistance improves health outcomes for those with long-term illnesses and lessens the burden on the healthcare system.[7]
Monitoring and Evaluation of program	• **Quality control mechanisms:** Only manufacturers accredited by WHO Good Manufacturing Practices (GMP) are used to source medicines. NABL-accredited labs evaluate every batch of medications to make sure they adhere to safety and effectiveness regulations. This rigorous testing ensures that the medicines available at Janaushadhi Kendras are of high quality.[8] • **Data management systems:** A data assembling system run by the Pharma and Medical Bureau of India (PMBI) monitors a number of indicators, such as the quantity of Janaushadhi Kendras in operation, the variety of medications offered, sales information, and consumer financial savings. This data is crucial for assessing the impact of the scheme and making informed decisions for improvement. • **Performance indicators:** Certain criteria are set up, like the quantity of medications available, the number of Kendras in operation, and the savings that citizens have made. The initiative's efficacy is measured by ongoing evaluation of these indicators.

> - **Feedback mechanisms:** Feedback from users, including patients and healthcare professionals, is encouraged by the program. Understanding user satisfaction and pinpointing areas where service delivery and product offerings need to be improved depend heavily on this input.
> - **Regular reporting:** The PMBI is in charge of creating frequent reports on the PMBJP's performance and results. Stakeholders can better grasp the initiative's problems and success thanks to these reports.
> - **Collaboration with state governments:** Cooperation with state governments supports monitoring initiatives and improves the reach and efficacy of awareness programs.

References

1. Ministry of Chemicals and Fertilizers. Pradhan Mantri Bhartiya Janaushadhi Pariyojana (PMBJP) [Internet]. March 7, 2023. Available from.http://janaushadhi.gov.in/pdf/Presentation%20on%20PMBJP_15022022.pdf
2. Ministry of Chemicals and Fertilizers. Union Minister for Chemicals and Fertilizers Dr. Mansukh Mandaviya flags off Jan Aushadhi Rath to commence celebrations of Jan Aushadhi Jan Chetna Abhiyaan [Internet]. 2023 Mar 1 [cited 2024 Oct 6]. Available from: https://www.pib.gov.in/PressReleasePage.aspx?PRID=1903403
3. Singh P, Ravi S, Dam D. Medicines in India: Accessibility, Affordability and Quality. Brookings India Research Paper. 2020; (032020-01)ISBN:978-81-941963-6-5.Pharmaceuticals and Medical Devices Bureau of India [Internet]. Gov.in. [cited 2024 Oct 6]. Available from: https://janaushadhi.gov.in/
4. Notification/Circulars [Internet]. Gov.in. [cited 2024 Oct 6]. Available from: https://pharmaceuticals.gov.in/niper-notificatio
5. Pharmaceuticals and Medical Devices Bureau of India [Internet]. Gov.in. [cited 2024 Oct 6]. Availablefrom:https://janaushadhi.gov.in/annual_report.aspx
6. Ministry of Chemicals and Fertilizers. Under Pradhan Mantri Bhartiya Janaushadhi Pariyojana only quality medicines are supplied through Jan Aushadhi Kendras [Internet]. PIB Delhi; 2024 Aug 9 [cited 2024 Oct 6]. Available from: https://pib.gov.in/PressReleasePage.aspx?PRID=2043774
7. Government of India, Ministry of Chemicals and Fertilizers, Department of Pharmaceuticals. Jan Aushadhi Kendra in Jharkhand. Unstarred Question No. 848, answered on 26th July, 2024. Lok Sabha.
8. Pharmaceuticals and Medical Devices Bureau of India. Guidelines for opening of new Pradhan Mantri Bhartiya Janaushadhi Kendra (PMBJK). New Delhi: Pharmaceuticals and Medical Devices Bureau of India; 2021. Available from: https://janaushadhi.gov.in/

QUESTIONS

Long Answer Question (LAQ)

1. Discuss the objectives and impact of the Pradhan Mantri Bhartiya Janaushadhi Pariyojana (PMBJP) on the accessibility and affordability of generic medicines in India. How does this initiative aim to bridge the gap in healthcare services for economically disadvantaged populations, and what measures have been implemented to ensure the quality of the medicines provided through this program?

Short Answer Questions (SAQs)

1. What are the key features of the Pradhan Mantri Bhartiya Janaushadhi Pariyojana (PMBJP)?
2. How does PMBJP contribute to the reduction of healthcare costs for the average Indian citizen?

Chapter 72: Pradhan Mantri Bhartiya Janaushadhi Pariyojana

Multiple Choice Questions (MCQs)

1. Which of the following is a primary objective of the PMBJP?
   a. To promote the use of branded medicines
   b. To provide affordable generic medicines to the public
   c. To eliminate all pharmaceutical companies
   d. To increase the import of foreign medicines
2. What is the role of Janaushadhi Kendras in the PMBJP initiative?
   a. To manufacture medicines
   b. To sell branded medicines only
   c. To distribute generic medicines at affordable prices
   d. To provide health insurance

Answers

1. b
2. c

CHAPTER 73

Beti Bachao Beti Padhao

Abhishek Raut, Akhil Dhanesh Goel, Shaili Vyas

Need of program/Scheme	The Beti Bachao Beti Padhao (BBBP) Programme was launched to address the declining Child Sex Ratio (CSR) and promote gender equality in India.[1] • A significant decline in CSR (from 927 girls per 1000 boys in 2001 to 918 in 2011). • Prevalence of sex-selective abortion and female feticide. • Gender discrimination leading to poor education, health and economic opportunities for girls. The need for this scheme arose due to societal preference for male children, contributing to discrimination and neglect against girls. It seeks to promote gender equality and change societal attitudes by emphasizing the value of the girl child. It focuses on increasing school enrollment and retention of girls, thereby promoting their overall development.
Implemented since	The BBBP Programme was launched by Hon'ble Prime Minister Shri Narendra Modi on 22 January 2015 by the Government of India in Panipat, Haryana. The initial focus was on 100 districts with the lowest child sex ratio however later on has been expanded to cover all 640 districts across India.[2]
Goal	**Primary goal:** To save the girl child and ensure her education and overall development. **Long-term vision:** To create a societal environment where every girl child is valued, given equal opportunities, and empowered to contribute to the nation's progress.
Targets[1]	Achieve a shift in community attitudes toward the girl child, reducing gender biases. • Improve the Child Sex Ratio (CSR) across the country. • Increase awareness and advocacy for the rights of the girl child. • Ensure 100% enrollment and retention of girls in schools. • Strengthen enforcement of laws against gender discrimination and sex-selective abortion. • Promote value and respect for girls in society.
Objectives[1]	Collaborate across various departments (Women & Child Development, Education, Health, etc.) to implement the scheme in a coordinated approach. • Eliminate gender-based discrimination and violence. • Strict enforcement of the Pre-Conception and Pre-Natal Diagnostic Techniques (PCPNDT) Act, 1994. • Promote equal opportunities for education, health, and development of girls. • Engage communities in challenging gender biases and stereotypes.
Organogram	The BBBP Programme is implemented through a multi-tier structure involving: **Ministry level—Ministry of Women and Child Development (MoWCD):** Acts as the nodal agency coordinating policy formulation and oversight with support from the Ministry of Health & Family Welfare (MoHFW) and Ministry of Education (MoE). **State level:** State departments of women and child development responsible for tailoring and executing the program within their respective states. **District level—District implementation committees:** Led by the district magistrate/collector, these committees ensure on-ground execution and monitor progress. **Local level—Panchayats/municipal bodies and local NGOs:** Implement community-level initiatives, awareness drives, and monitoring activities.
Beneficiaries	• **Primary beneficiaries:** Girl children (0–18 years) with focus on newborns and school-going girls. • **Secondary beneficiaries:** Pregnant and lactating mothers parents and guardians of girl children. • **Tertiary beneficiaries:** Teachers, health workers (Asha, anganwadi workers), community leaders, and the general public.

Components	BBBP focuses on three major components: • **Awareness generation:** Mass media campaigns, school programs, community events, and cultural activities to sensitize society. • **Strategic communication:** Deploying targeted IEC campaigns to reshape societal attitudes and dispel myths about the girl child. • **Social mobilization:** Engagement of community leaders, NGOs, and local influencers to drive change. • **Inter-sectoral coordination:** Collaboration among government departments, local bodies, and educational institutions. • **Monitoring mechanism:** Systems to track progress on indicators, such as child sex ratio, enrollment rates, and community engagement. • **Capacity building:** Training of frontline workers (e.g., anganwadi workers, ASHAs) and local administrators to identify and address gender bias. • **Enforcement of laws:** Strengthening implementation of PCPNDT Act, POCSO Act, and Dowry Prohibition Act.[3]
Strategies/ Deliverables under the program	• Strengthening policy implementation for gender equality. • Engaging communities through local governance, NGOs, and civil society. • Conducting extensive IEC (Information, Education, and Communication) campaigns. • Providing incentives for girl child education and welfare. • Enhancing women's empowerment programs. • Incentive-based schemes, such as Sukanya Samriddhi Yojana for girl child savings.[4]
Activities at various level or package of services	A. **Awareness and advocacy:** • National media campaigns (TV, radio, social media). • Public awareness campaigns on gender equality. • Engaging religious and social leaders to promote positive gender norms. • School-based gender sensitization programs. • Community engagement through women's SHGs and local leaders. • Encouraging birth registration of girls. B. **Early intervention and support services:** • Strict enforcement of PCPNDT Act to prevent sex-selective abortion. • Ensuring proper healthcare and nutrition for girl children. • Providing scholarships and incentives for girls' education. • Promoting institutional deliveries and maternal care. C. **Rehabilitation:** • Legal action against offenders in gender-based violence cases. • Setting up one stop centers for women in distress. • Providing financial and social security for girls through schemes, such as Sukanya Samriddhi Yojana. • Support services for abandoned girls through child protection schemes. • Scholarships and financial incentives for girls to complete education. • Shelter homes for victims of gender-based violence and discrimination.
Monitoring and evaluation of program	• **Data collection and dashboards:** Use of digital platforms and dashboards to continuously track key performance indicators (e.g., child sex ratio, enrollment and retention statistics). • **Regular reporting:** Periodic progress reports at district, state, and national levels. • **Field visits and reviews:** Scheduled inspections and audits by government officials to assess on-ground implementation. • **Third-party evaluations:** Independent assessments and audits to ensure transparency and objectivity. • **Feedback mechanisms:** Incorporating inputs from beneficiaries and community stakeholders to refine and improve program strategies. • **Outcome indicators:** Measurable impact on the child sex ratio, improvement in education and empowerment indicators, and positive shifts in community attitudes. • The Beti Bachao Beti Padhao scheme has made significant progress in promoting the rights of the girl child and advancing gender equality and empowerment of girls in India.

References

1. Ministry of Women and Child Development (MWCD), Government of India. Beti Bachao Beti Padhao: https://www.india.gov.in/beti-bachao-beti-padhao-scheme-ministry-women-child-development?page=1
2. Ministry of Women and Child Development. Empowering India's Daughters. A Decade of Beti Bachao Beti Padhao's Success Posted On: 21 JAN 2025 8:10PM by PIB Delhi
3. Pre-Conception and Pre-Natal Diagnostic Techniques (PCPNDT) Act, 1994.
4. Sukanya Samriddhi Account Scheme. National Saving Institute. https://www.nsiindia.gov.in/(S(bmueq12eshumrcrn0nizzemo))/InternalPage.aspx?Id_Pk=89

QUESTIONS

Long Answer Question (LAQ)

1. Discuss the need, objectives, implementation strategies, impact and critical appraisal of the "Beti Bachao Beti Padhao" program.

Short Answer Questions (SAQs)

1. Critical appraisal of the "Beti Bachao Beti Padhao" program.
2. Comment on the statement—Beti Bachao Beti Padhao programs promote gender equality in India.
3. Explain in brief the need for the "Beti Bachao Beti Padhao" program.

Multiple Choice Questions (MCQs)

1. When was the "Beti Bachao Beti Padhao" program launched?
    a. 2013
    b. 2014
    c. 2015
    d. 2016
2. Which of the following is NOT a key component of the "Beti Bachao Beti Padhao" initiative?
    a. Providing livelihood to girls
    b. Promoting the education of girls
    c. Ensuring better healthcare for girls
    d. Saving the girl child from gender-based violence
3. The "Beti Bachao Beti Padhao" program was initially launched in how many districts in India?
    a. 100
    b. 150
    c. 250
    d. 300
4. What is one of the significant challenges addressed by the "Beti Bachao Beti Padhao" program?
    a. Child labor
    b. Female infanticide and sex-selective abortion
    c. Unemployment for women
    d. Lack of sanitation facilities for girls
5. Which of the following states was initially part of the "Beti Bachao Beti Padhao" program's pilot phase?
    a. Maharashtra
    b. Haryana
    c. Uttar Pradesh
    d. Rajasthan

Answers

1. c   2. a   3. a   4. b   5. b

CHAPTER 74

Kayakalp

Suraj Kapoor, Shaili Vyas, Ashwin Ramana

Background/Need of scheme	The Swachh Bharat Abhiyan campaign was launched by the Prime Minister of India on October 2, 2024, to promote cleanliness in public spaces. Kayakalp is a continuation of this initiative aimed at promoting cleanliness, hygiene, and infection control in public health facilities across India.[1]
Implemented since	The Kayakalp Yojna was introduced in India on May 15, 2015, by Union Health Minister Shri JP Nadda.[1]
Goal	Enhancing the operation of public healthcare facilities by offering cash incentives and rewards to facilities that exhibit a high level of compliance with specified criteria, with the aim of improving cleanliness and hygiene in healthcare facilities.[1]
Targets	• Ensure 100% compliance with cleanliness and hygiene standards in all public health facilities. • Reduce healthcare-associated infections by 50%. • Achieve 100% compliance with biomedical waste management rules • Ensure all healthcare facilities have access to safe drinking water and adequate sanitation. • Maintain a high standard of infrastructure upkeep in all health facilities. • Achieve active community participation in cleanliness and hygiene activities. • Train 100% of healthcare staff in hygiene, infection control, and waste management practices. • Conduct regular audits and assessments to ensure compliance with Kayakalp standards. • Recognize and reward healthcare facilities that demonstrate exceptional hygiene and cleanliness standards.
Objectives	• To promote cleanliness, hygiene, Infection control, and environment-friendly practices in public health facilities. • To incentivize and recognize public healthcare facilities that show exemplary performance in adhering to standard cleanliness and infection control protocols. • To inculcate a culture of ongoing assessment and peer review of performance related to hygiene, cleanliness, and sanitation. • To create and share sustainable practices related to improved cleanliness in public health facilities linked to positive health outcomes.[2]
Organogram	Ministry of Health and Family Welfare (MoHFW) 2 National Kayakalp Steering Committee (Under Chairpersonship of AS and MD of NHM and Members) ↓ State Health Department State Kayakalp Steering Committee (Under Chairpersonship of Health secretary and MD of NHM and Members mostly senior health authorities, such as SQAC, Nodal Officer of NUHM, MHO, Superintendents of medical college, Head of NGO working in health and sanitation scheme, etc.) ↓ District Health Office District Kayakalp Implementation Committee (Under Chairpersonship of DM/Chief Medical Officer and Members of the Zila Panchayat Health Committee, DQAC, District CPHC Nodal Officer, etc.) ↓ Hospital/Health Center Administration Facility Kayakalp Committee (Head of health center and People from Rogi Kalyan samiti and Members)

Beneficiaries	The beneficiaries of the Kayakalp Health Scheme encompass a broad spectrum of stakeholders within the healthcare system. The beneficiaries and potential benefits are discussed below:
	• Patients
	  + Improved health outcomes
	  + Better experience.
	  + Increased trust:
	• Healthcare staff
	  + Safer work environment
	  + Training and development
	  + Enhanced reputation
	  + Recognition and incentives
	• Community
	  + Public health improvement
	  + Increased awareness
	  + Economic benefits
	• Government and policymakers
	  + Achievement of health goals
	  + Policy implementation
	  + Public trust
	• Environment
	  + Sustainable practices
	  + Pollution reduction

Components	The Kayakalp scheme comprises six components or parameters. Facilities undergo ranking based on percentage scores obtained during assessments of these parameters, determining eligibility for awards and incentives. The scheme emphasizes critical components to achieve its objectives. Here are the key components of the Kayakalp Health Scheme:[1,3]
	• **Sanitation and hygiene**
	  + *General cleanliness:* Implement regular cleaning schedules using standardized methods, materials, and equipment across healthcare facilities, including patient wards, outpatient departments (OPDs), emergency rooms, and administrative offices.
	  + *Sanitation facilities:* Ensure adequate maintenance and availability of toilets and washrooms for patients and staff.
	  + *Hand hygiene:* Promote hand hygiene practices with handwashing stations and sanitizers for healthcare workers, patients, and visitors.
	• **Infection control**
	  + *Sterilization and disinfection:* Ensure regular sterilization of medical instruments to prevent healthcare-associated infections.
	  + *Disinfection of surfaces:* Regularly disinfect surfaces and high-touch areas within healthcare facilities.
	  + *Isolation protocols:* Implement proper procedures in isolation rooms to prevent cross-contamination.
	  + *Personal protective equipment (PPE):* Ensure proper supply and use of PPE for healthcare workers to minimize infection risks.
	• **Waste management**
	  + *Biomedical waste management:* Segregate and handle biomedical waste at the source according to regulatory guidelines.
	  + *Disposal systems:* Ensure proper disposal methods, including incineration, for biomedical waste.
	  + *Training on waste management:* Regularly train healthcare workers on waste management protocols for compliance and safety.
	• **Water, sanitation, and hygiene promotion (WASH)**
	  + *Safe drinking water:* Provide safe and potable drinking water for patients, staff, and visitors.
	  + *Water quality testing:* Conduct regular testing of water quality.
	• **Hospital support services**
	  + *Laundry services:* Ensure availability of clean linen and textile materials to prevent infections among patients and staff.
	  + *Kitchen services:* Provide quality and safe food to aid in patients' recovery, free from microbiological, chemical, and physical hazards.

	✦ *Security and outdoor services management:* Maintain proper hygiene and sanitation standards among security personnel, manage crowds, and ensure quality services, such as housekeeping, laundry, diagnostics, and laboratory services.
	• **Improving hospital/Facility upkeep**
	  ✦ *Maintenance of general physical structure:* Develop adequate infrastructure, manage pests, maintain proper landscaping, and ensure grading around the hospital.
	  ✦ *Illumination and lighting:* Provide adequate lighting in patient wards, operating theaters (OT), OPDs, and outdoor areas of the hospital.
	  ✦ *Water conservation:* Ensure adequate quality and quantity of water with proper roof and rainwater harvesting systems in each healthcare facility.

Strategies/ Deliverables under the program	

Activities at various level or package of services	Developing a robust strategy for the Kayakalp scheme involves critical components to ensure its effectiveness and sustainability:
	• **Awareness and education**
	  ✦ Conduct campaigns, workshops, and awareness programs to educate healthcare professionals and the public on the importance of hygiene and sanitation.
	  ✦ Distribute educational materials, such as brochures, posters, and digital content to highlight best practices, using effective Information, Education, and Communication (IEC) activities.
	  ✦ Implement regular training programs for healthcare staff to reinforce proper sanitation practices and emphasize maintaining a clean environment.
	• **Infrastructure development**
	  ✦ Upgrade existing infrastructure to incorporate improved waste management systems, clean water supply, and adequate sanitation facilities.
	  ✦ Develop and implement maintenance schedules to ensure ongoing upkeep of facilities.
	  ✦ Allocate sufficient resources to support infrastructure enhancements and maintenance efforts.
	• **Incentives and recognition**
	  ✦ Recognize and reward healthcare facilities and staff that demonstrate exemplary hygiene and sanitation standards.
	  ✦ Create incentive programs to motivate staff and facilities to maintain high cleanliness standards.
	  ✦ Publicly acknowledge top-performing facilities and staff to inspire broader participation and commitment.
	• **Community engagement**
	  ✦ Involve local communities in cleanliness drives and awareness initiatives to promote hygiene practices beyond healthcare settings.
	  ✦ Establish partnerships with local NGOs, community groups, and stakeholders to support and advocate for the Kayakalp scheme.
	  ✦ Organize public events, such as cleanliness drives and health camps to encourage community participation and awareness.
	• **Policy and governance**
	  ✦ Develop and enforce Standard Operating Procedures (SOPs) for hygiene and sanitation in all healthcare facilities.
	  ✦ Set clear compliance standards and ensure adherence by all facilities through regular monitoring and evaluation.
	  ✦ Establish a regulatory body to oversee the implementation and enforcement of the scheme's guidelines and standards.
	• **Technology integration**
	  ✦ Implement a digital reporting system to monitor hygiene practices and address sanitation issues in real-time.
	  ✦ Develop mobile applications to provide hygiene guidelines, report sanitation issues, and offer access to educational resources for staff and patients.
	  ✦ Utilize data analytics to identify trends, areas for improvement, and measure the impact of hygiene initiatives on healthcare facilities.

Monitoring and evaluation of program	Monitoring and evaluation can be done in three steps[2] • **Step 1—Internal assessment:** Conducted quarterly by the Chief Medical Officer using a standardized tool based on the six components of the Kayakalp scheme. • **Step 2—Peer assessment:** Conducted annually by health staff from different blocks/districts. Facilities with an internal assessment score above 70% are eligible. • **Step 3—Nomination of facilities:** ✦ Facilities with a peer assessment score above 70% are nominated for national-level assessment. Apart from these, regular audits, collect feedback and tracking of key performance measure can be done.

Incentives based on national level assessment under Kayakalp scheme	• **District hospital:**
	  ✦ *Winner:* Cash award of ₹ 50 Lakhs
	  ✦ *1st runner-up (Districts ranked 26–50 in the state):* Cash award of ₹ 20 Lakhs
	  ✦ *2nd runner-up (Districts ranked >50 in the state):* Cash award of ₹ 10 Lakhs
	• **Sub-District Hospital (SDH)/Community Health Center (CHC):**
	  ✦ Two SDH/CHC selected if the state has more than 10 districts:
	    – Winner: Cash award of ₹ 15 Lakhs
	    – 1st runner-up: Cash award of ₹ 10 Lakhs
	• **Primary Health Center (PHC):** One PHC selected in each district: Cash award of ₹ 2 Lakhs
	• **Sub-Center (SC):**
	  ✦ *Winner:* Cash award of ₹ 1 Lakh
	  ✦ *1st runner-up (SCs ranked 26–50 in the district):* Cash award of ₹ 50,000
	  ✦ *2nd runner-up (SCs ranked >50 in the district):* Cash award of ₹ 35,000

References

1. Tiwari A, Tiwari A. (2016). Kayakalp: Impact of Swachh Bharat Abhiyan on cleanliness, infection control and hygiene promotion practices in District Hospitals of Chhattisgarh, India. IOSR Journal of Environmental Science, Toxicology and Food Technology. 2016; 10, 55-58. https://doi.org/10.9790/2402-1009015558.
2. Kayakalp-Swacchta Guidelines for Public Health Facilities
3. Chaudhary A, Mahajan A, Barwal V, Gautam P, Rattan S, Chamotra S. Kayakalp Utility of a novel Indian tool for the assessment of biomedical waste management in a district hospital of Northern India. CHRISMED Journal of Health and Research. 2019; 6, 93-96. https://doi.org/10.4103/cjhr.cjhr_130_18.

QUESTIONS

Long Answer Question (LAQ)

1. Describe in detail about Kayakalp scheme, its objective, strategy, monitoring and evaluation.

Short Answer Questions (SAQs)

1. What are the primary objectives of the Kayakalp scheme?
2. How are healthcare facilities evaluated and recognized under the Kayakalp scheme?

Multiple Choice Questions (MCQs)

1. What is main purpose of Kayakalp scheme?
   a. Improve quality of labor room
   b. Ensure cleanliness, hygiene in public place
   c. Ensure cleanliness, hygiene and infection control in public health facility
   d. Ensure cleanliness, hygiene and infection control in private health facility
2. Following is/are target of Kayakalp scheme:
   a. Ensure 100% compliance with cleanliness and hygiene standards in all public health facilities.
   b. Reduce healthcare-associated infections by 50%.
   c. Access to safe drinking water in health facility
   d. All of above
3. How many components of Kayakalp scheme?
   a. 3 b. 4
   c. 5 d. 6
4. Following is/are components/themes of Kayakalp scheme:
   a. Hospital/facility upkeep b. Sanitation and hygiene
   c. Infection control d. All of above
5. How much cash intensive has been given to winner primary health center?
   a. ₹ 1 lakh b. ₹ 2 lakhs
   c. ₹ 3 lakhs d. ₹ 4 lakhs
6. Scheme related to cleanliness, hygiene and sanitation of public health facility:
   a. Kayakalp b. Swachh Bharat Abhiyan
   c. Ujala d. None of the above

Answers

1. c   2. d   3. d   4. d   5. b
6. a

CHAPTER 75

National Jal Jeevan Mission

Vikram Kumar Gupta, Shaili Vyas, Rupesh Kumar

Background/Need of program/Scheme	Water is one of the most essential requirements of life. Our country India is home to 18% of global human population, 15% of the global livestock population, but with only 4% of global freshwater resources. Access to safe potable water is a basic human survival need. Sustainable Development Goals declared by the United Nations which are to be achieved by 2030 have Goal Number 6 related to access to safe water, sanitation and hygiene. Demand for water is rising owing to rapid population growth, urbanization and increasing water needs from agriculture, industry, and energy sectors. The demand for water has outpaced population growth. Half of the world's population is already experiencing severe water scarcity at least one month in a year. As a result of climate change, water scarcity is projected to increase further with the rise of global temperatures.[1] Hence, a dedicated program is a must to serve this important aspect in India. The Central Government assistance to states for rural water supply began in 1972 with the launch of Accelerated Rural Water Supply Programme. In 2009, it was renamed as National Rural Drinking Water Programme (NRDWP), a centrally sponsored scheme with fund sharing between the Center and the states. Later, Government of India restructured and subsumed the ongoing NRDWP into Jal Jeevan Mission program with ambition to provide Functional Household Tap Connection (FHTC) to every rural household, i.e., Har Ghar Nal Se Jal (HGNSJ) by the year 2024. The total budgetary allocation to the scheme is over ₹3 lakh crore. The fund sharing pattern between the Center and states is 90:10 for Himalayan and North-Eastern States, 50:50 for other states, and 100% for union territories. The 73rd Amendment to the Constitution of India has placed the subject of drinking water in the Eleventh Schedule and has assigned its management to Gram Panchayats.[2]
Implementation	Jal Jeevan Mission (JJM), is a flagship program of the Government of India, was launched by Hon'ble Prime Minister Narendra Modi on August 15th, 2019.
Goal	To provide piped drinking water, Har Ghar Nal Se Jal (HGNSJ) by 2024 to all rural households.[3]
Targets	To provide tap water connection to 14.60 Crore households to those who are without it, in partnership with states/Union territories under the mission by 2024.
Objectives	• To achieve by Year 2024 to enable all households to have access to and use of safe and adequate drinking water within premises to the extent possible. • JJM aspires to establish a Jan Andolan for water, making it a top priority for every rural household in the country. • To supply 55 liters of water per person per day to every rural household through Functional Household Tap Connections (FHTC) by 2024. • Planning and putting into action how essential water is for a better quality of life. • Assistance from states and UTs in organizing their financial funds and resources for the mission. • To provide functional tap connection to schools, anganwadi centers, health centers, wellness centers and community buildings, etc. • To monitor functionality of tap connections. • To promote and ensure voluntary ownership among local communities by way of contribution in cash, kind and/or labor and voluntary labor (**Shramdaan**). • To assist in ensuring sustainability of the water supply system, i.e., water source, water supply infrastructure, and funds for regular operation and maintenance (O&M).

	• To empower and develop human resources in the sectors such that the demands of construction, plumbing, electrical, water quality management, water treatment, catchment protection, O&M, etc., are taken care of in short and long-terms. • To bring awareness on various aspects and significance of safe drinking water and involvement of stakeholders in a manner that makes water everyone's business.
Structural organization	**National level:** National Jal Jeevan Mission **State level:** State Water and Sanitation Mission (SWSM) **District level:** District Water and Sanitation Mission (DWSM) **Gram Panchayat Level:** Paani Samiti/Village Water and Sanitation Committee (VWSC)/User group
Beneficiaries	• 14.60 Crore rural households • Village panchayat • Village water bodies • Farmer community with more availability of water bodies due to rainwater harvestation
Components	• In-village water supply (PWS) infrastructure for tap water connection to every household. • Reliable drinking water source development/augmentation of existing sources. • Transfer of water (multi-village scheme, where quantity and quality issues are there in the local water sources). • Technological intervention for treatment to make water potable (where water quality is an issue, but quantity is sufficient). • Retrofitting of completed and ongoing piped water supply schemes to provide FHTC and raise the service level. • Grey water management. • Capacity building of various stakeholders and support activities to facilitate the implementation.
Strategies/Deliverables for JJM program	• Labor, especially those working in the construction sector (skilled, unskilled and semi-skilled), may be deployed to expedite the completion of works under the scheme. • More funds allocation under the Mahatma Gandhi National Rural Employment Guarantee Act (MGNREGA) along with more funds in Jal Jeevan Mission. • Under the Jal Jeevan Mission, tap water is given to every rural household, even those in SC/ST-dominated villages in Tamil Nadu and Maharashtra, so that "no one is left out." Also, tap water is given top priority in places where the water quality is bad, such as deserts and drought-prone areas, SC/ST majority villages, aspirational and JE-AES affected districts, Saansad Adarsh Gram Yojana villages households in the country by 2024. • The Paani Samitis plan has village water supply systems in good shape also, wherein they operate the system in an organized way. At least half of these associations have between 10 and 15 members, at least half of whom are women. Other members come from self-help groups, accredited social and health workers, anganwadi teachers, and other places. • Every functional tap connection is to be linked with the Aadhar number of the head of the household subject to statutory provisions. Every asset created under JJM will be geo-tagged. • The provision of water will be for both domestic and industrial needs in rural. In rural areas, bulk water will be made available at the boundary of the village.[3] **100% Functional Household Tap Connections (FHTC)** If a census coded revenue village achieves provision of 100% FHTC to all its households located in all of its wards/habitations/Mohallas/Faliya/Majra/Chord/Palli/Kheda/tola, etc., then it would be declared as 100% FHTC village. If a district achieves provision of 100% FHTC to all households in all its census coded revenue villages, then it would be declared as 100% FHTC district. If a state achieves provision of 100% FHTC to all households in all its districts, then it would be declared as 100% FHTC.
Activities at various level or package of services	• The mission is based on a community approach to water and includes extensive Information, Education and Communication (IEC) as a key component of the mission. • Rainwater harvesting and water conservation are also the most important aspects of the mission. • Using recycled water and recharging structures. • Development of the watercourse. • Focus on planting trees (Afforestation). • Renovation of traditional and other water bodies. • Groundwater recharge and management of household wastewater for reuse. • Local management of both how much water is used and how much is available.

Section III: National Health Mission

Monitoring and evaluation of program	• JJM will significantly improve quality of life, particularly of women and children and assist in ODF-sustainability as water is important to sustain Swachh Bharat Mission's gains. • There will be procurement of various materials for water supply systems. This will generate employment and boost India's economy. • M&E will be done by third party independent survey agencies. Geocoding will help in identifying correct village and beneficiaries.

References

1. Operation Guidelines for the Implementation of Jal Jeevan Mission, Ministry of Jal Shakti, 2019. https://jalshaktiddws.gov.in/sites/default/files/JJM_Operational_Guidelines. (pdf)
2. Answer to Parliament Questions on JJM. No. 46/RN/Ref./Dec/2020
3. Website of Jal Jeevan Mission. https://jaljeevanmission.gov.in/.

QUESTIONS

Long Answer Question (LAQ)

1. Write in detail about the evolution of Jal Jeevan Mission program over the years. How it will help India in achieving few of the Sustainable Development Goals?

Short Answer Questions (SAQs)

1. Mention the objectives of Jal Jeevan Mission.
2. Explain briefly the components and organizational structure of Jal Jeevan Mission.

Multiple Choice Questions (MCQs)

1. The percentage of global freshwater resources available in our country India is:
    a. 2
    b. 4
    c. 6
    d. 10
2. As per Sustainable Development Goals declared by UNO, the access to safe water, sanitation and hygiene is to be met by year:
    a. 2025
    b. 2028
    c. 2030
    d. 2035
3. National Rural Drinking Water Programme was launched in which year by Central Government?
    a. 2000
    b. 2005
    c. 2009
    d. 2015
4. The year in which Jal Jeevan Mission was launched in our country by Central Government is:
    a. 2014
    b. 2017
    c. 2019
    d. 2022

5. Functional Household Tap Connection (FHTC) is a part of which national program?
   a. Accelerated Rural Water Supply Programme
   b. National Rural Drinking Water Programme
   c. Jal Jeevan Mission
   d. National Health Mission
6. The amount of water to be supplied per person per day to every rural household through Functional Household Tap Connections is:
   a. 30 Liters
   b. 45 Liters
   c. 50 Liters
   d. 55 Liters
7. The targeted number of beneficiaries of rural households as per Jal Jeevan Mission (JJM) is:
   a. 12. 60 Crore
   b. 14.60 Crore
   c. 16.50 Crore
   d. 18.5 Crore
8. Which of the following activity is not a part of Jal Jeevan Mission?
   a. Rainwater harvesting
   b. Ground water recharge
   c. Deforestation
   d. Recycling of water
9. Which number of amendment to the constitution of India placed the subject of drinking water in Eleventh Schedule and was assigned its management to Gram Panchayats?
   a. 67th
   b. 69th
   c. 73rd
   d. 75th
10. Har Ghar Nal Se Jal (HGNSJ), a centrally sponsored scheme is to be achieved by year:
    a. 2020
    b. 2024
    c. 2030
    d. 2034

Answers

1. b	2. c	3. c	4. c	5. c
6. d	7. b	8. c	9. c	10. b

CHAPTER 76

Swachh Swasth Sarvatra (SSS) Initiative

Deepak Upadhyay, Shaili Vyas, Bharti Koria

Background/Need of program/Scheme	The Swachh Swasth Sarvatra (SSS) initiative, a collaborative effort between the Ministry of Drinking Water and Sanitation (MoDWS), the Ministry of Health and Family Welfare (MoHFW), and the Ministry of Housing and Urban Affairs (MoHUA), aims to promote cleanliness and hygiene in urban health facilities. The initiative builds on the Kayakalp guidelines and involves coordination with States, Union Territories (UTs), and Urban Local Bodies (ULBs). At present its applicable to both rural and urban area healthcare facilities.[1]
Implemented since	The primary goal of the SSS initiative is to strengthen Community Health Centers/Primary Health centers in open defecation free (ODF) blocks to achieve higher levels of cleanliness and hygiene with the goal of making India free of open defecation. Three main Objectives of the SSS initiative are:[1,2] • Enabling Gram Panchayat/ULBs where Kayakalp awarded PHCs are located to become ODF. • Strengthening Community Health Center (CHC) and PHCs in ODF blocks to achieve higher level of cleanliness to meet Kayakalp standards through a support of ₹ 10 Lakh/₹ 5 lakh under NHM. • Build capacity through training in Water, Sanitation and Hygiene (WASH) Of nominees from covered PHC and CHC. • To enable grass root health workers in understanding the importance of elimination of Open Defecation
Strategies	The initiative focuses on making health facilities clean, hygienic, and improving waste management to induce behavioral changes in community for converting the block Open Defecation Free (ODF). It includes: • Providing training to health facility staff and nominees. • Ensuring facilities meet Kayakalp criteria and receive assessments. • Allocating funds for specific health and sanitation improvements.[1,2]
Key Activities	**At the State Level:** • Conduct training programs on Water, Sanitation, and Hygiene (WASH) components. • Support Gram Panchayat and ULBs in attaining and maintaining ODF status. **At the District/City Level:** • Planning and monitoring of SSS activities, trainings and meetings of MO-ICs by a nodal person. • Conduct assessments of facilities based on Kayakalp and WASH checklists. **At the Facility (CHC/PHC) Level:** **A Nodal Officer will be do** • Plan, Implementing and found gaps in WASH activities as per Kayakalp checklist. • IEC activities to raise awareness about sanitation and waste management among staff as well as community members visiting health facilities. • Promote community participation in cleanliness drives and the construction of toilet facilities.[1,3]
Roles and responsibilities of Ac ASHA and ANM	• Provide stewardship at local level in facilitating ODF free status • Conduct household visits and promote hygiene practices. • Assist in the construction of household toilets and discuss disease prevention during community meetings.[1,3]

Framework to achieve ODF Gram panchayat in under the PHC achieve Swachh Ratna[2,3]	1. Best PHC in district under kayakalp designated as 'Swachh Ratna' PHC 2. Nodal person identifed by PHC for cleaniness and hygiene activites 3. Nodal person trained by UNICEF (wash) 4. Trained person function as trainer for ASHA and PR members 5. ASHA and PR members motivate community members for ODF 6. The Gram Panchayat decleared ODF
Framework to achieve Swachh Ratna CHC in ODF Block[2,3]	1. ODF block 2. Identify CHC score less than 70% 3. Incentive of 10 lakh for addressing gaps under kayakalp and WASH 4. Reassessment of facility (state, district and facility level) 5. Achieved 70% oscore in kayakalp external assessment 6. Named as 'Swachh Ratna" CHC
Utilization of funds	Funds allocated under the SSS initiative are to be used for: • Repair and maintenance of health facilities. • Improvement of waste management systems. • Enhancing cleanliness and hygiene practices through IEC activities. The Swachh Swasth Sarvatra initiative is a comprehensive effort to improve sanitation and hygiene in health facilities through coordinated actions between various governmental bodies, training of

	staff, community involvement, and structured monitoring and funding mechanisms. The initiative aims to create cleaner, healthier environments and practices among community members under the stewardship of health centers, thereby reducing disease incidence and promoting overall public health.[4]
Monitoring and training	• A structured monitoring mechanism involves visits and assessments by state and city-level officers. • Training programs are organized at state and district levels to ensure effective implementation of the initiative.[4,5]

References

1. Ministry of Health and Family Welfare, Government of India. Operational Guidelines for Swachh Swasth Sarvatra. [Internet]. 2024 [cited 2024 Jul 22]. Available from: https://www.mohfw.gov.in
2. Ministry of Drinking Water and Sanitation, Government of India. Guidelines for Swachh Bharat Mission (Gramin). [Internet]. 2024 [cited 2024 Jul 22]. Available from: https://jalshakti-ddws.gov.in
3. Ministry of Housing and Urban Affairs, Government of India. Kayakalp Guidelines for Urban Health Facilities. [Internet]. 2024 [cited 2024 Jul 22]. Available from: https://mohua.gov.in
4. National Health Mission, Government of India. Framework for Implementation of Swachh Swasth Sarvatra. [Internet]. 2024 [cited 2024 Jul 22]. Available from: https://nhm.gov.in
5. UNICEF India. Enhancing Public Health through Sanitation: Swachh Swasth Sarvatra Initiative. [Internet]. 2024 [cited 2024 Jul 22]. Available from: https://unicef.in

QUESTIONS

Long Answer Question (LAQ)

1. Comment on Swachh Swasth Sarvatra (SSS) initiative? Write in detail about the initiative.

Short Answer Questions (SAQs)

1. Write the objectives, strategies of Swachh Swasth Sarvatra (SSS) initiative.
2. Write the role of ANM and ASHA in Swachh Swasth Sarvatra (SSS) initiative.

Multiple Choice Questions (MCQs)

1. How does the Swachh Swasth Sarvatra (SSS) initiative contribute to strengthening public health infrastructure in ODF (Open Defecation Free) blocks?
    a. By constructing new health facilities in ODF blocks
    b. By providing financial support and training to Community Health Centers (CHCs) and Primary Health Centers (PHCs)
    c. By focusing solely on the construction of toilets in ODF blocks
    d. By establishing international partnerships for health facility upgrades
2. What is the primary role of Accredited Social Health Activists (ASHAs) and Auxiliary Nurse Midwives (ANMs) within the SSS initiative?
    a. Managing waste segregation systems in health facilities
    b. Conducting assessments of health facilities to ensure they meet Kayakalp standards
    c. Facilitating Open Defecation Free (ODF) status by promoting hygiene practices at the community level
    d. Overseeing the allocation of funds for health facility improvements

3. **Which of the following is a key strategy under the SSS initiative aimed at inducing behavioral changes in the community?**
   a. Providing financial rewards for maintaining cleanliness in health facilities
   b. Conducting IEC (Information, Education, and Communication) activities among staff and community members visiting health facilities
   c. Outsourcing sanitation responsibilities to private agencies
   d. Promoting government-sponsored health programs without community involvement
4. **What monitoring mechanisms are employed in the SSS initiative to ensure the effective implementation of health and sanitation goals?**
   a. Independent assessments conducted by international health agencies
   b. Regular facility assessments by state and city-level officers, along with structured training programs
   c. Involvement of private contractors in the monitoring process
   d. Public voting and feedback through mobile applications
5. **How does the Swachh Swasth Sarvatra initiative ensure the proper utilization of funds allocated to health facilities?**
   a. By dedicating all funds to constructing new health facilities in urban areas
   b. By using funds for maintenance, waste management systems, and cleanliness improvements in existing health facilities
   c. By transferring funds directly to health workers for personal use
   d. By relying on external auditors to ensure transparency

Answers

1. b
2. c
3. b
4. b
5. b

CHAPTER 77

Pradhan Mantri Ujjwala Yojana

Suraj Kapoor, Akhil Dhanesh Goel, Bharti Koria, Ashwin Ramana

Implemented since	Launched on May 1, 2016.
Goal	• To provide LPG connections to women from Below Poverty Line (BPL) households • Improving health, reducing environmental pollution, and empowering women in rural and urban areas across India.[1]
Objectives	• To promote women empowerment • To provide a healthy cooking fuel • To prevent hazards-health related issues among the millions of rural population due to use of fossil fuel.
Targeted beneficiary	• Beneficiaries were to be identified using the Socio-Economic Caste Census (SECC) 2011 data. • The scheme also included provisions to extend the benefits to SC/ST households, forest dwellers, beneficiaries of the Pradhan Mantri Awas Yojana (Gramin), Antyodaya Anna Yojana, Most Backward Classes, tea and ex-tea garden tribes, people residing in islands, and riverside areas.
Organogram	Ministry of Petroleum and Natural Gas ↓ Implementing agencies (OMCs) ↓ State level coordinators ↓ District nodal officers ↓ LPG distributors ↓ Beneficiaries (BPL households)
Strategies/ Deliverables under the scheme	**Targeted Beneficiary Identification**[2] • **Data utilization:** Utilizing the Socio-Economic Caste Census (SECC) 2011 data to identify eligible BPL households. • **Inclusive approach:** Ensuring inclusion of marginalized groups, such as Scheduled Castes (SC), Scheduled Tribes (ST), Antyodaya Anna Yojana (AAY) families, forest dwellers, and most backward classes. **Financial Assistance and Support** • **Subsidy provision:** Providing a subsidy of ₹ 1600 per LPG connection to cover the security deposit for the cylinder, pressure regulator, safety hose, installation charges, and the first refill. • **EMI options:** Offering an EMI facility to cover the cost of the LPG stove and the first refill, which is deducted from the subsidy on subsequent refills to ease the financial burden on beneficiaries.

	Infrastructure expansion • **Distributor network:** Expansion especially in rural and remote areas • **Supply chain management:** Strengthening the supply chain to maintain a consistent and reliable supply of LPG. **Awareness and education campaigns** • **Information dissemination:** For widespread awareness • **Safety Training:** To ensure the safety of handlers, beneficiaries their families. **Technological Integration** • **Digital platforms:** For the efficient management of beneficiary data, subsidy distribution, and monitoring. • **Cashless transactions:** To reduce leakage and ensure transparency. **Collaboration and Coordination** • **Multi-stakeholder engagement:** Coordinating with state governments, district administrations, and local bodies • **Public-private partnerships:** Encouraging partnerships with private sector **Special Initiatives for Vulnerable Groups** • **Focused outreach:** to reach out to the most vulnerable and remote communities. • **Customized support:** to help these groups transition smoothly to using LPG. **Environmental and Health Focus** • **Promotion of clean energy:** To reduce indoor air pollution and associated health risks. • **Sustainability goals:** Broader environmental sustainability goals by reducing traditional fuel and deforestation **Policy and Regulatory Support** • **Government backing:** Strong policy support and regulatory measures from the central and state governments to facilitate • **Legislative framework:** To support the objectives of PMUY and ensure compliance among stakeholders.

Monitoring and evaluation	**Monitoring Components**[3]
	• **Real-time data tracking**
	  + Digital platforms
	  + Beneficiary tracking
	• **Periodic reports**
	  + Regular reporting
	  + State and district level reports
	• **Field visits and inspections**
	  + Random inspections
	  + Third-party audits
	• **Grievance Redressal Mechanism**
	  + Helplines and portals
	  + *Timely resolution:* Evaluation components
	Evaluation Component
	• **Impact assessment**
	  + Health impact
	  + Economic impact
	  + Environmental impact
	• **Beneficiary feedback**
	  + Surveys and interviews
	  + Focus group discussions
	• **Performance metrics**
	  + *Key performance indicators (KPIs):* Such as connections, refill rates, and the reduction in the use of traditional fuels.
	  + *Targets vs. achievements:* Comparing the targets to actual achievements
	• **Data analysis**
	  + Statistical analysis
	  + Geospatial analysis
	• **Reporting and dissemination**

References

1. https://www.india.gov.in/spotlight/pradhan-mantri-ujjwala-yojana#tab=tab-1
2. Deshpande R, Tillin L, Kailash K. The BJP's Welfare Schemes: Did They Make a Difference in the 2019 Elections. Studies in Indian Politics. 2019; 7, 219 - 233. https://doi.org/10.1177/2321023019874911.
3. Kar A, Pachauri S, Bailis R, Zerriffi H. Using sales data to assess cooking gas adoption and the impact of India's Ujjwala programme in rural Karnataka. Nature Energy. 2019; 1-9. https://doi.org/10.1038/s41560-019-0429-8

QUESTIONS

Long Answer Question (LAQ)

1. Describe in detail about Pradhan Mantri Ujjwala Yojana its objective, strategy, monitoring and evaluation.

Short Answer Questions (SAQs)

1. What is the primary goal of the Pradhan Mantri Ujjwala Yojana (PMUY)?
2. How does PMUY contribute to women's empowerment?

Multiple Choice Questions (MCQs)

1. When was the Pradhan Mantri Ujjwala Yojana launched?
   a. 2014
   b. 2015
   c. 2016
   d. 2017
2. Which ministry is responsible for implementing the PMUY?
   a. Ministry of Health and Family Welfare
   b. Ministry of Rural Development
   c. Ministry of Petroleum and Natural Gas
   d. Ministry of Finance
3. What is the primary benefit provided under the PMUY?
   a. Free LPG connections to BPL households
   b. Subsidized food grains
   c. Cash transfers
   d. Free medical care
4. How does PMUY contribute to women's empowerment?
   a. By providing them with financial independence
   b. By reducing their workload
   c. By improving their health
   d. All of the above
5. Which of the following is NOT a key component of the PMUY?
   a. Targeted beneficiary identification
   b. Financial assistance and support
   c. Infrastructure expansion
   d. Food security programs

Answers

1. c
2. c
3. a
4. d
5. d

CHAPTER 78

Ujjawala Scheme for Prevention of Trafficking and Rescue, Rehabilitation and Reintegration of Victims of Trafficking

Suraj Kapoor, Akhil Dhanesh Goel, Bharti Koria, Ashwin Ramana

Background/Need of scheme	Preventing trafficking and providing support to victims, especially women and children who have been subjected to commercial sexual exploitation and trafficking.
Implemented since	Since 2007
Goal	Strive to offer a range of support services, such as shelter homes, counseling, medical assistance, legal aid, vocational training, education, and others, in order to combat trafficking.
Objectives	The primary objective is to rehabilitate and reintegrate victims into society while also working on prevention measures to combat trafficking.[1]
Organogram	Ministry of Women and Child Development ↓ Coordinators National State/UT District Community ↓ NGOs, law enforcement, agencies, healthcare social Workers, legal aid vocational training providers, survivors
Beneficiaries	Victim and vulnerable population for sex trafficking and exploitation, such as children, woman
Components cum objectives	• **Prevention:** Educational programs, community outreach activities, and advocacy efforts to address the root causes of trafficking. • **Rescue and rehabilitation:** Shelter homes, counseling, medical assistance, legal aid, vocational training to address the immediate needs of victims and help them recover from the trauma of exploitation. • **Reintegration:** Reintegrating victims into society by providing them with opportunities for education, skill development and livelihood support to empower survivors to rebuild their lives and become self-reliant. **Capacity Building:** The law enforcement agencies, social workers, and community organizations. capacity-building initiatives, such as training programs, workshops, and the development of guidelines and protocols for stakeholders to tackle trafficking cases effectively
Monitoring and evaluation	The Ujjawala Scheme is equipped with comprehensive mechanisms for monitoring and evaluation (M&E) to guarantee the efficacy of its interventions and to continually enhance its implementation. The M&E framework concentrates on monitoring progress, evaluating impact, and making essential adjustments to strategies and activities. Here are the key components of the monitoring and evaluation process under the Ujjawala Scheme:[1] **Monitoring Mechanisms:** **Regular Reporting:** • **Monthly and quarterly reports:** Implementing agencies, such as NGOs and state governments, are required to submit regular reports detailing the activities carried out, the number of beneficiaries, and the progress of various components of the scheme.

- **Annual reports:** Comprehensive annual reports summarizing the yearly achievements, challenges, and learnings are also mandated.

Field Visits:
- **Inspections by officials:** Regular field visits and inspections by government officials and designated monitoring bodies to oversee the activities at the ground level, ensuring that the services provided meet the required standards.
- **Third-party evaluations:** Independent third-party organizations may conduct evaluations to provide an unbiased assessment of the implementation and impact of the scheme.
- **Management information system (MIS)—Data collection and analysis:** An MIS is employed to systematically collect, store, and analyze data related to the beneficiaries, activities, and outcomes. This helps in tracking progress and identifying areas needing attention.

Beneficiary Feedback—Surveys and Feedback Mechanisms: A system of regular surveys and feedback channels has been put in place to obtain input from beneficiaries regarding their experiences with the services provided, their satisfaction levels, and any challenges they come across.

Evaluation Mechanisms:

Impact Assessments:
- **Baseline and endline surveys:** Conducting baseline surveys at the beginning of interventions and endline surveys after a specified period to measure changes and assess the impact of the scheme on the beneficiaries.
- **Case studies and success stories:** Documenting detailed case studies and success stories to highlight the positive impacts and identify best practices.

Periodic Reviews:
- **Internal reviews:** Regular internal reviews by implementing agencies and stakeholders to assess the progress and effectiveness of the scheme's components.
- **External evaluations:** Engaging external evaluators to conduct periodic evaluations, providing an objective assessment of the scheme's performance and suggesting improvements.

Performance Indicators:
- **Key performance indicators (KPIs):** Defining specific KPIs, such as the number of victims rescued, rehabilitated, and reintegrated, the number of awareness campaigns conducted, and the participation levels in skill development programs.
- **Outcome metrics:** Evaluating long-term outcomes, such as the reduction in trafficking cases in targeted areas, improved socioeconomic status of beneficiaries, and successful reintegration into society.

Stakeholder Consultations:
- **Workshops and meetings:** Regular workshops and meetings with stakeholders including government officials, NGOs, law enforcement, and beneficiaries to review progress, discuss challenges, and plan future actions.
- **Advisory committees:** Forming advisory committees comprising experts, stakeholders, and community representatives to guide the implementation and evaluation processes.

Continuous Improvement:

Feedback Loop:
- **Incorporating findings:** Using the findings from monitoring and evaluation activities to make informed decisions and adapt strategies to improve the effectiveness of the scheme.
- **Responsive adjustments:** Making responsive adjustments based on real-time data and feedback to address emerging challenges and optimize interventions.

Capacity Building:
- **Training and development:** Ongoing training and development programs for staff and stakeholders to enhance their skills in monitoring, evaluation, and implementation.
- **Resource allocation:** Ensuring adequate resources and support for effective monitoring and evaluation activities

Reference

1. Ujjawala Scheme. Available on: https://wcd.nic.in/sites/default/files/Ujjawala%20New%20Scheme.pdf

QUESTIONS

Long Answer Question (LAQ)

1. Discuss objectives, key components, strategies for prevention of Ujjawala Scheme.

Short Answer Questions (SAQs)

1. What is the primary objective of Ujjwala Scheme?
2. Name three key components of Ujjwala Scheme.

Multiple Choice Questions (MCQs)

1. When was the Ujjwala Scheme launched in India?
   a. 2005
   b. 2007
   c. 2010
   d. 2012
2. Which of the following is NOT a key objective of the Ujjwala Scheme?
   a. Prevention of trafficking
   b. Rescue and rehabilitation of victims
   c. Reintegration of victims into society
   d. Providing free education for all beneficiaries
3. What are the primary beneficiaries of the Ujjwala Scheme?
   a. Children only
   b. Women only
   c. Children and women
   d. All individuals affected by human trafficking
4. Which of the following is NOT a component of the Ujjwala Scheme's prevention efforts?
   A. Educational programs
   b. Community outreach activities
   c. Law enforcement training
   d. Providing shelter homes
5. What is the role of monitoring and evaluation in the Ujjwala Scheme?
   a. Ensuring the effective implementation of the scheme
   b. Identifying new victims of trafficking
   c. Providing legal aid to victims
   d. Raising awareness about the dangers of human trafficking

Answers

1. b   2. d   3. c   4. d   5. a

CHAPTER 79

National Programme on Climate Change and Human Health

Harshal Ramesh Salve, Girish Jeer, Anjali Modi, Parul Sharma

Background/Need of the program	India launched its National Action Plan on Climate Change (NAPCC) in June 2008, which outlines comprehensive policies and programs aimed at climate mitigation and adaptation. The NAPCC's key initiatives include the designation of the Ministry of Environment, Forest and Climate Change as the Nodal Ministry, the formulation of the National Environmental Policy, and the establishment of the Prime Minister's Council on Climate Change. Initially comprising eight missions, the NAPCC later expanded to include four additional missions (including a Health Mission). In alignment with these efforts, the Ministry of Health and Family Welfare introduced the National Programme for Climate Change and Human Health (NPCCHH) in the year 2019. **National Action Plan on Climate Change** Eight missions to address climate change concerns and promote sustainable development 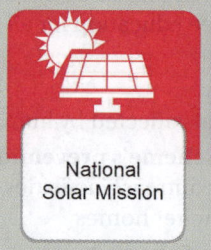 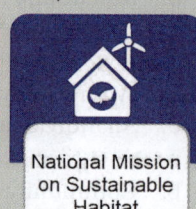  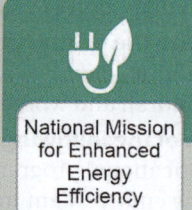 National Solar Mission · National Mission on Sustainable Habitat · National Mission for Sustaining the Himalayan Ecosystem · National Mission for Enhanced Energy Efficiency  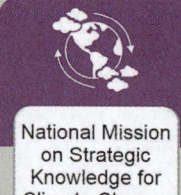   National Water Mission · National Mission on Strategic Knowledge for Climate Change · National Mission for a Green India · National Mission for Sustainable Agriculture
Goal	To reduce morbidity, mortality, injuries, and health vulnerability to climate variability and extreme weather.
Objectives	The program envisages to reach the targets as listed below: • **Awareness and education:** To create awareness among general population (vulnerable community), healthcare providers and policy makers regarding impacts of climate change on human health. • **Strengthening healthcare capacity:** To strengthen capacity of healthcare system to reduce illnesses/diseases due to variability in climate. • **Health preparedness and response:** To strengthen health preparedness and response by performing situational analysis at national/state/district/below district levels. • **Partnerships and synergy:** To develop partnerships and create synchrony/synergy with other missions and ensure that health is adequately represented in the climate change agenda in the country. • **Research and innovation:** To strengthen research capacity to fill the evidence gap on climate change impact on human health.

Health impact due to climate change	Health impacts are broadly categorized into:[1-7] • **Direct health impacts:** Resulting from increased frequency and intensity of extreme weather events, such as heatwaves, floods, heavy rainfall, cyclones, droughts, and cold waves. • **Indirect health impacts:** Including waterborne, vector-borne, and nutrition-related illnesses. Under NPCCHH, 17 Climate Sensitive Diseases (CSDs) or health issues are identified for focused action and integration are: 1. Air pollution-related illnesses 2. Heat-related illnesses 3. Vector-borne diseases 4. Extreme weather events-related health issues 5. Green and climate resilient infrastructure 6. WASH and water-borne diseases 7. Zoonotic diseases and one health 8. Cardiopulmonary diseases 9. Allergic health issues 10. Nutrition-related diseases, food security 11. Mental health issues 12. Coastal climate sensitive diseases 13. Hilly region and mountainous climate sensitive diseases 14. Mental health 15. Occupational health 16. Vulnerability assessment 17. Health information system 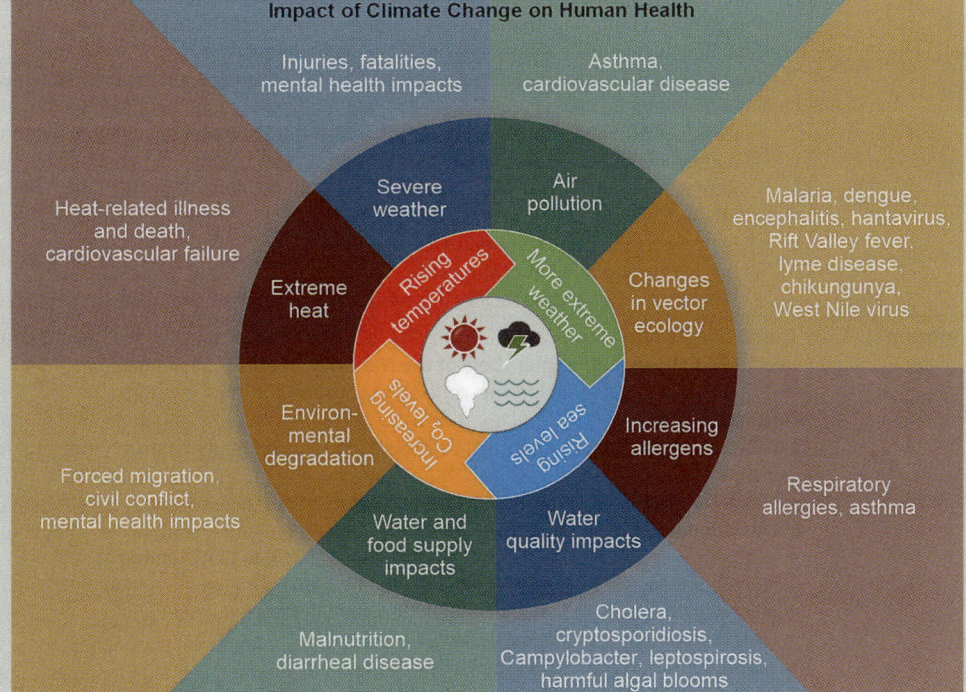 Five priority areas at present under NPCCHH at District level are: **1. Air pollution-related illnesses** ✦ The primary objective of ARI surveillance is to identify trends in air pollution-related illnesses concerning outdoor air quality in specific areas. The findings from this surveillance are shared with relevant authorities, including public health officials, to mitigate the impact of air pollution through timely and appropriate intervention measures.

	+ Designated sentinel hospitals, mainly consisting of medical colleges, district hospitals, and other hospitals with substantial patient inflow, are tasked with collecting daily data. This data is then shared with the District Nodal Officer (DNO). The DNO is responsible for analyzing the ARI surveillance data in conjunction with Air Quality Index (AQI) levels obtained from local air quality monitoring centers. Throughout the year, the DNO sends a monthly surveillance analysis report to both the state authorities and the National Centre for Disease Control (NCDC). Districts are also required to gather air quality data from the State Pollution Control Board (SPCB) and issue warnings to healthcare facilities. 2. **Heat-related illnesses** + Heat-related illness (HRI) surveillance is conducted to establish a baseline of HRI morbidity and mortality and to improve the health system's preparedness for extreme heat exposure. All health facilities within a district are required to implement the National Action Plan on Heat-related Illnesses (NAPHRI). NAPHRI is designed to guide state and district authorities in developing and executing action plans. + NAPHRI includes the development of heat stroke rooms and the preparedness of ambulances. Districts are responsible for collecting information on weather parameters and heatwave predictions from the state meteorological department during the summer months and issuing warnings to healthcare facilities about impending heatwaves. 3. **Vector-borne diseases:** Aligned with existing health program on vector-borne diseases, i.e., National Vector-borne Disease Control Programme (NVBDCP) to understand distribution of vector-borne disease pattern and identify shifting disease patterns in the district with changing climate. DAPCCHH are required to enlist vulnerable areas and population based on existing and projected disease distribution patterns and to support/implement existing vector control, disease prevention and management activities. 4. **Extreme weather events-related health impacts:** With support from the District/State Disaster Management Authority (DDMA/SDMA), the District Nodal Officer (DNO) is required to identify areas and populations vulnerable to prevalent climate change-related extreme weather events, such as extreme heat, floods, drought, cyclones, landslides, and sea level rise. 5. **Green (environmentally friendly and sustainable measures) and climate resilient infrastructure.** Key activities include: + Conducting energy audits of healthcare facilities to assess energy efficiency levels and implement carbon emission reduction measures. + Replacing existing non-LED lighting with LED lighting in healthcare facilities to enhance energy efficiency and reduce carbon emissions. + Installing solar panels in healthcare facilities. + Implementing rainwater harvesting systems in healthcare facilities. + Retrofitting healthcare facility infrastructure to make it climate and disaster resilient.
Organogram	The National Centre for Disease Control (NCDC) hosts the program,[2] overseen by the Additional director and Head, NPCCHH and other members of the National Steering Committee. NAPCCHH—Organizational framework (Organogram) for implementation **National Level** **National Level Advisory Committee:** Acts as the nodal body to policymaking, implementation and roll-out of the NAPCCHH. • Secretary Health and Family Welfare Chairman • Additional Secretary, Health, MoHFW, GoI Member • Secretary Health Research cum Director General- ICMR, GoI Member • Director General Health Services, GOI Vice-Chairman • Director, NCDC, DGHS, MOHFW, GOI Member Secretary • Director, NVBDCP, DGHS, MOHFW, GOI Member • Representation from other Ministries/departments: + Director General, National Disaster Management Authority Member + Secretary, Ministry of Environment, Forest and Climate Change Member + Secretary, Ministry of Earth Sciences Member + Secretary, Ministry of Agriculture Member + Secretary, Central Ground Water Board, Ministry of Water + Resources, Rural Development and Ganga Rejuvenation • Member: + Chairman, Central Pollution Control Board Member + Representation from Department of Science and Technology Member

National Level: Centre for Environmental and Occupational Health Climate Change and Health (CEOH and CCH) at National Centre for Diseases Control. This center is nodal agency for climate change and human health and will provide technical inputs and support to Environmental Health Cell at state and UTs regarding the capacity building, implementation, monitoring, supervision and evaluation of the NAPCCH program. It also strengthens surveillance of climate sensitive diseases and healthcare systems by involving premier institutes.

Structure:
- Director, NCDC Nodal Person and Member-Secretary
- Additional Director and Head (Public Health) 1
- Joint Director (Public Health) 3
- Deputy Director (Public Health) 3
- Assistant Director (Public Health) 6
- Senior Consultant—Capacity building/Training 2
- Senior Consultant—Environmental Health Specialist 2
- Senior Consultant—Monitoring and Evaluation 1
- Senior Consultant—Public Health Informatics Specialist 1
- Consultant—Finance and Admin 1
- Consultant—Communication/Advocacy 1
- Technical Officer—Data Management 3
- Secretarial Assistants cum Data Entry Operators 3

State Level: Each state has a State Nodal Officer (SNO) responsible for the NPCCHH
- **State Level—Governing Body**
  - Hon'ble State Health Minister Chairman
  - Principal Secretary (Health) Vice Chairman
  - Director Health Services/Head of Health System Member Secretary
  - Mission Director—National Health Mission Member
  - Director Medical Education Member
  - Regional Director—Health and Family Welfare Member

State Level Task Force: It is organized under the guidance of Principal Secretary (Health) of the state to implement the State Action Plan for Climate Change and Human Health (SAPCCHH) in their state/UT. SLTF is advised to have inter-ministerial members and public health expert as follows:
- Public Health Expert from State Health Department Nodal Officer
- Director, ICMR Institute/Center (If any branch in the State/UT) Member
- Director, Meteorological department of State/UT Member
- Chairman, State Pollution Control Board Member
- Chairman, State Disaster Management Authority Member
- State Surveillance Officers Member
- Environmental Engineer/Scientist from MOEFCC Member
- Secretary, State Agriculture Ministry Member
- Secretary, State Ground Water Board Member

At the **district level,** the program prioritizes the establishment of:
- **District Multi-sectoral Task Force (DTF)**
  - District Magistrate/District Commissioner Chairman
  - Chief Medical Officer/CDHO Member Secretary
  - Deputy CMO (Admin) Member
  - Senior Deputy CMO Member
  - DMO/DVBDOPO Member
  - District Health Education Information Officer Member
  - District Coordinator Member
- District Environmental Health Cell with a District Nodal Officer-Climate Change (DNO) should be constituted.
  Structure at District Environment Health Cell:
  - District Coordinator 1
  - Data entry operator 1

	The DNO and DEHC are important for timely implementation and adequate attention to local vulnerabilities. **Roles and Responsibilities of the District Environmental Health Cell:** • Prepare and implement the DAPCCHH • Conduct IEC campaigns and sensitization workshops • Conduct Sub-District/CHC/Block/PHC/SC level training for healthcare professionals and Panchayati Raj Institutions (PRI) • Implement healthcare strengthening measures and ensure health facility preparedness for prevalent climate-sensitive illnesses (CSI) in the District • Maintain and update District database of illnesses • Maintain District level data on physical, financial, epidemiological profile for these illnesses. • Conduct vulnerability assessments and risk mapping for commonly occurring climate sensitive illnesses • Supervise, monitor, and report program-related activities at every level.
Activities under the program	**Activities under the program have been planned and desired to be achieved in time-wise phases and manners. The Requested initial inputs for the first two years.** • Create an 'Environmental Health Cell' within the State Health Department. • State Health Department's State Nodal Officer for Climate Change Identification. • Notification of a Task Force comprising representatives from other health programs, specifically those related to vector-borne diseases, multiple sectors and departments, such as disaster management, Health Information System, Departments of Meteorology and other entities including the Control Board, Water and Sanitation Department, Public Works Department, and civil society. • Vulnerability Assessment for the baseline incidence rate of Climate Sensitive Illnesses • A state health adaptation plan must be developed to address extreme occurrences, specifically heat-related illnesses and air quality, environmental pollution and its impact on human health, infections transmitted by vectors, and illnesses caused by contaminated water sources. • The state health department should identify and enhance the capacity of departmental, institutional, and organizational health resources. • Collaborate with esteemed institutions or organizations, such as the Center of Excellence to establish training programs. Integration of mitigation and adaptation measures into the curriculum of students, together with the provision of guidance. • Create, merge, and execute a media communication strategy for widespread CSDs related to health. **Processes: Two to five years** • Create a framework specifically for implementing climate-sensitive diseases. • Backup plans for climate-sensitive diseases: competent and effective medical staffing, planning, and resource distribution. • Developing the skills and knowledge of medical professionals about policies and methods of treating climate-sensitive illnesses at the district level in every state. • Creation of mathematical or prediction models for population and healthcare system readiness, or early detection tools for CSDs (quick diagnoses, surveillance). • Regular evaluations to see if the indicators—vulnerability, preparedness, response capability, and environmental determinants—identified for every CSD have improved or deteriorated. • Raising awareness: Incorporate IEC; involve community members and local leaders; hold annual "Advocacy network meetings" and health lectures; celebrate particular days; hold health melas, etc. • Take into account the predicted risks associated with climate change when designing new healthcare facilities. If such facilities currently exist, make the necessary modifications in accordance with approved building codes. • Establish links between meteorological data, climate-sensitive disease data, environmental elements that impact health, and outcomes, such as morbidity and death. • A multi-sector management method for risk mapping and seasonal trends in CSDs. • Research, epidemiology research, and surveys on populations at risk for illnesses related to climate change.
Expected outputs of the NAPCCHH	• Awareness and behavior modification of general population for impact, illnesses, prevention and adaptive measures for climate sensitive illnesses. • Increase in trained healthcare personnel and equipped institutes/organization towards achievement of climate resilient healthcare services and infrastructure at district level in each state.

	• Integrated monitoring system for collection and analysis of health related data with meteorological parameters, environmental, socioeconomic and occupational factors • Regulation on key environmental determinants of health: Air quality, water quality, food, waste management, agriculture, transport. • Evidence-based support to policy makers, program planners and related stakeholders
National action plan for climate change and levels of prevention	The NAPCCHH has planned various activities for prevention and control at primary, secondary and tertiary levels. • **Focusing on primary prevention:** Awareness generation among health professionals, school children and general populace regarding health impact of climate change and mitigation measures. The special focus for school children to make them change agents in the community for propagating environment protect measures. Environment protective measures include tree plantation and protection, car/vehicle pooling, promotion of clean fuel, use of energy efficient appliances. Lifestyle modification such as promoting physical activities, no substance use, limiting consumption of HFSS food items, increasing vegetable and fruit consumption remains the cornerstone for prevention of noncommunicable diseases in the community. • **Focusing on secondary prevention:** Health system preparedness using heat action plan, state level health system action plan to ensure availability of skilled manpower, functional equipment and supplies helps in the management of climate sensitive illness at all levels of health care. Population-based screening under NP-NCD remains an important intervention for screening of NCDs and common cancers at the community level. • **Focusing on tertiary prevention:** Integration of actions with the national palliative care program is essential at secondary and tertiary level of health facilities. Medical colleges/institutes plays important in this integrated action.

Monitoring and evaluation	The monitoring and evaluation of the implementation of NAPCCH has been established using a combination of internal and external methods. The Ministry of Health and Family Welfare (MoHFW), State Department of Health and Family Welfare (DoHFW), District Health Officers, and individual health facilities will participate in frequent internal monitoring. An impartial agency will conduct external monitoring.
	  The District Nodal Officer (DNO) and District Environmental Health Committee (DEHC) members are responsible for visiting villages and health facilities to monitor IEC activities. They compile quarterly reports and share them with NPCCHH-HQ. The State Nodal Officer-NPCCHH (SNO) and Consultant-NPCCHH compile the minutes of District Task Force (DTF) meetings conducted each financial quarter and share them with NPCCHH-HQ.
	  The development of guidelines, training modules, and surveillance for the program is carried out by centers of excellence in collaboration with the NPCCHH of the National Centre for Disease Control (NCDC). The Center for Excellence on Air Pollution and Health at AIIMS, New Delhi plays a key role in this initiative.

References

1. Climate change. [cited 2024 Jul 19]. Available from: https://www.who.int/health-topics/climate-change
2. National Programme on Climate Change and Human Health. National Centre for Disease Control (NCDC). Available from: https://ncdc.mohfw.gov.in/national-programme-on-climate-change-human-health/
3. IPCC. Summary for Policymakers. In: Edenhofer O, Pichs-Madruga R, Sokona Y, Farahani E, Kadner S, Seyboth K, et al. (Eds). Climate Change 2014, Mitigation of Climate Change Contribution of Working Group III to the Fifth Assessment Report of the Intergovernmental Panel on Climate Change. Cambridge, United Kingdom and New York, NY, USA.: Cambridge Univ Press; 2014.
4. IPCC. Glossary. In: Field CB, Barros VR, Dokken DJ, Mach KJ, Mastrandrea MD, Bilir TE, et al. (Eds). Climate change 2014: impacts, adaptation, and vulnerability. Part A: Global and Sectoral Aspects Contribution of Working Group II to the Fifth Assessment Report of the Intergovernmental Panel on Climate Change. Cambridge, UK and New York, USA: Cambridge University Press; 2014.
5. Bush KF, Luber G, Kotha SR, Dhaliwal RS, Kapil V, Pascual M, et al. Impacts of climate change on public health in India: future research directions. Environ Health Perspect. 2011 Jun;119(6):765-70. doi: 10.1289/ehp.1003000. Epub 2011 Jan 27. PMID: 21273162; PMCID: PMC3114809.
6. Desai VK, Patel U, Rathi SK, Wagle S, Desai HS. Temperature and Humidity Variability for Surat (coastal) city, India; International Journal of Environmental Sciences. Volume 5 (5) 2015.
7. National Centre for Epidemiology and Population Health, The Australian National University, Canberra 0200, Australia (Prof A J McMichael PhD, RE Woodruff PhD); and University of Otago, Wellington School of Medicine and Health Sciences, Wellington, New Zealand (S Hales PhD). Lancet 2006;367:859–69 Published Online February 9, 2006 DOI:10.1016/S0140-6736(06) 68079-3

QUESTIONS

Long Answer Question (LAQ)

1. Discuss the objectives, strategies, and challenges of the National Programme on Climate Change and Human Health (NPCCHH) in India. How does the program aim to mitigate the impact of climate-sensitive diseases and improve healthcare infrastructure in the face of climate change?

Short Answer Questions (SAQs)

1. Explain the significance of the District Action Plan on Climate Change and Human Health (DAPCCHH) and its role in enhancing local healthcare preparedness in India.
2. Describe the five priority areas identified under NPCCHH at the district level and their relevance to public health in the context of climate change.

Multiple Choice Questions (MCQs)

1. What is the main goal of the National Programme on Climate Change and Human Health (NPCCHH)?
    a. To reduce the impact of climate change on wildlife
    b. To enhance economic growth
    c. To reduce morbidity, mortality, injuries, and health vulnerability due to climate variability and extreme weather
    d. To promote industrial development
2. Which organization is responsible for hosting the NPCCHH?
    a. Ministry of Environment, Forest, and Climate Change
    b. National Centre for Disease Control (NCDC)
    c. Indian Meteorological Department
    d. World Health Organization (WHO)
3. What is the primary focus of air pollution-related illness surveillance under NPCCHH?
    a. Tracking wildlife health
    b. Surveillance of acute respiratory illnesses (ARI)
    c. Monitoring heat-related illnesses
    d. Identifying malnutrition trends
4. Which of the following is NOT one of the 17 climate-sensitive diseases (CSDs) identified under NPCCHH?
    a. Vector-borne diseases
    b. Cardiopulmonary diseases
    c. Heat-related illnesses
    d. Cancer
5. What type of infrastructure does the NPCCHH emphasize for better preparedness against climate change impacts?
    a. High-rise buildings
    b. Smart cities
    c. Green and climate resilient healthcare infrastructure
    d. Conventional healthcare facilities

Answers

1. c
2. b
3. b
4. d
5. c

80 CHAPTER

Voluntary Blood Donation Programme

Rudresh Negi, Malatesh Undi, Bhautik Modi

Background/Need of program	Family/replacement donors are responsible for more than 45% of blood collected in India. These donors are more likely to be associated with a higher prevalence of transfusion-transmissible infections. In a resource restricted country like India, where comprehensive laboratory tests are not possible or practical, 100% voluntary blood donation is the way forward.[4] Also, voluntary blood donation ensures safe, reliable and adequate supply of blood and blood products.[4] Thus the safest blood donors are voluntary, non-remunerated and from low-risk populations. The World Health Organization also recommends 'for all countries to obtain all their blood supplies through voluntary unpaid donors' as per the adopted World Health Assembly resolution 28.72 of 1975.[1] 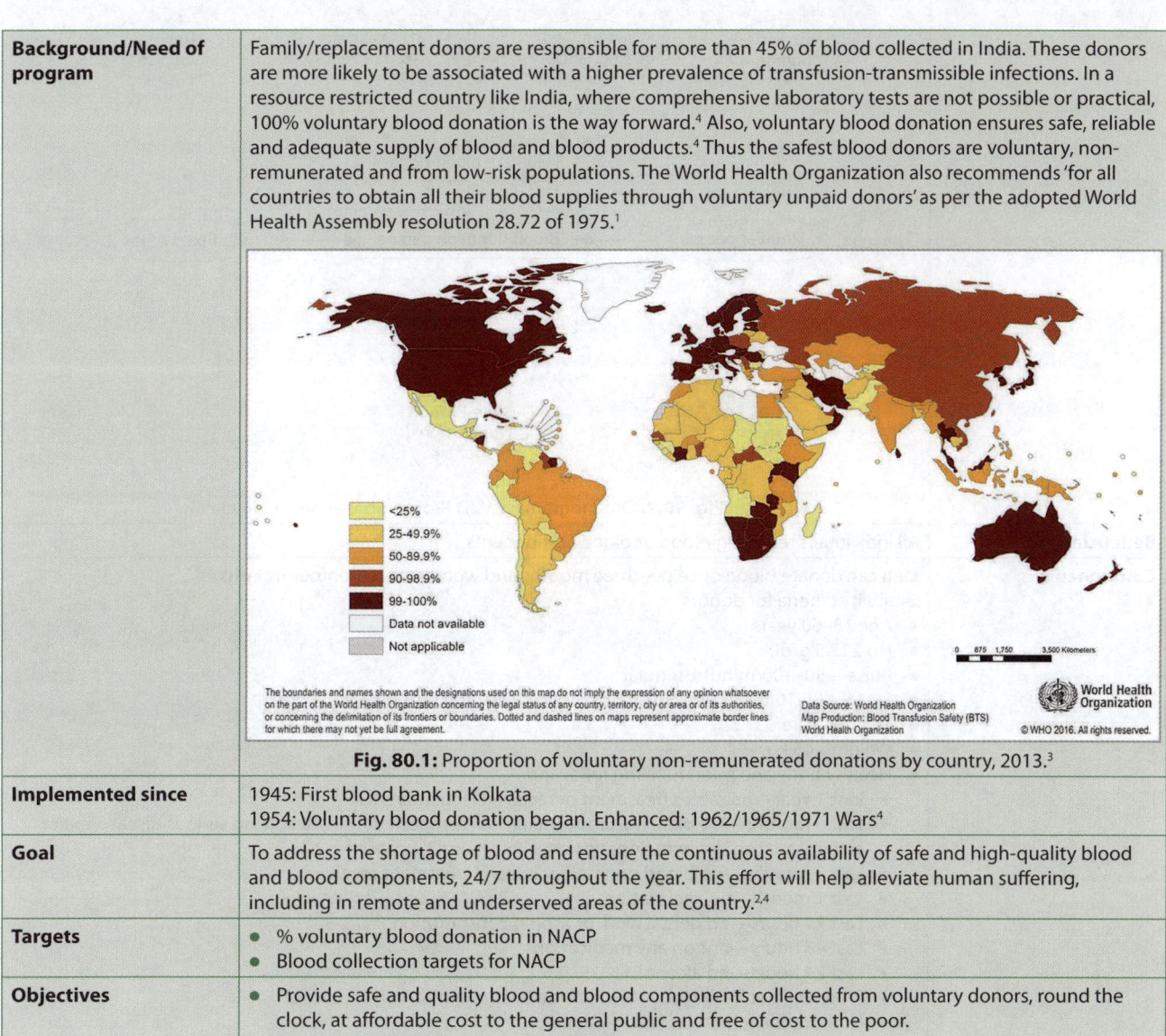 **Fig. 80.1:** Proportion of voluntary non-remunerated donations by country, 2013.[3]
Implemented since	1945: First blood bank in Kolkata 1954: Voluntary blood donation began. Enhanced: 1962/1965/1971 Wars[4]
Goal	To address the shortage of blood and ensure the continuous availability of safe and high-quality blood and blood components, 24/7 throughout the year. This effort will help alleviate human suffering, including in remote and underserved areas of the country.[2,4]
Targets	• % voluntary blood donation in NACP • Blood collection targets for NACP
Objectives	• Provide safe and quality blood and blood components collected from voluntary donors, round the clock, at affordable cost to the general public and free of cost to the poor. • Ensure safety and quality of blood.

	• Motivate and maintain a permanent well-indexed record of voluntary blood donors. • Educating the community on the beneficial aspects of blood donation and harmful effect of collecting blood from paid donors. • Actively encourage voluntary blood donation and gradually eliminate professional blood donors. • Promote AIDS awareness and education to the general public. • Assists the various organizations, clubs, colleges, public and private institutions and the public to conduct voluntary blood donation drives and arrange for motivational talks to enable progressively increase the number of voluntary non-remunerated blood donors every year.[2]
Organogram	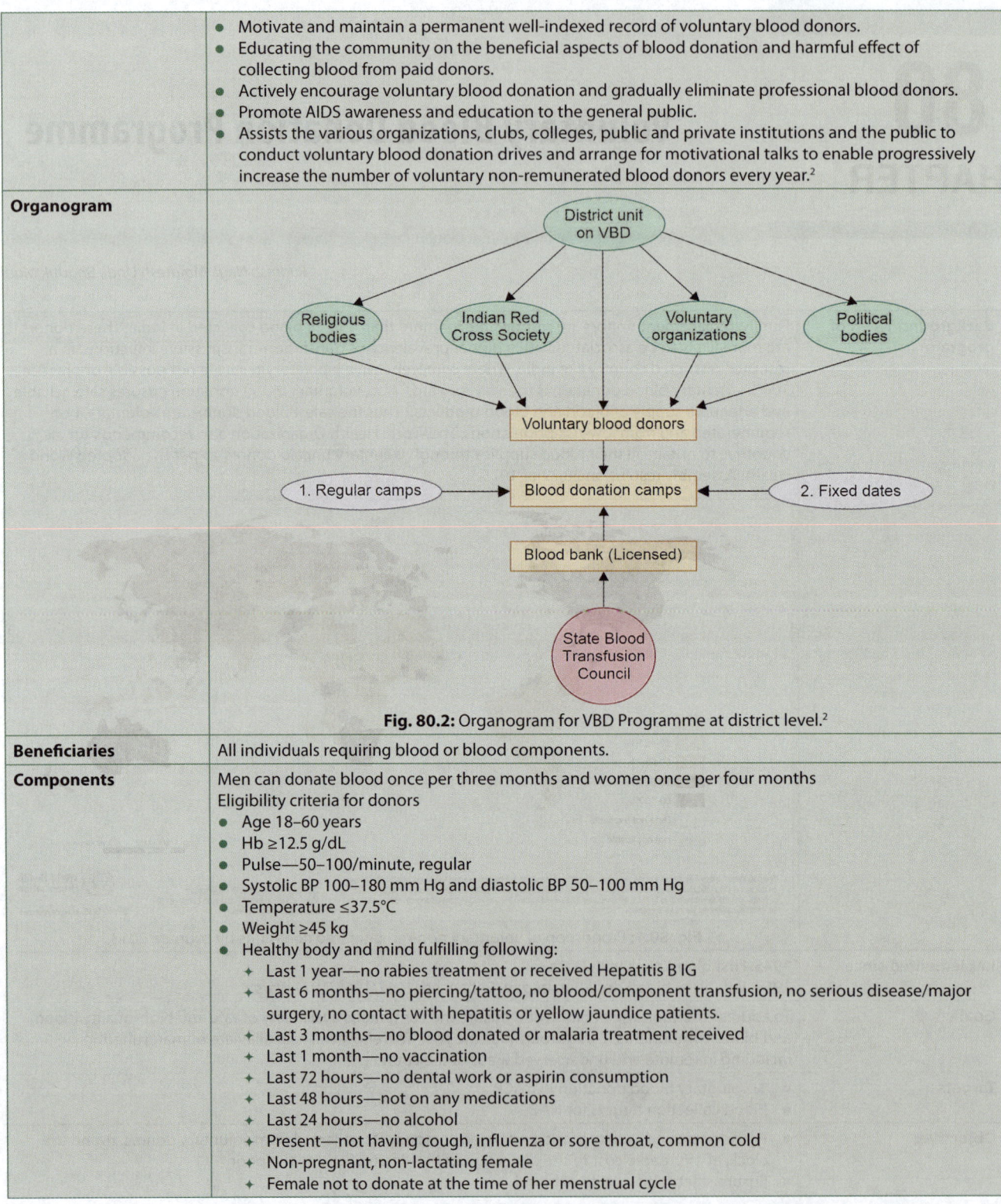 Fig. 80.2: Organogram for VBD Programme at district level.[2]
Beneficiaries	All individuals requiring blood or blood components.

Components	Men can donate blood once per three months and women once per four months
	Eligibility criteria for donors
	• Age 18–60 years
	• Hb ≥12.5 g/dL
	• Pulse—50–100/minute, regular
	• Systolic BP 100–180 mm Hg and diastolic BP 50–100 mm Hg
	• Temperature ≤37.5°C
	• Weight ≥45 kg
	• Healthy body and mind fulfilling following:
	  ✦ Last 1 year—no rabies treatment or received Hepatitis B IG
	  ✦ Last 6 months—no piercing/tattoo, no blood/component transfusion, no serious disease/major surgery, no contact with hepatitis or yellow jaundice patients.
	  ✦ Last 3 months—no blood donated or malaria treatment received
	  ✦ Last 1 month—no vaccination
	  ✦ Last 72 hours—no dental work or aspirin consumption
	  ✦ Last 48 hours—not on any medications
	  ✦ Last 24 hours—no alcohol
	  ✦ Present—not having cough, influenza or sore throat, common cold
	  ✦ Non-pregnant, non-lactating female
	  ✦ Female not to donate at the time of her menstrual cycle

- Not suffering from diabetes, chest pain, heart disease or high BP, cancer, blood clotting problem or blood disease, unexplained fever, weight loss, fatigue, night sweats, enlarged lymph nodes in neck or groin, white patches in the mouth, etc.
- Never had tuberculosis (TB), bronchial asthma, allergic disorders, liver or kidney disease, seizures or fainting episodes, blue or purple spots on the skin or mucous membranes, or received human pituitary growth hormones, etc.[2,4]

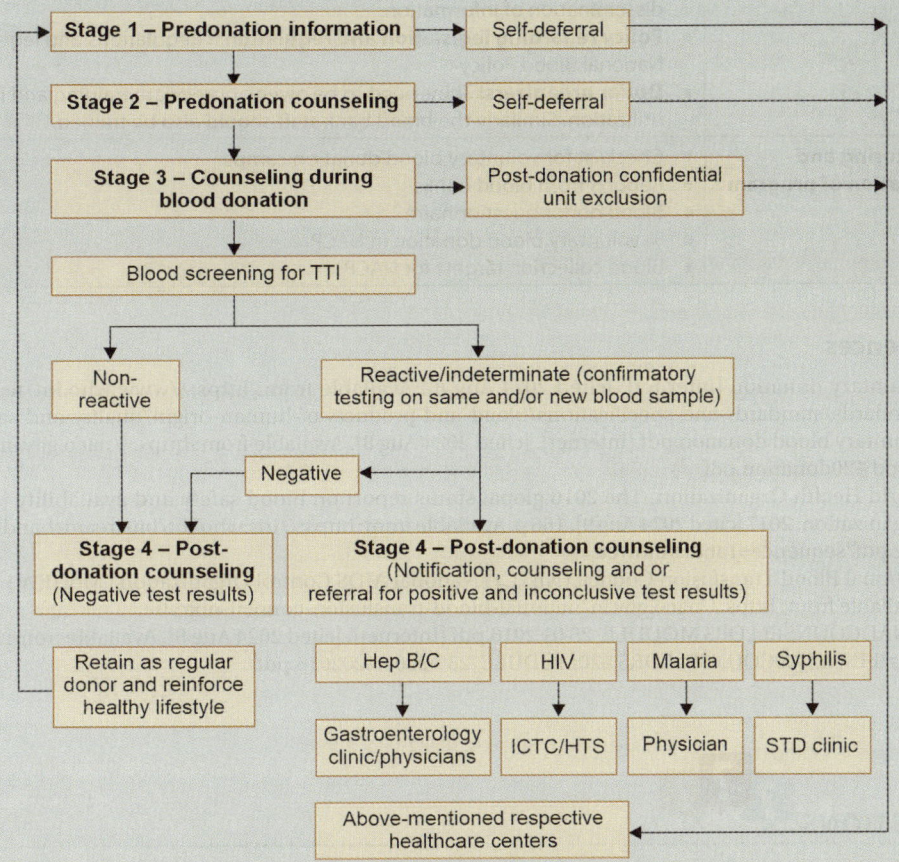

Fig. 80.3: Cascade of blood donor counseling.[4,5]

Activities at various level or package of services	The program is implemented by blood banks, state blood transfusion councils and recognized voluntary blood donor organizations, IRCS, CBOs, NGOs and includes the following activities: • **Need assessment:** To narrow the demand and supply gap. • **Education:** To spread awareness in general public prevent shortages of blood and its components in supply. The donor information material should be in simple local language. • **Awareness campaigns for the people:** To be conducted in schools for grooming the next generation of blood donors. Short courses for trainers and volunteers to be conducted. • **Donor motivation:** Can be done through seminars, talks, posters, hoardings, public exhibitions and competitions. • **Donations:** The underlying principle is "to go to the donors" rather than waiting for them to come to blood banks. This can be accomplished through blood donation camps and drives in areas of public gatherings, such as colleges, factories, workplaces, etc. • **Recognition:** Blood donors and donor organizations should be valued and honored with awards and certificates. List of donors can be maintained and preference given in hospitals and banks. • **Media:** The mass media can be efficiently utilized through a three pronged strategy of mass approach, group approach and individual approach.

	• **Database of donors:** A comprehensive database of blood donors and donor organizations would enable its prompt and time use. Sharing of this database with state governments and donor organizations would be helpful. • **Interaction and sharing of experiences:** Can be done through conferences and workshops and would enable mutual and multilateral exchange of information and experiences. • **Publications:** Through State Blood Transfusion Council, NACO and SACS would enable wider dissemination of information. • **Policy regarding legislation and regulations:** Regulations and legislations should follow the National Blood Policy • **Donor organizers:** They need to be given appropriate training and infrastructure for proper utilization. Similarly the blood bank staff should also be trained.[2]
Monitoring and evaluation of program	• Checklist for voluntary blood donation camps • Reports from blood banks • Blood donor questionnaire • % voluntary blood donation in NACP • Blood collection targets for NACP[2]

References

1. Voluntary donation [Internet]. [cited 2024 Aug 8]. Available from: https://www.who.int/teams/health-product-policy-and-standards/standards-and-specifications/blood-and-products-of-human-origin/quality-and-safety/voluntary-donation
2. voluntary blood donation.pdf [Internet]. [cited 2024 Aug 8]. Available from: https://naco.gov.in/sites/default/files/voluntary%20blood%20donation.pdf
3. World Health Organization. The 2016 global status report on blood safety and availability [Internet]. Geneva: World Health Organization; 2017 [cited 2024 Aug 9]. 166 p. Available from: https://iris.who.int/bitstream/handle/10665/254987/9789241565431-eng.pdf?sequence=1andisAllowed=y
4. National Blood Transfusion Council (NBTC) | National AIDS Control Organization | MoHFW | GoI [Internet]. [cited 2024 Aug 9]. Available from: https://naco.gov.in/national-blood-transfusion-council-nbtc-0
5. FINAL COUNSELLORS MODULE_25 01 2016.pdf [Internet]. [cited 2024 Aug 8]. Available from: https://naco.gov.in/sites/default/files/FINAL%20COUNSELLORS%20MODULE_25%2001%202016.pdf

QUESTIONS

Long Answer Question (LAQ)

1. Using the SWOT format critically analyze the status of Voluntary Blood Donation Programme in India.

Short Answer Questions (SAQs)

1. Comment on the Goal and objectives of Voluntary Blood Programme in India.
2. You as the Medical Superintendent of a District Hospital are planning a blood donation program. Mention the eligibility criteria to be set for blood donation.

Multiple Choice Questions (MCQs)

1. In post-blood donation counseling if the individual was reactive for syphilis, what will be the next step?
   a. Do nothing
   b. Refer to STD clinic
   c. Retain as regular donor
   d. None of the above
2. Ramesh has come to donate blood. What makes him ineligible to do so?
   a. Age 70 years
   b. Hb 15 g/dL
   c. Afebrile
   d. No alcohol intake in last 24 hours
3. Program closely associated with Voluntary Blood Donation Programme is:
   a. NTEP
   b. IDSP
   c. IMNCI
   d. NACP

Answers

1. b
2. a
3. d

CHAPTER 81

National Organ Transplant Programme

Rohit Katre, Pallavi Singh, Jagruti Prajapati

Background/Need of program/Scheme	The shortage of organs is virtually a universal problem but Asia lags behind much of the rest of the world. There are enough organs to transplant in India. Nearly every person who dies naturally, or in an accident, is a potential donor. Even then, innumerable patients cannot find a donor. Hon'ble Prime Minister has highlighted the importance of organ donation in the Mann Ki Baat Programme broadcast in October and November 2015. This has given impetus to the Organ Donation in the country.
Scenario of organ transplantation in India[1]	• There is a wide gap between patients who need transplants and the organs that are available in India. India is the country that performs the third most transplants globally. • In 2022, approximately 17.8% of all transplants used organs from deceased donors. • By 2022, there will have been 2,765 deceased organ transplants, up from 837 in 2013. • From 4,990 in 2013 to 15,561 in 2022, more organs from both deceased and living donors were transplanted overall. • An estimated 1.5–2 lakh people require kidney transplants annually. • In 2022, only 10,000 or so received one. Less than 3,000 of the 80,000 patients in need of liver transplants in 2022 actually received one. • Only 250 of the 10,000 people in need of a heart transplant in 2022 actually received one.
Implemented since	The Government of India is implementing National Organ Transplant Programme for carrying out the activities as per Amendment Act, training of manpower and promotion of organ donation from deceased persons. Organ donation and transplantation is a government regulated activity in India as per the provisions of the Transplantation of Human Organs and Tissues Act 1994 (as amended in 2011) • The Transplantation of Human Organs Act (THOA), 1994 was enacted in the year 1994 and was adopted in all States except erstwhile State of JandK and Andhra Pradesh which have their own legislation in this regard. • The Act was amended in 2011 and the Transplantation of Human Organs (Amendment) Act 2011, has come into force on 10-1-2014 in the States of Goa, Himachal Pradesh, West Bengal, and Union Territories. Other States who have adopted the amendment Act till date are Rajasthan, Sikkim, Jharkhand, Kerala, Odisha, Punjab, Maharashtra, Assam, Chhattisgarh, Haryana, Manipur, Gujarat, Bihar, Uttar Pradesh, Tamil Nadu and Madhya Pradesh. The amended Act is now named Transplantation of Human Organs and Tissues Act (THOTA), 1994. After reorganization of erstwhile State of Jammu and Kashmir, the THOTA 1994 is now also applicable in the Union Territories of Jammu and Kashmir and Ladakh. • Other States, namely Andhra Pradesh, Telangana, Karnataka, Uttarakhand, Arunachal Pradesh, Mizoram, Meghalaya, Nagaland and Tripura have not yet adopted the Transplantation of Human Organs (Amendment) Act 2011. • **Important amendments under the (Amendment) Act 2011:** Amendments for increasing the pool of organ donors are as under: **Living Donation** • Near relative "definition has been expanded to include grandchildren, grandparents. • Swap Donation (Donor Exchange) included.

	Cadaveric donation • Tissue donation, tissue transplantation and tissue banking included. • Mandatory transplant coordinators in transplant and retrieval hospitals • Registration of retrieval only centers • Mandatory request for donation from potential donors in intensive care units (ICU) • Brain stem death certification permitted by Anesthetist/intensivist if neuro experts are not available • National networking between retrieval centers, transplant centers, tissue banks, networking organizations at state, regional and national level for establishing an efficient organ procurement and distribution system in the country (Mandate given to Central Government) • National Registry for organ donation and transplantation (Mandate given to Central Government) • Eye/Cornea retrieval permitted from trained technicians **Other Amendments** • To protect vulnerable and poor there is provision of higher penalties has been made for trading in organs (imprisonment up to 10 years and fine up to ₹ one crore) • Act has made provision of greater caution in case of minors and foreign nationals and prohibition of organ donation from mentally challenged persons In November 2010, the National Organ Transplant Programme (2010-2012) approved NOTTO's creation (formerly termed MOPDO). After developing additional components, the NOTP scheme was approved for four years (2013–2014 to 2016–2017) and then underwent a three-year revision (2017–2018 to 2019–2020). As of right now, the program is extended through 2025–2026.
Aim	The National Organ Transplant Programme aims to improve access to the life transforming transplantation for needy citizens of our country by promoting deceased organ donation.[1]
Objectives	• To organize a system of organ and tissue procurement and distribution for transplantation. • To promote deceased organ and Tissue donation. • To train required manpower. • To build new infrastructure facilities for organ and tissue retrieval and transplantation, as well as to reinforce the ones that already exist, particularly in public sector hospitals and institutes. • To locate and create skill centers in NOTTO/ROTTO/SOTTO/Medical colleges/Institutes that are relevant for the training of transplant and retrieval surgeons, physicians, anesthetists, immunologists, nurses, transplant coordinators, etc. • To create and implement the Digital National Registry for Organ and Tissue Donation and Transplantation. • To protect vulnerable poor from organ trafficking. • To monitor organ and tissue transplant services and bring about policy and program corrections/changes whenever needed.
Organogram	NOTTO: National Organ and Tissue Transplant Organization ↓ ROTTO: Regional Organ and Tissue Transplant Organization (Chandigarh, Mumbai, Chennai, Kolkata, and Guwahati) ↓ SOTTO: State Organ and Tissue Transplant Organization (12 states)
Strategies/Deliverables under the program	• Promoting organ and tissue donation through advocacy and implementing different IEC initiatives to raise awareness among stakeholders and the general public. • Encouraging people to indicate that they are willing to donate when they pass away. • Create a network at the state, regional, and national levels for the removal, allocation, and transplantation of organs and tissues. • Developing the skills of those working in organ and tissue donation and transplantation. • To open new skill centers in NOTTO and a few national medical colleges to teach doctors, surgeons, immunologists, and other professionals. • Create and keep up a nationwide database for transplants and donations of organs and tissues. • Create the infrastructure needed for transplantation and organ and tissue donation at different levels.

	• Creating a reliable method of transportation for the quick and secure movement of tissues and organs throughout cities. (Air, train, surface, and metro transportation, including security, etc.) • Offering a system of insurance support and other forms of assistance to living donors. • Assisting in setting up a strong support network to guarantee the best possible graft results (such as immunosuppressive medications for those who cannot afford them and prompt, sufficient medical care).
New guidelines[2]	• **Age cap removed:** Since individuals are living longer, the highest age limit has been abolished. Previously, end-stage organ failure patients who were older than 65 could not register to receive an organ, according rules from the National Organ and Tissue Transplant Organization (NOTTO). • **No requirement for domicile:** As part of the "One Nation, One Policy," the ministry has eliminated the need to register as an organ recipient in a state of residence. A patient in need can now register to receive an organ in any state of their choosing, and they can even have the surgery performed anywhere. • **No registration fee:** The Center has requested that states that previously charged for this type of registration refrain from doing so. There will be no registration fee that states previously charged for this reason. A few of the states that requested funding for registration were Kerala, Gujarat, Telangana, and Maharashtra. A patient's registration on the organ recipient queue was required in some states to cost anything from ₹5,000 to 10,000.
Monitoring and evaluation of program	Monitoring of transplantation activities in the regions and states and maintaining databank by NOTTO.

References

1. National Organ Transplant Programme. Available on: https://dghs.gov.in/content/1353_3_NationalOrganTransplantProgramme.
2. Guidelines for implementation of national organ transplant program (period: 2021-22 to 2025-26)

QUESTIONS

Long Answer Question (LAQ)

1. Write a comprehensive overview of the National Organ Transplant Programme. What roles and responsibilities do NOTTO/SOTTO have for promotion of organ transplants in the country?

Short Answer Question (SAQ)

1. Write a short note on recent advances under the National Organ Transplant Programme.

Multiple Choice Questions (MCQs)

1. Consider the following statements regarding National Organ Transplant Programme (NOTP):
   Program will organize a system of organ and tissue procurement and distribution for transplantation.
   One of its aims is to protect vulnerable poor from organ trafficking.
   Which of the above statements is/are incorrect?
   a. 1 only
   b. 2 only
   c. Both 1 and 2
   d. Neither 1 nor 2

2. Where is the National Organ and Tissue Transplant Organization (NOTTO) is located?
   a. New Delhi
   b. Chennai
   c. Andhra Pradesh
   d. Jammu and Kashmir
3. When does NOTTO celebrate Indian Organ Donation Day?
   a. 1st December
   b. 27th November
   c. 21st November
   d. 24th March
4. Which ministry is responsible for organ transplantation in India?
   a. Ministry of Health and Family Welfare
   b. Ministry of Home Affairs
   c. Ministry of External Affairs
   d. Ministry of Civil Aviation
5. Who are the "near relatives" according to THOA Act?
   a. Only parents
   b. Parents, children and spouse
   c. Only brother and sister
   d. Grandparents and grandchildren in addition to parents, children, brother, sister and spouse.
6. According to the NOTTO (National Organ and Tissue Transplant Organization) guidelines which of the following is incorrect?
   a. The upper age limit has been removed
   b. No domicile requirement
   c. No fees for registration
   d. End-stage organ failure patient above 65 years of age was prohibited
7. India conducts which number of transplants in the world?
   a. Second highest
   b. First
   c. Third highest
   d. Fifth highest
8. Which of the following can be donated by live donor?
   a. Kidney
   b. Eye
   c. Heart
   d. Lung
9. The_____ regenerates in the donor after some time following transplantation.
   a. Kidney
   b. Liver
   c. Heart
   d. Lung
10. Which cells are transplanted to treat cancer like leukemia?
    a. Hematopoietic stem cells
    b. Red blood cells
    c. White blood cells
    d. Epithelial cells

Answers

1. d
2. a
3. b
4. a
5. d
6. d
7. c
8. a
9. b
10. b

CHAPTER 82: National Programme for Control and Treatment of Occupational Diseases

Swati Ghonge, Kajal Srivastava, Parul Sharma, Bharti Koria

Background/Need of program/Scheme	The United Nations estimates that nearly two million people die annually due to occupational risk factors, with over 2.78 million deaths worldwide and 374 million non-fatal injuries. The economic burden of occupational-related injury and death is nearly 4% of the global GDP.[1]
Implemented since	Ministry of Health and Family Welfare, Government of India has launched a scheme entitled "National Programme for Control and Treatment of Occupational Diseases" in 1998-99. The National Institute of Occupational Health, Ahmedabad (ICMR) is the nodal agency for the same.
Objectives	<ul><li>Maintenance and promotion of workers' health and working capacity</li><li>Improvement of working environment and work to become conducive to safety and health and</li><li>Development of work organizations and working cultures in a direction which supports health and safety at work.</li></ul>
Strategies/ Deliverables	<ul><li>It calls for providing a statutory framework on Occupational Safety and Health in respect of all sectors of industrial activities including the construction sector, designing suitable control systems of compliance, enforcement and incentives for better compliance.</li><li>To provide administrative and technical support services.</li><li>To provide a system of incentives to employers and employees to achieve higher health and safety standards.</li><li>To providing for a system of non-financial incentives for improvement in safety and health.</li><li>To establish and develop the research and development capability in emerging areas of risk and providing for effective control measures.</li><li>To focus on prevention strategies and monitoring performance through improved data collection system on work related injuries and diseases.[2]</li></ul>
Components	<ul><li>Continuous reduction in the incidence of work-related injuries, fatalities, diseases, disasters, and loss of national assets.</li><li>Improved coverage of work-related injuries, fatalities and diseases and provide for a more comprehensive data base for facilitating better performance and monitoring.</li><li>Continuous enhancement of community awareness regarding safety, health, and environment at workplace related areas.[3]</li><li>Continually increasing community expectation of workplace health and safety standards.</li><li>Improving safety, health, and environment at workplace by creation of "green jobs" contributing to sustainable enterprise development.</li></ul>

Chapter 82: National Programme for Control and Treatment of Occupational Diseases

Organogram	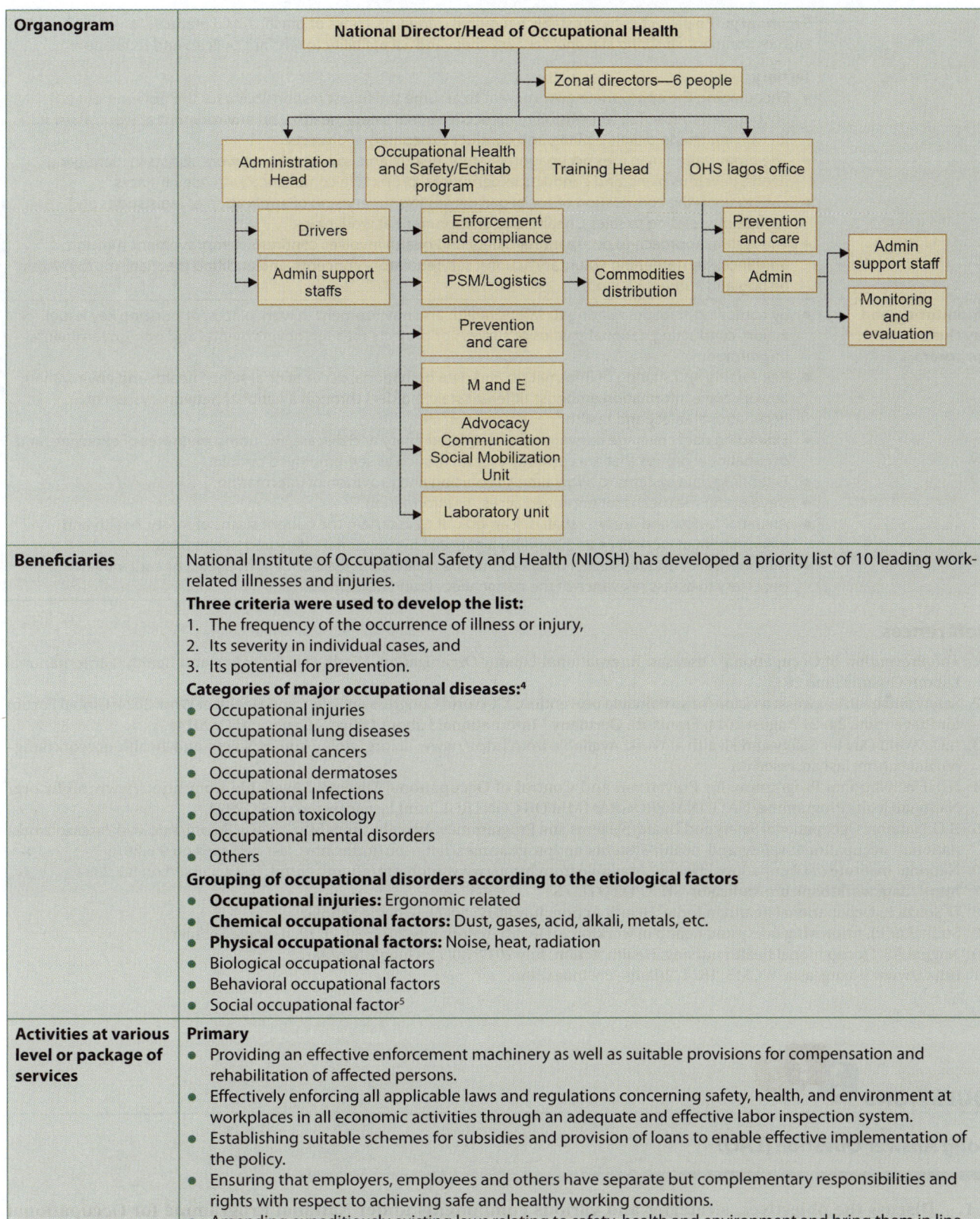
Beneficiaries	National Institute of Occupational Safety and Health (NIOSH) has developed a priority list of 10 leading work-related illnesses and injuries. **Three criteria were used to develop the list:** 1. The frequency of the occurrence of illness or injury, 2. Its severity in individual cases, and 3. Its potential for prevention. **Categories of major occupational diseases:**[4] - Occupational injuries - Occupational lung diseases - Occupational cancers - Occupational dermatoses - Occupational Infections - Occupation toxicology - Occupational mental disorders - Others **Grouping of occupational disorders according to the etiological factors** - **Occupational injuries:** Ergonomic related - **Chemical occupational factors:** Dust, gases, acid, alkali, metals, etc. - **Physical occupational factors:** Noise, heat, radiation - Biological occupational factors - Behavioral occupational factors - Social occupational factor[5]
Activities at various level or package of services	**Primary** - Providing an effective enforcement machinery as well as suitable provisions for compensation and rehabilitation of affected persons. - Effectively enforcing all applicable laws and regulations concerning safety, health, and environment at workplaces in all economic activities through an adequate and effective labor inspection system. - Establishing suitable schemes for subsidies and provision of loans to enable effective implementation of the policy. - Ensuring that employers, employees and others have separate but complementary responsibilities and rights with respect to achieving safe and healthy working conditions. - Amending expeditiously existing laws relating to safety, health and environment and bring them in line with the relevant international instruments.

	Secondary: The project aims to establish national standards, codes of practice, and manuals for safety, health, and environment, ensuring stakeholder awareness and accessibility to relevant policies and regulations.[6] **Tertiary** • Encouraging the appropriate government to assume the fullest responsibility for the government is encouraged to take full responsibility for occupational safety, health, and environment at work, assist in identifying needs, develop plans, and conduct experimental projects. • The organization manages occupational safety, health, and environment at work, assists in identifying needs, develops plans, and conducts experimental projects in compliance with relevant Acts.[7] • Calling upon the cooperation of social partners in the supervision of application of legislations and regulations relating to safety, health and environment at work place. • The system approach to occupational safety and health involves continuous improvement through guidance, strengthening voluntary actions, self-regulatory concepts, and auditing mechanisms for system testing and authentication.[8]
Monitoring and evaluation of program	• By compiling statistics relating to safety, health and environment at work places, prioritizing key issues for action, conducting national studies or surveys or projects through governmental and non-governmental organizations. • Reinforcing and sharing of information and data on national occupational safety, health and environment at work place information amongst different stake holders through a national network system on occupational safety and health.[9] • Extending data coverage relevant to work-related injury and disease, including measures of exposure, and occupational groups that are currently excluded, such as self-employed people. • Extending data systems to allow timely reporting and provision of information. • Developing the means for improved access to information.[10] • An initial review and analysis shall be carried out to ascertain the current status of safety, health and environment at workplace and building a national occupational safety and health profile. • National policy and the action program shall be reviewed at least once in five years or earlier if felt necessary to assess relevance of the national goals and objectives.[11]

References

1. The Prevention of Occupational Diseases. International Labour Organization. World Day for safety and health.© International Labour Organization 2023.
2. Safety and health at work: a vision for sustainable prevention: XX World Congress on Safety and Health at Work 2024: Global Forum for Prevention, 24 -27 August 2014, Frankfurt, Germany / International Labour Office. - Geneva: ILO, 2014.
3. ILO. World Day for Safety and Health at Work. Available from http://www.ilo.org/global/topics/safety-and-health-at-work/lang–en/index.htm, last accessed on
4. NIHFW. National Programme for Prevention and Control of Occupational Diseases. Available from http://www.nihfw.org/NationalHealthProgramme/NATIONALPROGRAMMEFOR CONTROL.html, last accessed on 9.7.2024
5. ILO. National Occupational Safety and Health Systems and Programmes. Available from http://www.ilo.org/safework/areasofwork/national- occupational-safety-and-health-systems-andprogrammes/lang--en/index.htm, last accessed on 9.6.2015
6. National Institute of Occupational Health. Available from http://www.nioh.org/aboutus.html, last accessed on 9.7.2024
7. http://data.worldbank.org/indicator/SH.XPD.TOTL.ZS.
8. D'Souza R. Occupational health in India. Health Action. July 2017; 30(7): [Google Scholar]
9. Sudhakar PJ. Improving safety and health of workforce. Health Action. July 2017; 30(7): 12. [Google Scholar]
10. Nagpal AS. Occupational health nursing, Health Action. July 2017; 30(7):[Google Scholar]
11. http://www.ilo.org/asia/WCMS_182422/lang--en/index.htm.

QUESTIONS

Long Answer Question (LAQ)

1. Discuss the objectives, strategies and various components under National Programme for Occupational Health in India.

Short Answer Questions (SAQs)

1. Draw-Organogram of National and Occupational Health Program in India.
2. You are appointed as Medical Officer at an Industrial Unit making Lead Batteries. Draft a occupational health program for workers at your work place.

Multiple Choice Questions (MCQs)

1. Following occupational diseases are notifiable under the Indian Factory Act, 1976, *except*:
   a. Silicosis
   b. Asbestosis
   c. Byssinosis
   d. Bagassosis
2. Ideal periodical examination of worker in an industry is done every:
   a. Day
   b. Month
   c. Year
   d. Depends on type of exposure
3. Indian constitution has declared that children less than _____ years should not be employed in factories or mines:
   a. 10
   b. 12
   c. 14
   d. 16
4. 'Safety officers' have to be appointed in factories where no. of workers is more than:
   a. 500
   b. 1000
   c. 2000
   d. 5000
5. Useful screening test for lead is measurement of:
   a. Coproporphyrin in urine
   b. Aminolevulinic acid in urine
   c. Lead in blood
   d. Lead in urine
6. Lead poisoning in industries commonly occurs by:
   a. Inhalation
   b. Ingestion
   c. Skin absorption
   d. Conjunctival route
7. Inhalation of sugarcane dust could cause:
   a. Bagassosis
   b. Byssinosis
   c. Tabacosis
   d. Farmer's lung
8. All are features of silico-tuberculosis, *except*:
   a. High sputum AFB^{+ve}
   b. Children of such cases do not get disease
   c. Impairment of total lung
   d. Nodular fibrosis
9. All are disease manifestations associated with low temperature, *except*:
   a. Chilblains
   b. Prickles
   c. Frostbite
   d. Trench foot
10. Periodic examination of factory workers is a type of:
    a. Primordial prevention
    b. Primary prevention
    c. Secondary prevention
    d. Tertiary prevention
11. With reference to lead poisoning, various parameters are given below with the levels:
    a. Coproporphyrin in urine
    b. Aminolevulinic acid in urine
    c. Lead in urine
    d. Lead in blood
    I. >70 mg/100 mL
    II. >5 mg/L
    III. >150 mg/L
    IV. >0.8 mg/L

Correct match is:
a. A-I B-II C-IV D-III
b. A-III B-IV C-II D-I
c. A-I B-IV C-II D-III
d. A-III B-II C-IV D-I

12. The minimum air space per worker prescribed by Indian Factory (Amendment) Act, 1987 is:
    a. 200 cu ft
    b. 300 cu ft
    c. 500 cu ft
    d. 700 cu ft
13. Maximum permissible level of whole body occupational exposure to ionizing radiation is:
    a. 1 rem per year
    b. 3 rem per year
    c. 5 rem per year
    d. 15 rem per year
14. "White Fingers" may result from which of the following occupational hazards:
    a. Heat
    b. Cold
    c. UV radiation
    d. Vibration

Answers

1. c
2. d
3. c
4. a
5. c
6. a
7. a
8. b
9. b
10. c
11. a
12. b
13. a
14. d

CHAPTER 83

National Programme on Containment of Anti-Microbial Resistance (AMR)

Nitesh Kumar, Rajendra Singh, Parul Sharma, Nilesh Fichdiya

Background/Need of program/Scheme	Antimicrobial resistance (AMR) can now be called a "silent pandemic" that threatens human health, animal health, and the environment. World Health Organization (WHO) has declared AMR as one of the major global health concerns. An estimated 1.27 million deaths were reported globally in 2019 owing to antimicrobial resistance. AMR is a problem for all countries of all income levels, but its drivers and consequences are accentuated by the poverty and inequality in health services. Thus, low-middle-income countries bear the major insult. The AMR has a multifaceted effect on the country. Baring the health sector's impact increases the country's economic burden. The World Bank estimates that AMR could result in an additional 1 trillion $ cost to the health sector by 2050 and a GDP yearly loss of 3.4 trillion US $ by 2030.[1,2] Inappropriate use of antibiotics is one of the most common causes of AMR. In addition, the development of newer antibiotics has decreased over the past three decades. Of the several antibiotics under clinical development, WHO has identified only six antibiotics as innovative for dealing with the priority list of pathogens suggested by it. Several studies have also shown the relationship between increased use of antibiotics and AMR. Thus, it is imperative for the countries to review their antibiotic policy.[3,4] India is one of the countries where bacterial illnesses are most common. In India, pneumonia claims the lives of 410,000 children under the age of five every year; pneumonia accounts for over 25% of all pediatric fatalities. Infectious disease-related crude mortality in India currently stands at 417 per 100,000 people. As a result, in the Indian context, the impact of AMR will probably be greater. Resistance has not only emerged to the more established and widely used medication classes; resistance to the more recent and costly treatments, such as carbapenems, has also rapidly increased. The data that is currently available shows that AMR rates are increasing nationally for a variety of infections that are clinically significant. The data on the prevalence of AMR in food animals and cattle in India is insufficient. There is hardly much data that can be generalized to the national level except for occasional research. Antibiotic resistance (AMR) resulting from antibiotic abuse in the livestock sector is expected to be an unmeasured burden in India because there are few laws prohibiting the use of antibiotics for reasons other than therapeutics. Owing to this, it was necessary for India to take an initiative on AMR containment, and thus the National Programme on AMR Containment was launched.[5,6]
Implemented since	**Historical trends** Acknowledging the threat of antimicrobial resistance, the Government of India has taken many initiatives. In 2010, it all began with the constitution of the National Task Force on AMR Containment, followed by the development of national policy on AMR containment in 2011. India pioneered organizing a summit of health ministers of the South-East Asian region in Jaipur in 2011. This summit prioritized AMR as a global health concern and mitigated a committed action. Then, under the 12th Five-Year Plan (2012-2017), MoHFW launched the National Programme on Containment of Antimicrobial Resistance. NCDC, New Delhi, is the nodal agency implementing and coordinating the AMR program. Under this program, initiatives were taken to open network laboratories nationwide to generate quality data on antimicrobial resistance for pathogens of public health importance. The "Global Plan of Action on Antimicrobial Resistance (GMR-AMR)" was endorsed in the 68th World Health Assembly, and all the member states were asked to implement this by 2017. This (GMR-AMR) set out 5 strategic objectives—improving awareness, surveillance, infection control, antimicrobial usage, and initiating innovative research. India adopted these strategies and added the sixth leadership strategy, and thus, "The National Action Plan on Antimicrobial Resistance (NAP-AMR) 2017-2021 was implemented.[7]

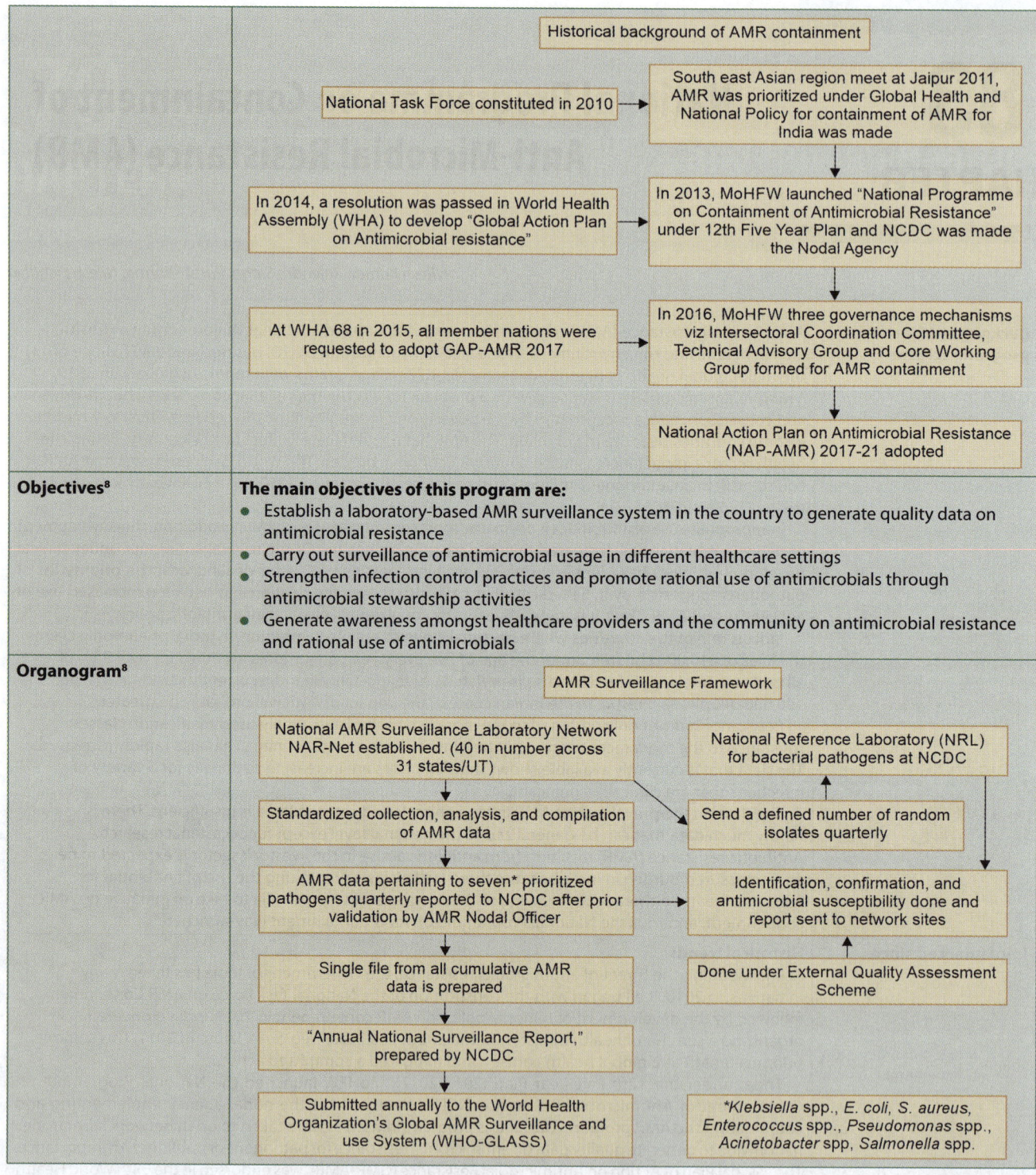

Key activities and components

Antimicrobial resistance surveillance
Under the National Programme on AMR Containment, one of the prime objectives was the capacity building of the medical colleges and large hospitals to generate quality AMR surveillance data so that the latest trends on AMR could be monitored. Under this initiative, a series of laboratories called the National AMR Surveillance Laboratory Network has been established. NARS-Net started the journey with eight medical college laboratories and has now been sequentially expanded to 40 laboratories (sentinel surveillance network sites) across 31 states/UT and the National Reference Laboratory (NRL) for bacterial pathogens at NCDC. The surveillance activities of NARS-Net involve the standardized collection, analysis, and compilation of AMR data from all network sites through open-source software, "WHO NET.[9]" WHONET is a free desktop Windows application developed and supported by the WHO Collaborating Centre for Surveillance of Antimicrobial Resistance. This application can be used to manage and analyze microbiology laboratory data with a particular focus on antimicrobial resistance surveillance. It has various modules in 44 languages, which aids in training and provides technical assistance.[9]

The participating sites report the AMR data pertaining to seven prioritized pathogens to NCDC. The data are submitted within 15 days of each quarter (data between 1st January to 31st March should be submitted by 15th April). The respective AMR nodal officer validates this quarterly data at the sites, which is submitted to network sites after validation. Each network site has to send a defined number of random isolates for identification, confirmation, and antimicrobial susceptibility at the NRL at the Centre for Bacterial Disease and Drug Resistance (CBDDR), NCDC. These samples are part of the External Quality Assessment Scheme (EQAS).

Then, a single file from all cumulative AMR data is prepared, and proper care is taken to avoid data duplication. The "Annual National Surveillance Report," is generated using this aggregated data which is available at the public domain through the NCDC platform and shared with different stakeholders.

NCDC is the nodal center for the global dissemination of this AMR report. Since 2018, this data has also been submitted to the World Health Organization's Global AMR Surveillance and Use System (WHO-GLASS).

Apart from reporting the AMR data, the sites are also mandated to share all emerging AMR alert isolates for confirmation to NRL at NCDC.[10]

Infection prevention and control
For the containment of AMR, an effective infection control policy was mandatory. "National Guidelines for Infection Prevention and Control in Healthcare Facilities" have been developed with WHO support and disseminated to various stakeholders. The ICMR guidelines on infection control suggest the need to develop Hospital Infection Control Committees at each level of health care. ICMR has launched the program on "Antimicrobial Stewardship, Prevention of Infection and Control (ASPIC). Under this, capacity building is being done nationwide for antibiotic stewardship.

Moreover, National Treatment Guidelines for antimicrobial use in infectious diseases have been released and uploaded on the NCDC website, which brings uniformity and judicious use of antibiotic use.[10]

Awareness generation and understanding of AMR
Several IEC materials have been developed and disseminated. Various activities are conducted across different educational institutes all year round; these include quizzes, competitions, lectures, radio talks, etc.

Under the WHO initiative, every year from November 18 to 24, it is celebrated as **World AMR Awareness Week (WAAW).** This is taken as an opportunity to advocate for the judicious use of antibiotics for AMR containment. Various activities, such as health talks, quiz competitions, symposiums, and workshops are organized. For creating community awareness folk plays, nukkads are organized by various medical colleges and NGOs. The major areas of concern that are dealt with in the awareness campaign are avoiding the over-the-counter and self-medication of antibiotics, the importance of proper prescription by doctors, and knowing about the harmful effects of antibiotic misuse.[11]

The plan assumes that increasing awareness must happen simultaneously on multiple fronts. The target populations are from the agriculture, animal health, and human health sectors. On the one hand, it must use public communication campaigns to encourage behavior change in these groups. On the other hand, coordinated efforts are required to make AMR a fundamental part of medical and veterinary professionals' professional education.

Raising awareness about requirement of containing AMR at the highest levels of policy-making is also necessary in order for it to become a national health policy priority.

Use of antimicrobials[12,13]
- There is a need for stringently framed and implemented regulatory mechanisms to limit the use of antimicrobials in humans, livestock, and food animals, especially for non-therapeutic use, such as growth promoters. These factors are the prime drivers of AMR.
- The FSSAI under MoHFW is the main authority for laying down evidence-based standards for food articles and regulating their manufacture, storage, distribution, sale, and import to ensure the availability of safe and wholesome food for human consumption.
- Seeing this, the government has made different provisions for growth promoters:
- The limits of food additives, containments, pesticide residues, heavy metals, mycotoxins, antibiotics, and pharmacological substances should be specified (sec 16 [2][b], FSSA, 2006).
- No food article should have the above-mentioned substances over the tolerance limits specified. (Section 21(1))
- Section 2.3.2 of the Food Safety and Standards (Contaminants, Toxins and Residues) Regulations, 2011 of FSSA, 2006 specifies the limits for antibiotics and other pharmacologically active substances in seafood including a variety of fishes and fish products, shrimps, prawns, etc.
- In 2015, different directives limiting the use of antibiotics in livestock rearing, dairy, and fisheries have been laid down.
- The National AMR Containment Policy also highlighted the need to establish a separate schedule H1 under the Drugs and Cosmetics Rules to regulate the sales of antibiotics. The national policy also outlined the proposal for color-coded tagging antibiotics and newer molecules (carbapenems, tigecycline, daptomycin, etc.) to eliminate their use outside of tertiary care settings.
- One important strategy for combating the excessive and inappropriate use of antibiotics in the clinical context is the implementation of antibiotic stewardship initiatives. The program is multidisciplinary and offers a range of interventions to enhance the appropriate use of antibiotics. Additionally, the system incorporates monitoring and evaluation to estimate the program's impact on improving antibiotic prescription practices in the short-term and lowering resistance levels in index bacteria in the long-term. Reducing the inappropriate use of antibiotics; optimizing drug class selection, dose, route, and duration of treatment to achieve the best possible outcomes for the patients; minimizing adverse effects on drug use and medical costs; and preventing or controlling the emergence of antibiotic resistance in index bacterial species are the main goals of an antibiotic stewardship program.

National Action Plan 2017-2021 (NAP-AMR)[14]

Goal:
To combat antimicrobial resistance in India, and contribute towards the global efforts to tackle this public health threat. It shall establish and strengthen governance mechanisms and the capacity of all stakeholders to reduce the impact of AMR in India. The scope of the NAPAMR focuses primarily on resistance in bacteria.

Objectives:
- Define the strategic priorities, key actions, outputs, responsibilities, and indicative timeline and budget to slow the emergence of AMR in India and strengthen the organizational and management structures to ensure intra- and inter-sectoral coordination with a One Health Approach.
- Combat AMR in India through better understanding and awareness of AMR, strengthened surveillance, prevention of emergence and spread of resistant bacteria through infection prevention and control, optimized use of antibiotics in all sectors, and enhanced investments for AMR activities, research and innovations.
- Enable monitoring and evaluation (M&E) of the NAP-AMR implementation based on the M&E framework.

Governance mechanism:
The MoHFW has outlined three governance mechanisms for effective AMR containment. These are—the Intersectoral Coordination Committee, Technical Advisory Group, and Core Working Group.
- **Intersectoral coordination committee:** Oversees and coordinates policy decisions on AMR containment and facilitates and coordinates the AMR response to antibiotic threat.
- **Technical coordination committee:** Provides technical support and formulates new initiatives to combat AMR.

Chapter 83: National Programme on Containment of Anti-Microbial Resistance (AMR)

	• **Core working group:** Provides technical and operational inputs to the National Centre for Disease Control (NCDC), identifies and maps different stakeholders, and ensures effective data procurement and surveillance activities. **Strategies/activities**. In NAP-AMR, six strategic priorities have been set up, of which five are in conjugation with the Global Action Plan on MAR (GAP-AMR), and the last one highlights India's role as a leader in AMR containment at the international level. 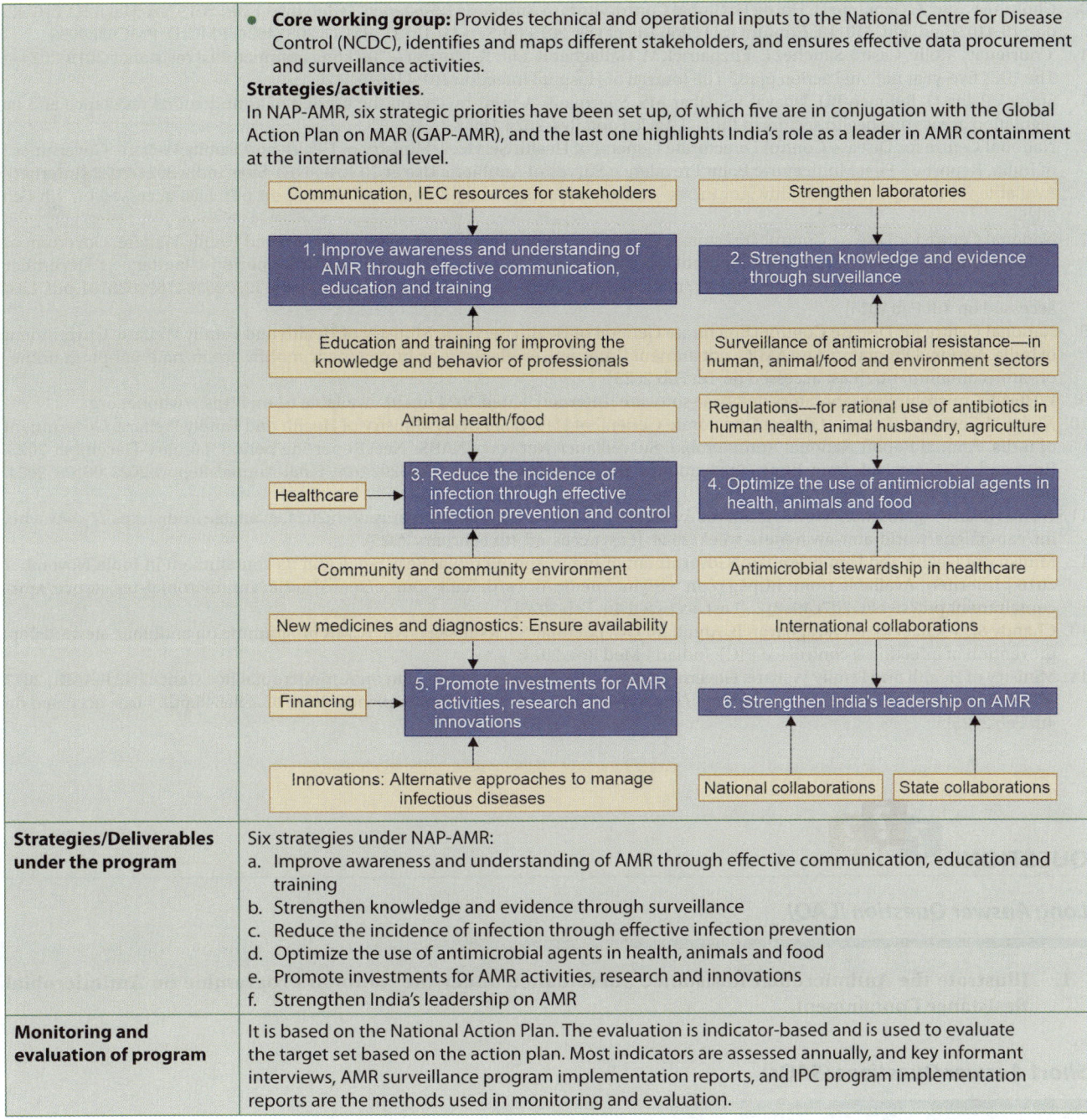
Strategies/Deliverables under the program	Six strategies under NAP-AMR: a. Improve awareness and understanding of AMR through effective communication, education and training b. Strengthen knowledge and evidence through surveillance c. Reduce the incidence of infection through effective infection prevention d. Optimize the use of antimicrobial agents in health, animals and food e. Promote investments for AMR activities, research and innovations f. Strengthen India's leadership on AMR
Monitoring and evaluation of program	It is based on the National Action Plan. The evaluation is indicator-based and is used to evaluate the target set based on the action plan. Most indicators are assessed annually, and key informant interviews, AMR surveillance program implementation reports, and IPC program implementation reports are the methods used in monitoring and evaluation.

References

1. World Health Organisation. Antimicrobial Resistance Fact Sheet. World Health Organisation;2023. Available from: https://www.who.int/news-room/fact-sheets/detail/antimicrobial-resistance [Last accessed 4th February 2025]
2. Fentie AM, Degefaw Y, Asfaw G, Shewarega W, Woldearegay M, Abebe E, et al. Multicentre point-prevalence survey of antibiotic use and healthcare-associated infections in Ethiopian hospitals. BMJ Open. 2022 Feb 11;12(2):e054541. doi: 10.1136/bmjopen-2021-054541. PMID: 35149567; PMCID: PMC8845215.

3. Chokshi A, Sifri Z, Cennimo D, Horng H. Global Contributors to Antibiotic Resistance. J Glob Infect Dis. 2019 Jan-Mar;11(1):36-42. doi: 10.4103/jgid.jgid_110_18. Erratum in: J Glob Infect Dis. 2019 Jul-Sep;11(3):131. PMID: 30814834; PMCID: PMC6380099.
4. Courtenay, Molly, Castro-Sánchez E, Fitzpatrick M, Gallagher R, Lim R, Morris G. "Tackling antimicrobial resistance 2019-2024—The UK's five-year national action plan." The Journal of Hospital Infection 101 4 (2019):426-7.
5. Singh VP, Jha D, Rehman BU, Dhayal VS, Dhar MS, Sharma N. A mini-review on the burden of antimicrobial resistance and its regulation across one health sectors in India. J Agric Food Res. 2024 Mar 1;15:100973.
6. National Centre for Disease Control Directorate General of Health Services, Ministry of Health and Family Welfare, Government of India. Report on First Multicentric Point Prevalence Survey of Antibiotic Use at 20 NAC-NET Sites India 2021-2022.[Internet]. Available from: https://ncdc.mohfw.gov.in/wp-content/uploads/2024/03/FinalNACNETReport.pdf. Last accessed on 4th Feb 2025]
7. National Centre for Disease Control Directorate General of Health Services, Ministry of Health and Family Welfare, Government of India.Annual Report National Antimicrobial Surveillance Network(NARS- Net) Reporting period 1 January-31 December 2022.[Internet].2023. Available from: https://ncdc.mohfw.gov.in/wp-content/uploads/2024/03/1257263841692628161.pdf. Last accessed on 4th Feb 2025]
8. National Centre for Disease Control Directorate General of Health Services, Ministry of Health and Family Welfare, Government of India. National Programme on AMR Containment.[Internet]. Available from: https://ncdc.mohfw.gov.in/national-programme-on-amr-containment/. [Last accessed on 4th Feb 2025]
9. WHONET microbiology laboratory database software [Internet]. [cited 2024 Jun 9]. Available from: https://whonet.org/
10. National Centre for Disease Control Directorate General of Health Services, Ministry of Health and Family Welfare, Government of India. Annual Report National Antimicrobial Surveillance Network (NARS- Net) Reporting period January-December 2023. [Internet].2024. Available from: https://ncdc.mohfw.gov.in/wp-content/uploads/2024/09/Final-Annual-Report-2023-06_08_2024.pdf. [Last accessed 4th Feb 2025]
11. World Health Organisation. World Antibiotic Awareness Week. World Health Organisation;2024. Available from: https://www.who.int/campaigns/world-amr-awareness-week/2024. [Last accessed 4th February 2025].
12. Ministry of Health and Family Welfare, Government of India. Antimicrobial Resistance and its containment in India November 2016.[Internet]. Available from: https://cdn.who.int/media/docs/default-source/searo/india/antimicrobial-resistance/amr-containment.pdf?sfvrsn=2d7c49a2_2. [Last accessed 4th Feb 2025]
13. Chandy SJ, Michael JS, Veeraraghavan B, Abraham OC, Bachhav SS, Kshirsagar NA. ICMR programme on antibiotic stewardship, prevention of infection & control (ASPIC). Indian J Med Res. 2014;
14. Ministry of Health and Family Welfare, Government of India. National Action Plan on Antimicrobial Resistance (NAP-AMR) 2017 – 2021.[Internet],2017. Available from: https://ncdc.mohfw.gov.in/wp-content/uploads/2024/03/File645.pdf. [Last accessed on 4th Feb 2025]

QUESTIONS

Long Answer Question (LAQ)

1. **Illustrate the Antimicrobial Resistance Surveillance under the National Programme on Antimicrobial Resistance Containment.**

Short Answer Questions (SAQs)

1. **Briefly describe WHO-NET.**
2. **Mention salient features of World AMR Week (WAAW).**

Multiple Choice Questions (MCQs)

1. What is "WHONET"?
    a. An open source software for management and analysis of AMR data
    b. A test to detect AMR at an early stage
    c. A centre of excellence established by WHO to monitor AMR
    d. A Network of WHO laboratories for AMR testing
2. Which is the nodal center for the implementation of AMR Programme in India?
    a. NHSRC—New Delhi
    b. NIE—Chennai
    c. NIV—Pune
    d. NCDC—New Delhi
3. The participating sites report the AMR data for how many prioritized pathogens to NCDC?
    a. Five
    b. Seven
    c. Nine
    d. Eleven
4. What is WHO-GLASS?
    a. A new technology to detect wide variety of anti-microbial resistance
    b. Global linezolid and other anti-microbial surveillance system by WHO
    c. Global antimicrobial resistance and use surveillance system by WHO
    d. Advanced microscope system invented with support of WHO
5. As per ICMR guidelines, where should the Hospital Infection Control Committee be formed?
    a. At each level of health care
    b. At all district level hospitals
    c. At all district level and super-specialty hospitals
    d. At all PHC and CHCs
6. Under the WHO initiative, when is World AMR Awareness Week (WAAW) celebrated?
    a. Every year from January 18 to 24
    b. Every year from April 18 to 24
    c. Every year from September 18 to 24
    d. Every year from November 18 to 24
7. Which of the following is/are major areas of concern to be dealt with in awareness campaign of World AMR Awareness Week (WAAW)?
    a. Avoiding the over-the-counter and self-medication of antibiotics
    b. The importance of proper prescription by doctors
    c. Knowing about the harmful effects of antibiotic misuse
    d. All of the above
8. All the following are among the six strategic priorities set up under NAP-AMR, *except:*
    a. Strengthen knowledge and evidence through surveillance
    b. Strengthen WHO's leadership on AMR
    c. Reduce the incidence of infection through effective infection prevention
    d. Optimize the use of antimicrobial agents in health, animals and food

Answers

1. a
2. d
3. d
4. c
5. a
6. d
7. d
8. b

CHAPTER 84

Social Security Schemes for Unorganized and Organized Sectors

Mohammad Waseem Faraz Ansari, Rudresh Negi, Praveena P

Background	India, being a socialist republic strives to provide its citizens, especially those employed with a "safety net" in the form of social security. These working men and women can be broadly categorized into the organized and unorganized sectors. The discussion will first focus on the organized sector where there are laws, such as The Employees' Provident Funds and Miscellaneous Provisions Act, the Employees' State Insurance Act, the Employee's Compensation Act the Industrial Disputes Act, the Maternity Benefit Act, and the Payment of Gratuity Act, 1972 (39 of 1972).
Need of program	**The Employees' Provident Funds and Miscellaneous Provisions Act** Social security is a needed bedrock of safety net especially required in the twilight years of life. In India the essence of social security laws originate from the Directive Principles of State Policy. Earlier due to prevalent local economy in India, social security was mostly provided by family and community. However, this changed dramatically with globalization, industrialization and liberalization. Thus, a need was felt to have solid social security measures in organized sector leading to passage of Employees' Provident Funds Ordinance on the 15th November, 1951 and finally the Employees' Provident Funds and Miscellaneous Provisions Act, 1952.[1,2]
Implemented since	1952
Goal	An innovation driven social security organization aiming to extend universal coverage and ensuring Nirbadh (Seamless and uninterrupted) service delivery to its stakeholders through state-of-the-art technology[2]
Targets	Financial security and social security for retirees, investment growth, financial awareness, long-term savings are key targets of the scheme
Objectives	• To meet the evolving needs of comprehensive social security in a transparent, contactless, faceless and paperless manner. • To ensure Nirbadh services with multilocational and auto claim settlement process for disaster proofing EPFO. • To ensure ease of living for members and pensioners, and ease of doing business for employers by leveraging Government of India's technology platforms for reaching out to millions[2]

Organogram

The Employees' Provident Fund Organization (EPFO) comes under the Ministry of Labour and Employment. It is responsible for the implementation, supervision and monitoring of this entire scheme.[2]

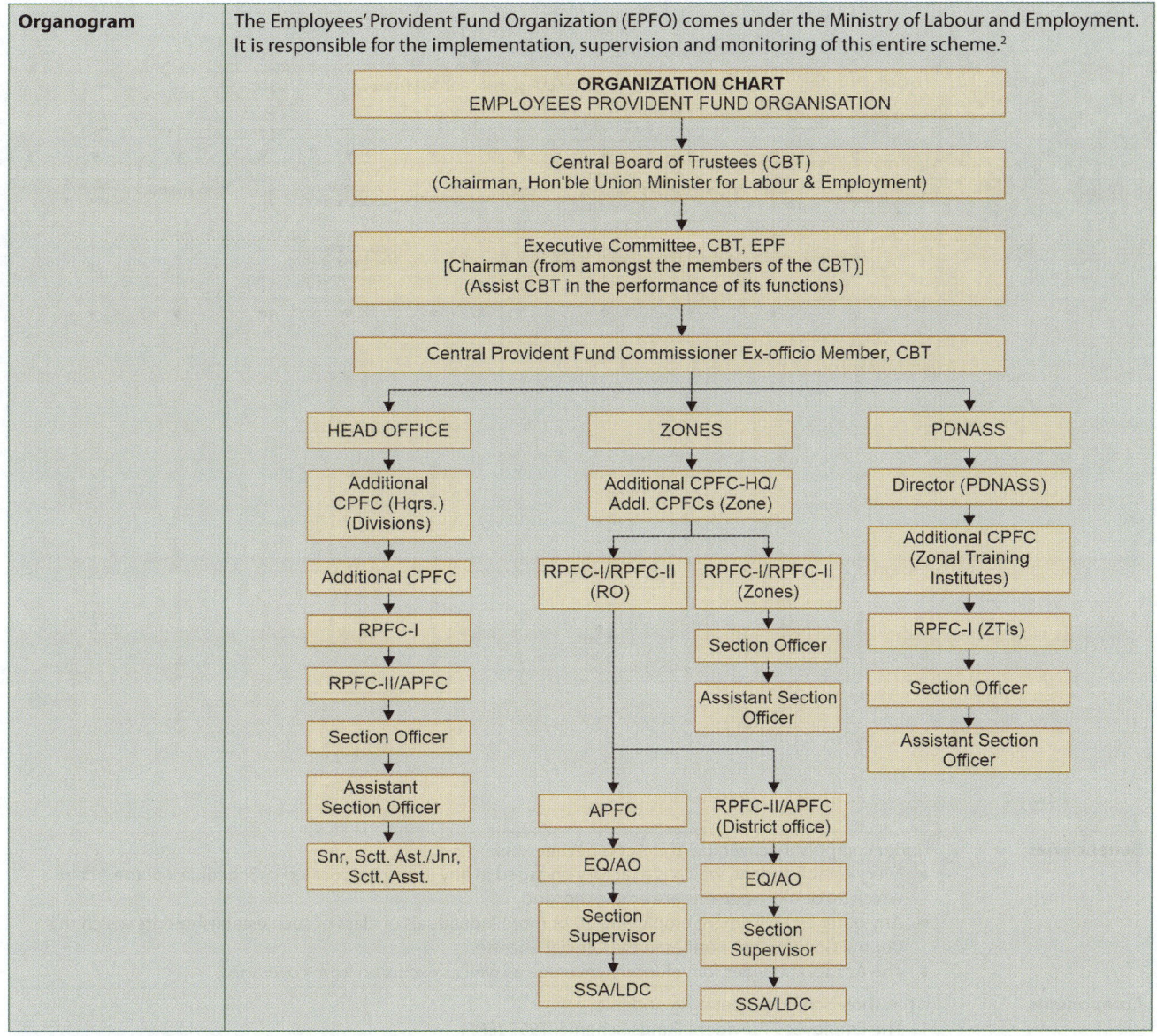

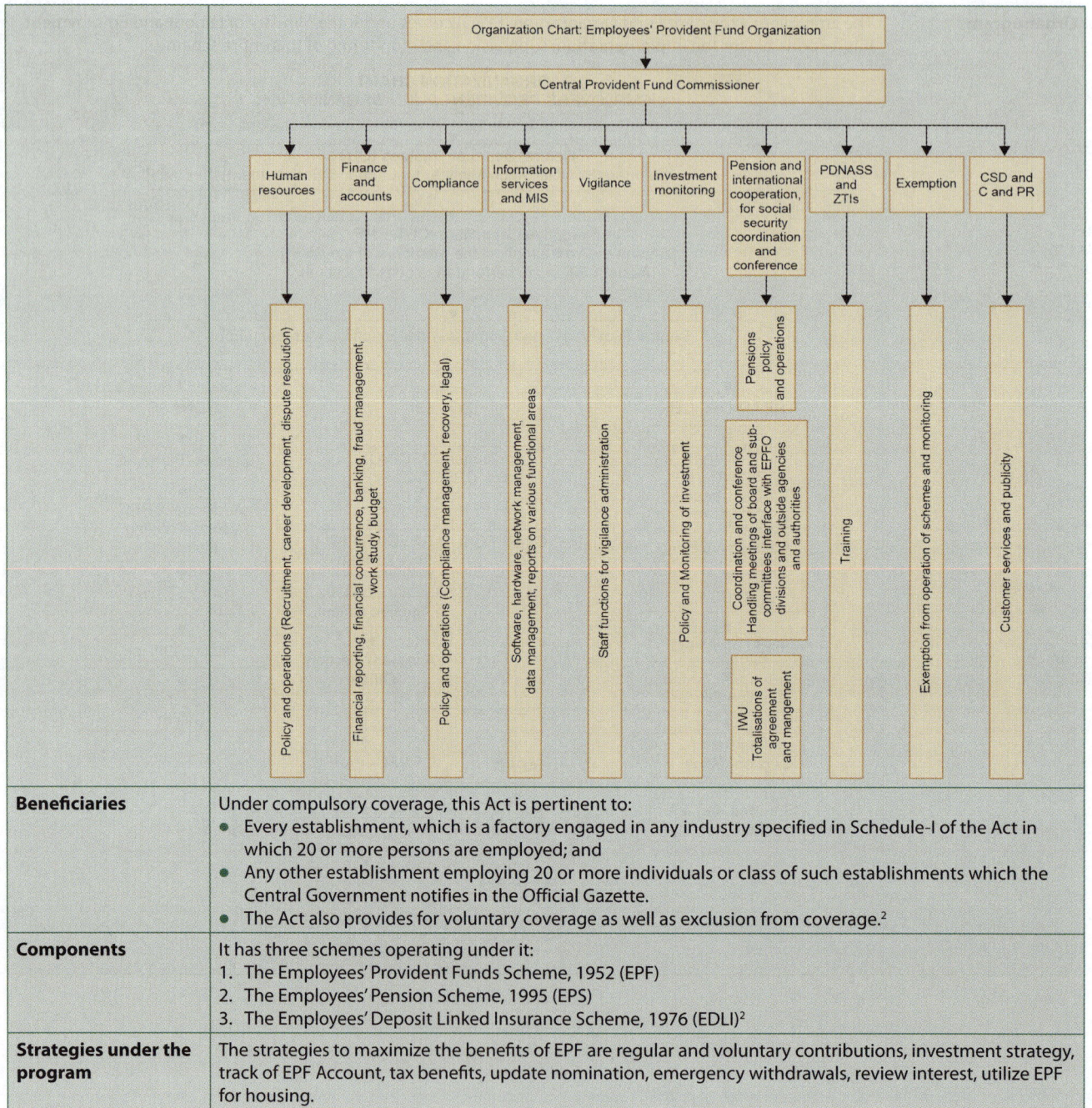

Beneficiaries	Under compulsory coverage, this Act is pertinent to: • Every establishment, which is a factory engaged in any industry specified in Schedule-I of the Act in which 20 or more persons are employed; and • Any other establishment employing 20 or more individuals or class of such establishments which the Central Government notifies in the Official Gazette. • The Act also provides for voluntary coverage as well as exclusion from coverage.[2]
Components	It has three schemes operating under it: 1. The Employees' Provident Funds Scheme, 1952 (EPF) 2. The Employees' Pension Scheme, 1995 (EPS) 3. The Employees' Deposit Linked Insurance Scheme, 1976 (EDLI)[2]
Strategies under the program	The strategies to maximize the benefits of EPF are regular and voluntary contributions, investment strategy, track of EPF Account, tax benefits, update nomination, emergency withdrawals, review interest, utilize EPF for housing.

Activities at various level	• The Employees' Provident Funds Scheme, 1952 (EPF)
	  ✦ Objective—to give after-retirement benefit for the employees or a group of employees or their legal heirs.
	  ✦ Coverage—establishments/factories with 20 people or more.
	  ✦ Membership—employees with monthly salary less than or equal to ₹15,000
	  ✦ Contribution—employee contribution 12% of salary and employer contribution 3.67%
	  ✦ Benefits:
	    – Accumulation of amount with interest on retiring or death to be paid as final settlement.
	    – Partial withdrawals are permitted for certain conditions, such as education, marriage, illness, natural calamities, unemployment, house construction, etc.
	    – Housing scheme for EPFO members
	• The Employees' Pension Scheme, 1995 (EPS)[2]
	  ✦ Based on the principle of "Defined Contribution-Defined Benefit" and based on actuarial principles for future financial viability.
	  ✦ Membership—limited to person with monthly salary of ₹15,000. At least 10 years of service. Age 58/50 years.
	  ✦ Contribution—employer contribution 8.33% of salary and central government contribution 1.16%
	  ✦ Benefits:
	    – Pension after retirement
	    – Disability pension due to total and permanent damage in service
	    – Children pension for 2 children till 25 years on death of member
	    – Orphan pension for 2 orphans till 25 years on death of member and no spouse
	    – Nominee pension
	    – Pension to dependent father/mother.[2]
	• The Employees' Deposit Linked Insurance Scheme, 1976 (EDLI)
	  ✦ Coverage-all factories/establishments under EPF Act 1952
	  ✦ Membership—all members of EPF
	  ✦ Benefits:
	    – Premature death of a member during service, an insurance of up to ₹7 lakhs is provided
	    – No premium is charged[2]

Activities at various level	• **Primary prevention:** Preventing financial instability and ensuring long-term savings through regular contributions, financial planning, education and awareness • **Secondary prevention:** Monitoring and tracking—regular reviewing of EPF account statements, advisory services that help the employees adjust their contributions or investments in response to changing financial situations • **Tertiary prevention:** Retirement planning, debt management, income replacement (Ensuring that EPF funds are used effectively to replace income in retirement and during financial difficulties).
Monitoring and evaluation of program	• **Reporting and documentation:** Through records and regular reports on the scheme's performance, contributions, and compliance. This is crucial for transparency and accountability. Regular communication helps ensure that employees are aware of their benefits and any potential issues • Conduct periodic internal or external audits to assess the accuracy and effectiveness of the EPF scheme's management. • Use audit findings to make improvements and address any discrepancies. • **Feedback and grievance redressal mechanism:** Implement a system for employees to provide feedback or raise concerns about the EPF scheme. • **Compliance check:** Verifying that contributions are made on time and in the correct amounts, and that records are accurately maintained. • Monitor contributions made by both the employer and employee. • **Fund performance:** Regularly review of performance • Analyze returns on investment and compare them with benchmarks or industry standards. • Monitor employees contributions and withdrawals • Online dashboard of key achievements[2,3]

EMPLOYEES STATE INSURANCE ACT (ESI ACT)

Need of program	Post-independence was a time when industry in India was in an embryonic stage and the country depended heavily on imports. However, a substantial number of manpower was engaged in industries, such as chemicals, jute and textiles. Being a socialist state, to develop a multi-pronged, comprehensive approach to reduce the health-related inequities, improve economic stability and ensure work place safety among the growing manpower working in industries the ESI Act 1948 was passed in the parliament. Thus, this was the first social security scheme in India.[4]
Implemented since	This ESI scheme was inaugurated by the Prime Minister of the country Pandit Jawaharlal Nehru on 24th February 1952 in Kanpur (hence forth celebrated as ESIC Day) in Kanpur. The first director of ESIC was Dr CL Katial. The ESI Act was implemented since 1948.[4]
Goal	The goal of the Employees' State Insurance (ESI) Act is to provide social security and health insurance benefits to employees.
Targets	It targets to protect labor rights and promote safe secure working environment for all workers
Objectives	To uphold human dignity in times of crises through protection from deprivation, destitution and social degradation while enabling the society the retention and continuity of a socially useful and productive manpower.
Organogram	Chairman, ESIC—Hon'ble Minister for Labour and Employment (I/c), Government of Indian Vice Chairman, ESIC—Secretary to the Government of India, Ministry of Labour and Employment Members of ESI Corporation[4]

Director General, ESIC
- FC → Addl. Comm. → Director/JD → DD/AD
- CVO → Addl. Comm. → Director/JD → DD/AD → Zonal vigilance (05) → Director → DD/AD
- IC (Rev. and Bft.) → Addl. Comm. → JD/DD/AD → Medical vigilance → Dy. Med Comm./Director → DD/AD
- IC (P and A) → Director → DD/AD
- IC (ICT) → Addl. Comm → Director → DD/AD
- IC (NTA) → Addl. Comm → Director (Admn./Medical) → DD/AD
- IC (Rectt.) → DD/AD → Chief Engineer → Zonal Supdt. Engg. (04) → Ex. Engg./Asstt. Eng./Jr. Engg.
- MC (MA) → DMC → JD/DD/AD
- MC (Ayush) → DMC → JD/DD/AD
- MC (ME) → DMC → JD/DD/AD
- JD/DD/AD

Regional office
- Addl. Commissioner/Director → JD/DD/AD
- Sub-Regional Office → Director/JD (Incharge) → DD/AD
- Branch office → Branch manager
- Dispensary cum branch office (DCBO) → IMO/AD

Beneficiaries	All establishments and factories that employ more than 10 employees and pay wages below or up to ₹21,000 per month and ₹25,000 per month for employees with disability Employees contribute 0.75% of the earning, while, the employers contribute 3.25% of the wages. Employees with wages up to ₹176/- a day are excused from payment[4]
Components	Coverage, contributions, administrative structure, appeals and redressal are the components of ESI Act. The major component is medical care, provided to insured person and his family members. There is no cap on treatment expenditure of an insured person or his family member. It is also provided to retired and permanently disabled insured persons and their spouses on payment of an annual premium of ₹120.
Deliverables under the program	• Sickness benefit is given as cash compensation at the rate of 70% of wages and is payable to insured workers during the periods of certified sickness for a maximum of 91 days in a year. In order to qualify for sickness benefit he/she is required to contribute for at least 78 days in a contribution period of six months. • Extended sickness benefit for two years in the case of designated 34 malignant and long-term diseases at a rate of 80% of wages. • Enhanced sickness benefit in the form of full wage is provided to insured persons undergoing sterilization for up to seven days and 14 days for vasectomy and tubectomy respectively. • Maternity benefit for confinement and pregnancy is paid for 26 weeks, which can be increased by one more month on medical advice at full wage subject to contribution for 70 days in the preceding Two contribution periods. • Temporary disablement benefit from day one is ensured irrespective of contribution status in case of employment injury. Temporary disablement benefit is given at the rate of 90% of wage till disability continues. • Permanent disablement benefit is paid at the rate of 90% of wage as monthly payment depending upon the extent of loss of earning capacity as approved by a medical board. • Dependent benefit—90% of salary as monthly payment to the dependents of a deceased, where death occured due to employment injury or occupational hazards. • Funeral expenses of ₹15,000 is payable from the first day of entering insurable employment. • Confinement expenses—benefits are given to an insured women or an IP in respect of his wife in case confinement happens at a place where needed medical facilities under ESI Scheme are not available. • Vocational rehabilitation and physical rehabilitation is also provided.[4]
Activities at various level	• **Primary prevention:** Implementation of safety standards and health regulations at workplace. • Ergonomic improvements, prevention of risk factors and promote lifestyle, regular health check-ups and immunization services, provision of health awareness programs through ESI hospitals. • **Secondary prevention:** Early diagnosis and treatment through annual health screening, early intervention programs to address emerging health conditions, timely medical consultations and emergency care through ESI hospitals and prompt usage of advanced technologies. • **Tertiary prevention:** Rehabilitation programs for employees recovering from injuries and illness disability limitation through physiotherapy and reconstructive surgeries, supportive services (counseling), vocational training.
Monitoring and evaluation of program	Administrative oversight for overseeing the administration and functioning of the ESI scheme. Periodic audits are conducted to assess the financial and operational aspects of the scheme. Maintaining and analyzing data related to contributions, claims, and benefits. Advanced data management systems help in tracking the status and effectiveness of the scheme. Regular reporting and feedback mechanism from beneficiaries and stake holders periodic monitoring through Hospital Development Committees and State Executive Committee. Online ESIC dashboard is available.[4,5]

SOCIAL SECURITY AND HEALTH SCHEMES IN UNORGANIZED SECTOR

The term 'unorganized worker' has been defined under the Unorganized Workers' Social Security Act, 2008 as 'a home based-worker, self- employed worker or a wage worker in the unorganized sector and includes a worker in the organized sector who is not covered by any of the Acts mentioned in scheduled II of Act, i.e., the Employee's Compensation Act, 1923 (3 of 1923), the Industrial Disputes Act, 1947 (14 of 1947), the Employees' State Insurance Act, 1948 (34 of 1948), the Employees Provident Funds and Miscellaneous Provision Act, 1952 (19 of 1952), the Maternity Benefit Act, 1961 (53 of 1961) and the Payment of Gratuity Act, 1972 (39 of 1972).[11] There are numerous schemes by the government for providing social security and health coverage umbrella to this group. Some of the prominent ones with brief description are as follows:

PRADHAN MANTRI SHRAM YOGI MAANDHAN (PM-SYM)[7,8]

Need for the scheme	It is a scheme for old age protection and social security.
Eligibility	Unorganized worker, age 18–40 years and monthly income till ₹15,000
Deliverables under the scheme	Pension of ₹3,000/month Voluntary and contributory scheme Contribution matched by the government

AAM AADMI BIMA YOJANA[6]

Need for the scheme	Implemented through LIC to provide death and disability cover for 48 identified vocational groups
Eligibility	Age 18–59, below poverty line
Deliverables under the scheme	Provides an insurance coverage of ₹30,000 for natural death, ₹75,000 death in accident, ₹37,500 for partial permanent disability due to accident and ₹75,000 for total permanent disability due to accident

PRADHAN MANTRI JEEVAN JYOTI BIMA YOJANA (PMJJBY)[8,9]

Need for the scheme	It is a 1-year life insurance scheme which can be reviewed every year at annual premium of ₹436 up to age of 55 years
Eligibility	Age 18–50 years and holding bank account
Deliverables under the scheme	Coverage of ₹2 lakhs in case of death due to any reason

PRADHAN MANTRI SURAKSHA BIMA YOJANA (PMSBY)[10]

Need for the scheme	It is a personal accident insurance scheme, renewable yearly with premium of ₹20
Eligibility	Age 18–70 years with bank account or post office account.
Deliverables under the scheme	Risk coverage of ₹2 lakhs for accidental death or total permanent disability and ₹1 lakh for partial permanent disability due to accident

AYUSHMAN BHARAT PRADHAN MANTRI JAN AROGYA YOJANA (AB-PMJAY)[8]

Need for the scheme	To provide secondary and tertiary hospitalization under universal health coverage
Eligibility	Families identified from Social Economic Caste Census (SECC) of 2011 based on six deprivation and 11 occupational criterias across rural and urban areas
Deliverables under the scheme	₹5 lakhs/family/year for secondary and tertiary care hospitalization corresponding to 1949 treatment procedures across 27 specialties

Other schemes and programs: Public Distribution System through One Nation One Ration Card scheme, Mahatma Gandhi National Rural Employment Guarantee Act, Deen Dayal Upadhyay Gramin Kausal Yojana, Pradhan Mantri Awas Yojana, Pradhan Mantri Gareeb Kalyan Rojgar Yojana, Mahatma Gandhi Bunkar Bima Yojana, Deen Dayal Antyodaya Yojana, PMSVA Nidhi, Pradhan Mantri Kaushal Vikas Yojana, etc., are also available.[8]

References

1. Employees' Provident Fund Organisation [Internet]. [cited 2024 Aug 12]. Available from: https://www.epfindia.gov.in/site_en/index.php

Chapter 84: Social Security Schemes for Unorganized and Organized Sectors

2. Annual_Report_2022-23.pdf [Internet]. [cited 2024 Aug 12]. Available from: https://www.epfindia.gov.in/site_docs/Annual_Report/Annual_Report_2022-23.pdf
3. EPFO|Chart Dashboard [Internet]. [cited 2024 Aug 12]. Available from: https://mis.epfindia.gov.in/ChartDashboard/
4. Employees' State Insurance Corporation, Ministry of Labour and Employment, Government of India [Internet]. [cited 2024 Aug 11]. Available from: https://www.esic.gov.in/
5. ESIC-Dashboard [Internet]. [cited 2024 Aug 11]. Available from: https://www.esic.in/Dashboard/Default.aspx
6. Aam Aadmi Bima Yojana | Labour Welfare | Government of Assam, India [Internet]. [cited 2024 Aug 11]. Available from: https://labour.assam.gov.in/scheme-page/aam-aadmi-bima-yojana
7. Maandhan [Internet]. [cited 2024 Aug 11]. Available from: https://maandhan.in/
8. New measures to protect interests of unorganised labour [Internet]. [cited 2024 Aug 11]. Available from: https://pib.gov.in/pib.gov.in/Pressreleaseshare.aspx?PRID=1986238
9. Pradhan Mantri Jeevan Jyoti Bima Yojana [Internet]. [cited 2024 Aug 11]. Available from: https://transformingindia.mygov.in/scheme/pradhan-mantri-jeevan-jyoti-bima-yojana/?share=81045
10. Pradhan Mantri Suraksha Bima Yojana (PMSBY) | Department of Financial Services | Ministry of Finance |Government of India [Internet]. [cited 2024 Aug 11]. Available from: https://www.financialservices.gov.in/beta/en/pmsby
11. Unorganized Worker Ministry of Labour and Employment| Government of India [Internet]. [cited 2024 Aug 11]. Available from: https://labour.gov.in/unorganized-workers

QUESTIONS

Long Answer Questions (LAQs)

1. Mention three schemes under Employees' Provident Funds and Miscellaneous Provisions Act. Describe any two.
2. Describe in detail the benefits ensured through ESI scheme. What other benefits could be supplemented?
3. Enumerate any six social security schemes for unorganized sector. Describe any two of them.

Short Answer Questions (SAQs)

1. Write a short note on monitoring and evaluation of EPS.
2. Critically analyze the "The Employees' Pension Scheme, 1995 (EPS)".
3. Mention the goal, target and objectives of workmen's compensation act.
4. How will you monitor the ESI scheme?
5. Justify the need of social security schemes for unorganized sector.
6. Compare and contrast Pradhan Mantri Shram Yogi Maandhan (PM-SYM) and Aam Aadmi Bima Yojana.

Multiple Choice Questions (MCQs)

1. The Employees' Provident Funds and Miscellaneous Provisions Act was passed in:
   a. 1948
   b. 1952
   c. 1965
   d. 1968
2. For Employees' Provident Funds Scheme employee contribution is:
   a. 5%
   b. 10%
   c. 12%
   d. 14%

3. **Employees contribution to ESI scheme is:**
   a. 0.75%
   b. 1.25%
   c. 3.25%
   d. 4.25%
4. **The chairman of ESIC is**
   a. Prime Minister
   b. President
   c. Minister for Labour and Employment
   d. Chief Secretary of Labour and Employment Department
5. **Pension under Pradhan Mantri Shram Yogi Maandhan (PM-SYM) is:**
   a. ₹10000/month
   b. ₹5000/month
   c. ₹3000/month
   d. ₹1000/month
6. **Per year per family coverage under Ayushmann Bharat is:**
   a. ₹1 lakh
   b. ₹3 lakh
   c. ₹4 lakh
   d. ₹5 lakh

Answers

1. b
2. c
3. a
4. c
5. c
6. d

CHAPTER 85

Schemes for Intellectual Disability

Lakshay Beri, Shaili Vyas, Akash Krishali, Padmaja Kanchi

Background/Need of the program/Scheme	There are 5,95,231 children in the 0–19 age range who have intellectual impairments, according to the 2011 Census. In the developing world, just 2% of disabled children receive any kind of schooling or therapy. In both developed and developing nations, the likelihood of unemployment and actual poverty is higher for working-age disabled individuals.[1]
Execution	The Rights of the Persons with Disabilities (RPwD) Act, 2016 was passed by the Central Government and went into effect on April 19, 2017.[1]
Objective	The Act gives people with disabilities rights and benefits to support their education, skill development, social security, health, rehabilitation, and leisure activities (PwD). The statute also guarantees seats in government-run or government-aided postsecondary educational institutions and government employment to those with qualifying impairments, including those with intellectual disability.

Different plans	• The following significant programs are carried out by the Department of Empowerment of Persons with Disabilities (DEPwD) for the welfare of PwD, especially children with intellectual disabilities:
	   ✦ Disabled Rehabilitation Scheme of Deendayal (DDRS)
	   ✦ Assistance with the Purchase and Fitting of Aids and Apparel Scheme for Disabled Persons (ADIP).
	   ✦ The Persons with Disabilities National Action Plan for Skill Development (PwD).
	   ✦ Educational Awards for Students with Disabilities.
	• Integrated Education for the Disabled Children Scheme: This federally funded program was first introduced by the Department of Social Welfare in 1974 and was then moved to the Department of Education in 1982.[2]

Strategies and deliverables under the schemes	**The Deendayal Disabled Rehabilitation Scheme (DDRS):** In order to help Persons with Disabilities (PwD), including children with intellectual disabilities, achieve and maintain their optimal levels of physical, sensory, intellectual, psychiatric, and sociofunctional functioning, Program Implementing Agencies (PIA) receive funding in the form of Grant-in Aid for their projects.[2] It is executed via the online e-Anudaan system. The program was updated on April 1st, 2018, and its cost standards were increased by 2.5 times to account for the expenses of rehabilitative therapies, assistive technology, instruction, and housing and lodging in special schools. Various model projects under DDRS: • Preschool, early intervention, and training are among the several DDRS model initiatives. • Children with intellectual, visual, speech, and hearing problems attend special schools. • Children with Cerebral Palsy Project. • The Rehabilitation Project for Leprosy Cure Patients. • Home-based Rehabilitation Program. • Community-based Rehabilitation Project. • The Low Vision Center Project. • Human Resource Development Project.

Assistance with the purchase and fitting of aids and apparel scheme for disabled persons (ADIP): Financial support is given to implementing agencies under this scheme in order to help eligible Divyangjan, including children with intellectual disabilities, acquire sophisticated, long-lasting, and modern, standard aids and appliances that reduce the effects of their disabilities and promote their physical, social, and psychological rehabilitation while also maximizing their economic potential. Between 2014 and 2021, the ADIP Scheme underwent modifications aimed at expanding its coverage and scope.[2]

The following are the key components of the updated ADIP Scheme, which is implemented from April 1, 2022.

- The price of assistive technology and assistance increased from ₹ 10,000 to ₹ 15,000.
- Raising the income ceiling to ₹ 22,500 per month for a 100% concession and ₹ 30,000 per month for a 50% concession from ₹ 15,000 per month to ₹ 22,500 per month respectively.
- High-end gadgets, such as digital hearing aids, artificial limbs, smart phones, smart canes, Daisy Players, Teaching Learning Material (TLM) kits, ADL kits for leprosy patients, etc., are available.
- A subsidy of ₹ 50,000 is available for Divyangjans with at least 80% impairment once every five years for motorized wheelchairs and tricycles.
- A high-end prosthesis with a maximum budget of ₹ 30,000 is available for individuals with disabilities of 80% or more.

For under five children with hearing disabilities, the cochlear implant program was created:
The following is the national action plan for the persons with disabilities (PwD) skill development:

- In March 2015, a Central Sector Scheme was introduced.
- As part of this program, individuals receive skill development through a network of government and non-government organizations that have been accredited as training partners. **Scholarships for Students with Disabilities:**

Prior to 2014: Only one scheme—National Fellowship for Persons with Disabilities.

New plans subsequent to 2014:[3]
- Pre-matriculation (for classes IX and X Only). The average scholarship award is ₹ 8,500 annually.
- Post-matriculation (from class XI to postgraduate diploma or degree). The average scholarship award is ₹ 35,000 year.
- First-rate instruction (for graduate or postgraduate degrees or diplomas in recognized centers of educational excellence). The average annual scholarship value is ₹ 1.75 lakh.
- National Overseas Scholarships (for Doctorates and Master's Degrees in foreign universities). The average annual scholarship amount is ₹ 20.00 lakh.
- National fellowship for persons with disabilities.
    + Complimentary coaching (for taking competitive exams to apply for government positions and to get into professional and technical courses). The average scholarship award is ₹ 85,000 year.
    + To expedite the implementation process, all six scholarship programs have now been combined into a single program called "Scholarships for Students with Disabilities."
    + The National Scholarship Portal is used to administer the pre-matric, post-matric, and top-class scholarship programs.
    + All scholarship programs release grants to recipients via Direct Benefit Transfer (DBT).

Additional changes made to the scholarship program as of April 1, 2018

Pre-matriculation
- The annual maintenance allowance rate was raised to ₹ 2,400.
- The annual ceiling on parental income was raised from ₹ 2.00 lakh to ₹ 2.50 lakh.
- Disability benefits vary based on the type of disability and might range from ₹ 2000 to ₹ 4000 annually.

After matriculation
- The annual maintenance allowance rate has been raised to ₹ 8,400.
- Disability benefits vary based on the type of disability and might range from ₹ 2000 to ₹ 4000 annually.

Top class
- Includes graduate-level coursework.
- There are now 300 spaces instead of 160.

Chapter 85: Schemes for Intellectual Disability   457

	Overseas scholarship • Applications are accepted all year long. • In light of the challenges faced by SwDs, the amount of the solvency certificate was reduced to ₹ 50,000. • DBT Mode is used to release scholarships: At a cost of ₹ 556.37 crore, scholarships for 1.84 lakh students with disabilities have been awarded during the past eight years.
	The Integrated Education Scheme for Children with Disabilities: The Integrated Education Scheme for Children with Disabilities: Covered are the following categories of impaired children: • Locomotor handicapped • Moderate-to-mild hearing loss. • Partially sighted children. • Groups of educable mentally disabled people (IQ 50–70) • Children with several disabilities. • Children with learning handicaps. Allowances given: • Stationery and books: ₹ 400 annually. • Monthly uniform cost: ₹ 50; • Monthly transportation cost: ₹ 50; • Monthly reader allowance: ₹ 50 in the case of blind students above class V. • Escort allowance: ₹ 75 per month (for children with lower extremity abnormalities who are seriously handicapped). • Children receive: Hostels with special amenities as well as remuneration for boarding and accommodation.
Monitoring and evaluation of program	The **Ministry of Social Justice and Empowerment** is in charge of all the aforementioned programs.

References

1. Schemes for intellectually disabled. Ministry of social justice and empowerment. GOI.[online]
2. Scheme of assistance to disabled persons for purchase/fitting of AIDS /appliances (ADIP scheme). Ministry of social justice and empowerment, GOI. [online]
3. Major achievement and initiative since 2014 . Department of empowerment of persons with disabilities. Ministry of Social justice and empowerment. GOI [online]

QUESTIONS

Long Answer Question (LAQ)

1. Describe in detail updates in various intellectual disability schemes.

Short Answer Questions (SAQs)

1. Mention the salient features of Deendayal Disabled Rehabilitation Scheme.
2. Enumerate various intellectual disability schemes.

Multiple Choice Questions (MCQs)

1. What is the percentage of disabled children in the developing world, who receive any education or rehabilitation?
    a. 2%
    b. 10%
    c. 17%
    d. 23%
2. Which of the following ministry monitors the schemes for PwD?
    a. Ministry of Social Justice and Empowerment.
    b. Ministry of Health and Family Welfare Ministry of Social Justice and Empowerment.
    c. Ministry of Education
    d. Ministry of Women and Child Development
3. The Rights of the Persons with Disabilities (RPwD) Act, 2016 which came into force on:
    a. 2016
    b. 2017
    c. 2018
    d. 2019
4. Which department carries out significant programs for the welfare of PwD, especially children with intellectual disabilities?
    a. Ministry of Social Justice and Empowerment.
    b. Department of Empowerment of Persons with Disabilities (DEPwD)
    c. Ministry of Education
    d. Ministry of Women and Child Development
5. Which scheme was applicable for Students with Disabilities Prior to 2014?
    a. National Overseas Scholarships
    b. Pre-matric and post-matric scholarships
    c. Top-class scholarship programs
    d. National fellowship for persons with disabilities
6. The Integrated Education Scheme for Children with Disabilities covers the people with following IQ.
    a. Under 29
    b. 30–49
    c. 50–70
    d. 71–100
7. What is the name of the scheme introduced by Government of India to help Persons with Disabilities (PwD)?
    a. Deendayal Disabled Rehabilitation Scheme (DDRS)
    b. E-Anudaan Scheme
    c. Pradhan Mantri Yojana
    d. National Scholarship Scheme
8. Which scheme was created for under five children with hearing disabilities, under Deendayal Divyangjan Rehabilitation Scheme (DDRS)?
    a. Antyodyay Parivar Suraksha Yojana
    b. Sparsh Yojana
    c. Cochlear Implant Program
    d. Manav Garima Yojana
9. Under Deendayal Disabled Rehabilitation Scheme (DDRS), all financial benefits are converged into the following heading:
    a. Scholarships for students with disabilities
    b. Pradhan Mantri Yojana
    c. Aadhaar Yojana
    d. Divyangjan Loan Yojana

10. "The Integrated Education Scheme for Children with Disabilities" covers following categories of impaired children, *except*:
    a. Locomotor handicapped
    b. Moderate to mild hearing loss
    c. Partially sighted children
    d. Children with mood swings

Answers

1. a	2. a	3. b	4. b	5. d
6. c	7. a	8. c	9. a	10. d

CHAPTER 86

Pradhan Mantri Swasthya Suraksha Yojana (PMSSY)

Abhishek Gope, Ranjana Singh, Santosh Kumar, Bharti Koria

Need of program/Scheme	The need for the PMSSY program arose from several key issues: • **Regional disparities in healthcare infrastructure:** India has significant inequalities in the distribution of healthcare facilities, especially tertiary care. Most advanced healthcare infrastructure is concentrated in urban centers, leaving rural and underserved areas with inadequate medical services. • **Shortage of medical professionals:** There is a persistent shortage of qualified healthcare professionals, particularly specialists and super-specialists, in many regions of the country. • **Improvement in medical education standards:** Many medical colleges in India suffer from outdated infrastructure and lack advanced training facilities. • **Need for affordable healthcare:** The private healthcare sector is often expensive and unaffordable for a large portion of India's population.
Implemented since	March 2006
Goal	The Pradhan Mantri Swasthya Suraksha Yojana (PMSSY) aims at correcting the imbalances in the availability of affordable healthcare facilities in different parts of the country in general, and augmenting facilities for quality medical education in the under-served States in particular.
Objectives	• Establish AIIMS as Centre of Excellence that can provide quality medical and nursing education • Quality tertiary healthcare facilities to the people
Components	The program has two components: 1. Setting up AIIMS institutions in different parts of the country 2. Upgrading existing government medical colleges/Institutions in a phased manner by constructing super-specialty blocks and trauma care centers, and procuring advanced medical equipment.
Strategies/Deliverables under the program	• **Phase I:** Six AIIMS-like institutes were established at Bhopal, Bhubaneswar, Jodhpur, Patna, Raipur, and Rishikesh, with full operational status since **2012–2013**. These institutions have a combined bed capacity of **5,764** beds.[1] • **Phase II to VII:** In addition to the six AIIMS institutes approved in phase I, sixteen more AIIMS institutes have been sanctioned in different parts of the country to render quality and affordable healthcare. The status of these institutes have been mentioned below **(Table 86.1)**

TABLE 86.1: Progress and functional status.[2]

Fully functional AIIMS	AIIMS where MBBS classes/ OPD services are functional	AIIMS where MBBS classes are functional	Others
1. Bhopal 2. Bhubaneshwar 3. Jodhpur 4. Patna 5. Raipur 6. Rishikesh	7. Raebaraeli# 8. Gorakhpur# 9. Mangalagiri# 10. Nagpur# 11. Bathinda# 12. Bibinagar# 13. Kalyani# 14. Deoghar# 15. Bilaspur# 16. Rajkot 17. Guwahati 18. Vijaypur (Jammu)#	19. Madurai	20. Awantipora (Kashmir)* 21. Majra, Rewari (Haryana)* 22. Darbhanga (Bihar)*

#Limited IPD services also started
*Construction ongoing

Monitoring framework

Output	Indicators	Target (2022–23)
Increased accessibility to AIIMS and AIIMS like institutes	1.1 Total bed capacity 1.2 Total number of specialty departments increased 1.3 Number of UG seats 1.4 Number of PG seats 1.5 Number of nursing seats	14500 595 1700 950 720
Availability of affordable tertiary care and medical institution	2.1 Number of super specialty departments created in GMC 2.2 Number of PG seats increased in GMC 2.3 Total number of super specialty beds	475 1230 16903

- **Upgradation of GMCIs**: A total of **75 upgradation projects** have been approved, out of which **60** projects were completed by **December 2022**. These projects added super-specialty departments and hospital beds, with an average of 8–10 departments and 150–250 beds per project.
- Fund allocation has been distributed between the center and state in ratio of 60:40.

Package of services
- Outpatient (OPD) and inpatient (IPD) services
- Emergency and trauma care units
- Blood bank facilities
- Intensive Care Units (ICU)
- Diagnostic services

References

1. Annual Report Pradhan Mantri Swasthya Suraksha Yojana 2022-2023; Ministry of Health and Family Welfare.
2. Pradhan Mantri Swasthya Suraksha Yojana; Ministry of Health and Family Welfare.

QUESTIONS

Long Answer Question (LAQ)

1. Discuss the key objectives, components, and strategies of the Pradhan Mantri Swasthya Suraksha Yojana (PMSSY). How has the program addressed the imbalances in healthcare facilities across India, and what progress has been made since its implementation in 2006?

Short Answer Questions (SAQs)

1. Pradhan Mantri Swasthya Suraksha Yojana.
2. Outline the objectives of Pradhan Mantri Swasthya Suraksha Yojana and the explain briefly the package of services provided.

Multiple Choice Questions (MCQs)

1. What is the primary goal of the Pradhan Mantri Swasthya Suraksha Yojana (PMSSY)?
    a. Increase the number of private hospitals in India
    b. Provide free healthcare to all citizens
    c. Correct the imbalance in the availability of affordable healthcare and improve medical education in underserved states
    d. Promote the export of healthcare services
2. Which of the following is NOT a component of the PMSSY program?
    a. Setting up AIIMS institutions
    b. Establishing free community health centers in rural areas
    c. Upgrading existing government medical colleges/institutions
    d. Improving tertiary healthcare infrastructure in underserved regions
3. How many AIIMS-like institutes were approved in Phase I of the PMSSY?
    a. 4   b. 6
    c. 10   d. 8

Answers

1. c   2. b   3. b

87 CHAPTER

Affordable Medicines and Reliable Implants for Treatment

Shaili Vyas, Niharika Verma, Parul Sharma

Background/Need of program/Scheme	• In India, over two-thirds (65%) of healthcare expenses are paid out-of-pocket (OOP), with 70% of these costs being spent on medicines. • To help reduce this financial burden on patients, particularly for pharmaceuticals, the Ministry of Health and Family Welfare (MoHFW) launched AMRIT (Affordable Medicines and Reliable Implants for Treatment), a nationwide network of retail pharmacy stores located in government hospitals.
Implemented since	• Launched in 2015, AMRIT is a major initiative by the Ministry of Health and Family Welfare designed to provide affordable medicines for a variety of diseases, including serious conditions, such as cancer and cardiovascular diseases. • AMRIT pharmacies are set up and operated by HLL Lifecare Ltd, a Central Public Sector Undertaking (CPSU) under the Ministry of Health and Family Welfare. • The first AMRIT outlet was opened on November 15, 2015, at AIIMS, New Delhi. • Currently, there are over 300 AMRIT pharmacies functioning across different states and union territories in India.[1]
Goal	To ensure that all medicines, implants, surgical products, and disposables are available and accessible at highly affordable prices.
Benefits	• AMRIT pharmacies provide both generic and branded life-saving medications under one roof, minimizing the need for patients to visit private chemists who sell at MRP. • The AMRIT pharmacy network offers access to over 5,200 medicines, implants, surgical disposables, and other consumables, with discounts of up to 60% off the Maximum Retail Price (MRP). • AMRIT also helps address shortages of essential medicines at government hospitals by supplying these items at significantly lower prices than local vendors.
Activities at various level or package of services	**AMRIT Outlets** • AMRIT retail outlets are established in partnership with both Central and State Government medical institutions. • These outlets serve both cash and credit customers. • They generally operate from 9:30 AM to 6:30 PM on weekdays, with flexible or 24/7 service depending on the requirements of the partner institution. • **Medicines/Items Available at AMRIT** The items available at AMRIT include: ✦ Medicines ✦ Implants ✦ Surgical products ✦ Ophthalmic items

Reference

1. HLL Lifecare - Amrit [Internet]. Lifecarehll.com. 2015 [cited 2024 Oct 23]. Available from: https://www.lifecarehll.com/page/render/reference/Amrit_Retail_Pharmacy_Stores_

QUESTIONS

Long Answer Question (LAQ)

1. How has AMRIT contributed to improving access to affordable medicines in India? What are the key strategies for ensuring the sustainability and scalability of the scheme?

Short Answer Questions (SAQs)

1. What is the primary goal of the AMRIT scheme?
2. What is AMRIT Pharmacy? Discuss their goals and strategies. What benefits do they provide for common man?

Multiple Choice Questions (MCQs)

1. When was the AMRIT scheme launched?
    a. 2013
    b. 2014
    c. 2015
    d. 2016
2. Which organization operates AMRIT pharmacies?
    a. HLL Lifecare Limited
    b. Indian Council of Medical Research
    c. National Pharmaceutical Pricing Authority
    d. World Health Organization
3. What is the primary source of medicines for AMRIT pharmacies?
    a. Private pharmaceutical companies
    b. Government-owned pharmaceutical companies
    c. Both A and B
    d. International pharmaceutical companies

Answers

1. c
2. a
3. b

CHAPTER 88

National Action Plan for Prevention and Control of Snakebite Envenoming

Anamika Tomar, Pragya Tripathi, Akhil Dhanesh Goel

INTRODUCTION

Snakebite envenoming is recognized as a neglected tropical disease, typically resulting from accidental bites by venomous snakes. This condition is a significant public health issue, particularly in tropical and subtropical areas. The World Health Organization (WHO) estimates that approximately 5.4 million snakebites occur globally each year, with 1.8 to 2.7 million resulting in envenoming. This leads to an estimated 8,000 to 130,000 deaths annually, alongside a considerable number of amputations and long-term disabilities.[1]

In 2017, the WHO classified snakebite envenoming as a priority neglected tropical disease and initiated a global strategy aimed at reducing snakebite-related deaths and disabilities by half by 2030. South Asia alone accounts for nearly 70% of worldwide snakebite fatalities, with India recording between 200,000 and 300,000 cases each year, which results in about 1,000 to 2,500 deaths.[1]

In India, snakebites are especially prevalent in rural and peri-urban areas, with high-risk states including Bihar, Jharkhand, West Bengal, Madhya Pradesh, Odisha, Uttar Pradesh, Andhra Pradesh, Telangana, Rajasthan, and Gujarat. Analyses from the Indian Million Death Study (2001–2014) and reviews of around 87,590 cases suggest that India experiences about 1.2 million snakebite deaths, averaging approximately 58,000 each year. Vulnerable populations include agricultural workers, herders, fishermen, children aged 10–14, and those living in substandard housing.[1]

The clinical repercussions of venomous snakebites can be severe, leading to paralysis, hemorrhage, tissue damage, and irreversible kidney failure. Pregnant women face heightened risks, as venom-induced hemorrhage can result in miscarriage. India is home to over 310 snake species, with 66 categorized as venomous or mildly venomous. Most bites are attributed to four main species known as the "Big Four": Russell's Viper (*Daboia russelii*), Spectacled Cobra (*Naja naja*), Common Krait (*Bungarus caeruleus*), and Saw-scaled Viper (*Echis carinatus*), with their distribution affected by environmental factors, such as habitat type and rainfall.[2]

According to the Central Bureau of Health Intelligence (CBHI), India records around 300,000 snakebite cases annually, leading to approximately 2,000 deaths. There is a significant discrepancy between reported fatalities and actual statistics, with research indicating that only about 7.23% of snakebite deaths are officially documented. Initiatives like the Integrated Disease Surveillance Programme (IDSP) and a case-based reporting system via the Integrated Health Information Platform (IHIP) have been introduced to enhance reporting and inform policy interventions.[1]

The National Action Plan for Snakebite Envenoming (NAPSE) in India is structured around four essential pillars crucial for effectively managing and preventing snakebite incidents nationwide.

KEY PILLARS OF NAPSE

- **Intersectoral coordination and collaboration:** This emphasizes the importance of cooperation among various sectors, including health, wildlife, and agriculture, to ensure a unified response to snakebite cases.[2]
- **Governance and management:** Effective governance is vital for NAPSE's implementation. This involves defining clear roles and responsibilities for stakeholders at both national and state levels to align efforts against snakebite envenoming.

- **Public awareness and education:** Raising awareness about snakebite prevention and treatment is essential. The plan includes initiatives to educate communities on snakebite risks and the necessity of seeking prompt medical attention.
- **Research and surveillance:** Continuous research and monitoring are required to understand snakebite epidemiology, track incidents, identify high-risk areas, and evaluate the effectiveness of interventions.[2,3]

Vision and Mission of NAPSE

- **Vision:** The primary goal is "to prevent and control snakebite envenoming to halve the deaths and disabilities caused by it by 2030."[3]
- **Mission:** The mission aims to progressively reduce morbidity, mortality, and complications associated with snakebites.[3]

Strategies in the Human Health Sector of NAPSE

The plan outlines several strategic actions to effectively manage and mitigate snakebite incidents, focusing on enhancing antivenom availability, improving surveillance, strengthening emergency care, establishing regional venom centers, and building capacity among health professionals.[3]

Ensuring Provision of Anti-Snake Venom (ASV) at Health Facilities
- **Financial support:** The Central Government will aid states in acquiring ASV through the National Free Drugs Initiative and ensure its inclusion in the essential drug list.
- **Trained personnel:** Healthcare staff must receive training to manage snakebites and administer ASV.
- **Supply chain management:** Continuous supply of ASV will be maintained, with monitoring to prevent shortages.
- **Cold chain facilities:** Adequate facilities will be established for proper ASV storage.
- **Monitoring adverse events:** A system will be developed to document and report adverse events related to snakebite treatments.

Strengthening surveillance of snakebite cases and deaths effective surveillance is critical for evaluating interventions and managing human exposures, including:
- **Snakebite notification system:** A web portal will be introduced for reporting snakebite victims within the health sector.[2]
- **Periodic reporting:** Strengthening of reporting through IDSP and IHIP.
- **Resource mapping:** Mapping healthcare facilities and laboratories equipped to manage snakebite cases and diagnose complications.[3]

Enhancing emergency care services: To improve emergency responses in district hospitals and community health centers (CHCs):
- **Ambulance services:** Ensure dedicated ambulances are available for snakebite cases.
- **Diagnostic tests:** Provide necessary tests for diagnosing snakebites, such as clotting tests and kidney function assessments.
- **Critical care facilities:** Ensure access to ventilator-equipped beds and strengthen ICU capacities for snakebite patients.
- **Dialysis units:** Establish units for patients needing dialysis.
- **Emergency medications:** Ensure essential emergency medications are available.[2]
- **Referral systems:** Implement protocols for managing and referring snakebite cases appropriately.[3]

Institutionalizing regional venom centers: At least five regional venom centers will be established, focusing on—
- **Research on regional venoms:** Studies on venoms from local species, particularly the "Big Four."
- **Biochemical studies:** Facilitating comprehensive research on various snake species and their venoms.
- **Production of ASV:** Development of region-specific ASV formulations based on local venom profiles.[3]

Capacity building through training
- **Training centers:** Existing institutions will be enhanced as training centers for snakebite management.
- **Professional development:** Healthcare professionals will be trained in effective snakebite management, including ASV administration.
- **Rural healthcare training:** Training will be provided for lower-level health facilities in rural areas to manage snakebite emergencies effectively.
- **Interdisciplinary training:** Joint training sessions for healthcare and veterinary professionals will be organized.
- **Laboratory training:** Enhanced training for laboratory professionals on diagnosing snakebites.[3]

Information, education, and communication (IEC): To promote awareness about snakebites:
- **Policy sensitization:** Engage policymakers and health professionals in discussions about snakebite management.
- **Targeted communication:** Assess specific communication needs for groups, such as agricultural workers in remote areas.
- **Development of IEC materials:** Create educational materials in multiple languages for diverse populations.
- **Community engagement:** Utilize media channels, such as community radio to spread information about snakebites.
- **24/7 snakebite helpline:** A dedicated helpline will provide immediate assistance and information regarding snakes and snakebites.
- **Education for traditional healers:** Programs will educate traditional healers to dispel myths about snakes and snakebites.[3]

Public-private partnerships: Collaborations with organizations, such as the Indian Medical Association (IMA) and NGOs will enhance activities related to snakebite prevention, research, and continued medical education.

Intersectoral coordination: Effective snakebite prevention will require engagement from sectors, such as vaccine manufacturers, wildlife organizations, tribal communities, and local governance.[3]

Strategies for the Agriculture/Animal Health Sector in NAPSE

Provision of ASV at Veterinary Facilities
- **Trained personnel:** Ensure veterinary facilities have trained staff for managing snakebites and administering ASV.
- **Supply management:** Maintain a steady supply of ASV and monitor demand to prevent shortages.[2]
- **Cold chain facilities:** Upgrade facilities for proper ASV storage.[3]

Prevention of Snakebites in Livestock
- **Risk area identification:** Identify high-risk areas near livestock and provide signage for preventive measures.
- **Natural barriers:** Create barriers to minimize contact between domestic animals and snakes.
- **Polyvalent antivenom provision:** Ensure veterinary facilities stock polyvalent antivenom with appropriate training.[3]

Strengthening Emergency Care Services
- **Mobile veterinary units:** Equip mobile units to respond to snakebite emergencies, ensuring ASV availability.
- **Basic diagnostic facilities:** Enhance veterinary hospitals with diagnostic tools for emergency treatment.[3]

Capacity Building for Veterinary and Agricultural Professionals
- **Training programs:** Conduct sessions on effective snakebite management and ASV administration.
- **Local management:** Train lower-level veterinary services for snakebite cases, especially in rural areas.
- **Training for various roles:** Provide training on diagnosis and antivenom administration.
- **Private sector engagement:** Involve private-sector professionals through workshops.[3]

- **Joint training initiatives:** Facilitate joint training for health and veterinary professionals.
- **Surveillance training:** Educate professionals on monitoring snakebite cases in animals.

IEC Initiatives
- **Community sensitization:** Collaborate with agricultural departments to educate animal owners about snakebite management.
- **Monitoring animal sheds:** Regularly inspect animal sheds for snakes and rodents.
- **Habitat management:** Clear vegetation around barns to reduce snake hiding spots.
- **Outreach programs:** Develop outreach through Krishi Vigyan Kendras (KVKs) to inform farmers.[3]

Strengthening surveillance of snakebite cases in animals: Effective surveillance is essential for evaluating interventions and managing human exposures.[3]

Production and Use of Antivenom
- **Supply and production:** Ensure adequate antivenom production for livestock and pets.
- **Training programs:** Provide training on intravenous antivenin administration based on various factors.

Strategies of the Wildlife and Forest Sector in NAPSE

Given that snakebites significantly affect rural communities, the wildlife and forest sectors can contribute significantly through:
- **Education and awareness:** Targeted campaigns will educate communities in forested and hilly regions on snakebite prevention.
- **Antivenom distribution:** Wildlife professionals will collaborate with health workers to distribute antivenom in remote areas.
- **Strengthening key stakeholders:** Engagement of local populations and stakeholders is essential for effective management strategies.
- **Systematic research and monitoring:** Research on snake behavior and habitat will inform strategies to reduce snakebites.
- **Snake venom collection and relocation:** Wildlife and forest departments will support research institutions in venom collection and safe snake relocation, helping to reduce bite risks and conserve snake species.[3]

References
1. WHO's Snakebite Envenoming Strategy for prevention and control.
2. Regional Action Plan for prevention and control of snakebite.
3. National Programme for Prevention and Control of Snakebite in India.

QUESTIONS

Long Answer Question (LAQ)

1. How does the National Action Plan for Prevention and Control of Snakebite Envenoming (NAPSE) aim to reduce snakebite-related morbidity and mortality in India by 2030, and what specific strategies does it propose to ensure the effective delivery of anti-snake venom, enhance public awareness, and engage various stakeholders in its implementation?

Short Answer Questions (SAQs)

1. What is the primary vision of the National Action Plan for Prevention and Control of Snakebite Envenoming (NAPSE)?
2. Which approach does NAPSE adopt to address the issue of snakebite envenoming in India?

Multiple Choice Questions (MCQs)

1. What is the main goal of the National Action Plan for Prevention and Control of Snakebite Envenoming (NAPSE)?
    a. To eliminate all snake species in India
    b. To halve snakebite deaths by 2030
    c. To increase snake farming
    d. To promote tourism in rural areas
2. Which of the following is a key feature of NAPSE?
    a. Establishing a national snake sanctuary
    b. Continuous access to anti-snake venom
    c. Banning all outdoor activities
    d. Promoting snake hunting
3. What is the Snakebite Helpline number introduced under NAPSE?
    a. 911
    b. 15400
    c. 108
    d. 100
4. Which stakeholders are involved in the implementation of NAPSE?
    a. Only government officials
    b. Key stakeholders, supporting stakeholders, and NGOs
    c. Only healthcare professionals
    d. International tourists
5. What approach does NAPSE utilize to formulate action plans?
    a. Traditional Medicine Approach
    b. One Health Approach
    c. Agricultural Development Approach
    d. Urban Planning Approach

Answers

1. b
2. b
3. b
4. b
5. b

Index

Page numbers followed by *f* refer to figure and *t* refer to table.

A

Aadhaar-based linkage 381
Aam Aadmi Bima Yojana 452
Aarogya Setu 367, 380
Accredited Social Health Activist 142, 196, 284, 343
    for breastfeeding, supporting 219
    for institutional delivery, cash assistance to 99
    home visits by 140
    incentive 91
    roles and responsibilities of 408
    training modules 322
    volunteer 99
    worker 20
        support to 135
Acquired immunodeficiency syndrome
    prevention and control 242
    response, progress of 242*f*
Active aging, promotion of 283
Activities 196
    across prevention levels 368
    structure of 189
Admission, strategies at time of 114
Adolescent Friendly Health Clinics 192, 193
    benchmark criteria for 192
    convergence approach of 193
    reporting mechanism for 193
    services, package of 192
Adolescent girls, scheme for 199, 215
Adolescent health
    care 387
    enhance 179
    interventions 191, 191*f*
Adolescent Health Day 182, 196
Adolescent Health Resource Centers 183
Adolescent population 179
Adolescent-Friendly Club 197
    Meetings 183, 197
Adolescent-Friendly Health Clinics 179, 183, 191
Adulthood, transition to 179
Advanced care, building expertise for 285
Advanced directive, provision of 304
Adverse event following immunization
    management 153
    types of 154
Adverse event management system 204
Advisory committees 416
Advocacy 187, 225, 230, 255, 322, 397
Affordable medicines 463
Agriculture, strategies for 467
Air pollution illnesses 419
Albendazole 203
All National Health Programs, logos of 5
All Training and Teaching programs 302
Ambulance services 466
Amoxicillin 171
Amrit outlets 463
Anemia 163, 201
    check for 168
    non-nutritional causes of 208
    prevalence of 206*t*
    screening 201
    severe 163
    testing and treatment of 209
Anemia Mukt Bharat 206
    dashboard and digital portal 209
    strategy 206
Anganwadi
    helper 343
    infrastructure 214
Anganwadi Center 139, 203
    screening 149
Anganwadi Services Scheme 214
    Team 340
Anganwadi worker 142, 219, 284, 343
    home visits by 140
Animal Birth Control Regulations 261
Animal health
    component 260
    sector, strategies for 467
Animal Welfare Board 260
Annual reports 416
Anti-bullying programs 187
Anti-larval measures 232
Antimicrobial
    resistance surveillance 439, 441
    use of 442
Anti-snake venom
    ensuring provision of 466
    production of 466
Antivenom
    distribution 468
    production and use of 468
Antyodaya Anna Yojana 10, 357
Artificial intelligence 374
    powered telehealth 375
Atal Pension Yojana 74
Audits 358
Auxiliary Nurse Midwife 343
    for breastfeeding, supporting 219
    online 379
    roles and responsibilities of 408
Awareness 70, 184, 188, 255, 397, 401, 413, 418
    and advocacy, increased 225
    campaigns for 237, 392, 427
    generation 441
    raise 106
    week 441
Ayushman Arogya Mandir 386
Ayushman Bharat 10
    Digital Mission 363, 369
    integration with 372
Ayushman Bharat Health Account 366
    registrations 364
Ayushman Bharat Health and Wellness Center 372, 375
Ayushman Bharat Pradhan Mantri Jan Arogya Yojana 24, 452
Ayushman Bharat Programme 385

B

Bacterial infection 164
Bajaj Committee 35
Baseline survey data 353
Batch size 131
Behavior change
    communication 170, 182, 210, 233, 319
    prevention through 277

Index

Beneficiaries 40, 54, 74, 255
   feedback 413, 416
   identification, targeted 412
   indirect 270
   under scheme 347
Beti Bachao Beti Padhao 199, 396, 397
   programme 396
Bhore Committee 35
Biannual deworming 201
Biochemical studies 466
Biological control 232
Bivalent oral polio vaccine 266
Blindness, reduce prevalence of 53
Block level monitoring 344
Block public health units 30
Brain stem death certification 431
Breast problem 160
Breastfeeding 165
   creating enabling environment for 220
   exclusive 224
   practices 138
   promoting exclusive 223
   rates, increased 225
Breathing, difficult 167
Bridge gap 138
Bridge population 244
Broadening product offering 392
Building capacity 56
Bungarus caeruleus 465
Burn
   care 325
      objectives 324
   injury management 325

C

Cable Television Networks (Amendment) Rules 313
Cadaveric donation 431
Cancer Day 277
Capacity building 55, 134, 141, 142, 148, 152, 182, 231, 233, 234, 247, 255, 269, 280, 296, 328, 333, 354, 367, 415, 416
   and training 130
   through training 467
Cardiovascular disease 275
Care
   continuum of 386
   improved quality of 385
   integrated 302
   quality of 57
   secondary 29
Caregiver's practice 166, 168
Case detection, enhanced 246
Case studies 416
Cash assistance provided for
   rural areas 99
   urban areas 99

Cashless transactions 413
Cataract 291
Central authority comprises 305
Central bureau of health intelligence 465
Central Mental Health Authority 305
   function of 305
Central mental health team 302
Central monitoring unit 344
Central public sector undertaking 463
Central sector components 26
Centrally sponsored components 25
Chadha Committee 35
Character education 187
Chemical occupational factors 435
Chief executive officer 39
Chikungunya 234
Child health and development, improving 223, 225
Child health
   priority of 138
   screening 147
Child malnutrition, reduced 223, 225
Child mortality
   and morbidity, reduce 139
   reducing 223
Child nutrition, promoting good 138
Child-friendly services, ensuring 174
Childhood
   blindness 291
   diseases 147
   health care 387
   illnesses, manage 138
Children's vision 290
Childs feeding 168
Childs immunization 168
Chronic disease management 373
Chronic Obstructive Pulmonary Disease Day 277
Cigarettes and other Tobacco Products Act, monitoring enforcement of 312
Citizens 366
Clean energy
   affordable and 43
   promotion of 413
Clean water and sanitation 43
Climate
   action 44
   change 20
   resilient infrastructure 420
Clinical skills training 31, 163
Cloud-based and mobile-friendly 372
Coaching team 94
Cold chain
   facilities 466, 467
   infrastructure, strengthening 152
   management 152

Collaboration 20, 187, 392
   and coordination 413
Color codes
   chart booklets 157
   different 157
Commodities 91, 142, 183
Common krait 465
Common ophthalmic care 387
Communicable diseases 85, 227, 387
   management 387
Communication 181, 230
   targeted 467
Community 181, 186, 224, 255, 400
   awareness 109, 170, 290
      guidelines for 314
   based Maternal and Child Death Surveillance and Response, steps for 119
   diagnosis 354
   engage influential members of 322
   engagement 20, 21, 401, 467
      and education 231, 257
      and social mobilization 153
   for mental health and development 303
   Health Center 124, 174, 192, 284, 285, 302, 402
   healthcare level 285
   leaders, promote involvement of 318
   mobilization and behavioral change 214
   participation 21, 55, 65, 271
   partnerships 187
   platforms 386
   sensitization 468
   support 224
Community-based
   events 214
   Infant and Young Child Feeding Programs 224, 225
   initiatives 182
   Maternal and Child Death Surveillance and Response 119
   newborn screening 148
   outreach 179
Community-level activities 220
Complementary feeding 138, 224
   practices, improved 225
   providing appropriate 223
Comprehensive management 353
Comprehensive primary healthcare 57
Comprehensive program management 319
Conducting screening camps and outreach activities 256
Conflict resolution 187
Convergence activity, platform for 216

Index

Convergence with development programs 348
Convergence within health and family welfare 182
Coordination and collaboration 314
Coordination with international agencies and stakeholders 256
Core technology 375
Core working group 443
Corneal transplantation 291
Cost
  norms 215
  savings 374
Cost-effectiveness 18
Counsel mother about
  development supportive practices 168
  feeding 168
  her own health 168
Counseling 181, 183
  for adolescents, facility-based 179
  services 187
Covid-19 374
  vaccination campaign 152
Critical care facilities 466
Critical lifeline 374
Curative services 183
  availability of 13
Current human resources, use of 321
Customized support 413
Customs duty exemptions 68
Cytochrome B 239

D

Daboia russelii 465
Dakshata 114
  training 7
Danger signs 166
Data
  analysis 413
  gaps 21
  reporting 326
  security, strengthening 374
  standardization and quality control 271
  transmission 120
  utilization 412
Data collection 277
  and analysis 416
  and dashboards 397
  and entry 143
  and program monitoring 140
  and research 325
Data management 182
  systems 393
Data-driven decision-making 363
Day care center 301, 302
Deaths and complications, preventable 93

Decentralization 58
Decentralized planning and implementation 65
Dedicated childcare services near maternal health departments 176
Deendayal Disabled Rehabilitation Scheme 455
Defects at birth 147
Deficiencies 147
Dehydration, severe 161
Delivery and postpartum care, gaps in 93
Demand generation 184
Dengue 234
Dental fluorosis 353
Department of food and public distribution, organization chart of 357*f*
Develop human resources 52
Deworming 210
  dose and regimen for 208*t*
Diabetes
  day 277
  type 2 275
Diabetic retinopathy 291
Diagnostic services 237
Dialysis units 466
Diarrhea 161
  management 215
Dietary diversification 210
Digital health
  adoption 365
  and innovations 58
  initiatives 361
  records 365
  solutions 257
Digital healthcare, revolution in 375
Digital infrastructure, expanding 374
Digital integration 387
Digital platforms 413
Digital public goods 367
Digital tools, use of 95
Digitalization and supply chain management 392
Direct beneficiaries 270
Direct financial assistance 68
Direct health impacts 419
Direct nutrition interventions 60
Direct service delivery
  screening 256
  treatment 256
  vaccination 256
Disability prevention and management 247
Disabled persons, apparel scheme for 455
Disabled Rehabilitation Scheme 455
Disaster preparedness 187
Discharge, strategies at time of 115

Disease
  burden 230
  burden of 13
  control programs, strengthening 55
  management 231
  monitoring, enhance 269
Distributor network 413
District early intervention center 149
District Environmental Health Cell, roles and responsibilities of 422
District health department 139
District hospital 124, 174, 276, 284
  level 285
District joint steering committee on rabies 260
District level
  activities 319
  monitoring 344
District Mental Health Program 301
District multi-sectoral task force 421
District oral health cell 318
District tobacco control cell 311
District Women and Child Development Department 139
District-level activities, monitoring and supervision of 256
District-specific action plans 256
Donated eyes, collection of 291
Donor
  database of 428
  motivation 427
  organizers 428
Dropouts and left-outs, reducing 152
Drug
  and insecticide resistance monitoring 233
  resistance patterns 238
Drug resistant-tuberculosis
  extensively 238
  management 237
  regimen 238, 239
Drug-susceptible tuberculosis 238
Dual-mode functionality 372

E

Ear, nose, and throat care 387
Early childhood care and education 214
Early detection and treatment 289
Early diagnosis
  and complete case management 230
  and prompt treatment 171, 233
Early intervention and support services 397
Early management and referral 147
E-bloodbank 380
Economic burden 310
Educating communities for supportive environment 285

Education 188, 401, 418
   and awareness 289, 468
   campaigns 413
   for traditional healers 467
E-health
   assistance and teleconsultation 380
   initiatives 378
E-hospital 380
Elderly and palliative care 387
Electronic cigarettes, prohibition of 313
Electronic health records 188, 372
Electronic vaccine intelligence network 152, 153
Emergency
   and critical care 373
   care services
      enhancing 466
      strengthening 467
   care, imparting skills of 188
   medical services 387
   medications 466
Emerging diseases, less focus on 385
Emerging health threats 52
Emotional health 187
Emotional intelligence 187
Emphasizing underserved and rural areas 392
Employees Provident Funds 446
Employees State Insurance Act 450
Empower
   adolescents 180
   committee 365, 368
   mothers 225
Empowered Programme Committee 83
Empowering frontline health service providers 125
Empowering mothers 223
Enable sexual and reproductive health 180
Enabled rural expansion 375
Enabling digital doctors 368
Enabling environment and demand generation 220
Encourage population stabilization 53
Encourage public health and preventative initiatives 52
Encourage research and development 53
Enhancing early detection and screening 68
Entrepreneurial incentives 392
Environment 400
Environmental and health focus 413
Environmental and Occupational Health Climate Change and Health 421
Environmental education 187
Environmental health 187
Environmental management 232

Epidemiological transition 52
Equipment availability 95
Equitable 183, 192
Equity 302
E-raktkosh 381
E-sanjeevani 367, 372, 373, 375
   evolution of 372
   impact of 374
Essential drugs, accessibility of 392
Ethambutol 238
Evaluations and audits, independent 233
Evidence-based
   care 302
   decision making 13
Excellence, centers of 69
Expectant mother 99
Expert team 321
Expertise and infrastructure 31
Eye
   diseases, treatment of 291
   surgeons, training of 291
Eye care services
   primary 291
   secondary 291

F

Facility-based approach, structure of 192f
Family planning 111, 387
Family-centric, respectful, and dignified care, providing 176
Feedback and grievance redressal 95
Feedback mechanism 277, 394, 397
Female sex workers 244
Fever 162
Field visits 416
   and inspections 413
   and reviews 397
Filariasis 232
Financial punishment, provision of 305
Financial assistance and support 412
Financial protection 385
Financial security 446
Financial support 466
   mechanisms 68
First aid training 187
First blood bank 425
First referral unit 124, 174
   at Community Health Centers 30
Fixed day approach 201
Fixed-dose combination 238, 239
Flexi pool at state level, use of 312
Fluorosis 353
Folic acid supplementation 184, 201
Food
   and public distribution 357f
   fortification 210
   grains 348
   security and nutrition 225

Food Adulteration Act, prevention of 313
Food Safety and Standards (Packaging and Labelling) Regulations 313
Foster behavior reshaping of community 333
Foster collaborative partnerships 180
Fragmented health data 363
Free cataract surgery 290
Frequent data collection 55
Frontline workers, capacity building of 140
Functional household tap connections 405
Funds 142
   pattern 340
   raising 318
   utilization of 409

G

Gender equality 43
Gender-based violence 179
General danger signs, check for 167
Generic medicines, providing 392
Geographic coverage 130
Geriatric specialists, lack of 283
Glaucoma 291
Global adult tobacco survey 310
Global health
   priorities 13
   trends 21
Global polio eradication initiative 264
Global youth tobacco survey 310
Good health and well-being 43
Goods and Services Tax 313
Government and policymakers 400
Government backing 413
Government-aided schools 149
Grief counseling 187
Grievance redressal mechanism 111, 413
Growing elderly population 283
Growth
   measurement 215
   monitoring and promotion 140
Guidelines and protocols implementation 95

H

H monoresistant treatment 238
Habitat management 468
Health
   and hygiene promotion 188
   and wellness
      ambassadors 188
      ambassadors, capacity building of 189
      center 25, 285, 386
   assembly resolution 425

Index **475**

centers, upgrade 385
check-ups 140, 210, 342, 343
committees 35
    recommendations 35
coverage, provide 385
data consent managers, establishing 367
education 186, 187
expenditure, increase 53
facility registry 367
finance 57
ID for every citizen 365
impact on 230
    indirect 419
inequities 21
management information 57
policies 49
preparedness and response 418
records, blockchain-based 375
screening 188, 187
services 187, 215
status and program impact 56
workers, training of 152, 157
workforce 21
Health infrastructure 57
    improving 53
    strengthen 52
Health program 13
    evolution of 3
Health promotion 135, 280
    and education 55
    campaigns 280
    for behavior change 276
    including counseling, prevention and 276
Health system 223
    and capacity building, strengthening 171
    level 334
    performance 57
    strengthening 57, 85, 109, 223-225, 233
    support 224
Healthcare
    affordable 460
    delivery system 24
    divide, bridging 372
    facilities 231, 366
    infrastructure, regional disparities in 460
    preventive 53
    professionals registry 366
    services via mobile app and website, providing 368
    staff 400
    system 24
    to homes, bringing 373
    universal access to 53

Healthcare access
    disparities 385
    enhanced 385
    improved 365
Healthcare personnel 130
    training for 290
Healthcare provider 270, 366
    capacity building 220
    integration 364
    trained 93
Healthcare workers
    exposed to infectious materials 255
    training 374
Health-seeking behavior, promoting appropriate 139
Healthy nutrition 186
Healthy school environment 186
Hearing
    disabilities 456
    loss, prevent 294
Heat-related illnesses 420
Hematopoietic stem cell transplantation 68
Hepatitis B vaccine 151
High maternal
    and child mortality rates 52
    mortality on delivery day 93
Holistic development, promote 179
Holistic wellness model 32
Home and community level 334
Home visit 134, 142
Home-based care 140
    for newborn 134
        and young child 174
    for young child 6, 138
        program 138
Home-Based Newborn Care 6
    kit 135
    promoting 130
Honorarium to cook-cum-helpers 348
Hospital support services 400
Hospital/facility upkeep, improving 401
Hub-and-spoke model 372, 375
Human health sector, strategies in 466
Human immunodeficiency virus
    prevention and control 242
    response, progress of 242*f*
Human papilloma virus vaccine 152
Human resource 57, 319, 321
    for health 57
    gaps 20
    strengthening 95
Hygiene 186, 224
Hypertension 275
    day 277

I

Identify treatment 158-163
Idiopathic dysplasia 244

Illness care, minor 387
Immune deficiency disorders 68
Immunization 140, 215, 342, 343
    coverage 152
    ensuring age-appropriate 139
    essential 266
    programs 187
    routine 152
    services, types of facilities 125
Implementing agency 129
Inadequate feeding practices 138
Inadequate health
    care infrastructure 52
    infrastructure 283
Incentive
    and awards 214
    and recognition 401
    mechanisms 140
India fights dengue 378
Indian Medical Association 467
Indian Standards Sets, bureau of 353
Indigenous research, promoting 68
Industry, innovation, and infrastructure 43
Infant and young child feeding 223, 224
    practices, improving 223
Infant mortality rate 53
Infection
    control 400
    prevention and control 441
Information 192
    and awareness 183
    availability, enhance 180
    dissemination 413
Information, education and communication 312, 319, 354, 467
    initiatives 468
    materials, development of 467
    use of 65
Infrastructure 318
    and resource gaps 93
    development 325, 401
    expansion 413
    maintenance 86
    strengthening 280
    upgradation 95
Injuries and violence 179, 180
    prevent 180
Innovation and flexibility 348
Insecticide resistance 20
Institutional deliveries, promote 106
Institutionalizing regional venom centers 466
Integrate different medical systems 52
Integrated Child Development Services Scheme 9, 339, 340
Integrated Disease Surveillance Programme 8, 269

Integrated Health Information Platform 269, 465
Integrated Management of Neonatal and Childhood Illness 6, 156, 158
 facility-based 124
 package, implementation of 157
Integrated programme for senior citizens, scheme of 75
Integrated vector management 233, 234
 and vector surveillance 230
Intellectual disability, schemes for 455
Intensified behavior change communication campaign 208
Interdisciplinary training 467
Internal assessment 402
Internal reviews 416
Internet of things (IoT) 374
 integration 374
Interoperability standards 367
Interrupting poliovirus transmission, milestones for 265
Intersectoral collaboration 171, 269, 271, 467
 and coordination 465
Interventions under scheme 199
Intra-ministerial coordination 209
Iodine 350
 deficiency disorders control cell, establishment of 350
Iron and folic acid
 fortified foods, mandatory provision of 208
 supplementation, regimen for 208t
Isoniazid 238
 preventive therapy 238, 239

J

Jal Jeevan Mission 404
Jan Andolan 214
Janani Shishu Suraksha Karyakram 5, 101
Janani Suraksha Yojana 5, 98
 benefits of 99
 scheme, eligibility for 99
 target groups of 99
 vision of 98
Janaushadhi Suvidha Sanitary Napkin 392
Japanese encephalitis 231
 incidence, reduce 231
 vaccine 151
Jaundice 164
Joint
 action plan, developing 142
 training initiatives 468
Joint Monitoring Missions 232
Jungalwalla Committee 35
Juvenile diabetes 275

Juvenile Justice (Care and Protection of Children) Act 313

K

Kala-azar 230
 control efforts 230
Kanya Shiksha Pravesh Utsav Campaign 199
Kartar Singh Committee 35
Kayakalp 11, 399
 scheme 400, 402
Keratoplasty 291
Key health issues 179
Kilkari 379
Kitchen devices 348
Kitchen-cum-stores 348
 repair of 348
Knowledge and innovation hub 40

L

Labor
 and complications, management of 95
 room
  certification of 95
  quality improvement initiative 93
Laboratory network, strengthening 237
Laboratory training 467
Landless agriculture laborers 358
LaQshya 5, 93
Laws, enforcement of 397
Learning, ensure transfer of 114
Legislative framework 413
Lentin commission 36
Leprosy
 elimination of 246
 program, history of 246
Leprosy-free India 246
Levofloxacin 238
Life below water 44
Lifestyle trends 21
Liver transplantation 68
Living donation 430
Local awareness campaigns 256
Logistic support 319
Logistics management 152
Lower maternal mortality ratio 53
Low-priced medications 392

M

Malaria 162, 233
Malnutrition 162
Management information system 416
Mandatory transplant coordinators 431
Manpower training and development 296
Manual data collection approach 143
Married adolescents 181

Mass awareness campaign 171
Mass drug administration 232
Mass Media Campaigns 311
Maternal and Child Death Surveillance and Response 6, 117
 facility based 120
 process for migrant death 121
Maternal and child health
 care 373
  enhance 52
 initiatives 55
 services 225
Maternal and infant mortality, reduce 106
Maternal care 134
Maternal death
 notification of 119
 surveillance and response organogram 118
Maternal health, improve 106
mCessation 313, 379
mDiabetes 379
Meals during summer vacation 348
Measles vaccine, second dose of 151
Measles-rubella vaccine campaign 151
Media campaign 312
Medical education standards, improvement in 460
Medical needs 130
Medical professionals, shortage of 460
Medical system 392
Medicines 57, 463
Menstrual health education 186
Menstrual Hygiene Scheme 184, 186
 components of 188
Mental health 179, 180, 187
 awareness 187
 conditions, caregivers of person with 306
 delivery mechanisms for 303
 enhance 180
 helpline 302
 holistic approach to 302
 information system 302
 network, building comprehensive 306
 promotion of 303
 services 374, 387
  universal access to 303
 support 186
Mental Healthcare Act 304
Mental illness, prevention of 303
Mental-wellbeing 306
Menu under scheme 348
Mera Aspataal 378
Micronutrient 60
Mid-day meal scheme 10, 347
Mission Indradhanush 7, 151, 152

Mission Parivar Vikas 89-91
  coverage of 90
  implementation 91
  strategy of 90
Mission Poshan 2.0 339
Mission steering group 365, 368
Mobile
  academy 379
  eye units 290
  health team 148
  veterinary units 467
Module construction 321
Monitor whether maternal deaths 117
Monitoring
  and reporting 109
    accountability mechanisms 45
  and supervision 204
  and surveillance 233
  and training 410
  animal sheds 468
  steps of 136
Monovalent oral polio vaccine type 2 266
Mother and child tracking system 379
Mother newborn care unit 174
Mothers absolute affection 7, 219
  program, components of 219f
Mothers and caregivers 139
Mudaliar Committee 35
Mukherjee Committee 35
Multidrug-resistant TB 238
Multilingual support 372
Multi-purpose workers 322
Multi-stakeholder
  collaboration 45
  engagement 413
MusQan
  certified facility 176f
  initiative
    government health facilities 174t
    sustenance under 177f
  scheme 174f, 175f

N

National action plan for antimicrobial resistance 439
National Action Plan for
  Climate Change and Human Health 422
  climate change and levels of prevention 423
  dog mediated rabies elimination 261
  prevention and control of snakebite envenoming 465
  snakebite envenoming 465
    key pillars of 465
    mission of 466
  welfare of senior citizens 75

National AIDS Control Organisation, organogram of 243
National AIDS Control Programme 8, 241
National Anemia Mukt Bharat Unit 209
National Ayush Mission 31
National Center of Excellence and Advanced Research on Anemia Control 209
National Centre for Disease Control 260, 421
  Hosts 420
National Commission on Macroeconomics and Health 36
National Council of Senior Citizens 74
National Deworming Day 201, 203, 204
National Digital Health Ecosystem 25
National Digital Health Mission 25, 363
National Family Health Survey 206
National Family Planning Indemnity Scheme 89
National Fellowship for Persons with Disabilities 456
National Health Analytics Platform 367
National Health Authority 24, 365, 368
National Health Electronic Registries 367
National Health Mission 3, 5, 25, 79, 83
  components 85
  integration 284
  Steering Committee 329
  under umbrella of 319
National Health Policy 51, 52, 56, 129
  formulation of 18
National Health Portal 378
National Health Program 17, 18, 31
  framework 1
  integrating with 392
National Health Registries 365
National Health Systems Resource Centre 25
National Institute of Occupational Health 434
National Institution for Transforming India Aayog 38
National Iodine Deficiency Disorder Control Programme 10, 350
National Jal Jeevan Mission 12, 404
National Leprosy Eradication Programme 8, 246
National Level Advisory Committee 420
National Mental Health Policy 302
National Mental Health Programme 9, 301
National Mentoring Group 94
National Networking 431
National Nutrition Mission, Poshan 2.0 213
National Nutrition Policy 60
National Nutrition Strategy 206

National Nutritional Programme 85
National Oral Health Cell 318
National Oral Health Programme 9, 318
National Organ and Tissue Transplant Organization 431
National Organ Transplant Programme 12, 430, 431
National Policy for Older Persons 73
National Policy for Rare Diseases 67
National Population Policy 64
  challenges and criticisms of 65
  impact and achievements of 66
  small family norm under 65
National Programme for
  Climate Change and Human Health 11, 418
  Containment of Anti-Microbial Resistance 439
  Control and Treatment of Occupational Diseases 434
  Control of Blindness 289
  Control of Blindness and Visual Impairment 12, 289
  Control of Non-Communicable Diseases 12, 21, 279
  Healthcare of Elderly 74, 283
  Palliative Care 12, 332
  Prevention and Control of Cancer, Diabetes, Cardiovascular Diseases and Stroke 15
  Prevention and Control of Deafness 9, 293
  Prevention and Control of Fluorosis 353
  Prevention and Control of Noncommunicable Diseases 275
  Prevention and Management of Trauma and Burn Injuries 324
National Quality Assurance Standards 174
National Rabies Control Programme 11, 260
National Registry 70
  for Organ Donation 431
National Rural Health Mission 25
National Sickle Cell Anemia Elimination Programme 9, 321
National Suicide Prevention Strategy 303
National Technical Advisory Committee on Rabies 260
National Telemedicine Service 372
National Tobacco Control Cell 311
National Tobacco Control Program 12, 310
National Tobacco Quitline Services 314
National Training and Capacity Building 256

National Tuberculosis Elimination
    Programme 8, 236
    newer initiatives in 239
National Urban Health Mission 25
National Vector Borne Disease Control
    Programme 7, 20, 229
National Viral Hepatitis Control
    Programme 8, 253
Natural Barriers 467
Navjaat Shishu Suraksha Karyakram 124,
    129, 130
    eligibility criteria for 130
Nayi Pehal 91
Neglected tropical disease 465
Neonatal and infant health care 387
New leprosy child cases 247
Newborn 111, 123
    care of normal 125
    screening, implementing 130
Newborn care 134
    and resuscitation 95
    corner 125
    existing gaps in 138
    facility-based 123, 124, 174
    practices, enhancing 130
    services, human resource for 124
Newborn deaths 129
    and stillbirths 93
Newborn stabilization unit 125, 174
    criteria for admission in 126
Newer initiatives 107
Newer strategies 58
Nidan Kendras 69
Nikshay Poshan Yojana 239
Nipple problem 160
Niti Aayog 5, 206
No more tension mobile app 378
Nominated representative, provision of
    304
Non-alcoholic fatty liver disease 275
    integration of 279
Noncommunicable disease 85, 179, 180,
    273, 387
    prevalence of 283
    prevention of 276
    type of 277
Non-first referral unit-community health
    center 30
Non-governmental organizations 224
Non-nutritional interventions 199
Non-skeletal fluorosis 353
Novel oral polio vaccine 266
Nutrition 179, 180, 187, 337
    and growth, promote 138
    and health education 342, 343
    and hygiene awareness 201
    education and counseling 224, 225

improve 180
intervention for especially vulnerable
    groups 60
rehabilitation center 174
status, improve 139
support for Poshan 214
Nutritional intake of calories and protein
    60
Nutritional interventions 140
Nutritional norms 215, 342
Nutritional Programs 62
Nutritional status
    enhance 106
    situational analysis of 60
Nutritional support 199

O

Occupational diseases, categories of
    major 435
Occupational injuries 435
One-time curative treatment, disorders
    with 68
Online registration system 380
Operation 366
    theater 124
Opioids, use of 333
Optimal early childhood development,
    ensuring 139
Optimal functioning, benchmarks for 183
Oral health care 318, 387
Oral health-promoting environment
    conducive 318
Oral polio vaccine 266
    global stockpile of 266
Oral-breast-cervical cancer 275
Organ transplantation 68, 430
Out-patient department 174, 373, 375
Outreach programs 468
Outreach services 183

P

Palliative care in private sectors,
    provision of 333
Palmar pallor 163
    severe 163
Panchayats Adhyaksh Sahakari Samiti 99
Parental and community engagement
    186
Partnerships 45, 182
    and synergy 418
Patient care services, guidelines for 314
Patient satisfaction, improving 93
Patient support systems 237
Pediatric care, advance quality of
    provisioned 174f
Pediatric drugs, essential 176
Pediatric tuberculosis 238

Peer education program 182, 196
Peer educators, role of 182
Peer mediation 187
Peer support programs 187
Pentavalent vaccine 151
Periodic evaluations 56
Periodic reporting 466
Periodic reports 413
Periodic reviews 231, 416
Periodic surveys 257
Personal health records framework 367
Pharmaceutical manufacturers, working
    together with 392
Physical achievements 184
Physical activity 187
    promote 186
Physical health 187
Physical occupational factors 435
Planning Health Program 14
Planning National Health Program 13, 14
Pneumococcal conjugate vaccine 151
Pneumonia 161
Policy
    advocacy 21
    analysis 18
    and coordination 231
    and governance 401
    and regulatory support 413
    changes 56
    development 225
    enactment 18
    formulation 322
        and strategic planning 255
    guidance, provide 40
    instruments, indirect 60, 61
    makers 270, 366
    regarding legislation and regulations
        428
    sensitization 467
Polio
    event, detecting and responding to 266
    vaccine, inactivated 266
    virus
        circulating vaccine derived 266
        type 2, vaccine derived 266
Polio Eradication Strategy 264
Poliomyelitis, endgame strategy for 264
Poliovirus 266
Polyvalent antivenom provision 467
Population growth and health resources 52
Population
    protect 266
    screening 290
    target 238, 239
Poshan 9
Poshan Abhiyaan 206, 214
    initiative 206

Poshan Scheme 347
Post-certification strategy 266, 266f
Pradhan Mantri Ayushman Bharat Health Infrastructure Mission 25
Pradhan Mantri Bhartiya Janaushadhi Kendra Network 392
Pradhan Mantri Bhartiya Janaushadhi Pariyojana 391
Pradhan Mantri Digital Saksharta Abhiyan 8
Pradhan Mantri Jan Arogya Yojana 74, 386
Pradhan Mantri Jan Aushadhi Yojana 11
Pradhan Mantri Jeevan Jyoti Bima Yojana 452
Pradhan Mantri Matru Vandana Yojana 106
  benefit of 107
  targets of 106
Pradhan Mantri National Dialysis Programme 328
Pradhan Mantri Poshan Shakti Nirman 347
Pradhan Mantri Shram Yogi Maandhan 452
Pradhan Mantri Suraksha Bima Yojana 452
Pradhan Mantri Surakshit Matritva Abhiyan 6, 103
Pradhan Mantri Swasthya Suraksha Yojana 460
Pradhan Mantri TB Mukt Bharat Abhiyaan 239
Pradhan Mantri Ujjwala Yojana 11, 412
Pregnancy
  and childbirth care 387
  promote early registration of 106
Pregnant woman
  eligibility of 101
  free entitlements for 101
Premature death worldwide, tobacco causes of 310
Prenatal screening 70
Preschool education 343
Preschool nonformal education 341, 342
Preventive healthcare, focus on 387
Preventive services, availability of 13
Primary health care 29, 52
Primary healthcare
  enhancing 53
  level 171, 255, 285
    activities 322
Primary Health Center 124, 139, 192, 204, 284, 285, 302, 402
Private sector engagement 467
Problem identification 18
  and selection of priorities 14

Productive referral system 52
Program implementation 14
Program indicators 121
Program management 230
Program objectives 17
Program performance monitoring and evaluation 322
Program, monitoring and evaluation of 41, 55, 76, 86, 96, 104, 107, 112, 115, 136, 143, 149, 153, 239, 244, 387, 393, 406
Programme on immunization, expanded 151
Progress and functional status 461t
Promote community involvement 52
Promote cooperative federalism 40
Prophylactic dose 208t
Prophylactic iron and folic acid supplementation 207, 210
Protein 215, 342
Public awareness 21, 311, 325
  and education 466
Public distribution system, functioning of 358f
Public health
  education and community mobilization 234
  impact 13, 231
    assessment 234
  importance days 277
  investment 52
  issue 201
  officials 270
Publicity and awareness campaigns 392
Public-private partnership 31, 55, 58, 65, 225, 237, 367, 413, 467
  model activities 302
Pulmonary tuberculosis 238
Pulse
  oximeter 171
  polio immunization 151

Q

Qualitative indicators 121
Quality 302
  care 328
  circles 95
  education 43
  healthcare infrastructure, lack of 385
Quality assurance
  interventions 95
  under suman 111
Quality control 392
  ensuring 392
  mechanisms 393
Quarterly reporting 184
Quaternary level 326

R

Rapid improvement cycles 95
Rare diseases
  categorization of 68
  classifications of 68
Rashtriya Bal Swasthya Karyakram 7, 146, 147
Rashtriya Kishor Swasthya Karyakram 7, 179
Rashtriya Varishth Jan Swasthya Yojana 284
Rashtriya Vayoshri Yojana 74
Rates-per day per beneficiary 215
Reaching vulnerable populations 306
Real-time data
  monitoring 230
  tracking 413
Real-time response 271
Recognition and awards 220
Referral and perioperative management 95
Referral pathways 280
Referral services 183, 342, 343
Referral systems 466
Regimen 239
Regional geriatric centers 284, 286
Registration and capacity building of volunteers 112
Regular health screenings 186
Regular monitoring 271
Regular reporting 355, 394, 397, 415
Rehabilitation 397, 415
  and support 210
Reintegration 415
Renal transplantation 68
Reporting 277
  and dissemination 413
  and utilization of data 114
  format 184
Reproductive Child Health application 379
Reproductive health 387
Reproductive maternal
  neonatal, child and adolescent health 85
  plus nutrition 87
Reproductive tract infection, prevention and control 242
Rescue and rehabilitation 415
Research 277
  and academic institutions 224
  and data collection 284
  and development 56
    promotion of 69
  and evidence generation 225, 226
  and innovation 20, 21, 31, 418
  and surveillance 280, 466

and survey 302
  on regional venoms 466
Resistance 439
Resource allocation 325, 416
  and financial management 255
Resource constraints 20, 21
Resource mapping 466
Respectful maternity care, ensuring 93
Responsibility 94, 182, 343
  and oversight 387
Responsible consumption and
    production 43
Responsive feeding 224
Rifampicin 238
Right of person with mental illness,
    provision for 305
Rights of Persons with Disabilities Act
    455
Rotavirus vaccine 151
Rural healthcare training 467
Russell's viper 465

S

SAARTHI 91
Saas Bahu Sammelan 91
Saathiyas, eligibility criteria for 196
Safe and healthy environment 187
Safe blood and blood products 254
Safe disposal facilities 186
Safe drinking water and sanitation 254
Safe injection practices 254
Safety training 413
Saksham Anganwadi 214
  and Poshan 2.0 339
Sanitary products 186, 188
Sanitation 186, 224
  and hygiene 400
  and safe drinking water, enhance 53
Saw-scaled viper 465
Scheme, components of 348
School Awareness Programs 312
School Eye Screening Program 291
School health
  component 348
  promotion activities 188
School Health and Wellness Program 184
School Health Program 186, 188
  components of 187
School nurse 187
School-based initiatives 182
Screening 322
  facility-based 148
  frequency of 277
  methods of 277
Senior Citizens Welfare Fund 74
Sensitization and community awareness
    322

Service 343
  at different levels, package of 125
  at subcenter 276
  at village level, convergence of 65
  guarantee 109
  models 375
  package of 107, 130, 163, 192, 201,
      203, 214, 285, 296, 461
  provider 216
  provision of 188
  under school health, package of 188
Service delivery
  enhancement 152
  framework 343
  levels 385
  platforms 209
Sexual and reproductive health 179
Sexually transmitted infection,
    prevention and control 242
Sick child 164
Sick newborn
  care of 125
  providing care for 130
  triage of 125
Sick Newborn Care Units, criteria for
    admission in 126
Skeletal fluorosis 353
Skill
  assessment and training 95
  imparted in training, types of 131
  of healthcare professionals, and
      paramedical staff 176
Skilled birth attendance, ensuring 130
Skin test 239
Snake venom collection and relocation
    468
Snakebite 465
  deaths 465
  envenoming 465
  helpline 467
  in livestock, prevention of 467
  notification system 466
  prevention 467
  strengthening surveillance of 466, 468
Social and behavior change
    communication 179
Social Awareness and Action to
    Neutralize Pneumonia Successfully
    6, 170
Social health 187
Social marketing and communication
    224
Social mobilization 182, 230
Social security 446
Social security and health schemes in
  organized sectors 446
  unorganized sector 446, 451

Social-emotional learning 187
Soil-transmitted helminth 203
Special newborn care unit 125, 174
Specialized care 285
  and capacity building 322
Specialized healthcare services 373
Specialized medical care 210
Specialized tertiary care 284
Spectacled cobra 465
Staff norms 341
Staff sensitization 95
Stakeholder
  consultations 416
  strengthening key 468
  training and capacity building of 311
State Action Plan for Senior Citizens 75
State and mental health authorities,
    support to 302
State Blood Transfusion Council 428
State Health Agencies 365
State Health Department 139
State Joint Steering Committee on Rabies
    260
State Mental Health Authority 305
  function of 305
State Mentoring Group 94
State Oral Health Cell 318
State Organ and Tissue Transplant
    Organization 431
State Tobacco Control Cell 311
State Women and Child Development
    Department 139
Stiff neck 162
Stigma, reduce 247
Strategic information management 244
Strategy and policy development 18
Strategy formulation 14
Strengthening healthcare
  capacity 418
  infrastructure 68, 387
  provider capacities 220
Strengthening primary
  care network 285
  healthcare 55, 372
Strengths, weaknesses, opportunities,
    threats analysis 19-21
Stress management 187
  techniques 187
Stroke 275
  day 277
Students with disabilities, scholarships
    for 456
Subsidy provision 412
Substance
  abuse 179, 180
  misuse, prevent 180

Suicide
    attempted 303
    provision of decriminalization of 305
    reduction of 303
Supervisory skills training 163
Supplementary food 342
Supplementary immunization activities 152
Supplementary nutrition 215, 341, 342, 343
Supplies and commodities, essential 114
Supply and production 468
Supply chain 152
    and logistics, strengthening 209
    management 413, 466
    strengthening 95
Supply management 467
Support early childhood development 138
Support exclusive breastfeeding 106
Support first-time mothers 106
Support services, availability of 95
Supportive supervision 141, 184
    and monitoring 140
Surakshit Matritva Aashwasan 6, 109
    initiative 109
    service guarantee packages 110, 111
    volunteer 112
Surveillance
    and data management 230, 231
    and epidemic preparedness 233
    and response 234
    systems 231
    training 468
Surveys and feedback mechanisms 416
Sustainable development
    goals 43, 369
        index 45
    importance for 179
Swachh Bharat Mission 10
Swachh Swasth Sarvatra 408
Systematic facility audits 95
Systematic research and monitoring 468

T

Technical skills 157
Technological advances 21
Technological integration 413
Technology 57
    integration 401
        and transparency 385
Tele manas 306
Tele-consultation 306
Tele-counseling 306
Telemedicine 367
Teleophthalmology network and mobile ophthalmic units 291

Tertiary care 30
Tertiary eye care services 291
Third-party
    audits 368
    evaluations 397, 416
Tissue donation 431
Tobacco 310
    and alcohol reduction 280
    cessation center 314
        setting and expansion of 312
    control laws, monitoring enforcement of 312
    control legislations 312
    free educational institutes 314
Traditional medical systems, integration of 53
Trafficking and rescue, prevention of 415
Trainers, role of 131
Training
    and capacity building 312, 325
    and development 416
    and research 326
    centers 467
    materials, availability of 322
    modules 285
    of manpower, types of 163
    package of 131
    place of 163
    programs 467, 468
    sites of 131
    type of 163
Transgenders 244
Transmission and ecology 231
Transparency and e-government 392
Transplantation of Human Organs Act 430
Trauma care 325
    objectives 324
Treatment costs, reducing 68
Tuberculosis
    care, universal access to 237
    preventive treatment 237, 238
    type of 238
Tuberculosis-mukt gram panchayat 239
Two-way referral criteria and functional linkages, establishing 176

U

Ujjawala scheme 415
Underlying conditions, management of 210
Undernutrition, impact of 138
Unified health
    interface 367
    ID, development of 367
Universal and inclusive nature 45
Universal drug sensitivity testing 239

Universal health coverage 25, 36, 385, 387
Universal Immunization Programme 7, 151, 153
Universal Vaccine Intelligence Network 153, 154
Unmodified electroconvulsive therapy, prohibition of 305

V

Vaccination 231
    and treatment access 231
    demand generation for 254
    efforts 231
Vaccine
    coverage, ensuring 171
    logistics management system 152
Vector control 230
    measures 231
Vector-borne diseases 420
Venomous snakebites, clinical repercussions of 465
Veterinary and agricultural professionals, capacity building for 467
Victims of trafficking, reintegration of 415
Vigilance committees 358
Village Health Sanitation and Nutrition Committee 196, 344
Viral hepatitis 255
    information and management system 254
    management of 254
    morbidity and mortality due to 254
Vision 56, 466
Visual impairment management 291
Visually appealing ambiance 176
Vital medicines 55
Vitamin A supplementation 215
Voluntary Blood Donation Programme 425, 426f
Voluntary non-remunerated donations, proportion of 425f
Vulnerable adolescents, target 180
Vulnerable groups, special initiatives for 413
Vulnerable populations, protect 231

W

Wage loss, financial assistance for 106
Waste management 400
Water 186
    quality monitoring, reporting format for 270
    sanitation, and hygiene 225
    promotion 140, 400
Weaknesses 20, 21

Web-based blood bank management system 381
Weekly iron 184, 201
　and folic acid supplementation program 201, 202, 209
Wellness and preventive care, promoting 385
Wild poliovirus 266
Wildlife and forest sector, strategies of 468
Workers' health, maintenance and promotion of 434
World Health Organization 332
World Heart Day 277

Y

Young infant's immunization status 166
Yuwa Samvad 182

Z

Zero disabilities 246, 247
Zero hunger 43